Atlas of
Dermatopathology

Atlas of Dermatopathology

George F. Murphy, MD
Herman Beerman Professor of Dermatology
Professor of Pathology
University of Pennsylvania
School of Medicine
Philadelphia, Pennsylvania

Arlene J. Herzberg, MD
Fellow in Dermatopathology
University of Pennsylvania
School of Medicine
Philadelphia, Pennsylvania

Present Affiliation
Department of Pathology
Peninsula Regional Medical Center
Salisbury, Maryland

W.B. SAUNDERS COMPANY
A Division of Harcourt Brace & Company
Philadelphia London Toronto Montreal Sydney Tokyo

W.B. SAUNDERS COMPANY
A Division of Harcourt Brace & Company

The Curtis Center
Independence Square West
Philadelphia, Pennsylvania 19106

Library of Congress Cataloging-in-Publication Data

Murphy, George F. (George Francis)
Atlas of dermatopathology/George F. Murphy, Arlene Herzberg.—
1st ed.

p. cm.

Includes bibliographical references and index.

ISBN 0–7216–4886–X

1. Skin—Diseases—Atlases. I. Herzberg, Arlene. II. Title.
[DNLM: 1. Skin Diseases—pathology—atlases. 2. Skin—pathology—atlases. WR 17 M978a 1996]

RL81.M87 1996 616.5′0022′2—dc20

DNLM/DLC 95-1014

Atlas of Dermatopathology ISBN 0–7216–4886–X

Printed in the United States of America

Last digit is the print number: 9 8 7 6 5 4 3 2 1

Preface

This Atlas is a companion to the text *Dermatopathology: A Practical Guide to Common Disorders.* In both works, we have sought to determine how written and graphic information may better serve diagnostic pathologists confronted with the types of skin biopsy specimens that predominate in daily practice. Students of dermatopathology consistently declare that textual and pictorial information are no substitute for actually examining slides directly, using the microscope. What, then, are the differences that make the use of books so poor a substitute for the actual practice of dermatopathology? One answer is that the examination of slides is a dynamic process, in which multiple views are made possible by the constant moving of the slide to scan different fields. Moreover, the fields examined are scrutinized at differing magnifications, adding a vertical as well as a horizontal dimension to this highly dynamic technique of compiling visual data. The result is an immense array of visual images that are presented to and processed by the cerebral cortex, sometimes within only a matter of seconds, in order to drive and direct a diagnostic algorithm. In the figures that accompany this Atlas, attempts are made to provide multiple fields and magnifications of the disorders under consideration in order to partially recapitulate this complicated and unique visual process.

The standard text format also lacks another important dimension readily available to the microscopist: the perception of color. Stained in red and blue, the basophilic and acidophilic molecules that constitute the cells within tissue sections are admixed in such a manner as to produce a remarkable and sometimes subtle spectrum of colors, which assists in the diagnostic evaluation of biopsy specimens. The diagnostic significance of tinctorial qualities in tissue sections was emphasized by Nathwani and coworkers* in 1986 in a chapter subheading concerning lymphoproliferative disorders entitled *Recognition of Cellular Constituents According to Colors and Tinctorial Properties at Low Magnification.* Here they wrote:

"Because diseases of lymph nodes generally result in alterations in the appearance of individual lymphoid cells, many pathologists feel that lymphoid disorders are recognized better at high than at low magnification. Although fine cellular details are best appreciated at high magnification, an indication of cell size, chromatin structure (clumped, blastic, vesicular), cell types (lymphocytes, plasma cells, eosinophils, epithelioid histiocytes, mummified cells), location of cells (follicles, interfollicular areas, sinuses, medulla), and the relationship of one cell type to another may be assessed at low magnification. One can make this assessment by determining the presence of one or multiple colors and the location and relationship of the colors to one another. Based on evaluation of color, one may conclude whether the proliferation is polymorphous (multiple colors) or monomorphous (one color). For example, if only one color is present, this, in our experience, almost invariably indicates lymph node involvement by malignant lymphoma. The recognition of tinctorial properties of different cells will facilitate identification of cellular details at both low and high magnifications."

---

* Nathwani BN, Burke JS, Winberg CD. Architectural features of normal, neoplastic, and nonneoplastic lymph nodes: A practical diagnostic approach. In: Murphy GF, Mihm MC, eds., *Lymphoproliferative Disorders of the Skin.* Boston, Butterworths, 1986:75.

In skin, tinctorial properties are enormously important in formulation of a correct diagnosis. Fibrinoid vessel necrosis, mucin deposition, forms of dermal "necrobiosis," amyloid deposits, spongiosis and morphea pallor, calcium deposition, altered matrix elements in perforating folliculitis, and many more important findings involve appreciation of color in formulating a definitive diagnostic impression. The creation of this Atlas is based on this belief that "seeing" diagnostic images, by scanning horizontal planes in multiple panels and zooming in and out in vertical planes (multiple magnifications), and "seeing" complex but reproducible color patterns are critical to bridging the gap between the didactic text and the dynamic microscope.

GFM
AJH

Acknowledgments

We are grateful to the following individuals for their contributions to the Atlas of Dermatopathology:

Rosalie Elenitsas, *Chapter 2*
Michael H. Goldschmidt, *Chapter 25*
Suzanne M. Jacques, *Chapter 22*
Christine Jaworsky, *Chapters 2, 20, and 21*
W. Dwayne Lawrence, *Chapter 22*
William C. Lloyd, III, *Chapter 24*
Kenneth L. Piest, *Chapter 24*
Neil W. Savage, *Chapter 23*
Laurence J. Walsh, *Chapter 23*
Allan E. Wulc, *Chapter 24*

Contents

V
Regional Dermatopathology, 279

I

Introduction to Basic Nomenclature, Structure, and Methods

1

Structure, Function, and Reaction Patterns

Normal skin is a remarkably complicated organ. The epidermal layer is composed of at least four cell types, three of which are known to subserve important protective functions. The underlying dermis is even more sophisticated, containing a myriad of cells and matrix molecules that collaborate to provide a microenvironment necessary for normal epidermal function, as well as to promote constant movement of cells, molecules, and signals essential to cutaneous integrity. The normal epidermal and dermal layers have ways of responding to internal abnormalities and external insults, and these responses are conventionally visualized by comparing structural alterations with what is known to be normal.

Tinctorial characteristics of normal, reactive, and neoplastic skin cells are different and, along with architecture, cytology, and correlative clinical information, contribute to routine diagnostic assessment. The epidermal layer is a good example. Although the normal epidermis at scanning magnification is dark pink as a result of color mixing of eosinophilic cytoplasm and basophilic nuclei, a spongiotic epidermis is pale pink, the result of the dilutional effect of widened intercellular spaces, which are colorless. Normal follicular infundibula, which stain in a manner similar to that for the surface epidermis, may appear to be pale blue when infiltrated by mucin in the setting of alopecia mucinosa. Dermal cells and elements also have characteristic coloration. Normal dermal mucin strands are pale blue-gray; mast cells may have a granular basophilic cytoplasm with some routine stains; and infiltrating cells such as eosinophils are identified by their typical eosinophilic cytoplasm.

Thorough appreciation of the normal tinctorial characteristics of skin is therefore essential to accurate recognition of structural elements and cells, to determination of whether such components are abnormally increased or decreased, and to comparison with reactive and neoplastic counterparts. Table 1–1 provides several common examples of how such comparisons are useful in normal practice.

The purpose of this chapter is to provide a basis of normal tinctorial characteristics for the evaluation of the lesional pathology represented in subsequent chapters. It must be remembered, however, that staining techniques and results may vary among laboratories. Therefore, comparisons are most accurately made when results are used from one laboratory that has standardized staining practices.

Table 1–1. Examples of Tinctorial Characteristics of Skin

Normal	Abnormal
Red-purple admixture of normal stratum granulosum	Superficial pink pallor of verruca plana
Pink hue of stratum basalis	Dark-blue hue of basal cell layer in lentigo maligna
Basophilic nuclei with pale-pink cytoplasm of normal Langerhans cells and melanocytes	Clear cytoplasm of pagetoid cells in extramammary Paget disease
Pink epithelium of normal adnexa	Blue/pink zonation of pilomatricoma
Pink-red hue of hair follicle epithelium	Blue-gray hue of follicular mucinosis
Pink quality of papillary dermis	Blue-gray quality of solar elastosis
Pale-red dermal collagen	Dark-red collagen in rheumatoid nodule

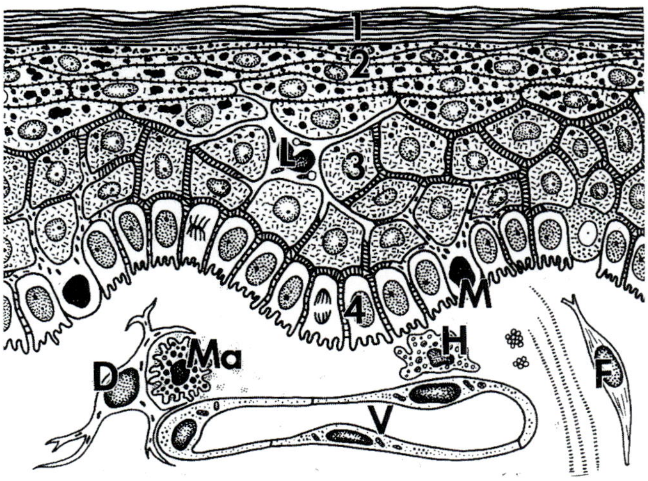

Figure 1–1. Normal human skin. The epidermis is composed of four layers of keratinocytes: the stratum corneum (1), the stratum granulosum (2), the stratum spinosum (3), and the stratum basalis (4). Within the midepidermis are dendritic Langerhans cells (L), and admixed within the stratum basalis are pigment-producing melanocytes (M). The underlying collagenous dermis contains microvessels (V), fusiform fibroblasts (F), histiocytes (H), dendrocytes (D), and granule-containing mast cells (Ma).

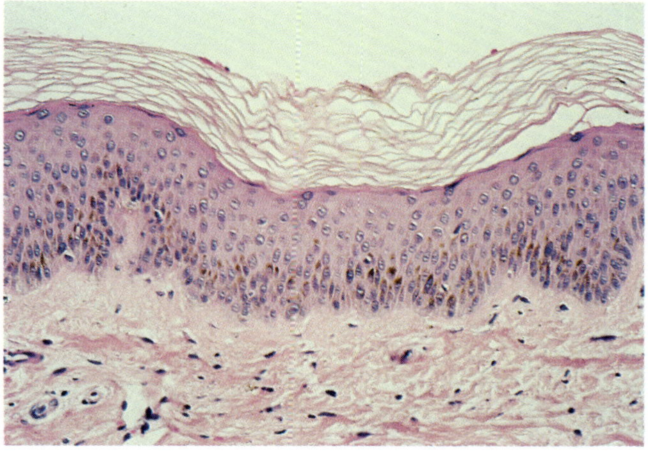

Figure 1–2. Normal human epidermis, truncal skin. The epidermal layer is composed of discrete cell populations that undergo orderly, gradual upward maturation from the stratum basalis to form the overlying stratum spinosum, stratum granulosum, and stratum corneum. Rete ridges undulate with underlying dermal papillae along the base of the epidermal layer.

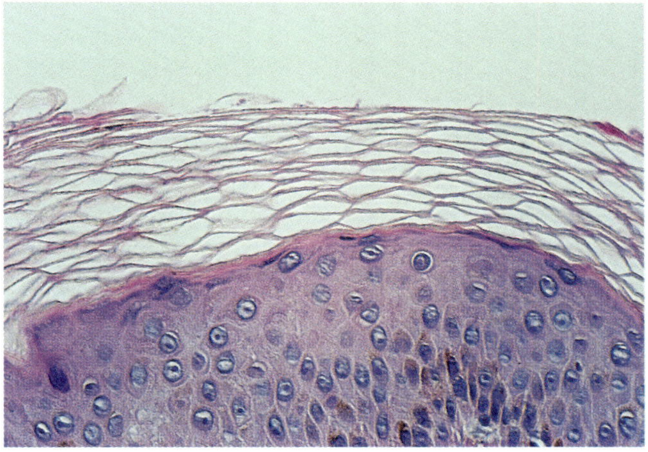

Figure 1–3. Normal human epidermis, truncal skin. The normally anucleate stratum corneum shows a characteristic basket-weave appearance, and subtle perturbations in underlying nucleated keratinocytes are translated into diagnostically informative abnormalities of this horny layer.

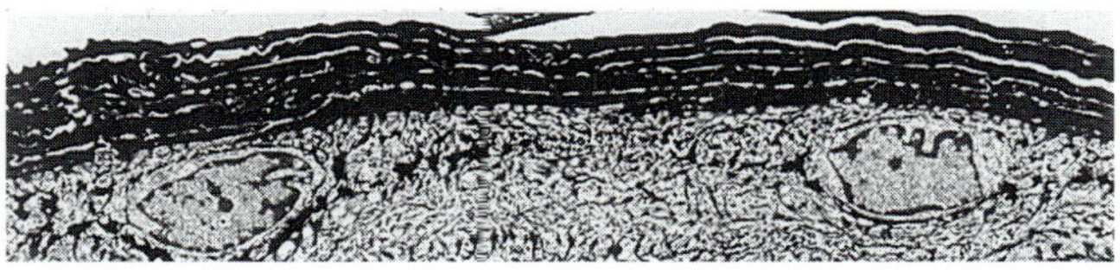

Figure 1–4. Normal human epidermis, truncal skin. Ultrastructurally, the transition from the stratum granulosum to the stratum corneum is quite dramatic and correlates with terminal differentiation and the formation of involucrin-rich cell envelopes.

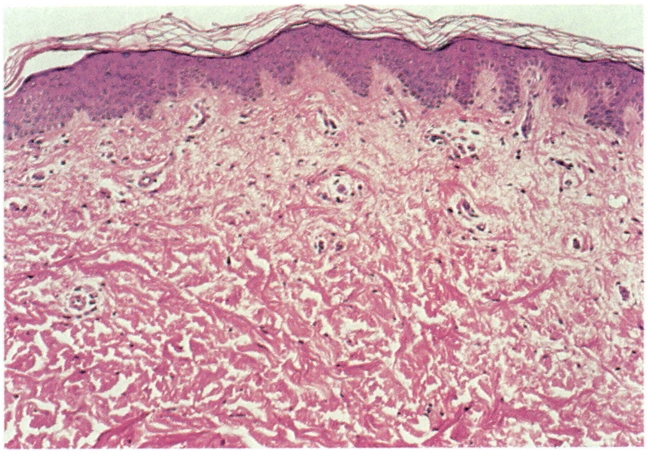

Figure 1–5. Comparison of normal cutaneous architecture in back (shown here) and palm (see Fig. 1–6). There are marked differences in epidermal and stratum corneum thickness, in degree of compaction of stratum corneum, and even in texture and vascularity of the underlying dermal connective tissue.

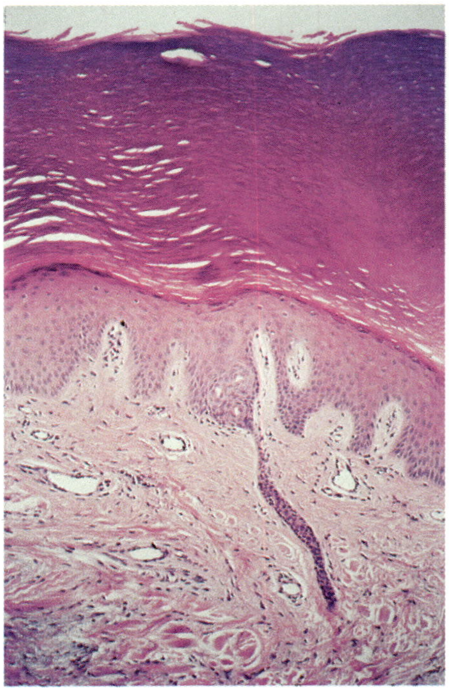

Figure 1–6. Comparison of normal cutaneous architecture in back (see Fig. 1–5) and palm (shown here). A longitudinally sectioned eccrine duct is observed; eccrine glands occur in much higher density on the palm than on truncal skin.

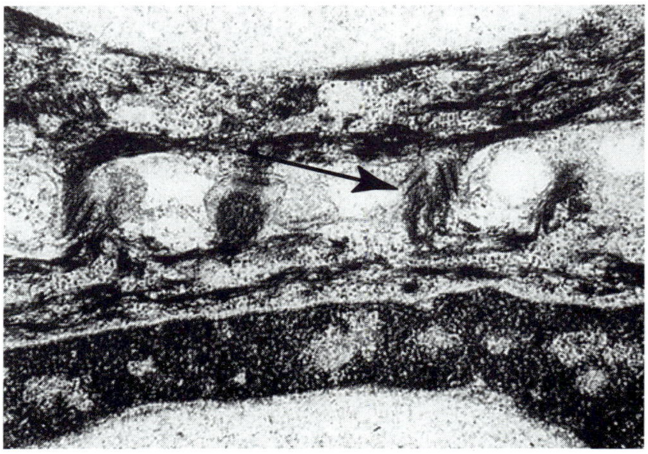

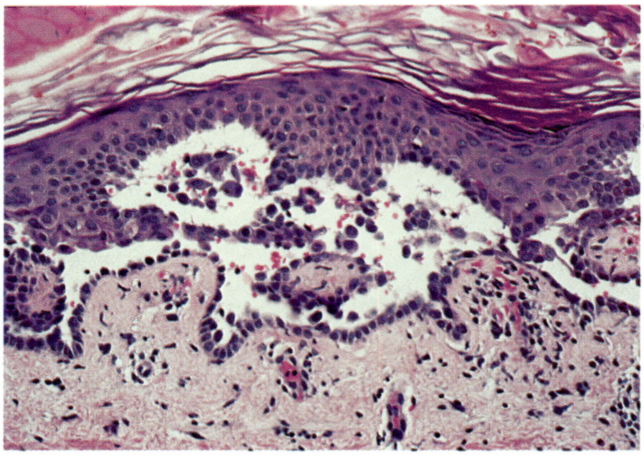

Figures 1–7 and 1–8. Structural-functional relations in epidermal cells. Keratinocytes are bound together by tonofilament-desmosome complexes (Fig. 1–7, *arrow*) that span the peripheral cytoplasm and plasma membranes of adjacent cells. Compromise of these adhesion sites results in cleft or blister formation due to dyshesion (Fig. 1–8), a process called acantholysis.

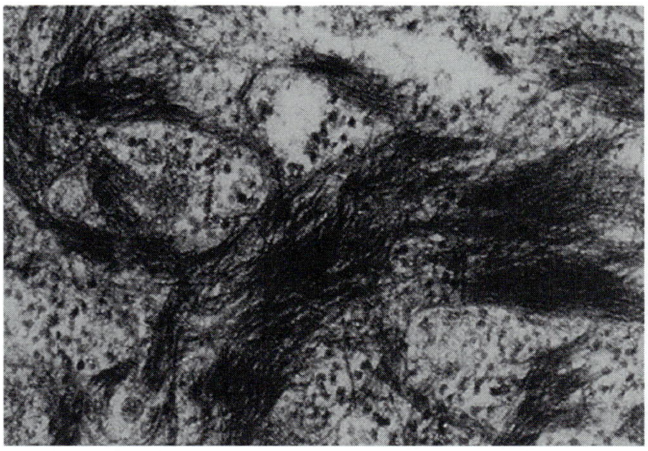

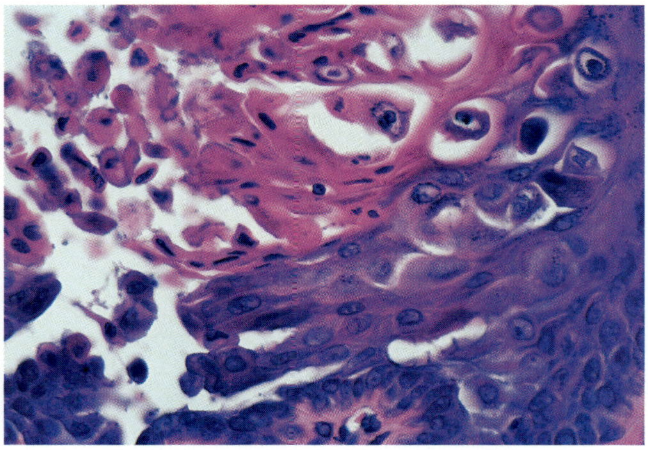

Figures 1–9 and 1–10. Structural-functional relations in epidermal cells. Keratinocyte cytoplasm is progressively filled with keratin intermediate filaments (*i.e.,* tonofilaments) as these cells mature (Fig. 1–9). Aberrant or premature expression of the structural proteins produces dense, hypereosinophilic cells, a process called dyskeratosis (Fig. 1–10).

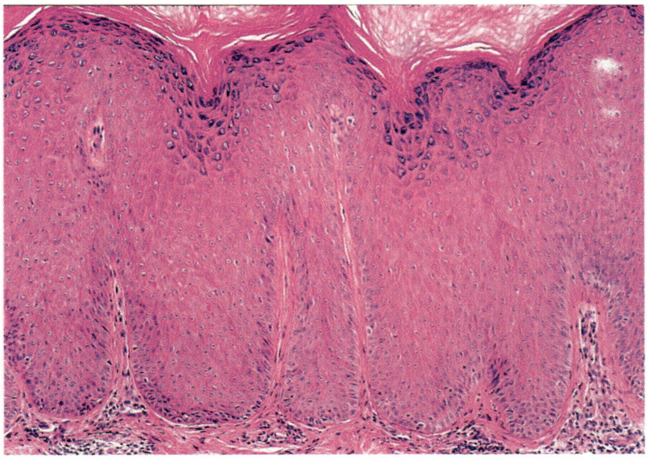

Figure 1–11. Epidermal hyperplasia, or acanthosis. As a result of chronic exogenous trauma (*e.g.,* rubbing, irritation), the stratum spinosum, stratum granulosum, and stratum corneum may become markedly thickened. Note the associated prominence of enlarged rete ridges.

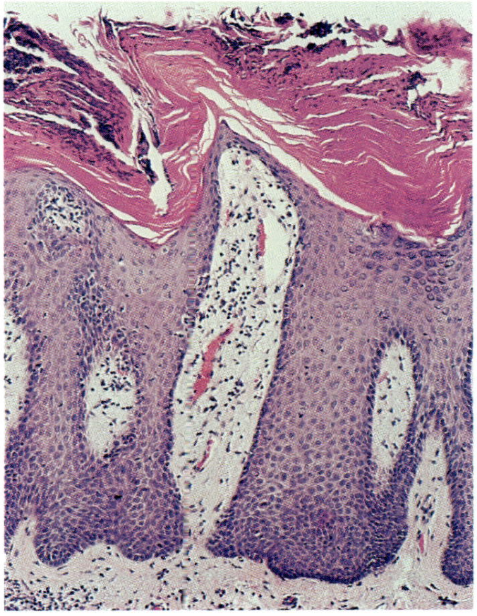

Figure 1–12. Epidermal hyperplasia, or acanthosis. In response to poorly defined endogenous stimuli, acanthosis is characteristic of established psoriasis, although in this case there is thinning and loss of the stratum granulosum and retention of pyknotic nuclei into the scale (*i.e.,* parakeratosis). There also is associated upward enlargement of dermal papillae.

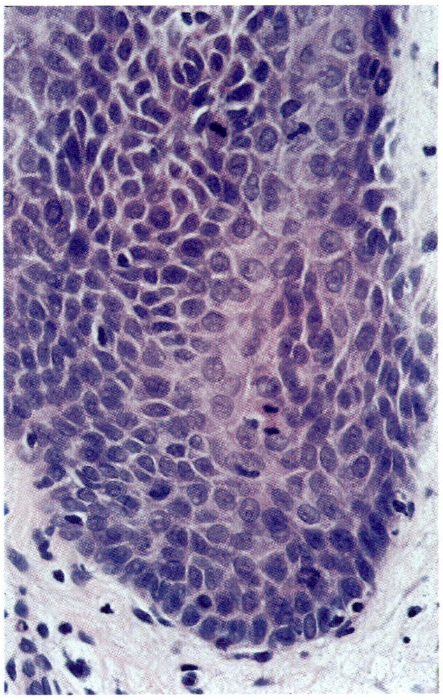

Figure 1–13. Epidermal hyperplasia, or acanthosis. Hyperplasia is often but not invariably associated with increased mitotic activity, particularly above the stratum basalis.

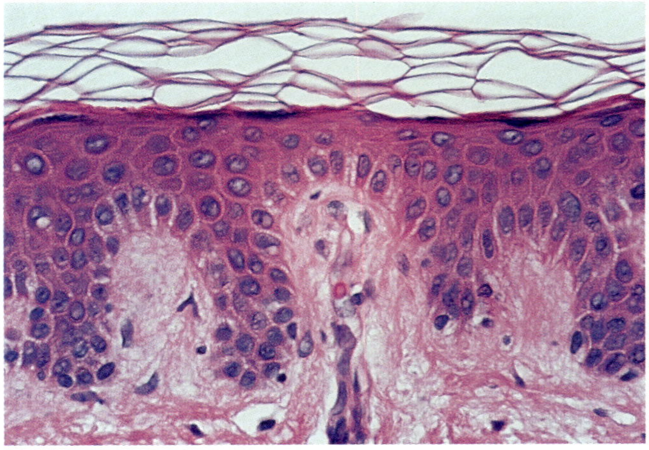

Figure 1–14. Comparison of normal and aberrant scale patterns. Normal epidermis shows a basket-weave stratum corneum and a well-developed pattern of interdigitating rete ridges and dermal papillae.

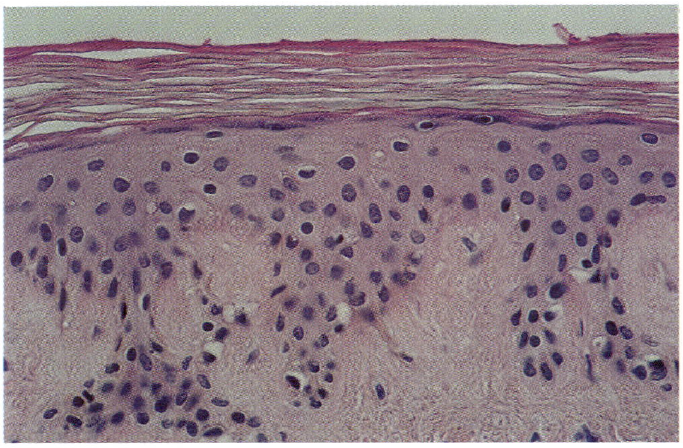

Figure 1–15. Comparison of normal and aberrant scale patterns. Poorly fixed skin may result in artifactual distortion of the normal scale pattern, producing compacted orthokeratosis similar to that seen in certain forms of ichthyosis.

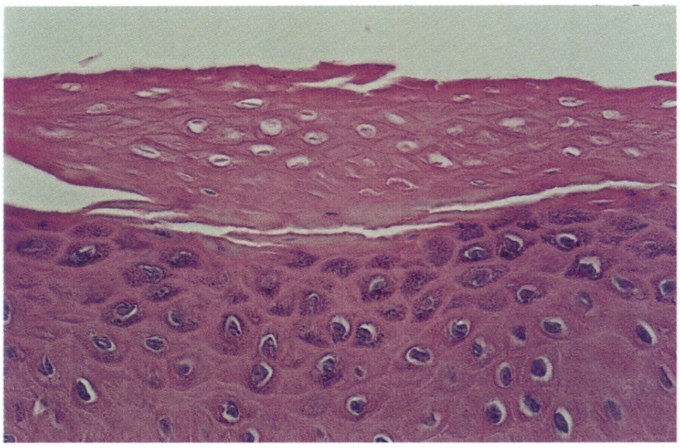

Figure 1–16. Comparison of normal and aberrant scale patterns. Early hyperkeratosis is characterized by compaction of scale and residua of degenerated nuclei.

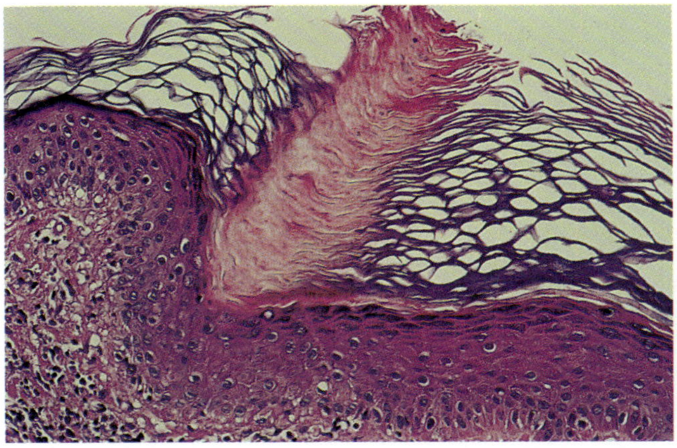

Figure 1–17. Comparison of normal and aberrant scale patterns. Parakeratosis is characterized by retention of pyknotic nuclei into the stratum corneum. Here, it is discretely localized to a small zone of underlying hypogranulosis, permitting side-by-side comparison with normal scale. This extremely focal, column-like zone of parakeratosis is referred to as a cornoid lamella.

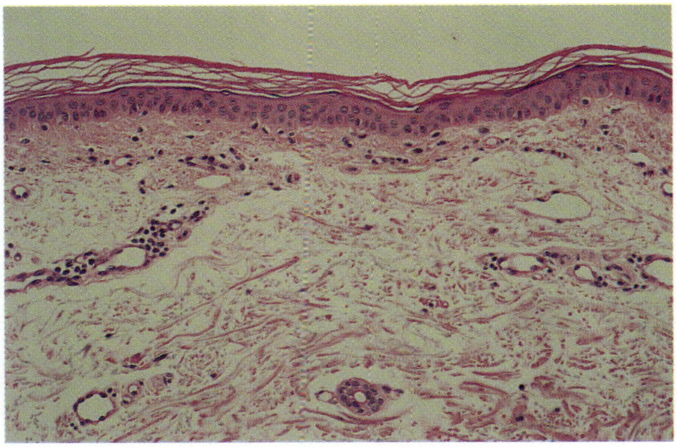

Figure 1–18. Epidermal and dermal atrophy. The epidermal layer is only three cells thick, and rete ridges are entirely absent. Dermal collagen fibers are abnormally thin and pale. These atrophic changes were elicited by chronic topical application of a potent fluorinated steroid; similar alterations are associated with senescence. Epidermal atrophy occurs independent of mesenchymal atrophy in certain cytotoxic dermatoses (*e.g.,* discoid lupus erythematosus).

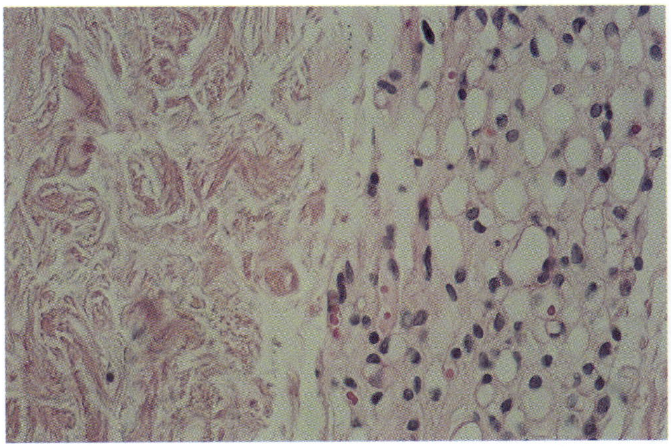

Figure 1–19. Subcutaneous atrophy. Note the small adipocytes separated by pale-pink spaces, indicating that the subcutaneous fat is atrophic. These atrophic changes were elicited by chronic topical application of a potent fluorinated steroid.

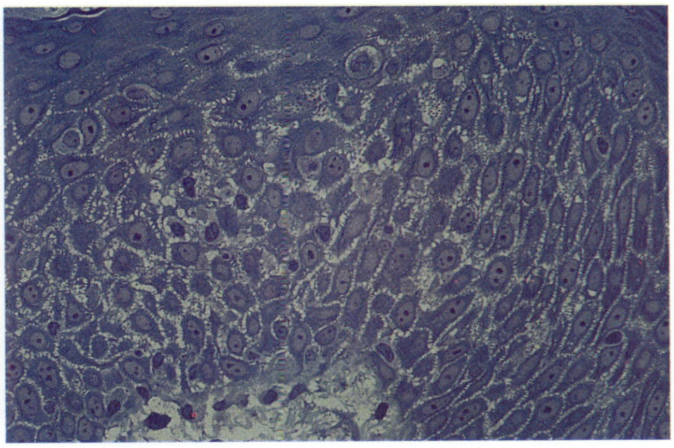

Figure 1–20. Spongiosis. The widened intercellular spaces and prominence of spiny intercellular attachment sites result in a spongy appearance. (Giemsa-stained, plastic-embedded specimen.)

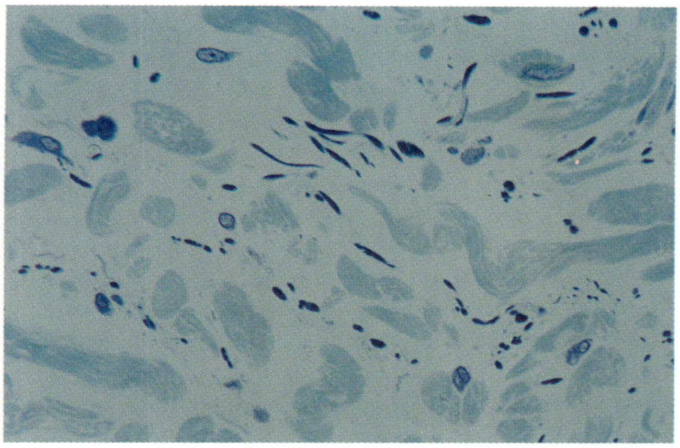

Figure 1–21. Dermal edema. Widening similar to that in Figure 1–20 of intercollagenous spaces occurs in the underlying dermis. Epidermal spongiosis and dermal edema are characteristic of acute contact hypersensitivity reactions, whereas pure dermal edema is more typical of urticaria. (Giemsa-stained, plastic-embedded specimen.)

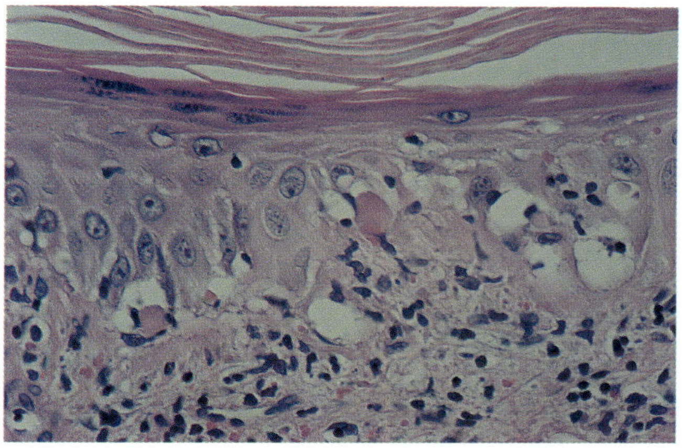

Figure 1–22. Cytotoxic alteration. Numerous degenerating and necrotic keratinocytes appear as hypereosinophilic bodies in the lower epidermal layers of the skin of this patient, who has dermatitis associated with an influx of lymphocytes with cytotoxic capabilities. Keratinocytes undergoing vacuolar degeneration are also prominent. Incorporation of apoptotic bodies into the superficial dermis (*i.e.,* colloid body formation) may occur in some dermatoses.

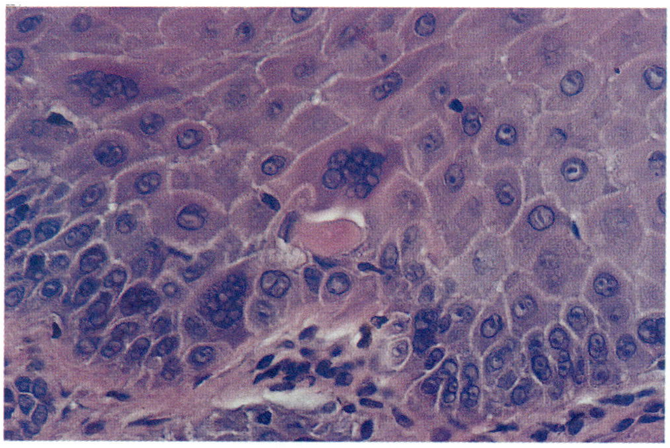

Figure 1–23. Cytotoxic alteration. Occasional apoptotic cells are observed within normal epidermis. Note the adjacent multinucleated keratinocyte, a phenomenon of no pathologic significance when not associated with evidence of causation (*e.g.,* herpesvirus).

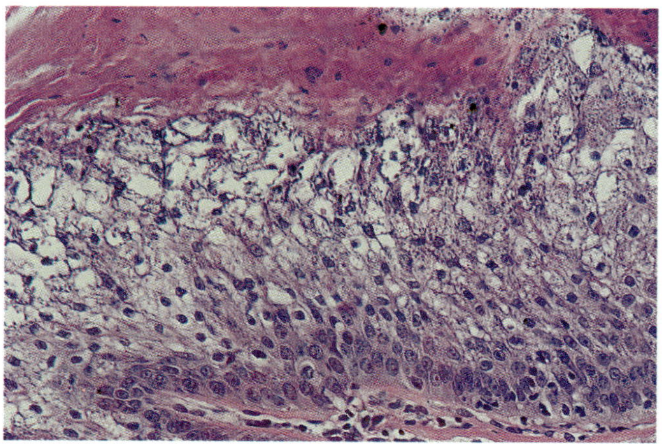

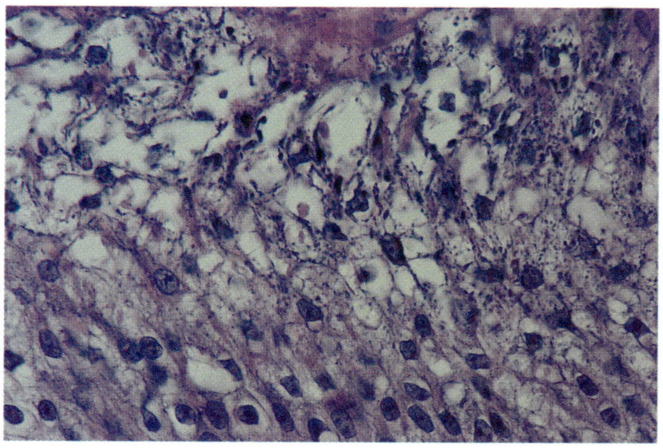

Figures 1–24 and 1–25. Keratinocyte lysis and swelling. In epidermolytic hyperkeratosis, there is ballooning and dissolution of upper epidermal cells as a result of faulty maturation.

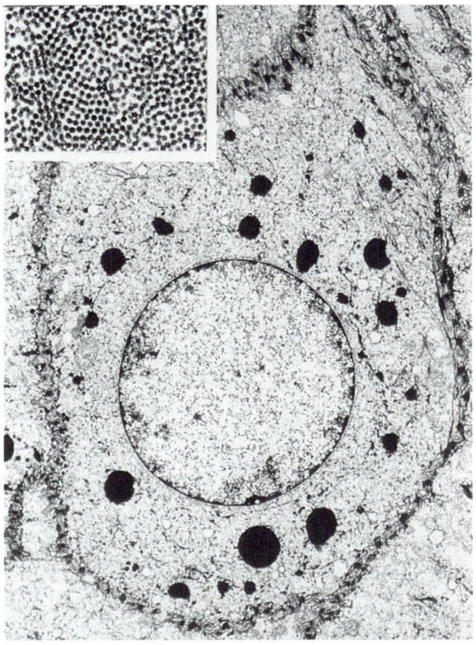

Figure 1–26. Keratinocyte lysis and swelling. In patients who have human papillomavirus infection, cells of the upper epidermal layers show electron-lucent cytoplasm and diminished tonofilament expression for this level by electron microscopy and are recognized as koilocytes by light microscopy. There are intranuclear viral inclusions *(inset)* and characteristically rounded contours of enlarged keratohyaline granules within the cytoplasm.

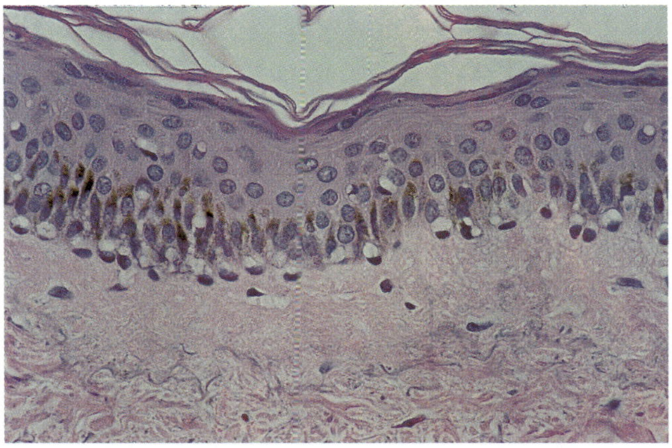

Figure 1–27. Routine histology of human melanocytes. In patients who have lentiginous melanocytic hyperplasia, melanocytes are prominently displayed along the stratum basalis as cells with ovoid, dense nuclei; unapparent cytoplasm; and pericellular clear spaces due to cytoplasmic contraction.

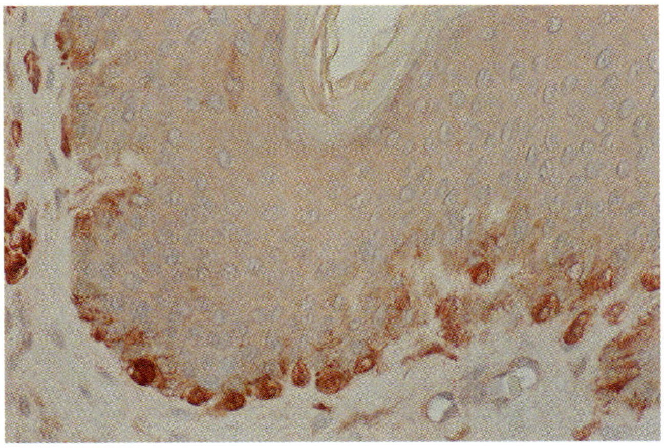

Figure 1–28. Routine immunohistochemistry of human melanocytes. Immunohistochemistry for S100 protein further defines the normal basal distribution of these cells.

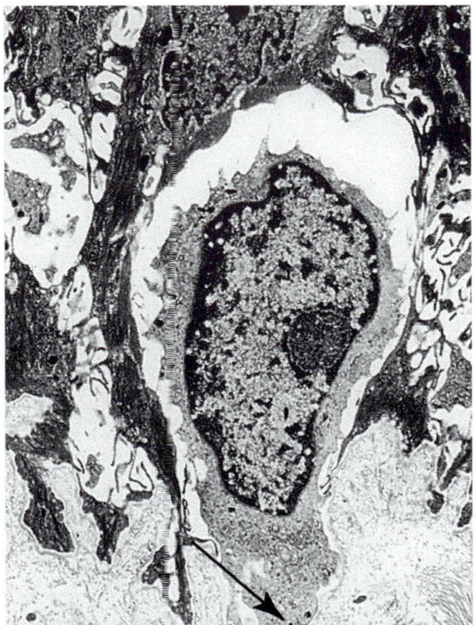

Figure 1–29. Routine ultrastructure of human melanocytes. Ultrastructural examination shows melanocytes have relatively electron-lucent cytoplasm devoid of tonofilaments; note solitary melanosome *(arrow)*.

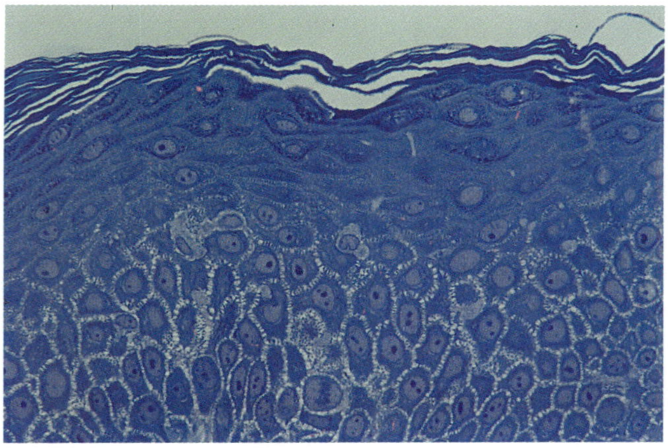

Figure 1–30. Structure and distribution of epidermal Langerhans cells. Although Langerhans cells are not apparent in routine hematoxylin and eosin–stained sections, in 1-μm-thick, plastic-embedded sections they appear as midlevel epidermal cells (with pale cytoplasm).

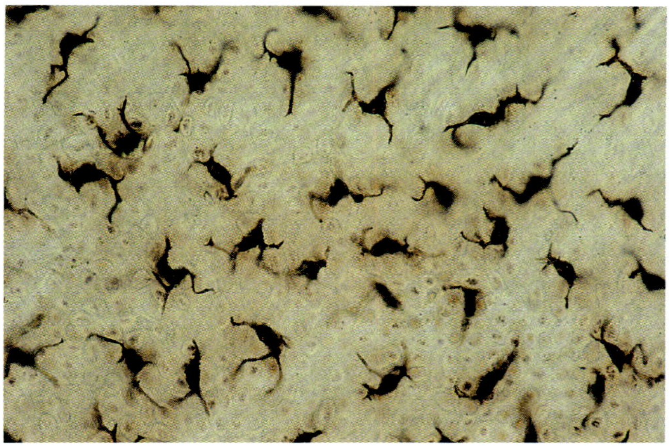

Figure 1–31. Structure and distribution of epidermal Langerhans cells. Like melanocytes, Langerhans cells and associated dendrites are uniformly distributed throughout the epidermal layer for efficient coverage of the epidermal surface. (ATPase enzyme histochemistry of epidermal sheet.)

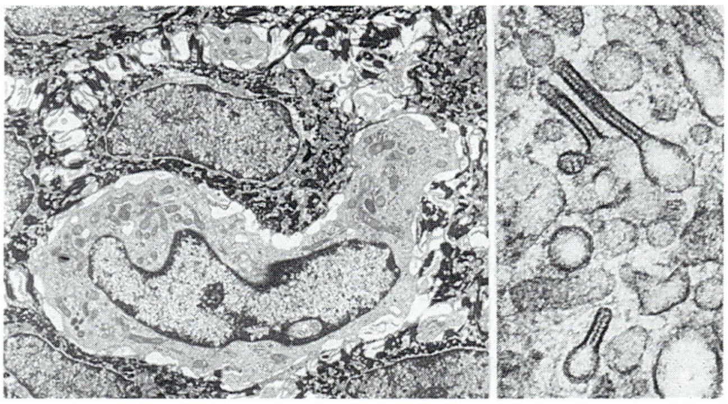

Figure 1–32. Structure and distribution of epidermal Langerhans cells. Ultrastructurally, Langerhans cells have relatively electron-lucent cytoplasm and vaguely infolded nuclear contours and contain tennis racket–shaped Birbeck granules.

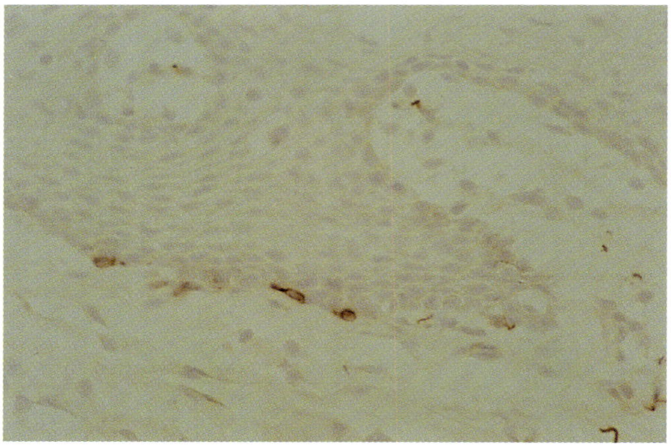

Figure 1–33. Epidermal neuroendocrine cells, or Merkel cells. Neuroendocrine cells are present in small numbers in normal epidermis and require immunohistochemical probes for their detection within the stratum basalis.

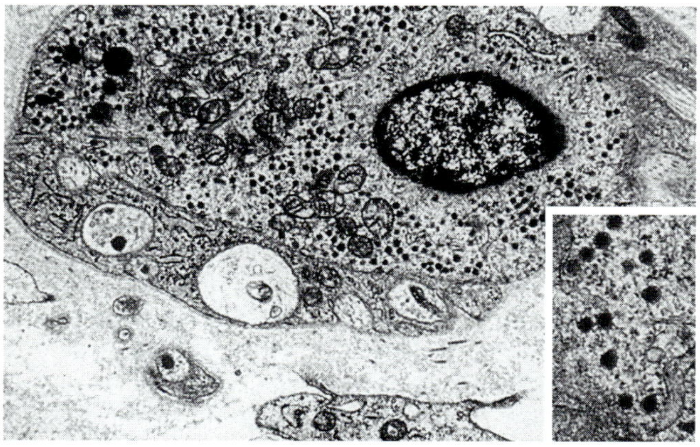

Figure 1–34. Epidermal neuroendocrine cells, or Merkel cells. These cells characteristically contain small, membrane-bound, dense-core granules *(inset)*.

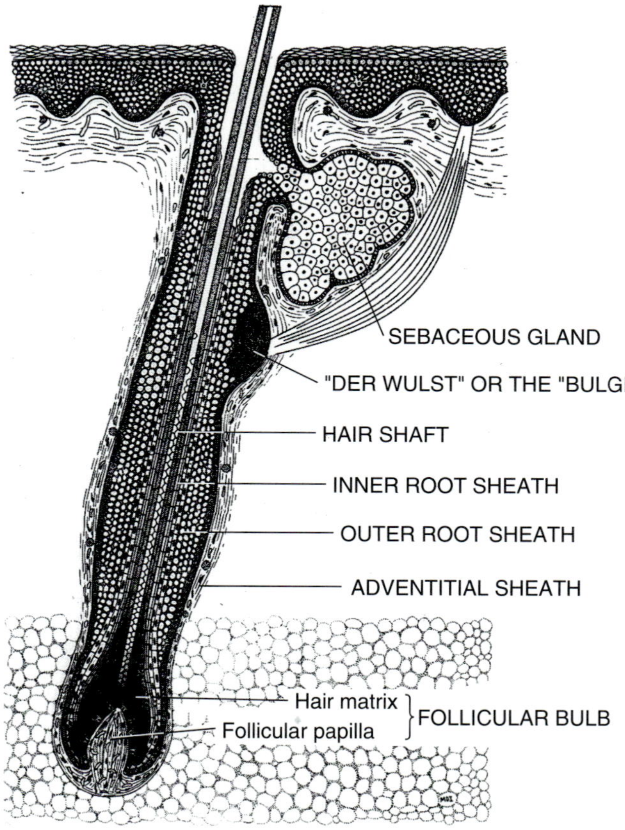

Figure 1–35. Schematic diagram of an adult human hair follicle. The follicle, an invagination of the surface epidermis, is characterized by an infundibulum that communicates directly with the epidermal layer and is delimited by the duct orifice of the sebaceous gland. Directly below the sebaceous duct is the bulge, a putative site of follicular stem cells. Along its midportion (*i.e.,* isthmus), the hair shaft is surrounded by eosinophilic inner root sheath epithelium and clear (*i.e.,* glycogenated) outer root sheath epithelium, as well as a mesenchymal adventitial sheath that is contiguous with the overlying papillary dermis. The terminal portion of the follicle is composed of the basaloid hair matrix and its mucinous stroma, the follicular papilla, both of which are commonly recapitulated in basal cell carcinoma.

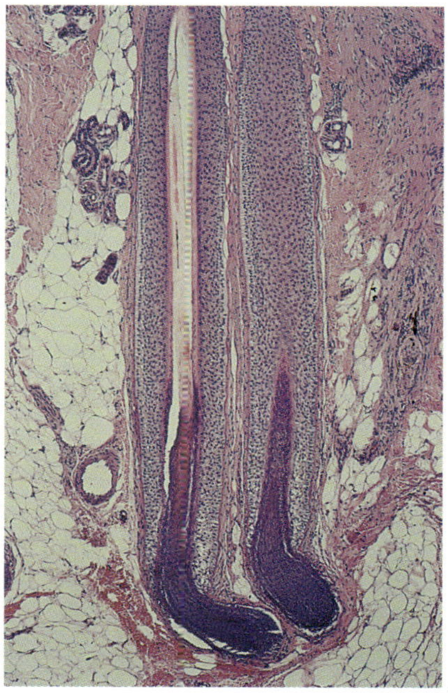

Figure 1–36. Epidermal adnexa. Hair follicles should be regarded as specialized downgrowths of the epidermis. At certain body sites (*e.g.,* scalp, axilla), adnexal epithelium may extend into subcutaneous fat.

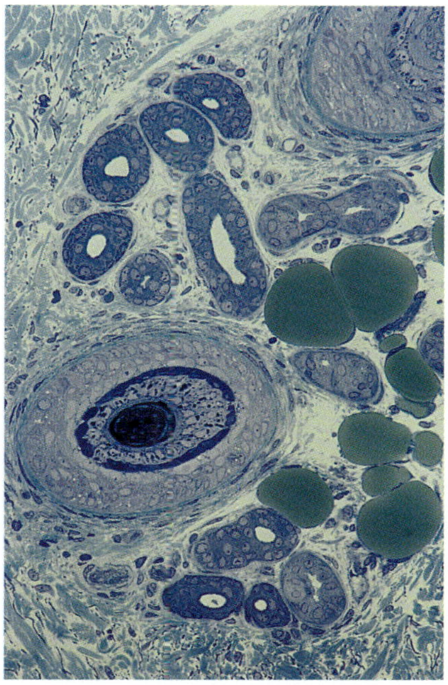

Figure 1–37. Epidermal adnexa. Sweat glands also should be regarded as specialized downgrowths of the epidermis. (Giemsa-stained, plastic-embedded section.)

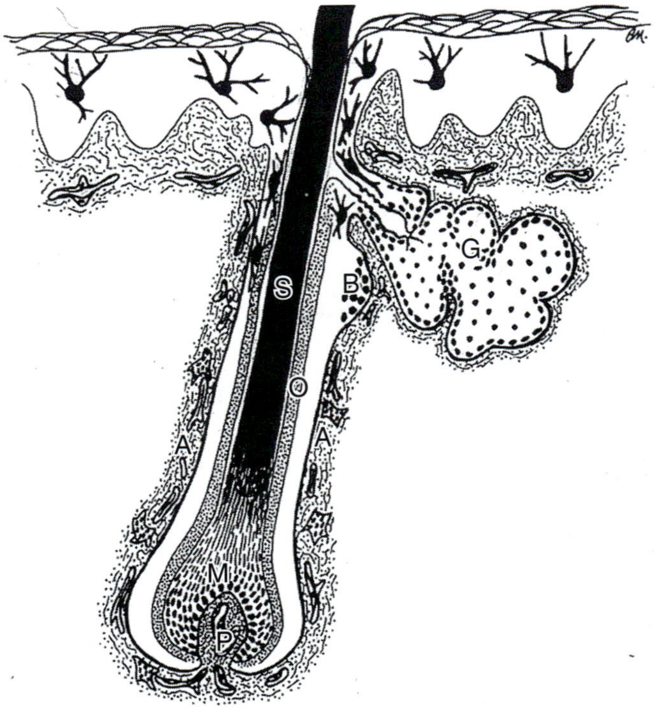

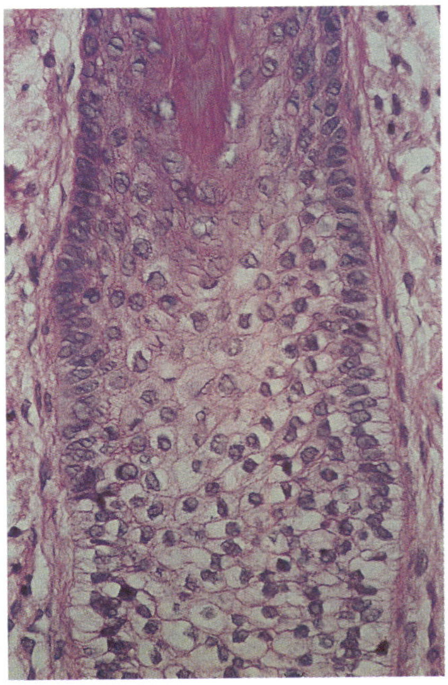

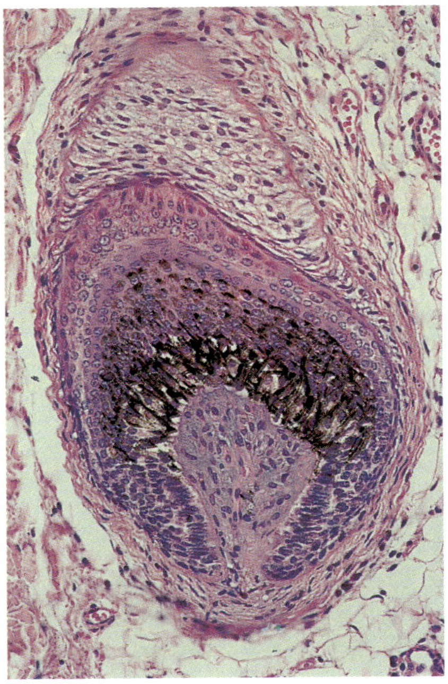

Figures 1–38 through 1–40. Schematic representation (Fig. 1–38, *top left*) and correlative histology (Figs. 1–39, *top right,* and 1–40, *bottom*) of human anagen hair follicle. Important features relative to common follicular tumors and inflammatory diseases include glycogenated outer root sheath (O; correlative histology shown in Fig. 1–39); hair papilla (P) and hair matrix cells (M) (correlative histology shown in Fig. 1–40); hair shaft (S); follicular stem cell bulge (B); sebaceous gland (G); perifollicular connective tissue adventitia (A) rich in blood vessels and mast cells and contiguous with papillary dermal collagen; and Langerhans cells that are concentrated within the infundibular epithelium as well as evenly distributed within the interfollicular epidermis.

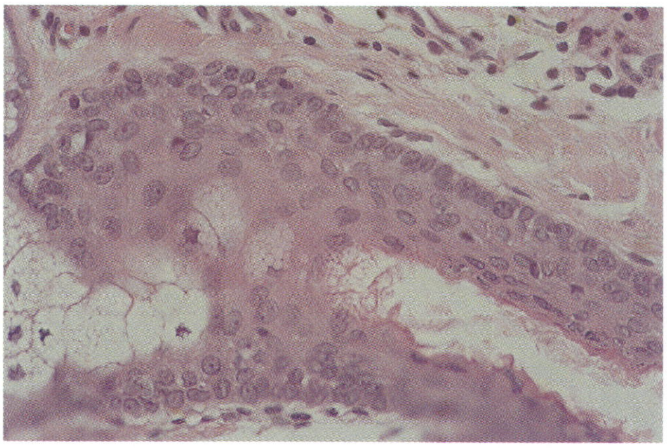

Figure 1–41. The sebaceous duct has a corrugated, eosinophilic lining that is recapitulated in the walls of steatocystomas.

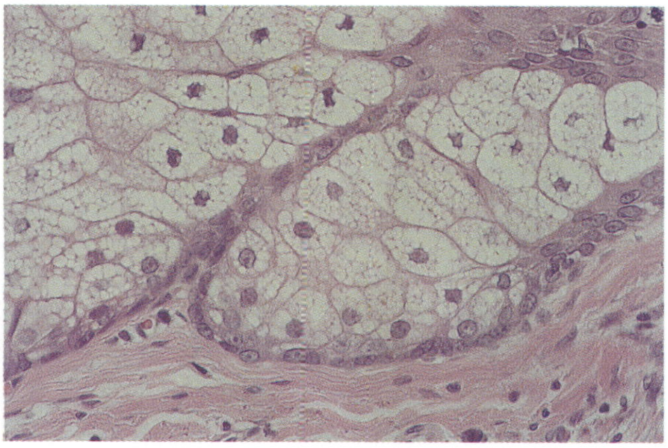

Figure 1–42. The sebaceous lobule is composed of large polyhedral epithelial cells containing clear lipid vacuoles bordered by a single layer of nonlipidized basaloid cells. Scalloped nuclear borders result from compression by vacuoles.

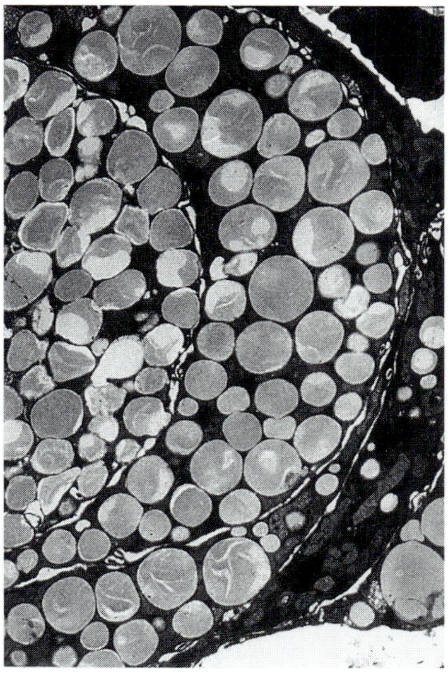

Figure 1–43. These vacuoles (see Fig. 1–42) contain homogeneous gray material on ultrastructural examination, a technique that may be helpful in evaluation of sebaceous carcinoma, even after retrieval from paraffin blocks.

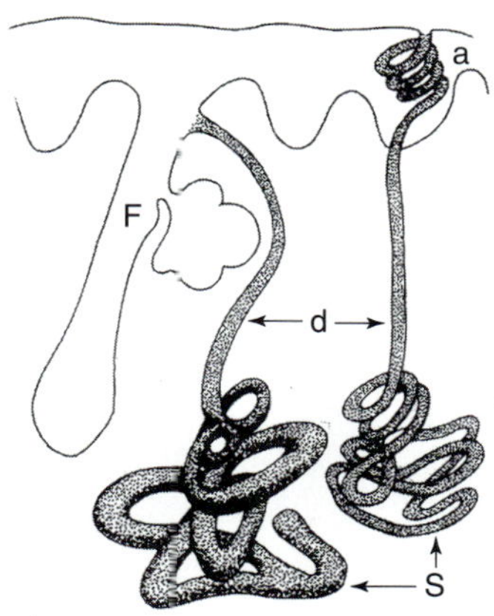

Figure 1–44. Schematic representation and correlative histology of the human eccrine and apocrine apparatuses. The eccrine gland to the right consists of a coiled secretory segment (S), a straight intradermal duct (d) that ascends toward the epidermal layer, and a coiled terminal duct or acrosyringium (a) that traverses the epidermal layer and terminates on the skin surface. The acrosyringium is lined by a thin mantle of eosinophilic material (*i.e.*, cuticle). The apocrine gland to the left has a larger secretory coil and a similar dermal duct segment and originates from a hair follicle (F).

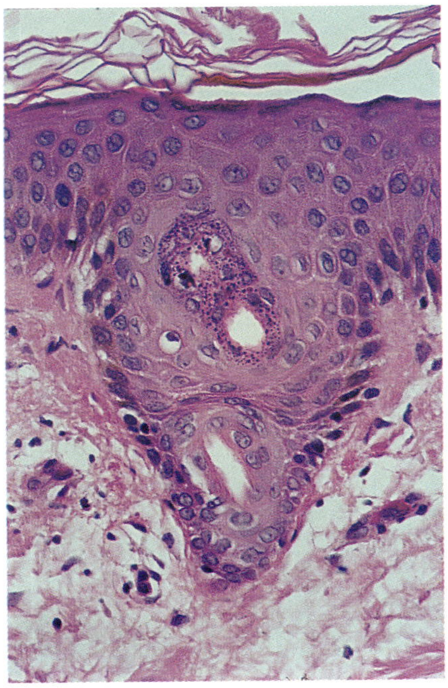

Figure 1–45. Correlative histology of the human eccrine apparatus—acrosyringium.

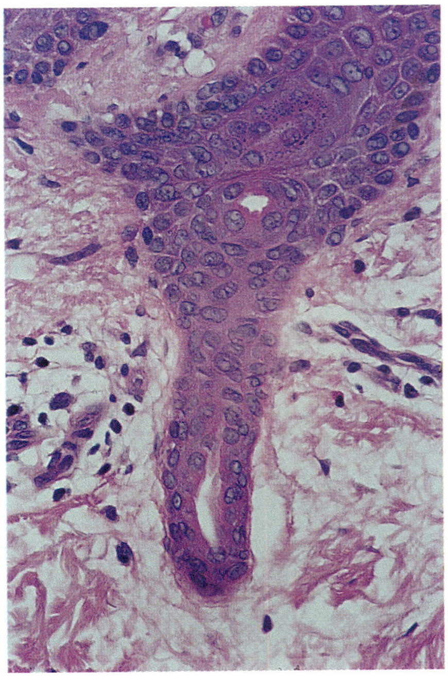

Figure 1–46. Correlative histology of the human eccrine apparatus—superficial portion of dermal eccrine duct.

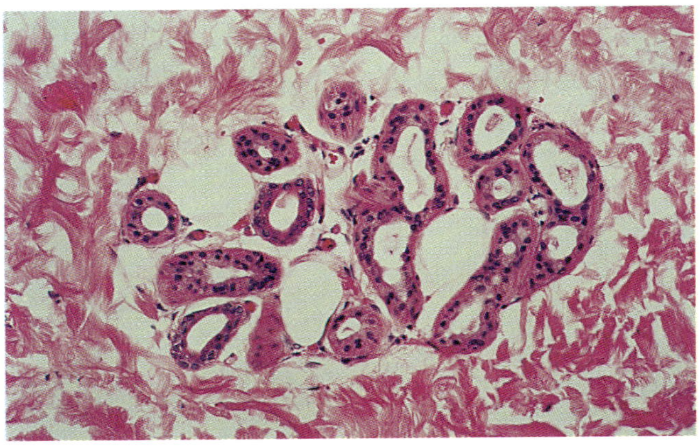

Figure 1–47. Correlative histology of the human eccrine apparatus—secretory coil.

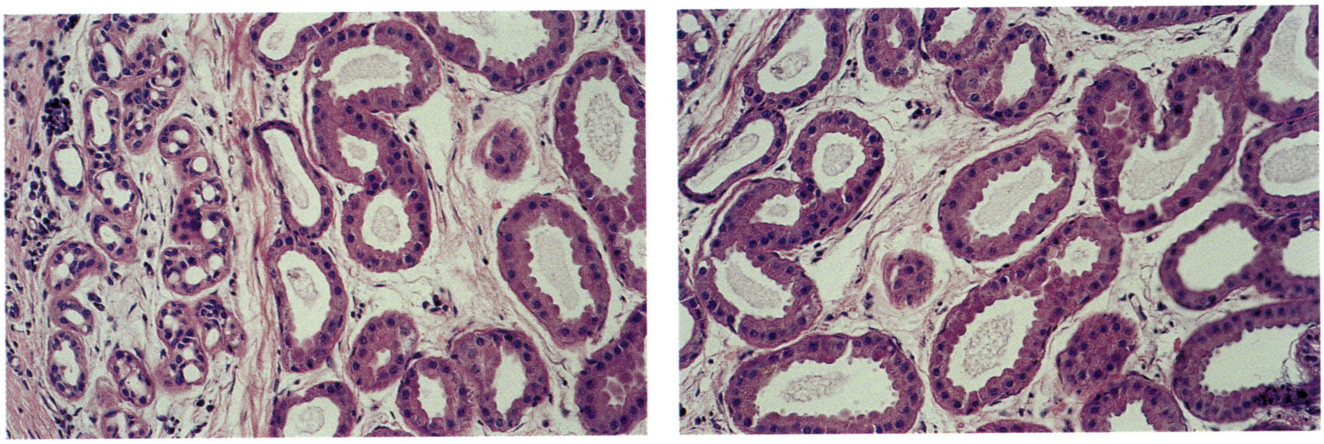

Figures 1–48 and 1–49. Correlative histology of the human apocrine apparatus. The apocrine secretory coil (Fig. 1–48, *left*) is larger and composed of more dilated glands than its eccrine counterpart (Fig. 1–48, *right*). In cross section, the apocrine duct resembles the eccrine duct, although the apocrine gland is distinguished by lining epithelial cells with eosinophilic cytoplasm and bulging luminal membranes (Fig. 1–49).

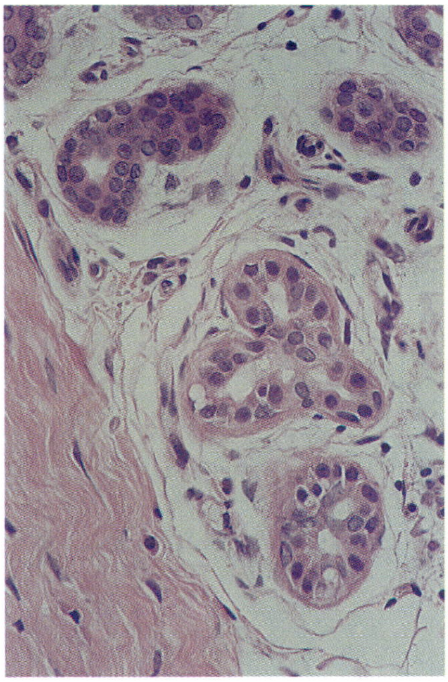

Figure 1–50. Unlike the eccrine duct, the eccrine secretory coil is lined by cuboidal epithelium with a pale, often vacuolated cytoplasm and surrounded by a thin mantle of myoepithelial cells. The vessels surrounding the duct and coil are contiguous with the superficial vascular plexus, which separates papillary from reticular dermis. (Compare with Figs. 1–51 and 1–52.)

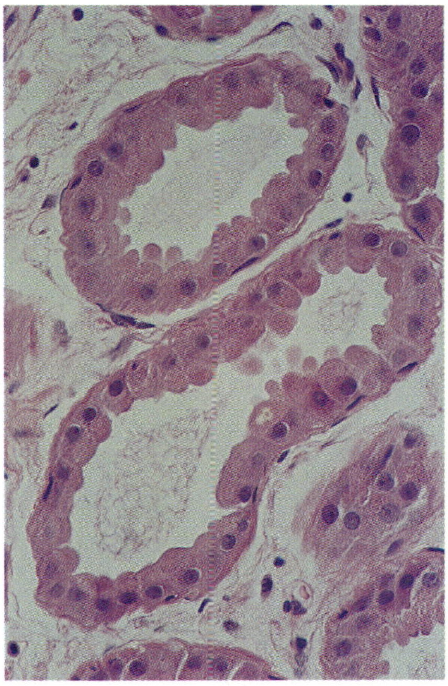

Figure 1–51. The epithelium lining the apocrine coil has granular, eosinophilic cytoplasm and protuberant luminal membranes that appear to bud into the lumen (decapitation- or apocrine-type secretion; *center*). (Compare with Figs. 1–50 and 1–52.)

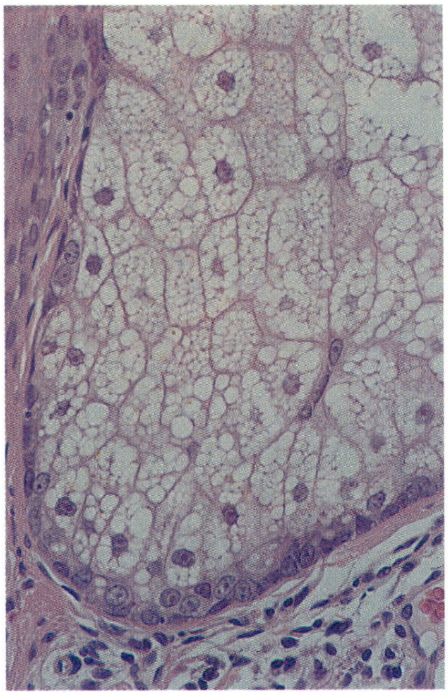

Figure 1–52. The sebaceous gland is composed of vacuolated, lipidized epithelial cells bordered by a single layer of nonlipidized basaloid cells at the perimeter. Lipid vacuoles characteristically indent the nuclear membrane, producing a scalloped nuclear contour. (Compare with Figs. 1–50 and 1–51.)

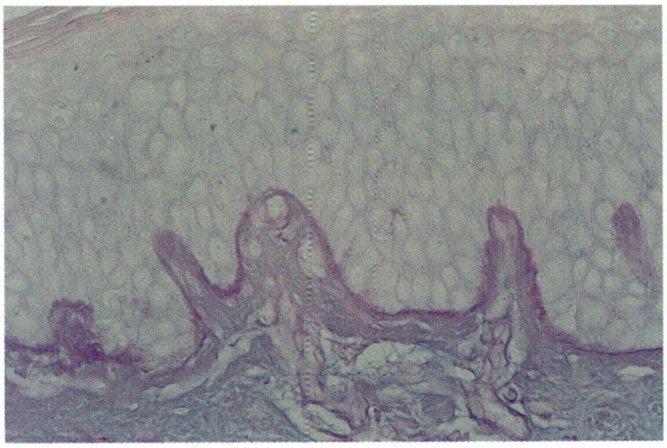

Figure 1–53. Normal epidermal basement membrane zone. This periodic acid–Schiff stain demonstrates the thin, uniform basement membrane that normally separates the epidermal and dermal layers.

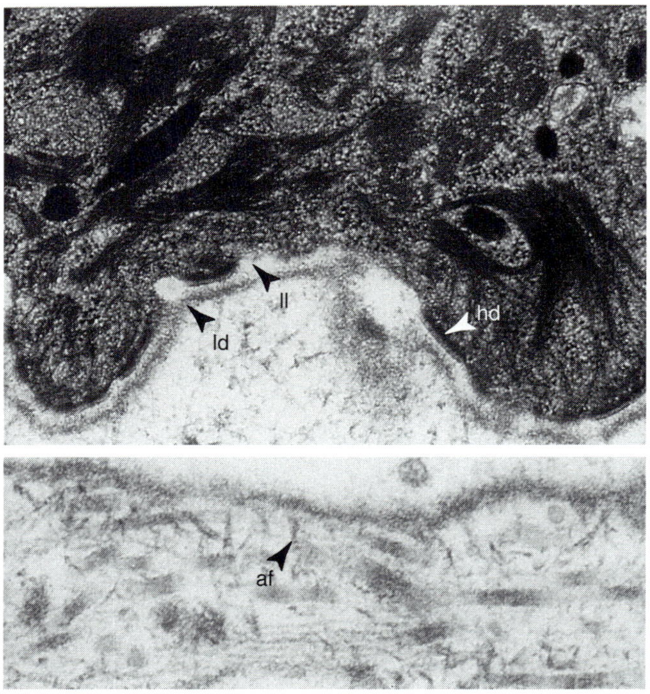

Figure 1–54. Normal epidermal basement membrane zone. Ultrastructurally, this membrane is composed of a lamina lucida (ll), lamina densa (ld), and anchoring fibrils (af). Hemidesmosomes (hd) bind basal keratinocytes to the basement membrane.

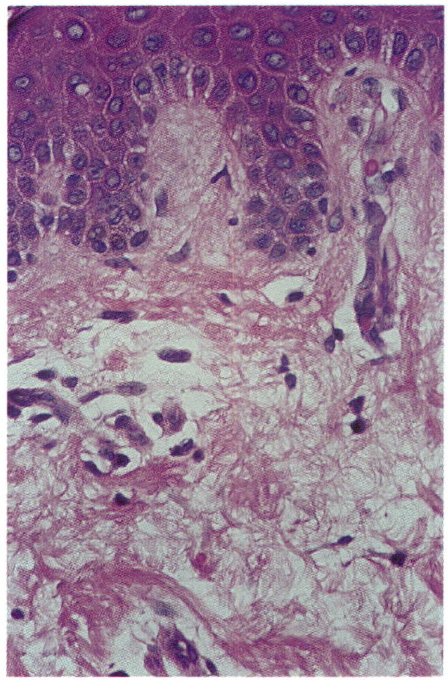

Figure 1–55. The superficial microvascular plexus represents an anatomic boundary between papillary dermis and reticular dermis. Cells that surround this plexus include mast cells (one to three per vessel profile), macrophages, and dermal dendrocytes. Capillary loops *(top right)* emanating from this plexus extend vertically into dermal papillae and are conduits for nutrients that supply the avascular epidermal layer.

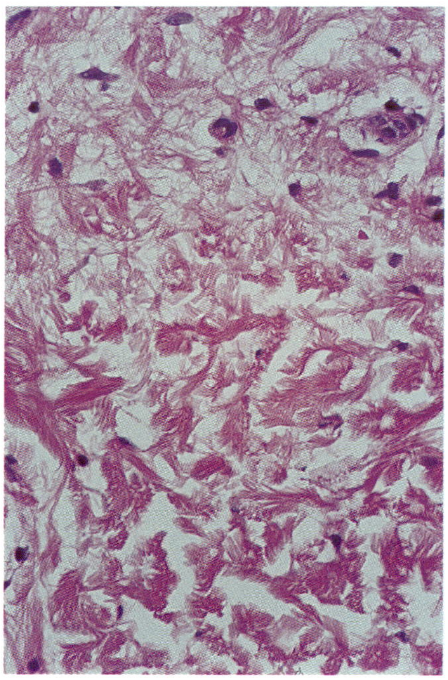

Figure 1–56. The papillary dermis *(top center)* is composed of type III collagen and is formed by thin, interwoven strands. The reticular dermis *(bottom center)* is composed of type I collagen and is formed by relatively thick collagen bundles.

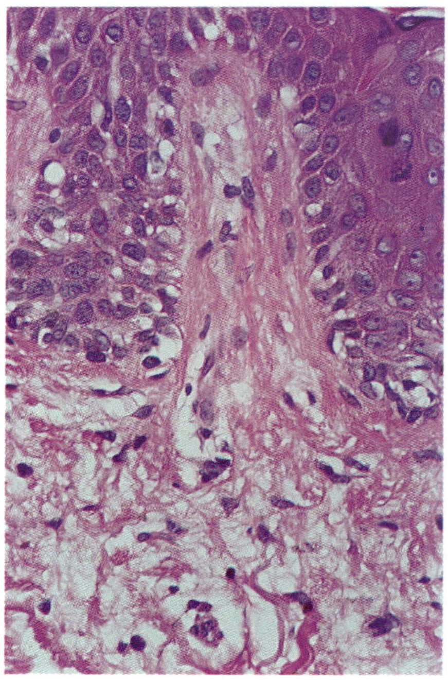

Figure 1–57. Dermal papillae and associated microvessels. The delicate capillary loops and surrounding papillary dermal collagen seen in routine sections of normal skin undergo dramatic alterations in patients with conditions such as stasis dermatitis (see Fig. 1–59) and lichen simplex chronicus (see Fig. 1–60).

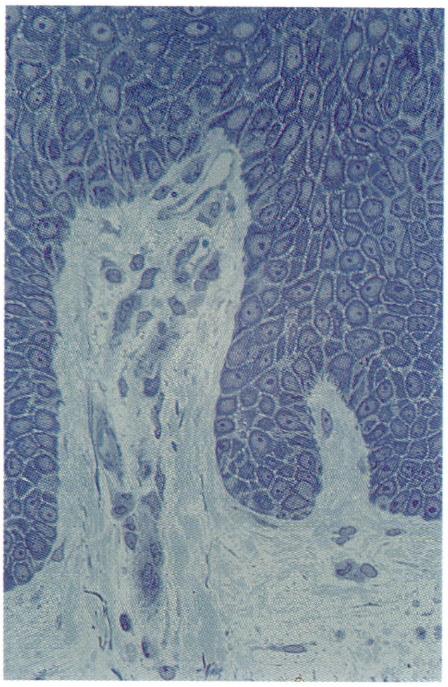

Figure 1–58. Dermal papillae and associated microvessels. Here, the delicate capillary loops and surrounding papillary dermal collagen are seen in 1-μm sections.

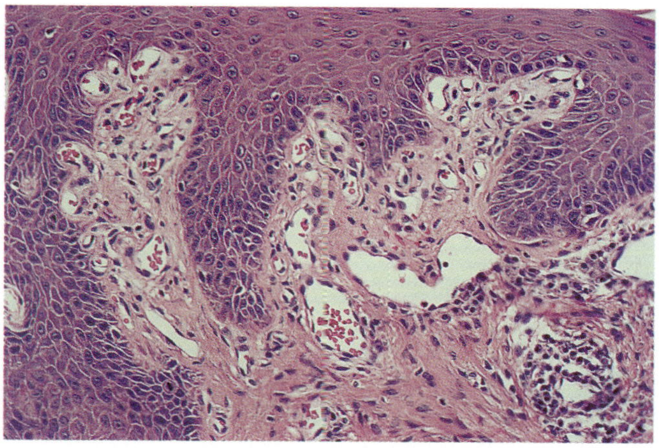

Figure 1–59. In stasis dermatitis, superficial vessels become ectatic and tortuous, and the delicate surrounding collagen assumes a coarse, fibrillar quality.

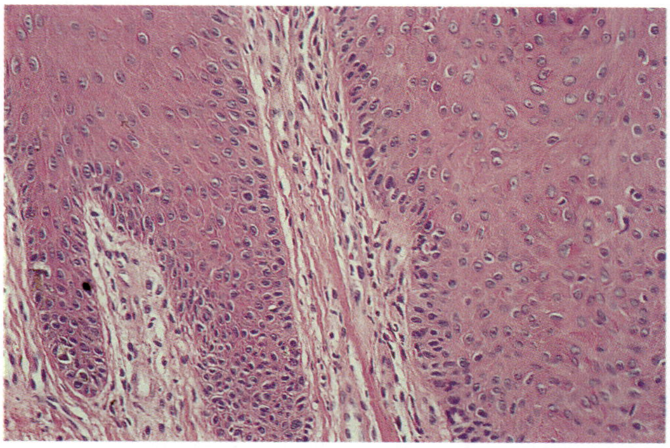

Figure 1–60. In lichen simplex chronicus, collagen within dermal papillae thickens and aligns in a vertical array.

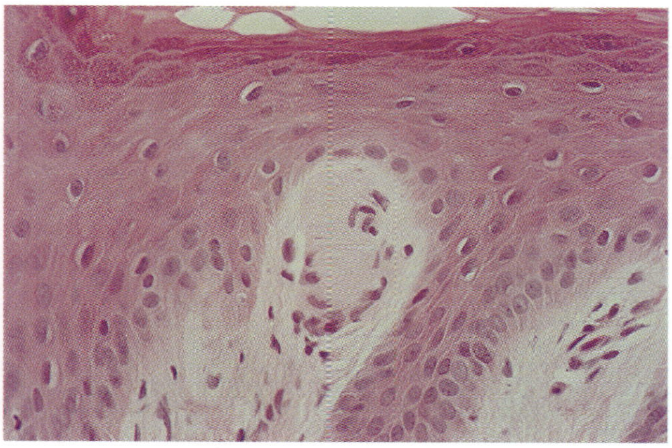

Figure 1–61. Meissner corpuscles within the superficial dermis represent touch receptors.

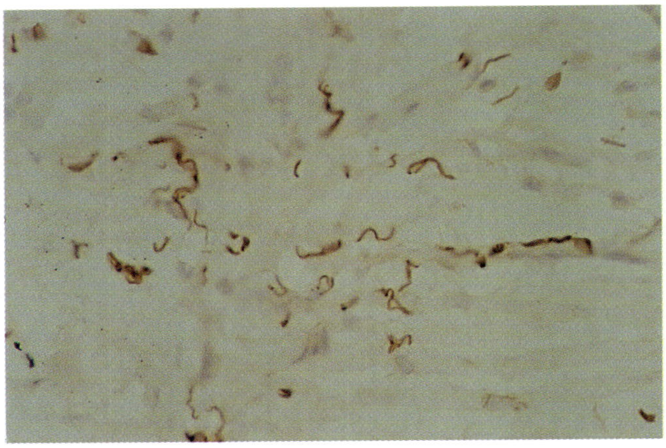

Figure 1–62. Unmyelinated nerve fibers, stained immunocytochemically for the neural cell adhesion molecule, are closely associated with vascular plexuses and adnexal structures.

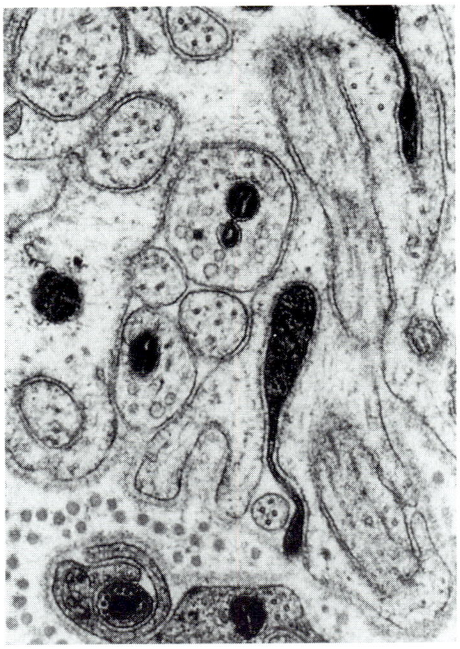

Figure 1–63. Ultrastructure of unmyelinated dermal nerve fibers. Axons *(center)* are enveloped by Schwann cell cytoplasm *(left).*

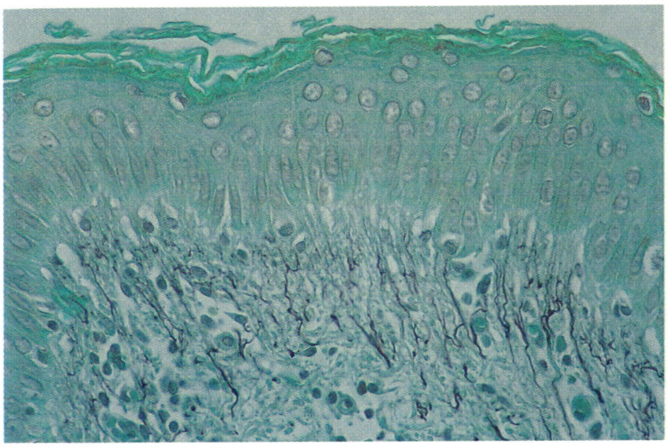

Figure 1–64. The normal human elastic fiber network (dark-gray, thin fibers) tethers the epidermis to the reticular dermis. (Elastic tissue stain.)

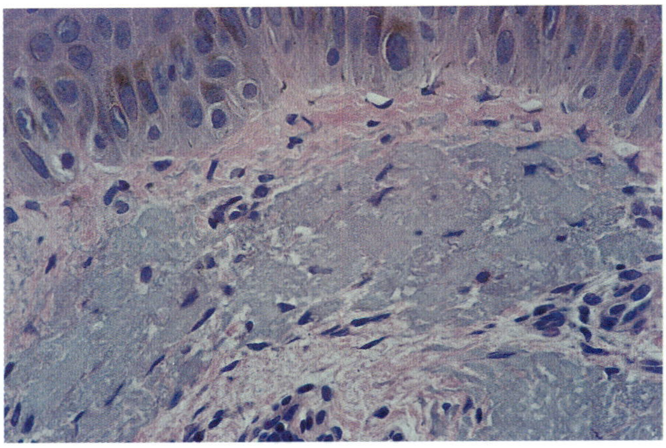

Figure 1–65. Solar elastosis (blue-gray material [*center*]) replaces the normal elastic fiber network. (Routine hematoxylin and eosin stain.)

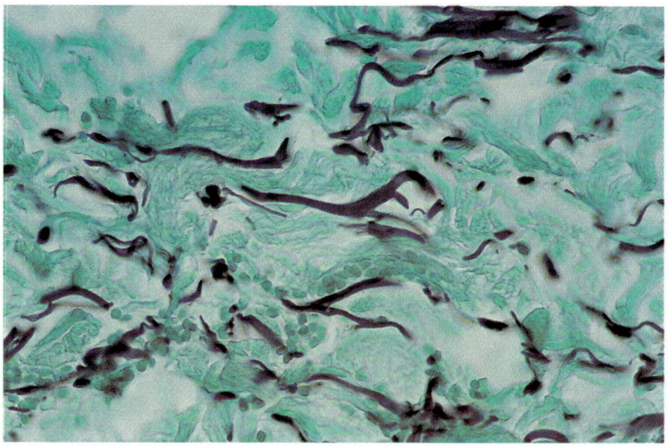

Figure 1–66. Reticular dermal elastic fibers normally are present amid collagen bundles. (Elastic tissue stain.)

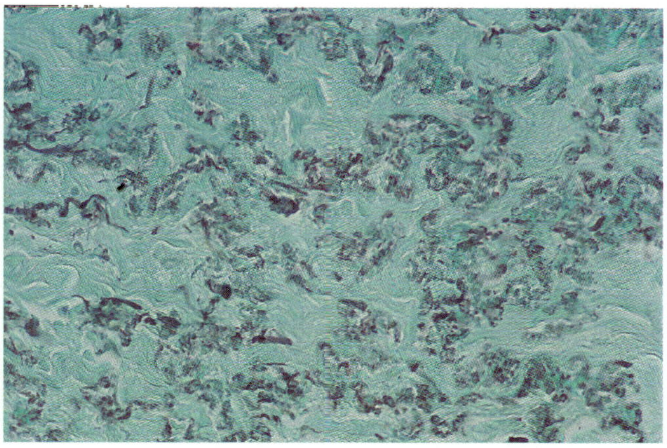

Figure 1–67. Pathologically altered reticular dermal elastic fibers are seen in a patient who has pseudoxanthoma elasticum. (Elastic tissue stain.)

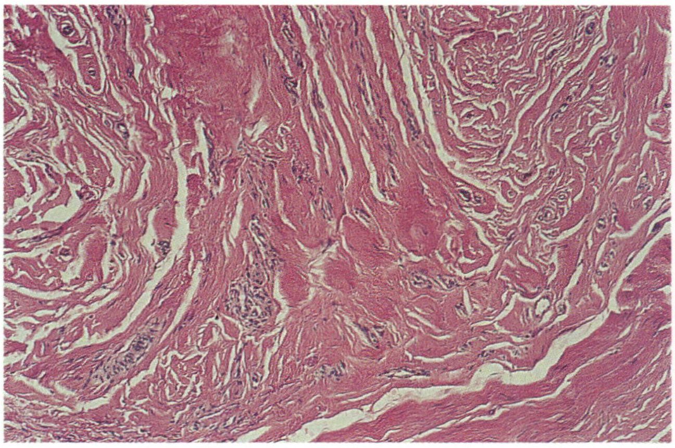

Figure 1–68. Common reaction patterns of dermal collagenous matrix: sclerosis and proliferation. In hypertrophic scars, dermal collagen is replaced by whirling parallel arrays of collagen fibers and proliferating vessels.

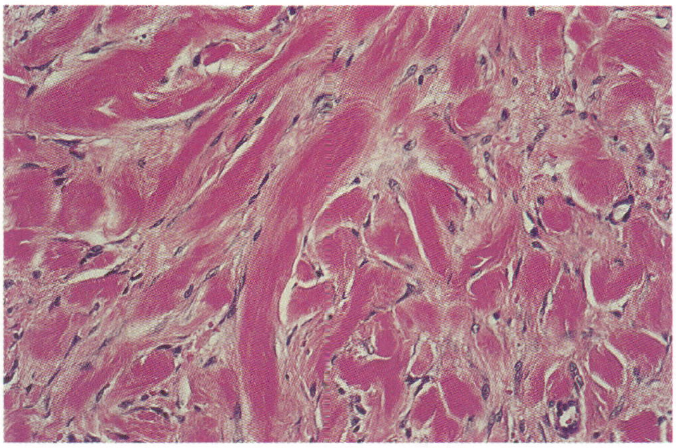

Figure 1–69. Keloids are characterized by glassy, intensely eosinophilic bands of collagen interspersed with pale, thin fibers.

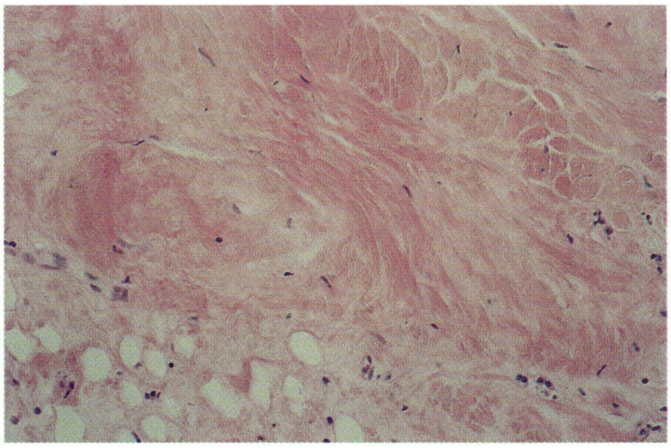

Figure 1–70. Scleroderma typically has pale-pink, homogenized collagen containing few nucleated cells.

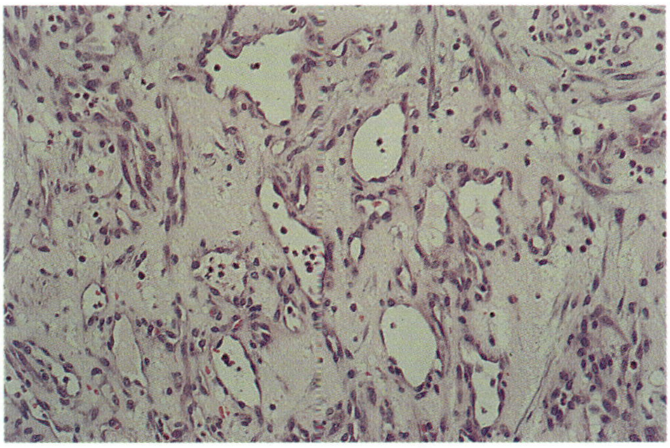

Figure 1–71. Pyogenic granulomas are typified by aggregates of dilated, proliferating vessels within a pale, edematous, often inflamed collagenous stroma.

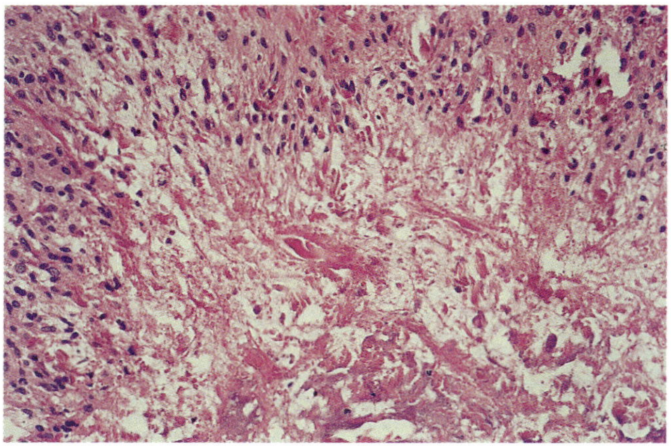

Figure 1–72. Common reaction pattern of dermal collagenous matrix: degeneration. Particulate, pink-blue, mucinous necrobiosis of collagen takes place in patients who have granuloma annulare.

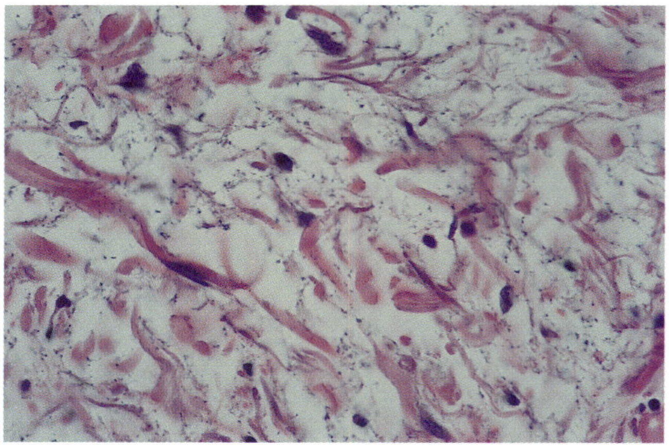

Figure 1–73. Higher magnification of Figure 1–72 shows stringy, pale-blue mucin strands admixed with thin collagen fibers.

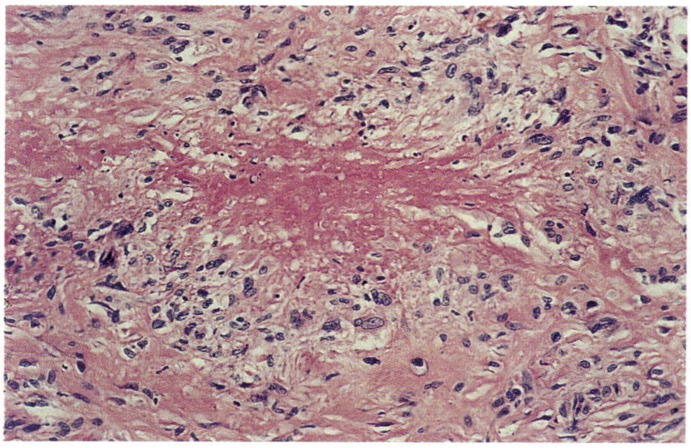

Figure 1–74. Granular (*i.e.,* fibrinoid) collagen degeneration of the rheumatoid nodule is present in the central portion of the panel.

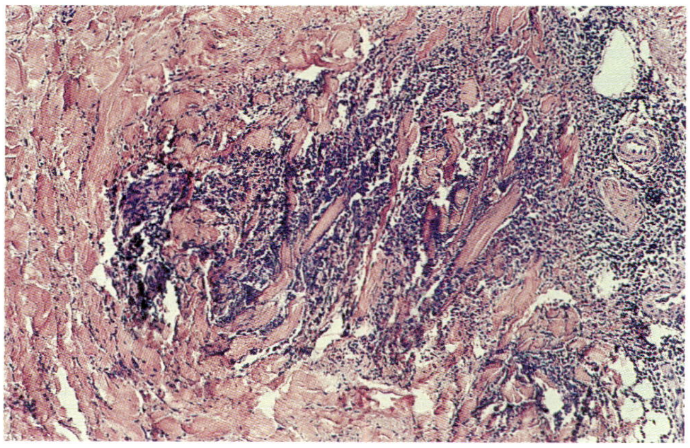

Figure 1–75. Glassy, red-orange collagen bundles entrapped in darkly stained aggregates of inflammatory cells (eosinophils) are known as flame figures.

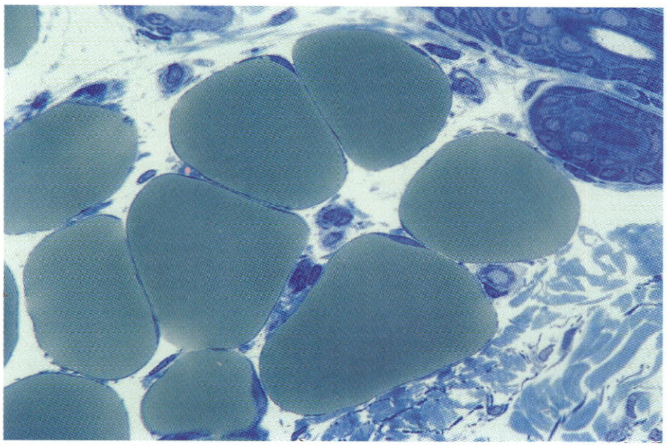

Figure 1–76. Subcutaneous fat: patterns of reaction and injury. A 1-μm section shows adipocytes as cells engorged with homogeneous blue lipid with compressed nuclei at the cell perimeter.

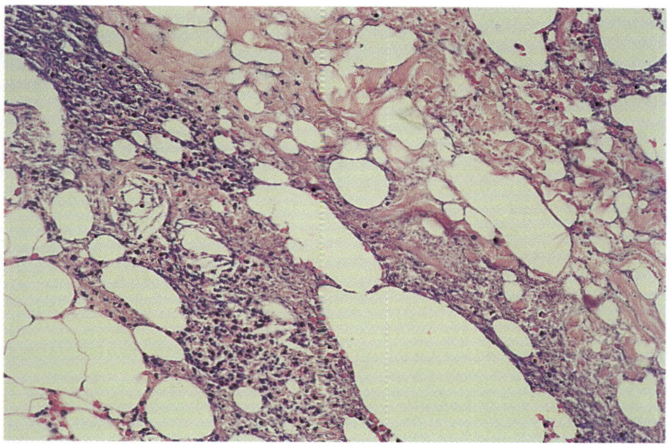

Figure 1–77. Atrophy and liquefactive necrosis of adipocytes within a lobule in lupus panniculitis.

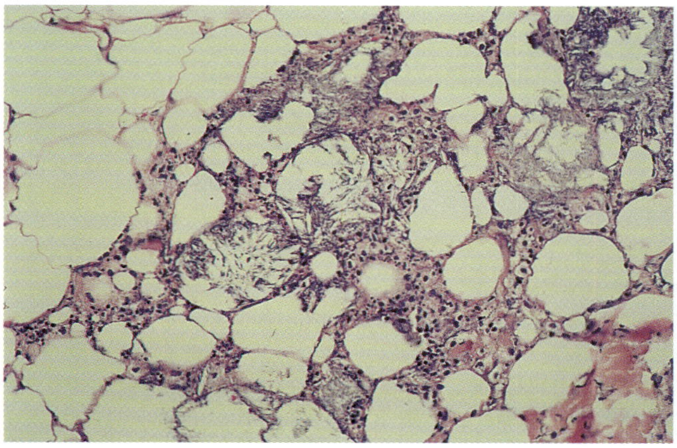

Figure 1–78. Aggregates of basophilic inflammatory cells are associated with crystallization of lipid within adipocytes in subcutaneous fat necrosis of the newborn.

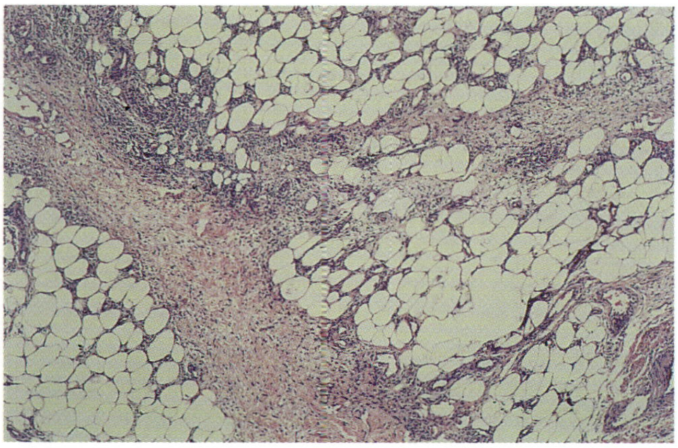

Figure 1–79. Septa that separate fat lobules are prominently infiltrated by basophilic aggregates of inflammatory cells in patients who have septal panniculitis (*i.e.,* erythema nodosum); the pale-pink zone in the involved septum represents early fibrosis.

2

Diagnostic Methodology: Special Techniques

The purposes of this chapter are to briefly depict available special diagnostic techniques and to provide a practical guide for more commonly encountered immunofluorescence patterns in skin. With the historical development of diagnostic immunofluorescence techniques for evaluation of lupus erythematosus and certain vesiculobullous disorders, dermatopathology has paved the way for the growing utilization of special diagnostic techniques in pathology as a whole. Although virtually all laboratories employ histochemistry as an adjunct to routine hematoxylin and eosin–stained sections, many do not have immunostaining or ultrastructural approaches readily available. However, growing numbers of referral laboratories provide these services on receipt of appropriately fixed or preserved tissue samples, making these specialized approaches readily available when problem situations arise.

Routine histochemical stains are generally used for detection of inorganic substances such as iron, calcium, and silver; polysaccharides (periodic acid–Schiff stain with and without diastase digestion); mucopolysaccharides (Alcian blue stain); mast cell metachromasia (Giemsa reagent); lipids (oil-red-O stain); extracellular matrix elements (Weigert stain for elastin); organisms (Ziehl-Neelsen stain for acid-fast bacilli); and certain enzymes (DOPA reagent). Figure 1–66 depicts histochemical stains for elastic fibers, and Figure 1–31 demonstrates enzyme histochemistry. By definition, appreciation of technical characteristics is critical to interpretation of routine histochemical stains. In a similar manner, immunohistochemistry that employs chromogenic substrates for antibody detection also requires careful evaluation of color and hue to differentiate true reactivity from endogenous pigment (*e.g.*, melanin or hemosiderin). Finally, immunofluorescence, which requires evaluation of the bright-green fluorochrome, fluorescein, may be difficult to interpret as a result of endogenous and background fluorescence characteristics of skin cells and matrix elements. In general, the green light attributed to excitation of the fluorescein molecule has a brighter, more glimmering quality than the dull glow of background images.

This chapter is intended primarily to provide a visual reference for specific and nonspecific immunofluorescence patterns in a manner in which color quality, hue, intensity, and architecture can be appreciated simultaneously.

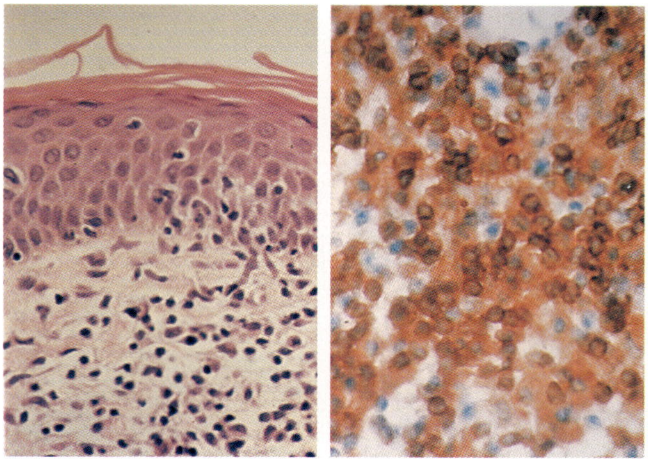

Figure 2–1. Cell typing by immunohistochemistry. In routine sections *(left)*, these relatively small lymphocytes appear bland, although they are diffusely infiltrating the papillary dermis and have begun to migrate into a relatively nonspongiotic epidermal layer. T-cell typing *(right)* reveals more than 90% of these cells to be of the CD4+ helper-inducer T-cell subset, consistent with a clonal proliferation of this functional class of T cells.

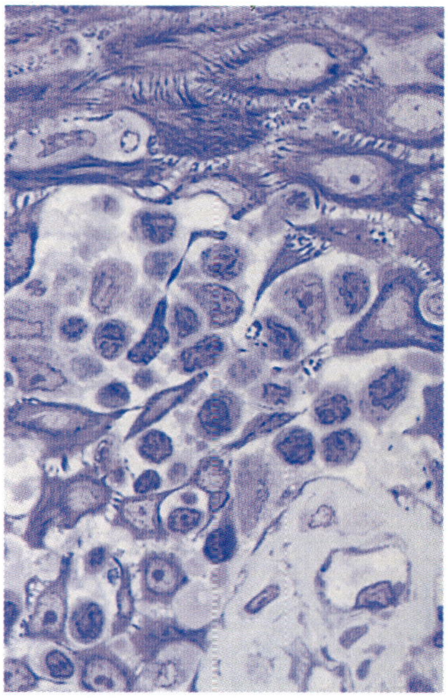

Figure 2–2. One-micron section. In early cutaneous T-cell lymphoma, lymphocytes infiltrating the epidermis display markedly infolded nuclear membranes when viewed in 1-μm sections.

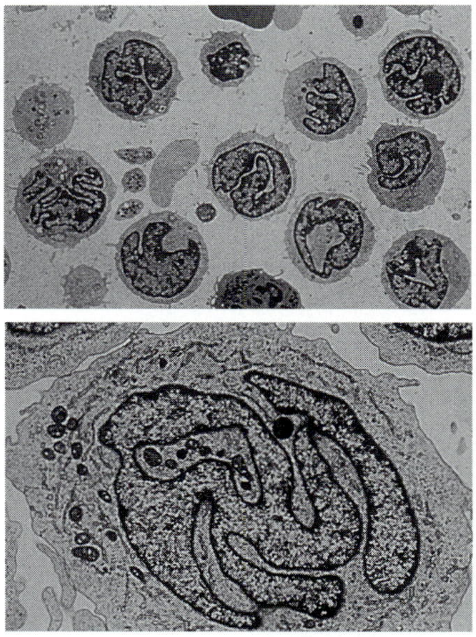

Figure 2–3. Transmission electron microscopy. These cells in buffy coat preparations from peripheral blood have characteristic cerebriform contours of Sézary-Lutzner cells. Computer-assisted image analysis of such ultrastructural images has been used to quantify the degree of nuclear complexity and to show that such cells are different from activated T cells, which also may exhibit some degree of nuclear irregularity.

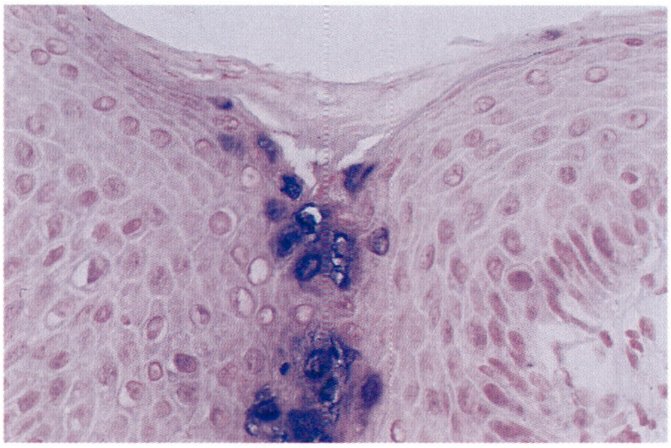

Figure 2–4. In situ hybridization for human papillomavirus. The labeled genomic probe is seen as zones of deep purple staining over virally infected nuclei. This probe was specific for human papillomavirus types 6 and 11, which are the common cause of condylomata.

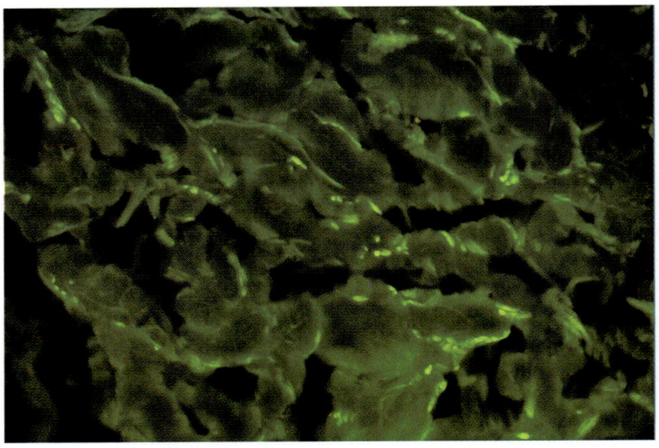

Figure 2–5. Autofluorescence for reticular dermal elastic fibers. Autofluorescence patterns are commonly confused with positive staining.

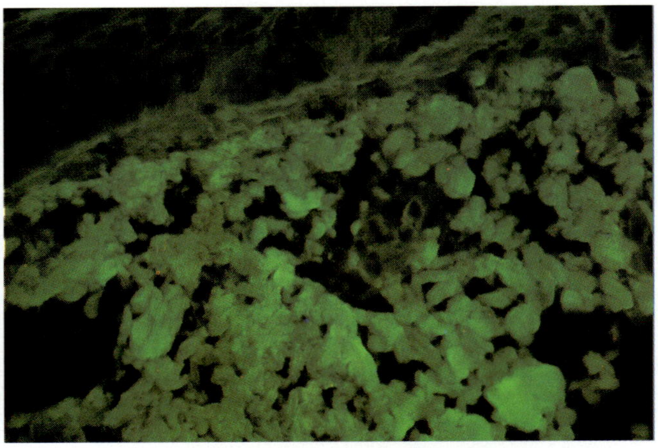

Figure 2–6. Autofluorescence for elastotic material in the papillary dermis of sun-damaged skin. The patchy autofluorescence of elastotic material is characteristic and should not be mistaken for colloid bodies or true antibody deposits.

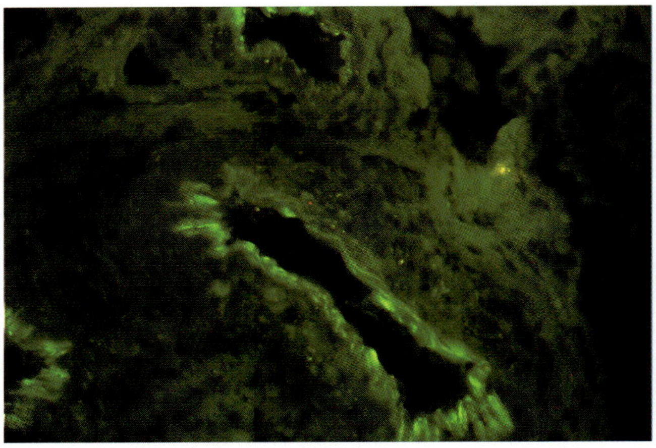

Figure 2–7. Autofluorescence for elastic lamina of a muscular dermal artery. The glassy quality of this vessel wall staining differentiates this pattern from true immune complex deposition, which tends to be granular.

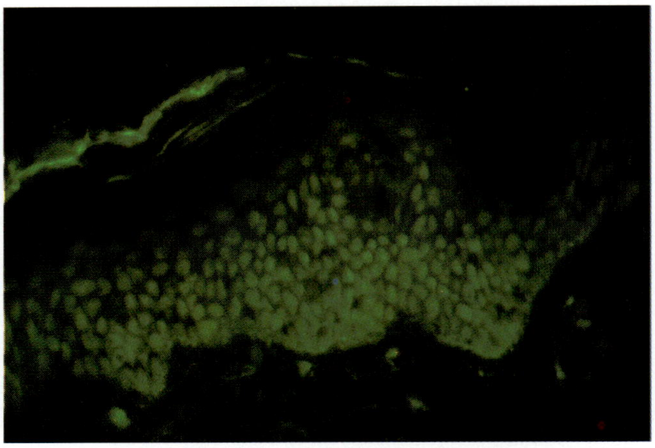

Figure 2–8. This pattern of nuclear fluorescence within the epidermal layer may be the result of intrinsic nuclear autofluorescence or specific or nonspecific binding of antibodies to nuclear proteins.

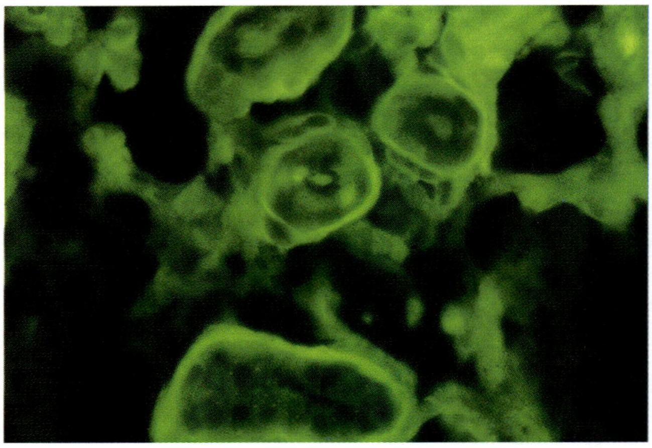

Figure 2–9. Basement membrane zone autofluorescence affecting the basement membranes of normal eccrine coils. Similar findings may be seen along the dermal-epidermal junction and around blood vessels. Weak linear basement membrane staining could be erroneously interpreted, although the universal expression of this pattern on all basement membranes, including those of dermal vessels, is an important clue indicating that this represents autofluorescence.

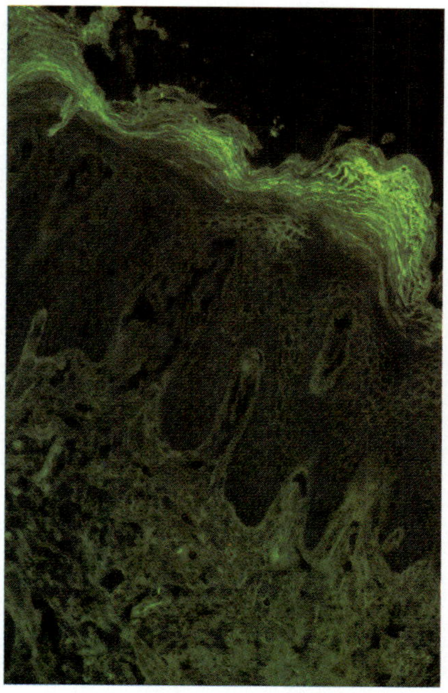

Figure 2–10. Although immunoglobulins and complement within the stratum corneum of the epidermis *(top)* may be associated with psoriasis, impetigo, scale or crust formation, and loculated serum transmitted into the scale in patients who have resolving spongiotic dermatitis, all may produce a similar nonspecific picture.

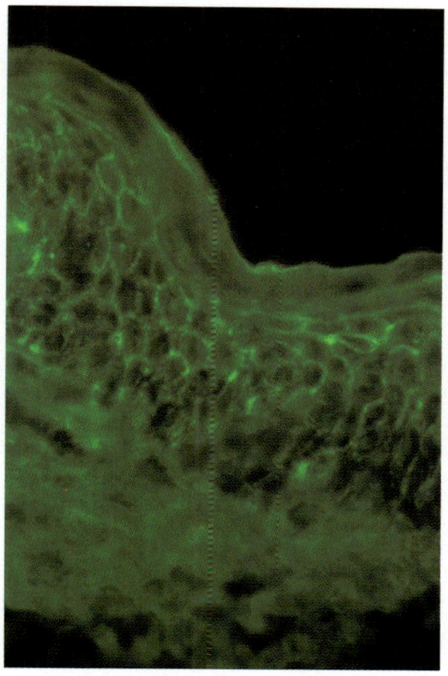

Figure 2–11. Active spongiotic dermatitis may result in nonspecific leakage of immune reactants into the intercellular spaces of the surface epidermis *(center)* or adnexal epithelium, resulting in a pattern that mimics cell membrane staining in patients who have pemphigus. In such instances, all antibody classes (*i.e.,* IgG, IgA, IgM) are generally detected, in contrast to preferential expression of one antibody class (*e.g.,* IgG), which suggests a specific reaction.

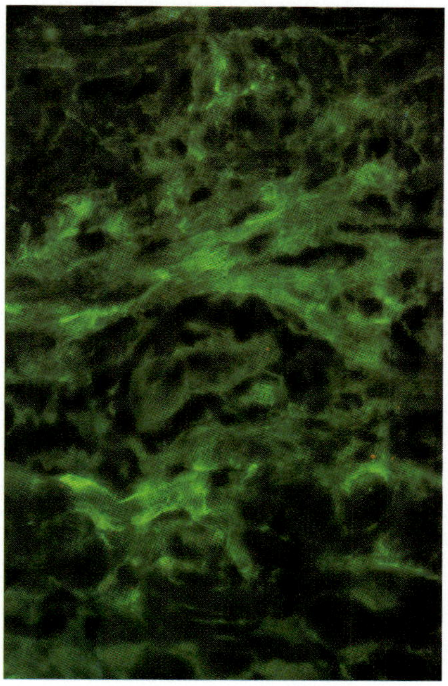

Figure 2–12. Immune reactants and fibrin commonly are deposited in the perivascular *(center)* space. This is indicative of increased vascular permeability but is not representative of a diagnostically specific pattern.

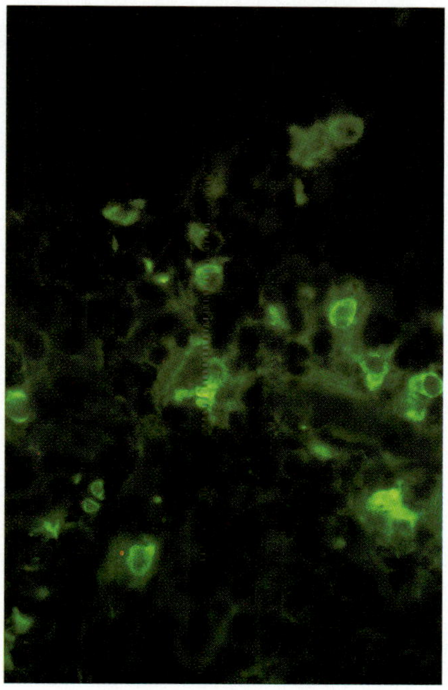

Figure 2–13. Nonspecific binding of immunoglobulins via Fc-receptor interactions with plasma membranes of inflammatory cells must be distinguished from specific staining of immune complexes in the walls of small venules.

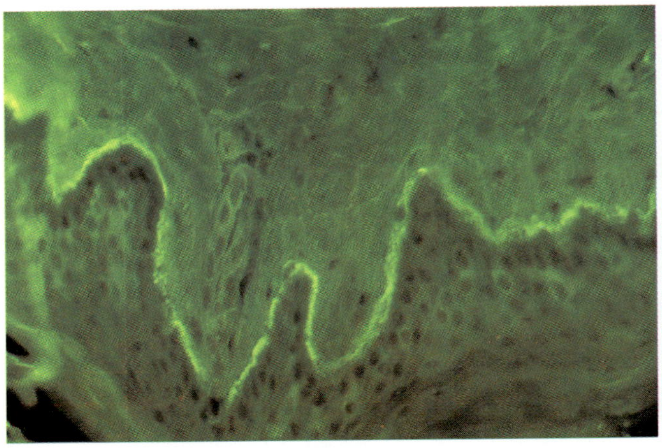

Figure 2–14. Linear basement membrane staining: pemphigoid. The linear staining seen in the subepidermal *(center)* basal lamina of perilesional skin is usually most intense for C_3 and has a glassy, ribbon-like quality. An identical pattern is present in herpes gestationis.

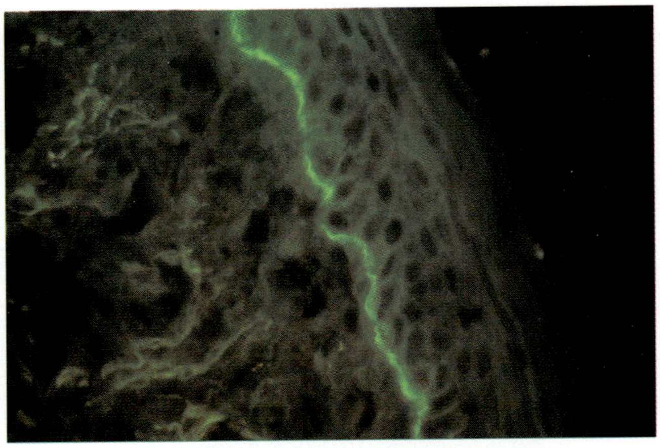

Figure 2–15. Similar staining may also be present about the adnexal epithelium (*center right:* follicular infundibulum).

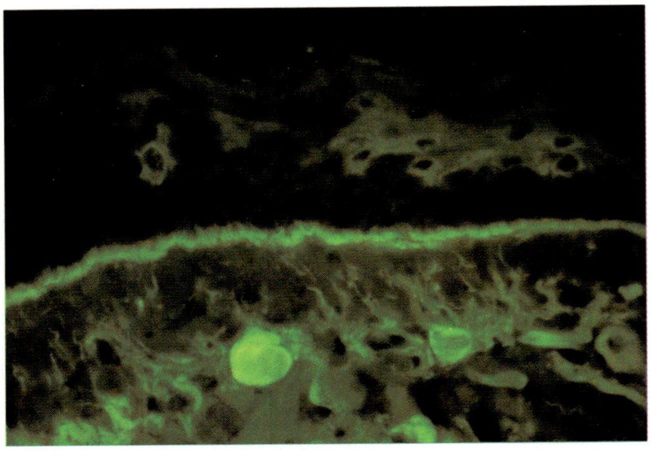

Figure 2–16. In pemphigus, recurrent involvement of a lesional site with repeated basal cell layer injury followed by re-epithelialization may result in colloid body formation *(bottom)* in addition to typical linear basement membrane zone reactivity *(center).* Colloid bodies characteristically stain diffusely for immunoglobulin (particularly IgM) and complement. In new lesions, the presence of colloid bodies in the setting of linear basement membrane zone staining for C_3 also raises the possibility of herpes gestationis.

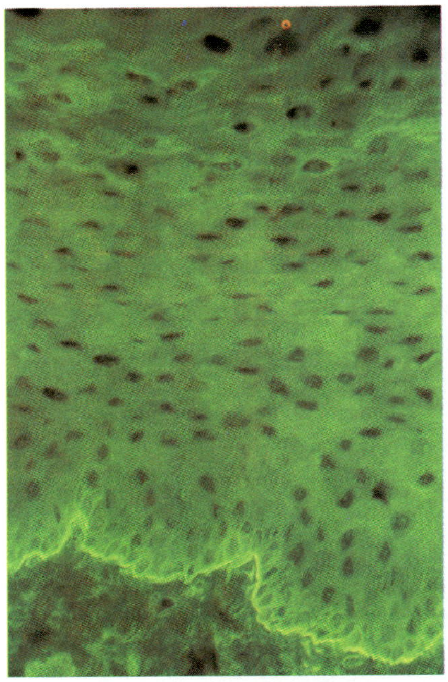

Figure 2–17. Indirect immunofluorescence in pemphigoid. Serum from patients with active pemphigoid may contain antibodies to the bullous pemphigoid antigen also expressed within the basal lamina of monkey esophagus. Serum incubated with sections of esophagus and then stained with fluorescein isothiocyanate (FITC)-labeled antibodies to human immunoglobulin produce a linear staining pattern *(bottom)* identical to that observed by direct immunofluorescence of lesional or perilesional skin.

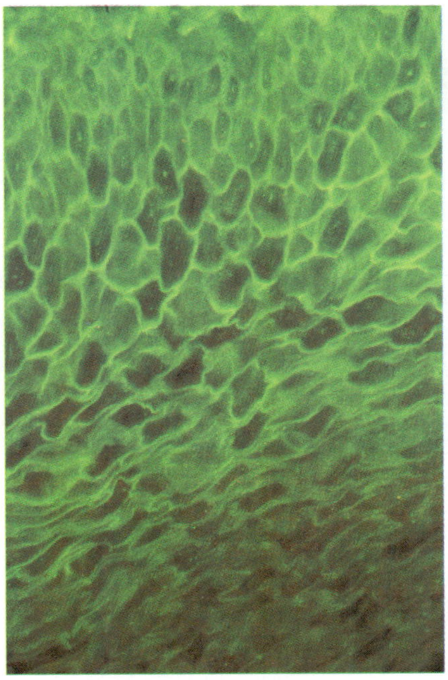

Figure 2–18. Indirect immunofluorescence in pemphigus. In pemphigus, circulating antibodies bind to intercellular spaces within the esophageal epithelium, resulting in a characteristic fish-net pattern.

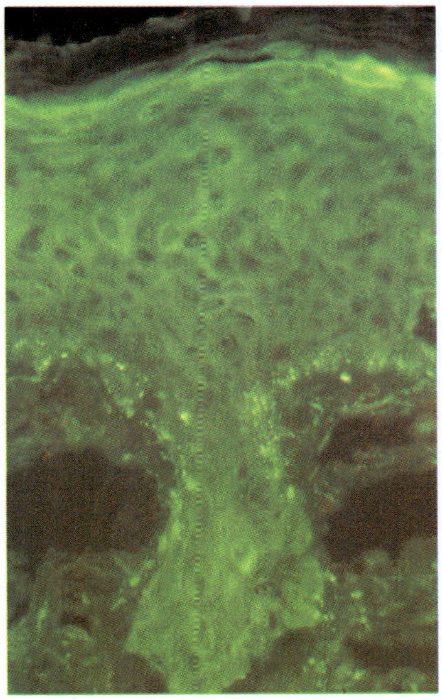

Figure 2–19. Lupus erythematosus. Although the epidermal layer shows homogeneous autofluorescence, the bright, shiny quality of the granular deposits of IgG at the dermal-epidermal junction in the biopsy specimen of nonlesional skin is easily discerned.

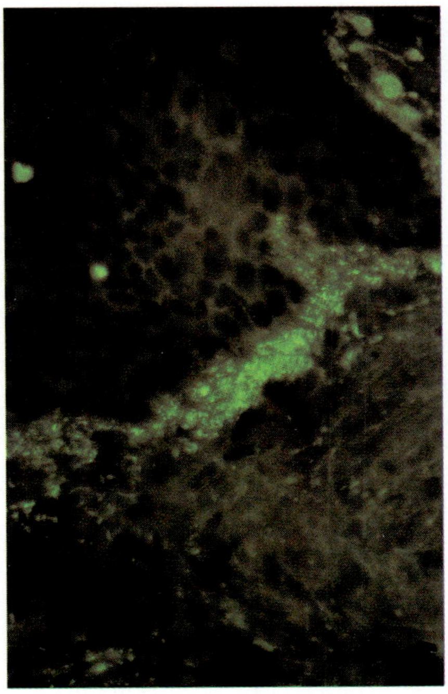

Figure 2–20. Lesional skin in lupus erythematosus shows even more pronounced granular deposits *(center)*. Other antibody classes and complement also may be present. Positive lupus band tests must show continuous, strong staining along the dermal-epidermal junction. The occurrence of a positive band in nonlesional skin is an indicator of systemic disease.

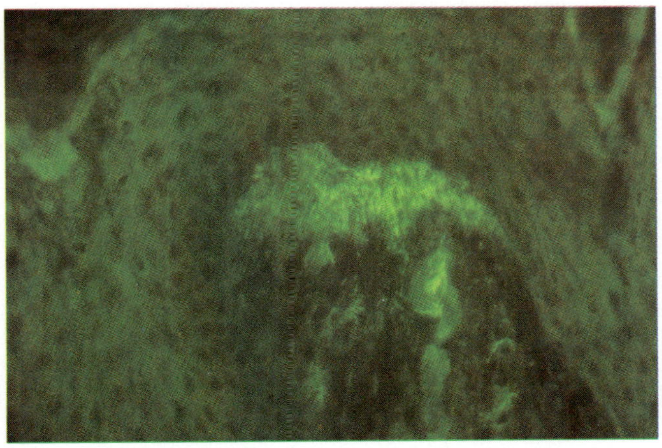

Figure 2–21. Dermatitis herpetiformis. Granular staining for IgA within the dermal papilla *(top center)* is readily observed in a developing lesion. At times, anchoring fibrils are outlined by the antibody deposits. In older lesions, granular staining may diffuse along the dermal-epidermal interface, mimicking a positive lupus band test. Unlike the pattern in lupus erythematosus, however, the granular pattern in dermatitis herpetiformis remains accentuated in the papillae and is predominated by antibody deposits of the IgA subclass.

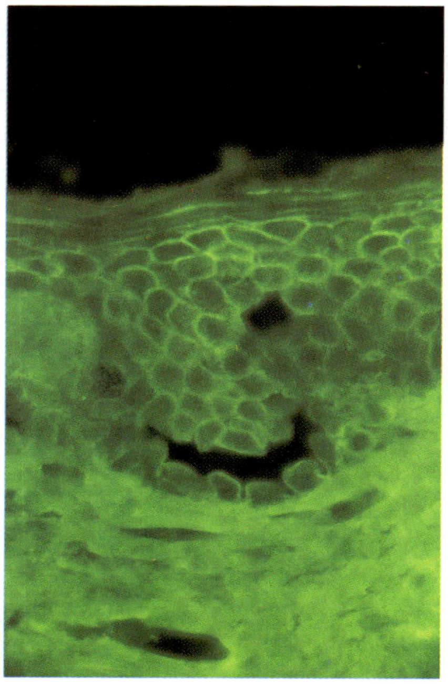

Figure 2–22. Pemphigus. A fish-net pattern of cell membrane IgG deposition preferentially stains the lower half of the epidermal layer in this characteristic biopsy specimen of experimentally induced pemphigus vulgaris. Note the early suprabasal acantholysis.

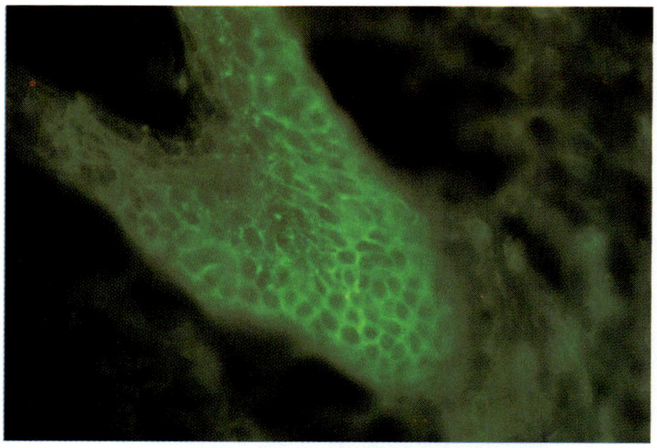

Figure 2–23. In pemphigus, follicular epithelium may show a similar staining pattern to that in Figure 2–22.

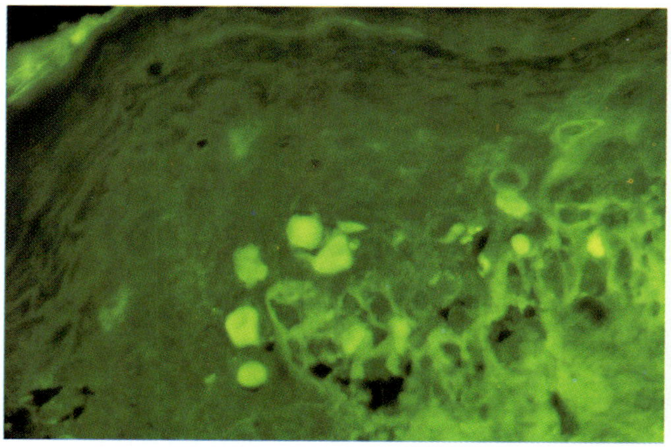

Figure 2–24. Colloid body formation: erythema multiforme. In acute cytotoxic dermatitis (*i.e.,* erythema multiforme), apoptotic cells within the epidermis take up immunoglobulin, particularly IgM, and are detected as intensely stained homogeneous round zones above a vacuolated basal cell layer *(center).*

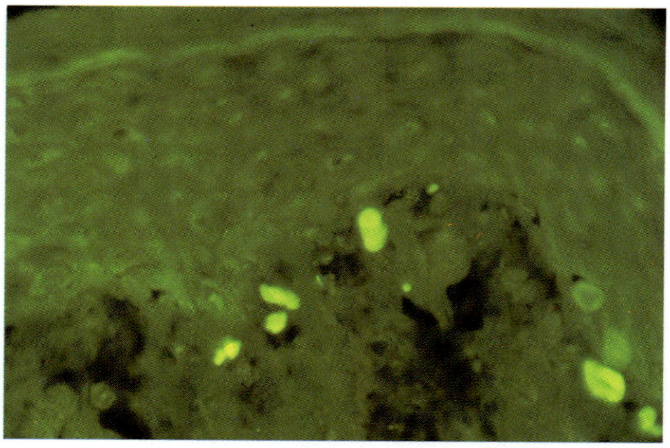

Figure 2–25. Colloid body formation: lichen planus. In chronic cytotoxic dermatitis (*i.e.,* lichen planus), such cells often are incorporated into the superficial dermis *(center);* colloid bodies are signified by globular zones of predominantly IgM deposition directly beneath the dermal-epidermal junction.

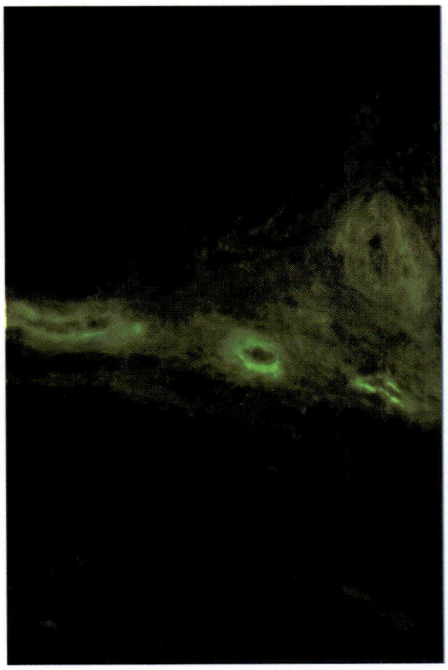

Figure 2–26. Vascular staining in necrotizing vasculitis. Small vessels within dermal papillae show granular deposits of IgG exclusively localized to their walls *(center).*

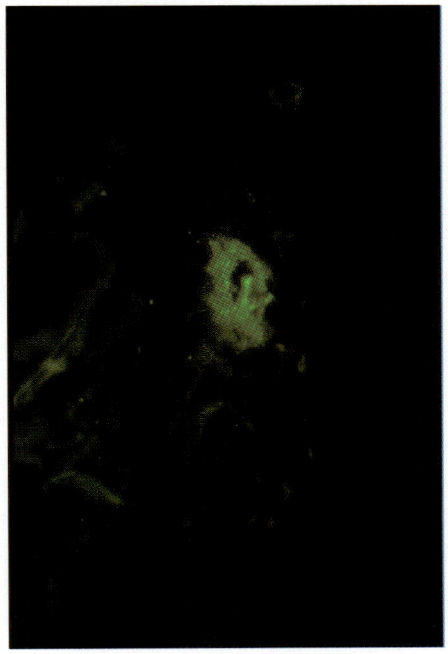

Figure 2–27. A similar pattern of deposition is seen for C_3 in an underlying superficial dermal venule.

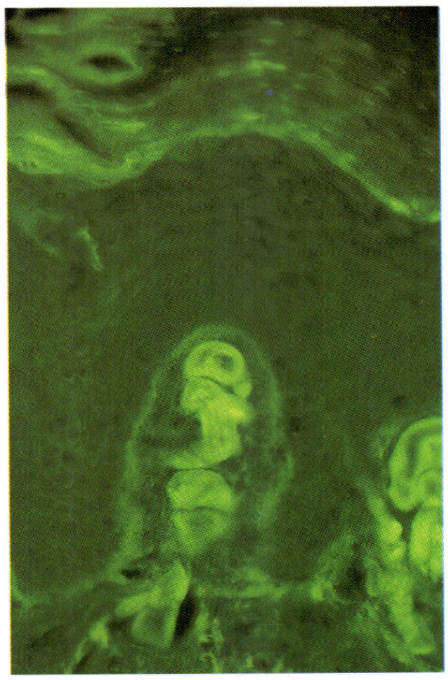

Figure 2–28. In porphyria, there is characteristic widening of small vessel walls *(center)* by homogeneous, glassy deposits of immunoglobulins (IgG) and albumen. As in vasculitis, the staining is localized precisely to vessel walls, as opposed to the vessel wall staining that accompanies increased permeability (*e.g.,* in urticaria or spongiotic dermatitis). The character of staining, however, is very different: granular in vasculitis and homogeneous in porphyria.

II

Inflammatory Dermatoses

3

Spongiotic Dermatitis

Spongiotic dermatitis is a category representing a diverse group of cutaneous disorders that share the finding of spongiosis within the epidermal layer. The term *spongiosis* derives from the absorbent sponge that originates from the porous connective tissue skeleton of marine animals of the phylum Porifera. In spongiotic dermatitis, the dermal-epidermal junction is abnormally permeable to plasma and proteins liberated from superficial venules, and as in a sponge, fluid accumulates predominantly within intercellular spaces separating keratinocytes. In early or mild spongiotic dermatitis, widened intercellular spaces within the epidermal layer impart a spongy appearance to the stratum spinosum, often accompanied by an intraepidermal accumulation of benign lymphocytes as they migrate from their initial perivenular location. From the standpoint of tinctorial change, this alteration results in pallor of the epidermal layer when viewed at scanning magnification. This reaction pattern contrasts with *urticaria,* in which the dermal-epidermal junction is not permissive to upward dissipation of occasionally pronounced dermal edema and inflammatory cell infiltration, and with *epidermotropic cutaneous T-cell lymphoma,* in which intraepithelial lymphocytic migration and proliferation occur in the relative absence of spongiosis. Interestingly, in urticaria, the same phenomenon that is seen in spongiosis (accumulation of extracellular fluid) produces pallor of the papillary dermis, resulting in a pale-pink hue.

The vague term *eczematous dermatitis* is frequently used to refer to spongiotic processes. Generally, this term refers to a clinical condition characterized by a pruritic, erythematous, oozing papulovesicular dermatitis that, with chronicity, may evolve to scaling, lichenified plaques. However, numerous disorders may show these features in the absence of the histologic finding of spongiosis. Eczematous dermatitis, therefore, fails to describe adequately temporal or clinicopathologic parameters required for its qualification as a meaningful descriptive term and is not used further in this chapter.

Subtle alterations in epidermal hue can represent the first indicator of a spongiotic process. In addition, at scanning magnification, a basophilia about superficial dermal vessels generally indicates an inflammatory component. Inflammatory cells often exhibit variations in coloration (*e.g.,* intense cytoplasmic redness of eosinophils versus pale-pink cytoplasm of neutrophils) that may be helpful in their rapid and accurate identification.

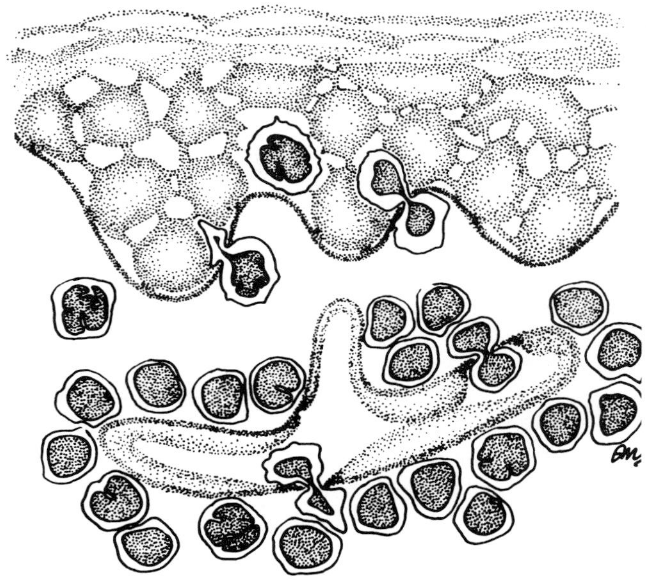

Figure 3–1. Structural-functional basis for spongiotic dermatitis. Early evolution of acute spongiotic dermatitis is characterized by lymphocyte epidermotropism. The intercellular spaces of the epidermis are widened by edema fluid derived from hyperpermeable venules within the underlying superficial vascular plexus. This vascular event is accompanied by initial accumulation of lymphocytes and other inflammatory cells within the perivascular space of superficial and sometimes deep dermal venules. Lymphocytes also characteristically migrate into the overlying spongiotic epidermal layer.

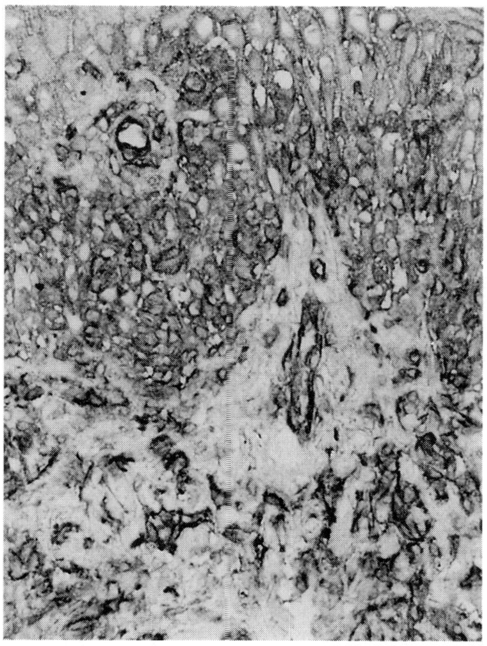

Figure 3–2. Patterns of lymphocytic trafficking in spongiotic dermatitis are partially determined by the expression of adhesion molecules by skin cells. An immunohistochemical preparation of a specimen from a patient who has early acute spongiotic dermatitis shows reactivity for intercellular adhesion molecule-1 (ICAM-1) by keratinocytes, endothelial cells, and dermal dendritic immune cells and fibroblasts. ICAM-1 binds lymphocytes, and its expression correlated precisely with sites of lymphocyte migration in this biopsy specimen.

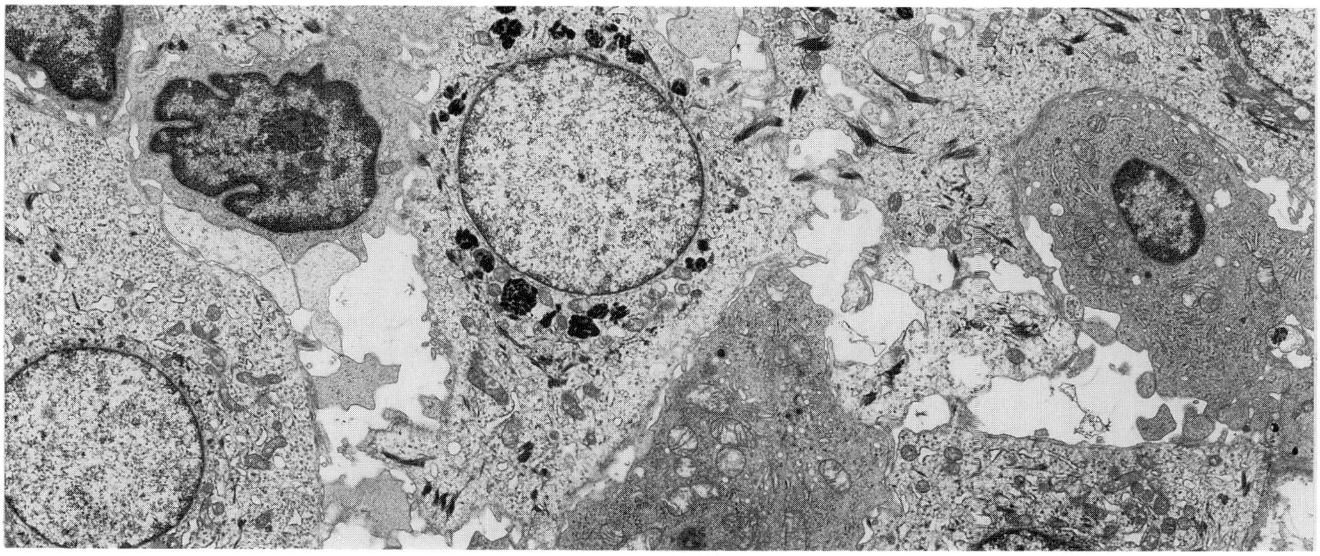

Figure 3–3. Ultrastructural studies confirm widened intercellular spaces within the epidermis in a patient who has spongiotic dermatitis. Several lymphocytes may also be seen within the prominent, expanded gaps separating adjacent keratinocytes. Disruption of intercellular junctions (*i.e.*, desmosomes) may eventuate in microvesicles and clinical blisters.

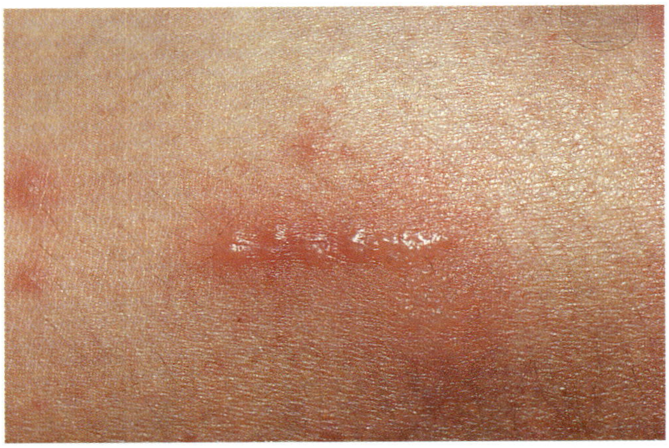

Figure 3–4. Clinical appearance of spongiotic dermatitis. Initial erythema and induration have evolved to form vesicles filled with clear yellow fluid. These vesicles resulted from intercellular edema within the epidermal layer (*i.e.*, spongiosis) that traumatically destroyed intercellular attachments. In time, the vesicles will rupture and dry, and if the inflammatory stimulus remains, persistent erythema and abnormal scale formation will supervene (subacute to chronic spongiotic dermatitis). Note the linearity of the lesion that corresponds to the zone of antigen contact.

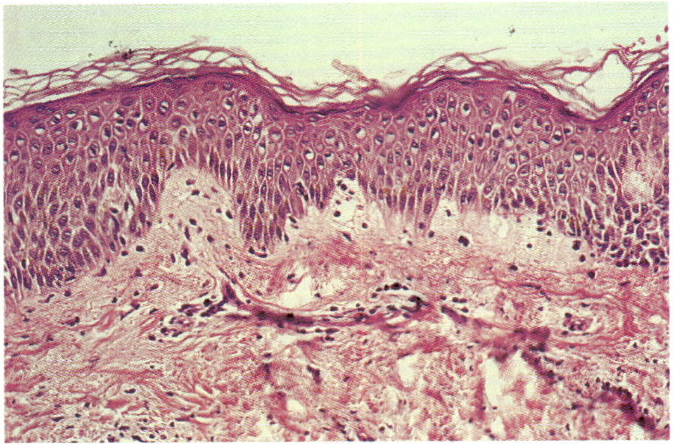

Figure 3–5. Temporal evolution of acute spongiotic dermatitis. Edema fluid initially accumulates within the papillary dermis, similar to urticaria. Edema within the dermis is subtle, but it may be appreciated as a band of pallor beneath the basement membrane zone of the epidermis.

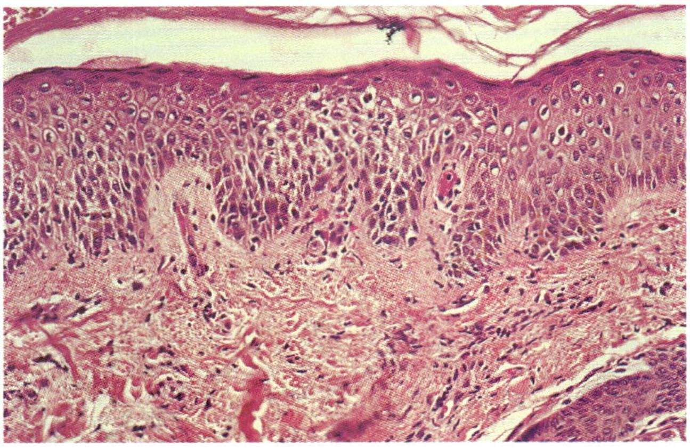

Figure 3–6. As lymphocytes begin to accumulate about superficial venules and migrate into the epidermal layer, associated spongiosis is observed as focal regions of epidermal pallor resulting from the increased area occupied by widened intercellular spaces.

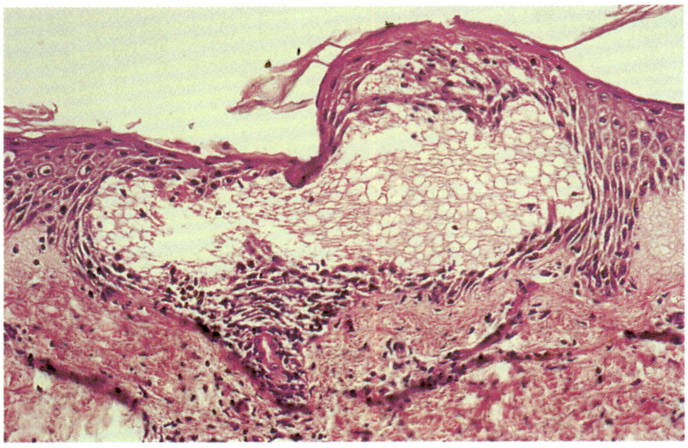

Figure 3–7. Traumatic lysis of intercellular junctions as spongiosis becomes more pronounced results in intraepidermal microvesicles filled with pink, proteinaceous, serum transudate.

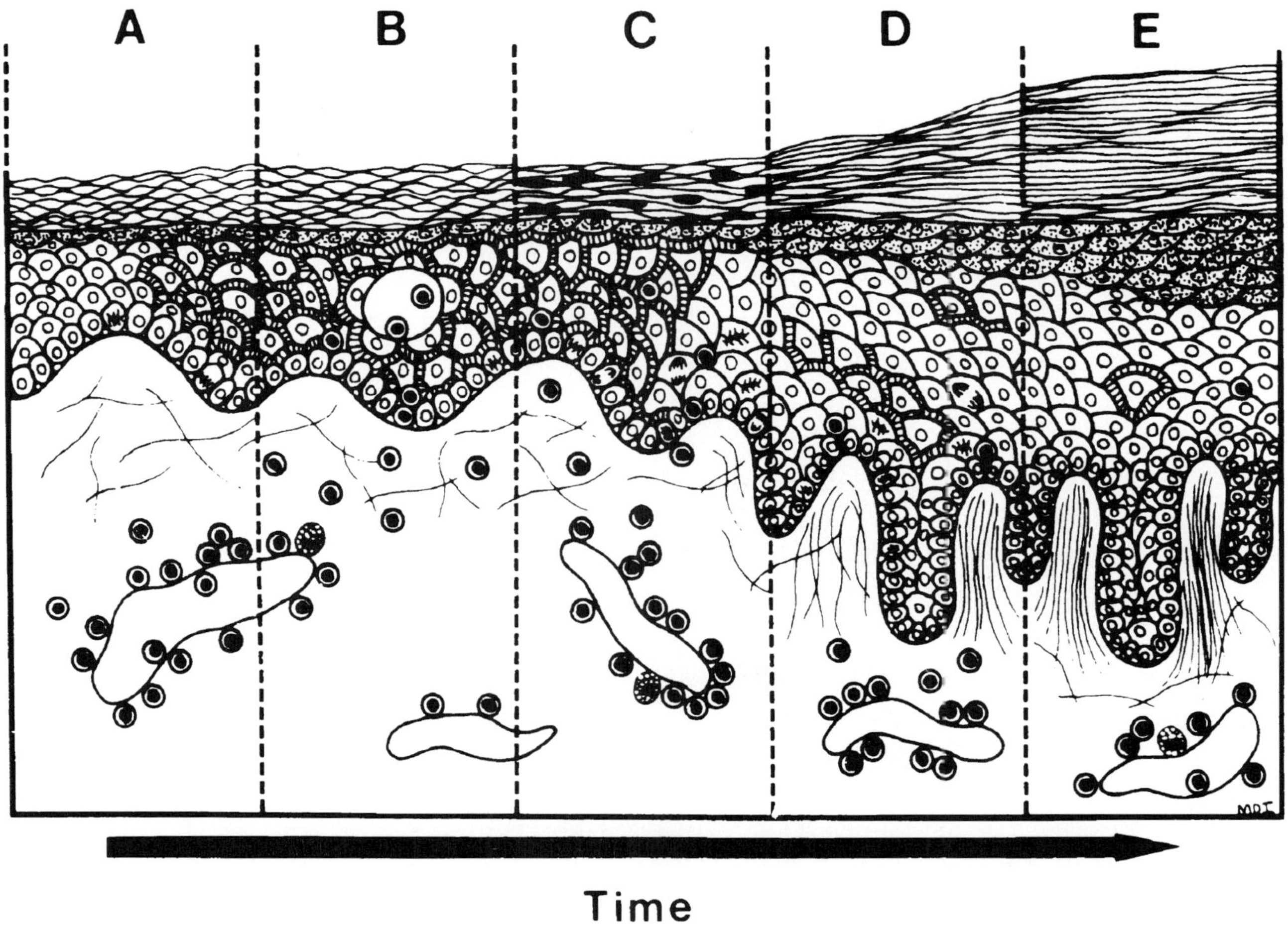

Figure 3–8. Evolutionary stages of spongiotic dermatitis. *A,* Initial perivascular infiltration is followed within 24 to 48 hours by papillary dermal edema and spongiosis with microvesicle formation *(B)*. *C,* Abnormal scale, including parakeratosis, follows, along with progressive epidermal hyperplasia *(D)* and hyperkeratosis *(E)*. Chronic excoriation results in vertically oriented fibrosis of dermal papillae (*i.e.,* lichen simplex chronicus).

Allergic Contact Dermatitis

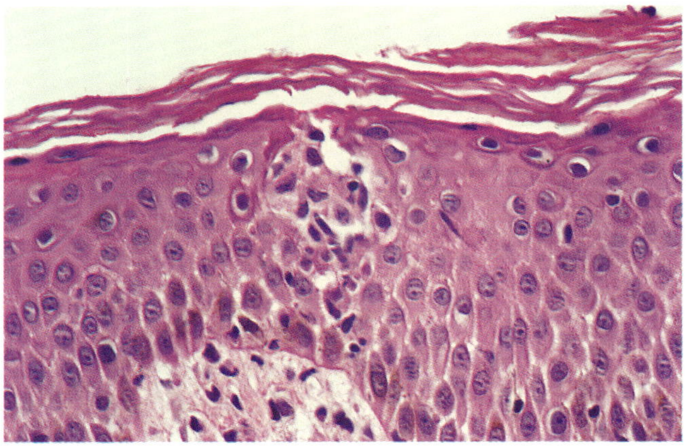

Figure 3–9. Allergic contact dermatitis (ACD). Epidermotropism of lymphocytes into spongiotic foci of the epidermal layer is observed at higher magnification. Several cells in this aggregate display infolded nuclear contours and abundant quantities of pale-pink cytoplasm. These foci represent hyperplastic aggregates of Langerhans cells (*i.e.,* Langerhans cell microgranuloma), a frequent finding in ACD.

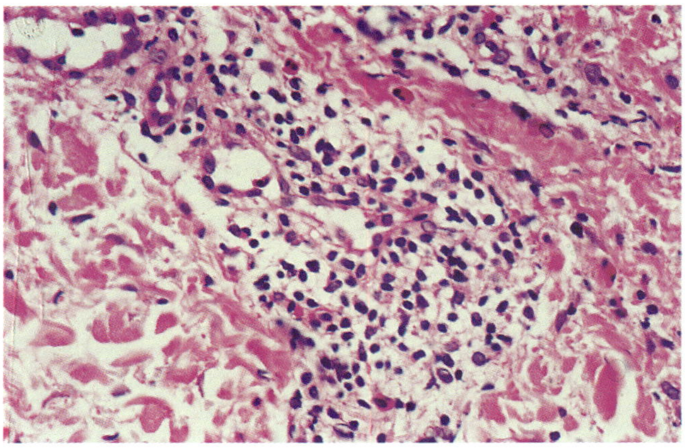

Figure 3–10. The perivascular inflammatory infiltrate in allergic contact dermatitis consists of lymphocytes, monocytes, and, often, eosinophils *(bottom right)* located about postcapillary venules. Spaces between perivenular collagen bundles are abnormally accentuated as a result of superficial dermal edema.

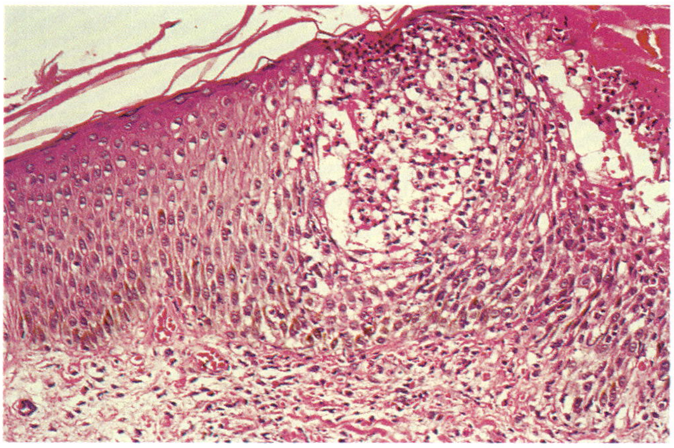

Figure 3–11. In some cases of allergic contact dermatitis, eosinophils may be so numerous as to form intraepidermal micropustules (*i.e.,* eosinophilic spongiosis). The finding of eosinophilic spongiosis itself, however, is not specific and has a broad differential diagnosis that includes certain insect-bite reactions, pemphigoid, and, rarely, pemphigus and the vesicular stage of incontinentia pigmenti.

Atopic Dermatitis

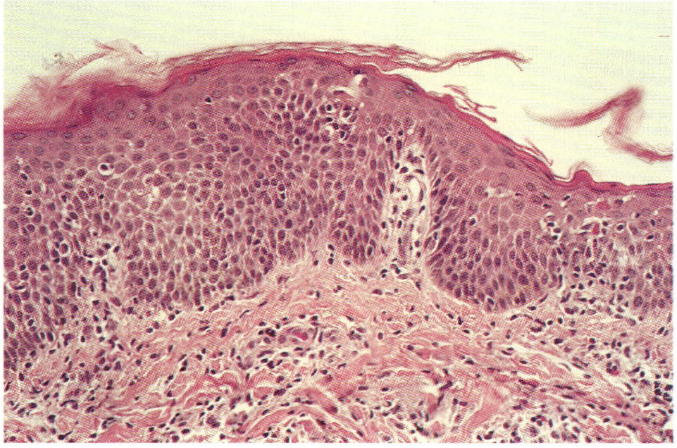

Figure 3–12. Atopic dermatitis. At low-to-medium magnification, the epidermis is focally hyperplastic and minimally spongiotic. The underlying papillary dermis contains a sparse, perivascular, lymphocytic infiltrate.

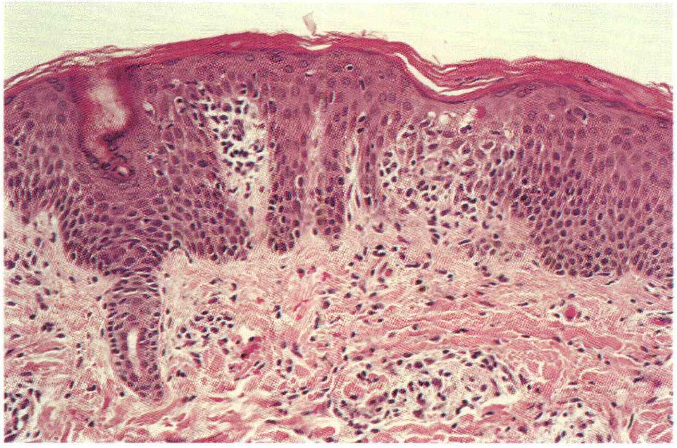

Figure 3–13. Single-cell epidermotropism by lymphocytes into a mildly and focally acanthotic and spongiotic epidermal layer is observed in this biopsy specimen from a patient who has atopic dermatitis. In this figure and Figure 3–12, the stratum corneum is diffusely abnormal, exhibiting compacted hyperorthokeratosis or parakeratosis. These features, within the context of a low-grade spongiotic process, indicate the chronicity that typifies the histology of atopic dermatitis.

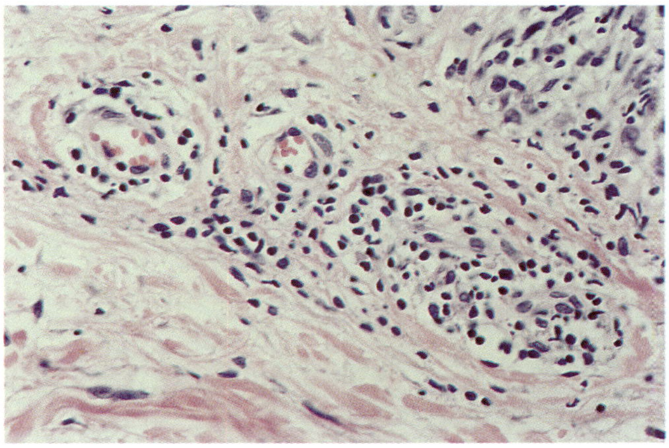

Figure 3–14. The inflammatory infiltrate about superficial venules is composed predominantly of lymphocytes and occasional monocytes; eosinophils are rarely encountered. As in allergic contact dermatitis, spaces separating perivenular co - lagen bundles are enlarged due to interstitial edema.

Primary Irritant Dermatitis

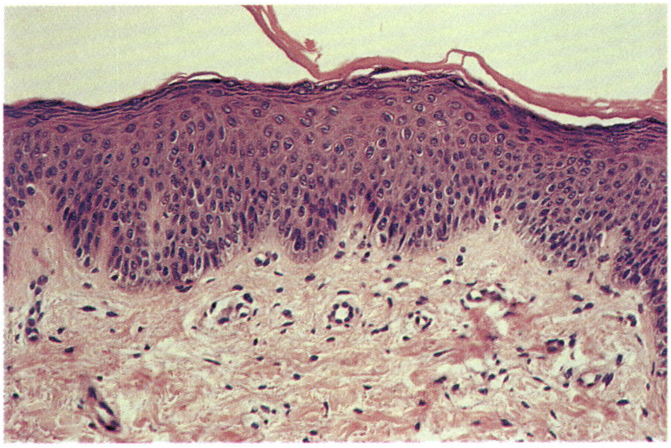

Figure 3–15. The features of low-grade irritant dermatitis at low magnification include superficial dermal pallor and vascular ectasia with sparse, associated mononuclear cell infiltration and an irregularly hyperplastic epidermis containing mildly spongiotic foci that are easily overlooked.

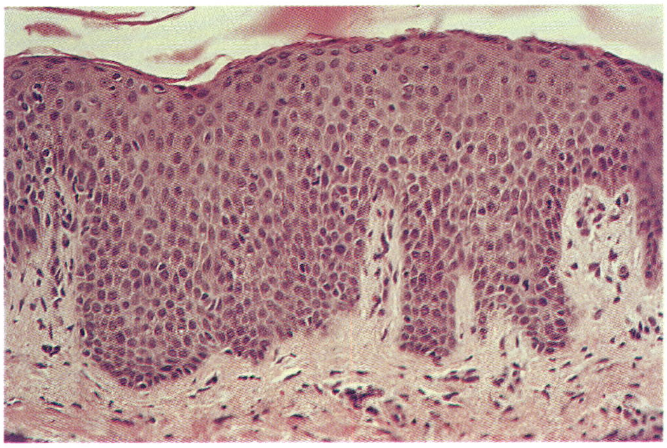

Figure 3–16. On closer inspection, uniformly widened intercellular spaces are observed within the lower two thirds of the epidermal layer. Epidermotropism is not a prominent feature of primary irritant dermatitis, and Langerhans cell microgranulomas and eosinophilic spongiosis are not encountered. Many biopsy specimens of irritant dermatitis without accompanying clinical data are indistinguishable from those of atopic dermatitis.

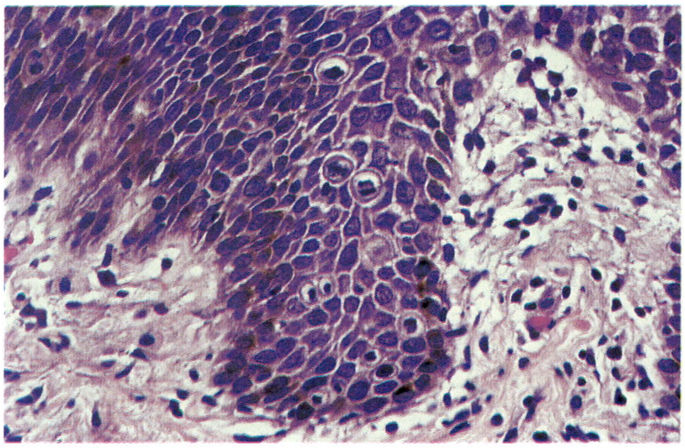

Figure 3–17. Numerous mitotic figures are present above the basal cell layer, which indicates the active proliferative component that typifies primary irritant dermatitis. There is a background of mild spongiosis.

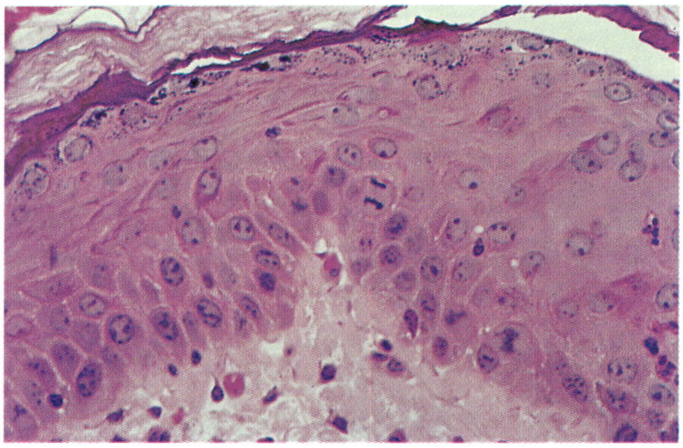

Figure 3–18. Reactive basaloid epidermal hyperplasia and enhanced mitotic activity characterize guinea pig epidermis 48 hours after application of chemical irritant. This hyperplastic response during the acute stages of lesion evolution is a helpful feature in differentiating early primary irritant dermatitis from forms of acute spongiotic dermatitis resulting from cutaneous hypersensitivity.

Nummular Dermatitis

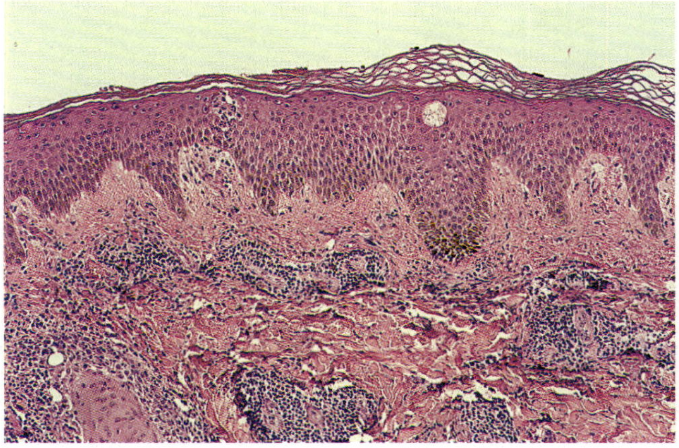

Figure 3–19. Scanning magnification of a coin-like plaque of nummular dermatitis demonstrates epidermal hyperplasia within the setting of diffuse, mild spongiosis. As in allergic contact dermatitis, there is a superficial, perivascular, mononuclear cell infiltrate with occasional foci of epidermotropism.

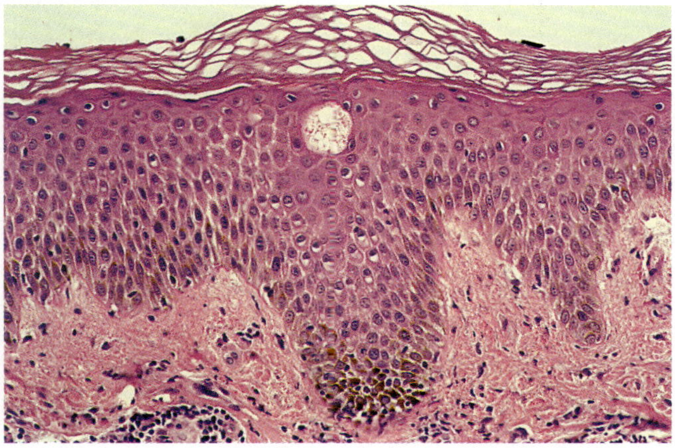

Figure 3–20. At higher magnif cation, zones of spongiosis may be associated with minute intraepidermal microvesicles, which correlate with pinpoint vesicles observed clinically.

Seborrheic Dermatitis

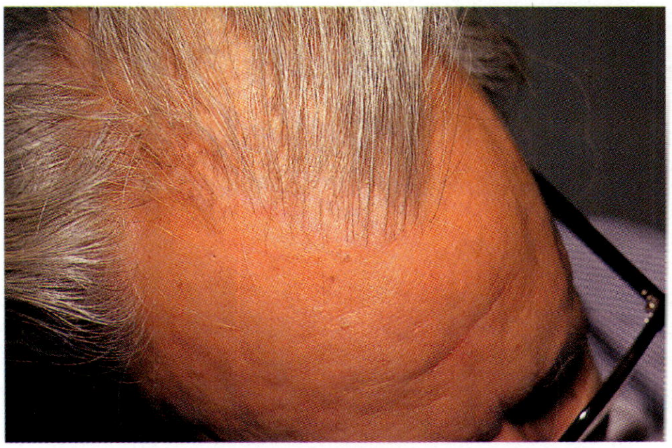

Figure 3–21. The gross pathology of seborrheic dermatitis, a common condition, typically is observed as subtle zones of erythema and scaling involving hair-bearing skin (edges of this subtle plaque defined at hairline). The scale has an oily consistency and a tan-yellow color, a helpful feature in differentiating this condition from psoriasis.

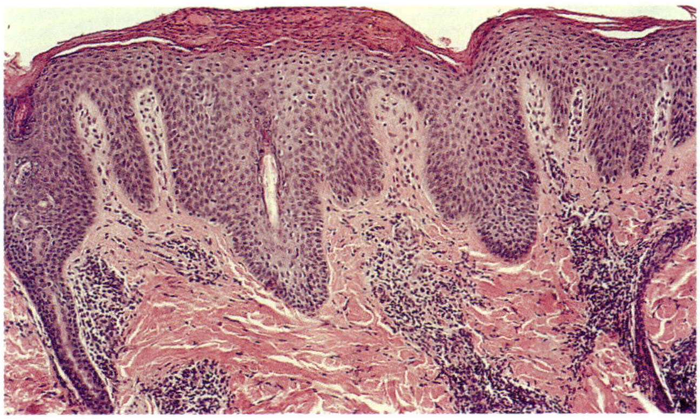

Figure 3–22. An active lesion of seborrheic dermatitis demonstrates an admixture of mild spongiosis and irregular psoriasiform hyperplasia, broad zones of parakeratotic scale containing occasional neutrophils, and a superficial perivascular inflammatory infiltrate within an edematous papillary dermis.

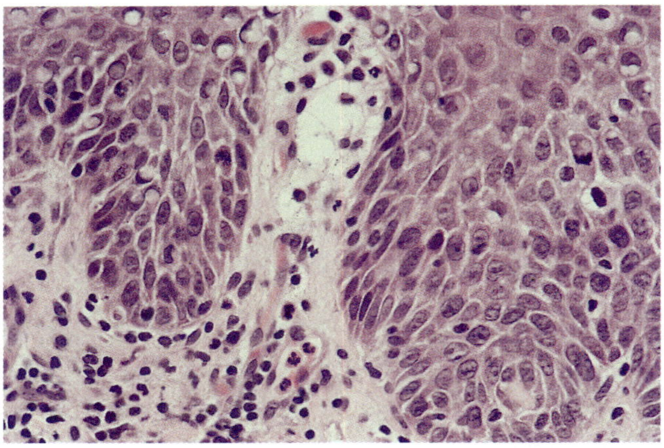

Figure 3–23. On closer inspection, scattered neutrophils *(center)* may be identified within pale dermal papillae expanded by interstitial edema.

Dyshidrotic Eczema

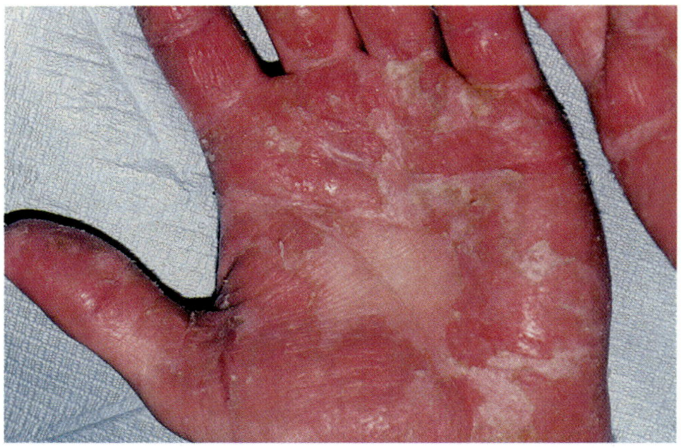

Figure 3–24. Dyshidrotic eczema. Hand eczema involving palmar skin is evidenced as zones of erythema and scaling in a setting of superimposed atrophy resulting from chronic steroid use. Small vesicles are present in the erythematous regions.

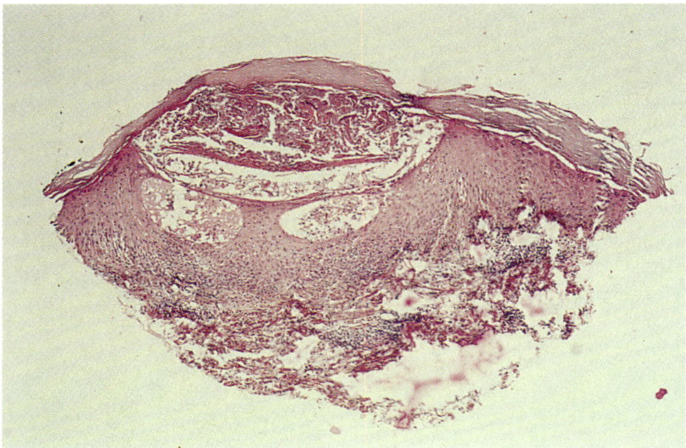

Figure 3–25. A typical biopsy specimen of dyshidrotic eczema demonstrates a well-formed intraepidermal fluid-filled vesicle that is readily appreciated at scanning magnification. The acral origin of the skin sample is indicated by the uniformly thick, compacted stratum corneum that extends to cover adjacent, relatively uninvolved skin.

Pityriasis Rosea

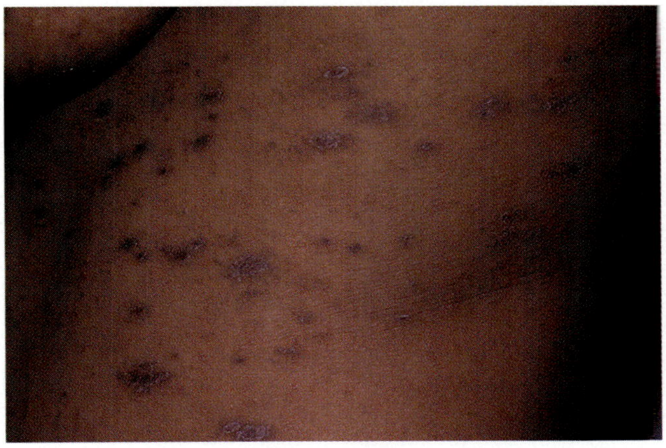

Figure 3–26. Comparison of pityriasis rosea (Figs. 3–26 through 3–28) and guttate parapsoriasis (Figs. 3–29 through 3–31). Oval plaques of pityriasis rosea are in a typical parallel arrangement along axes of skin folds, as if along the branches of a fir tree, when viewed sagittally from the back. Each plaque is pale-pink to orange and has delicate, adherent scale, which is often most pronounced at the periphery.

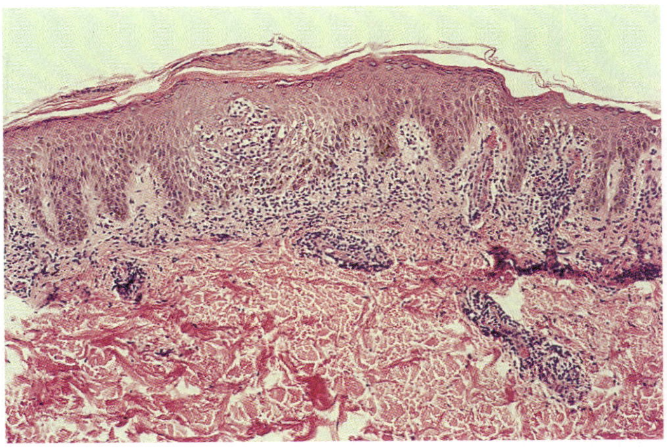

Figure 3–27. Scanning magnification of pityriasis rosea demonstrates the characteristic superficial perivascular lymphocytic infiltrate underlying a mildly hyperplastic and spongiotic epidermal layer. Discrete pulses of parakeratotic scale are evident at this level of magnification.

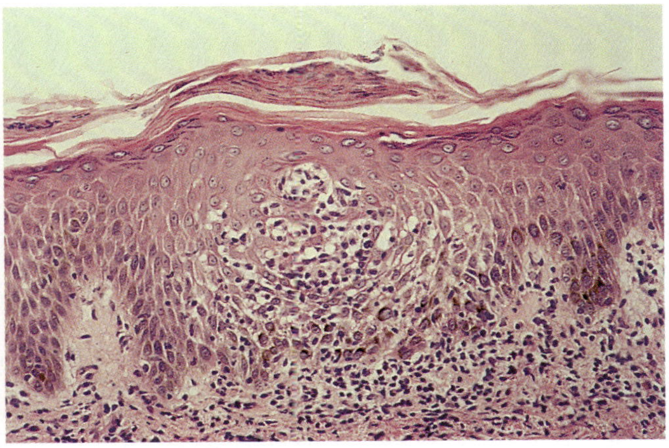

Figure 3–28. Higher magnification of pityriasis rosea. Note the zone of lymphoid epidermotropism associated with overlying, tightly compacted parakeratotic scale. Free erythrocytes within the papillary dermis are frequently associated with such zones of epidermotropism and assist in differentiating pityriasis rosea from its close mimic, guttate parapsoriasis.

Guttate Parapsoriasis

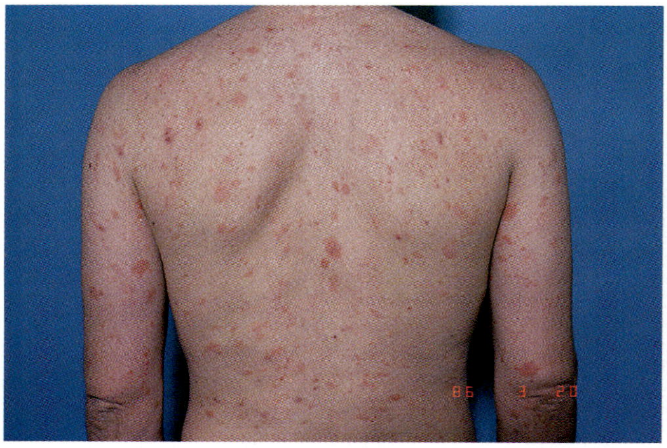

Figure 3–29. The gross pathology of guttate parapsoriasis closely resembles that of pityriasis rosea, although a tree-like distribution pattern is not characteristic of guttate parapsoriasis. Individual plaques are small and digitate and should not be confused with the ambiguously named yet unrelated large-plaque parapsoriasis, which is a dysplasia of T-cell lineage.

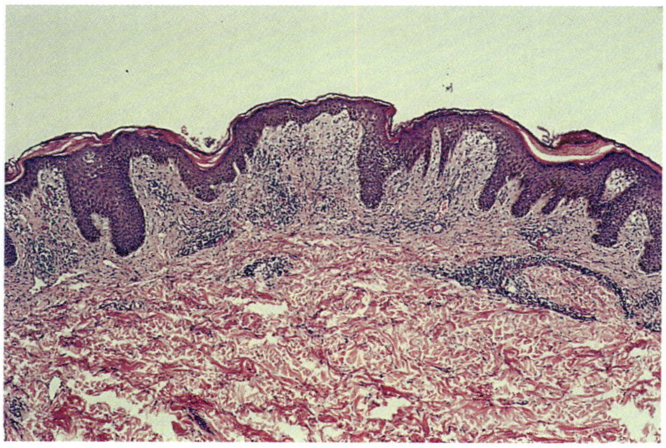

Figure 3–30. At low power, guttate parapsoriasis has an appearance that is difficult to distinguish from pityriasis rosea. There is a superficial perivascular lymphocytic infiltrate, irregular epidermal hyperplasia with mild spongiosis, and mounds of parakeratotic scale.

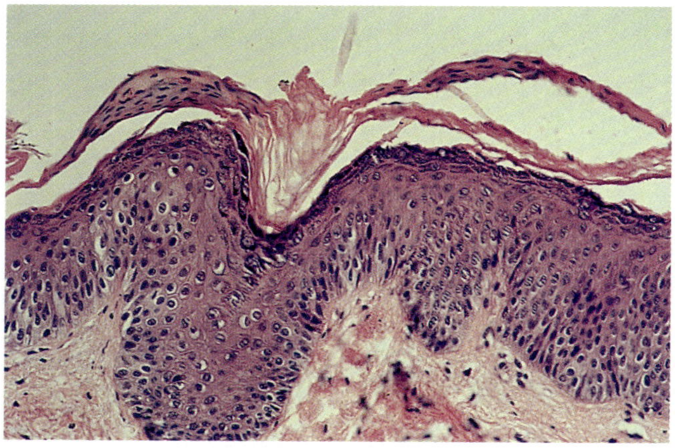

Figure 3–31. Changes within the epidermis and stratum corneum in guttate parapsoriasis are nearly identical to those in pityriasis rosea. Epidermotropism is minimal, however, and primary papillary dermal hemorrhage is not observed. Nonetheless, the two disorders often require persistent clinical observation for differentiation; guttate parapsoriasis is a chronic disorder, whereas pityriasis rosea usually resolves within months after onset.

Photoallergic Spongiotic Dermatitis

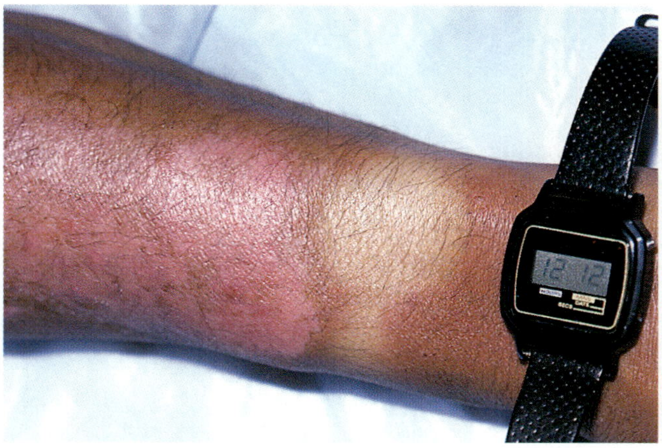

Figure 3–32. In this clinical example of photoallergic dermatitis, induration, erythema, pruritus, and early vesiculation occurred 24 hours after modest exposure to sunlight. Skin remains normal only in protected regions such as the zone shielded by the wristwatch.

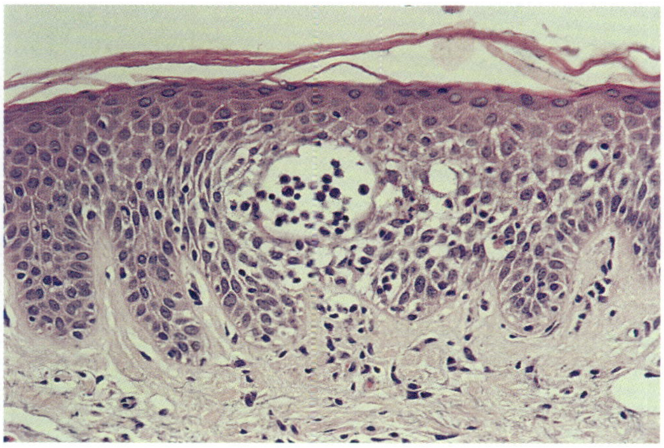

Figure 3–33. Spongiosis and lymphoid epidermotropism are similar to those encountered in allergic contact dermatitis; the former is an important discriminating feature in excluding polymorphous light eruption and photoexacerbated lupus erythematosus, which generally are devoid of spongiosis.

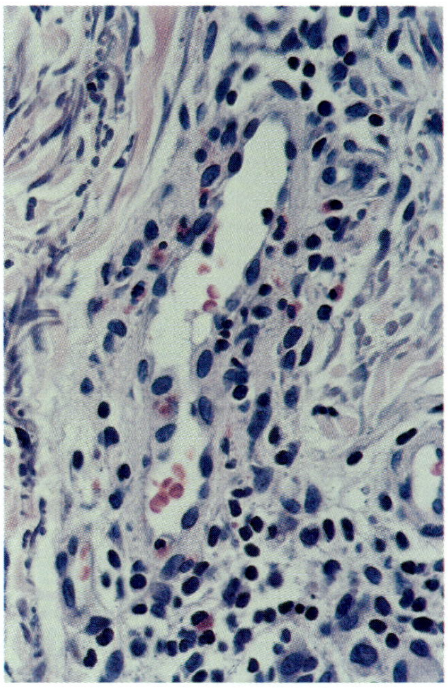

Figure 3–34. A helpful feature in the diagnosis of photoallergic dermatitis is prominent endothelial cells with apparently vacuolated cytoplasm.

Spongiotic Drug Eruption

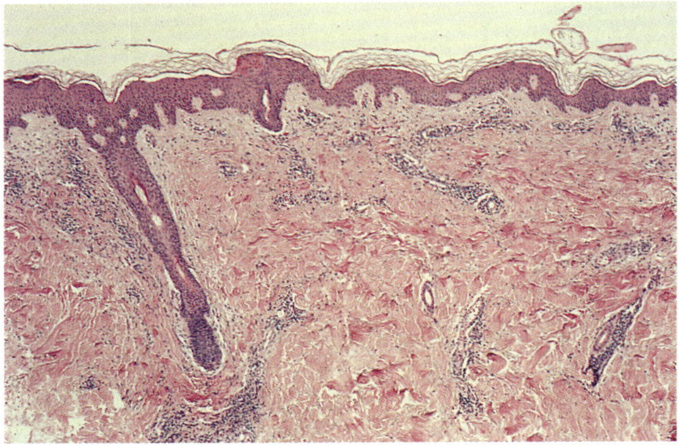

Figure 3–35. At scanning magnification, the inflammatory infiltrate in many spongiotic drug eruptions involves both superficial and deep dermal vessels. As opposed to photoallergic dermatitis, the degree of angiocentric infiltration does not diminish with increasing depth.

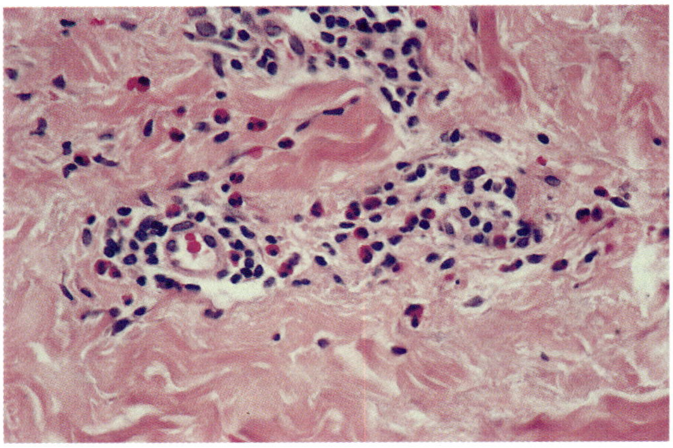

Figure 3–36. Eosinophils are often numerous within the mononuclear cell infiltrates of spongiotic drug eruptions.

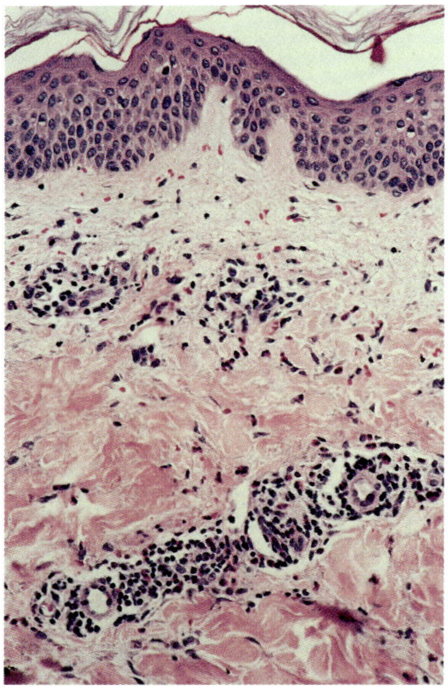

Figure 3–37. The epidermis is minimally spongiotic in this early lesion of a drug eruption; in time, focal microvesiculation indistinguishable from that seen in allergic contact dermatitis may develop in some lesions, although many lesions show only slight spongiotic change during their entire evolution. Note that the cuff of inflammatory cells about the lowermost vessel in the reticular dermis is actually more pronounced than that surrounding the more superficial vessel within the pale, edematous papillary dermis.

Spongiotic Insect-Bite Reaction

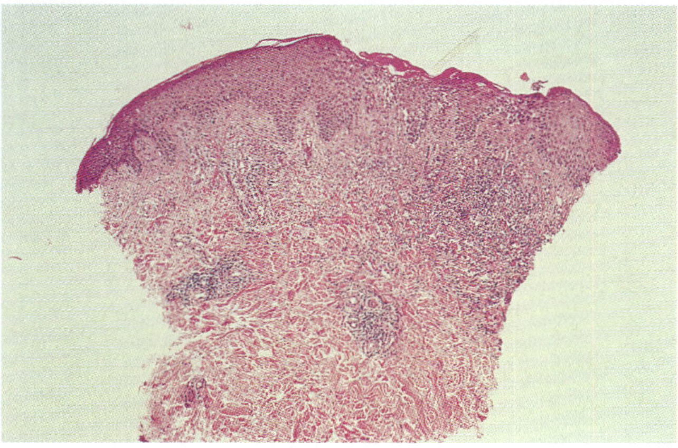

Figure 3–38. The architecture of this spongiotic insect-bite reaction is angiocentric at the edge *(left)* and confluent in the center *(right)*. This, combined with the depth of infiltration (frequently into the subcutis), imparts a wedge-like shape that is helpful in making this diagnosis at scanning magnification.

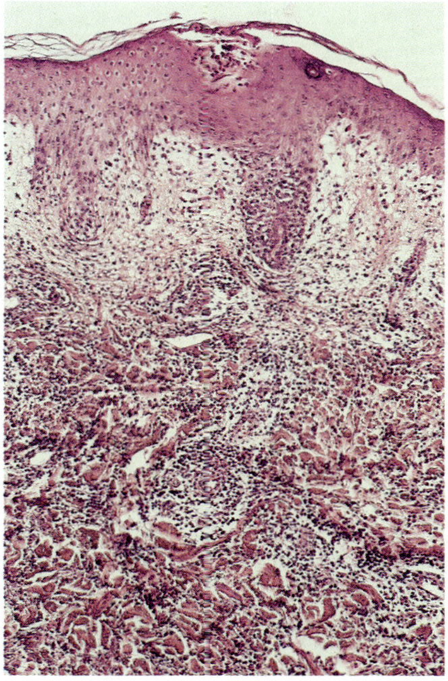

Figure 3–39. The central portion of an insect bite may contain a dell lined by necrotic and inflammatory cells and represents a residual punctum through which foreign protein was injected. Note the spongiosis, papillary dermal edema, and almost tumoral (*i.e.*, lymphocytoma-like) confluent inflammatory infiltrate composed of activated mononuclear cells, eosinophils, and, occasionally, granulomas reacting to retained birefringent chitinous fragments.

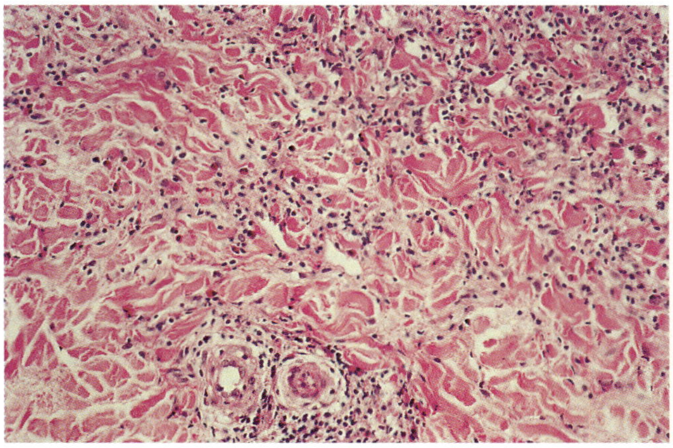

Figure 3–40. At the edge of the infiltrate depicted in Figure 3–39, inflammatory cells infiltrate the dermal matrix as streams of cells, a pattern reminiscent of granuloma annulare and focally observed in many insect-bite reactions.

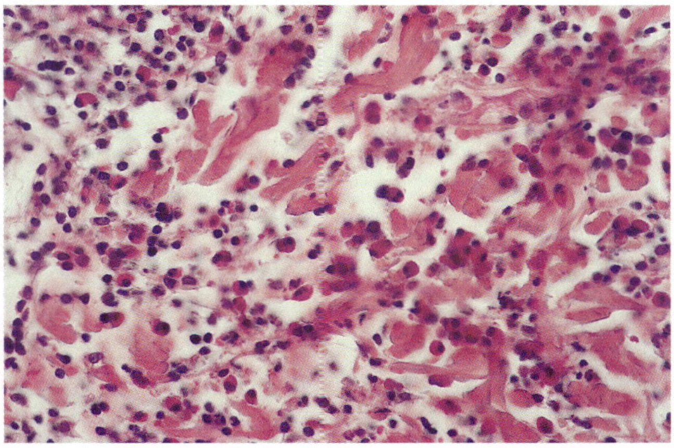

Figure 3–41. Numerous eosinophils are present among the inflammatory cells that infiltrate the intervenular connective tissue. This loss of angiocentric distribution by eosinophils is a helpful feature in the diagnosis of insect-bite responses.

Dermatophytosis

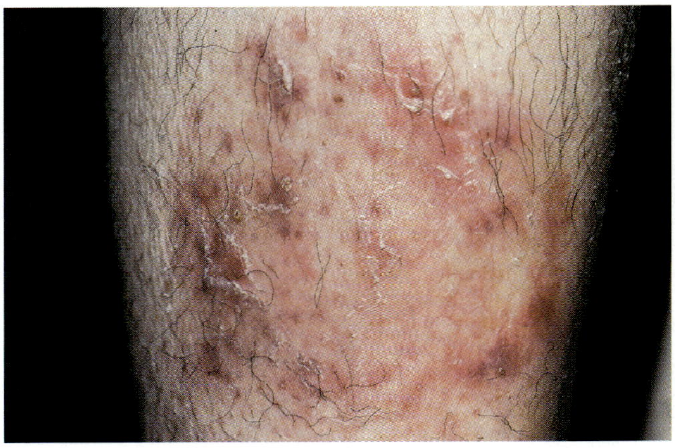

Figure 3–42. Dermatophytosis. An eczematous clinical appearance was caused by a superficial fungal infection (*i.e.*, tinea corporis). There is peripheral erythema, scaling, and intermittent pruritus, leading to confusion with contact dermatitis. Note, however, the characteristic central clearing.

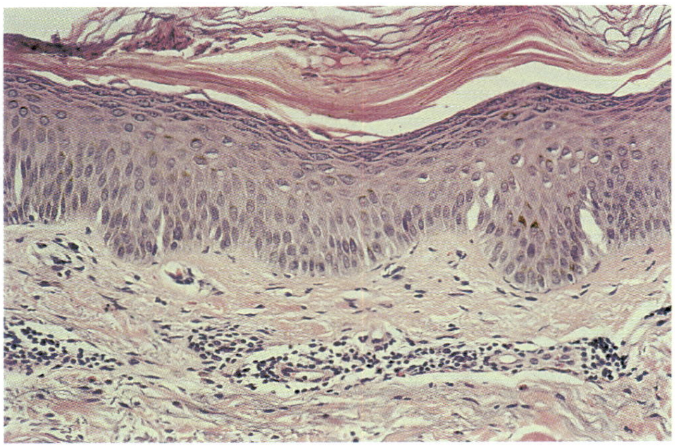

Figure 3–43. Biopsy of the plaque depicted in Figure 3–42 shows a nonspecific, mild spongiotic dermatitis. The zones of vertically alternating parakeratosis and compacted orthokeratosis, giving a laminated "sandwich-like" appearance to the stratum corneum, provide a clue regarding the underlying cause of these apparently nondiagnostic changes.

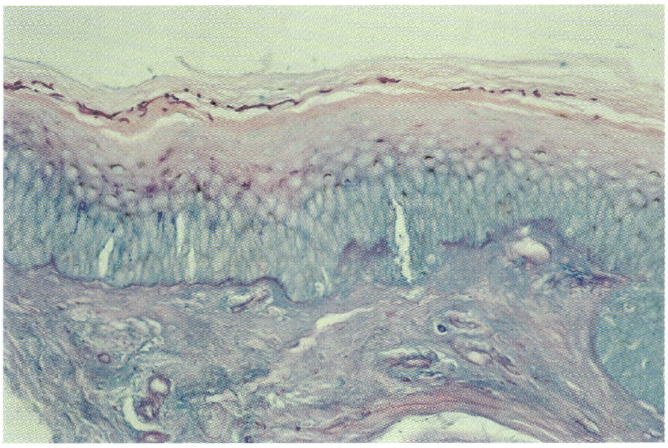

Figure 3–44. Periodic acid–Schiff stain reveals numerous hyphal forms within the stratum corneum, confirming the diagnosis of low-grade spongiotic response evoked by dermatophytosis.

Incontinentia Pigmenti, Spongiotic Stage

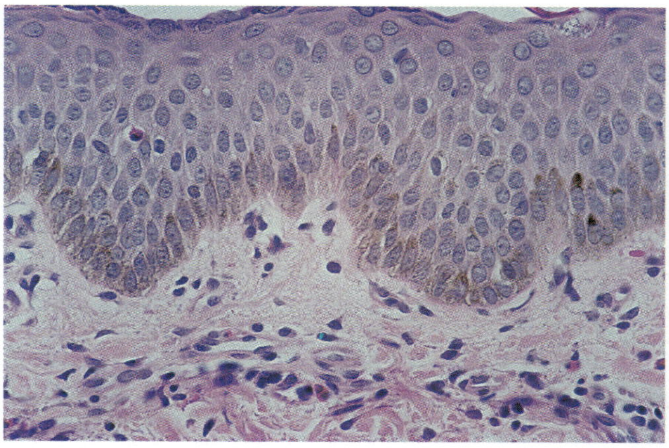

Figure 3–45. Incontinentia pigmenti, spongiotic-vesicular stage. An early lesion shows only mild spongiosis and a nonspecific superficial lymphocytic infiltrate.

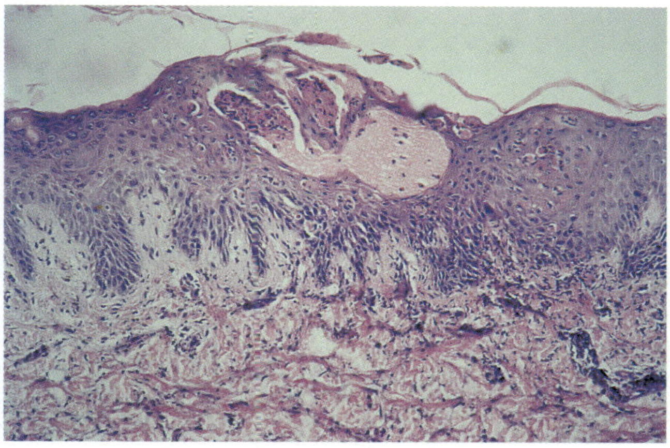

Figure 3–46. An advanced lesion has a typical, well-formed intraepidermal vesicle overlying a superficial infiltrate composed of mononuclear cells, eosinophils, and rare basophils.

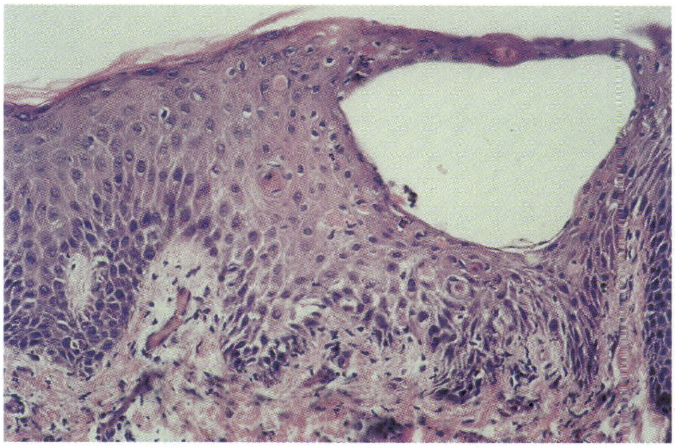

Figure 3–47. A clue to the diagnosis of incontinentia pigmenti is the finding of early zones of dyskeratosis within the vesiculated epidermal layer *(to left of vesicle).*

Spongiotic Dermatitis: Diagnostic Pitfalls

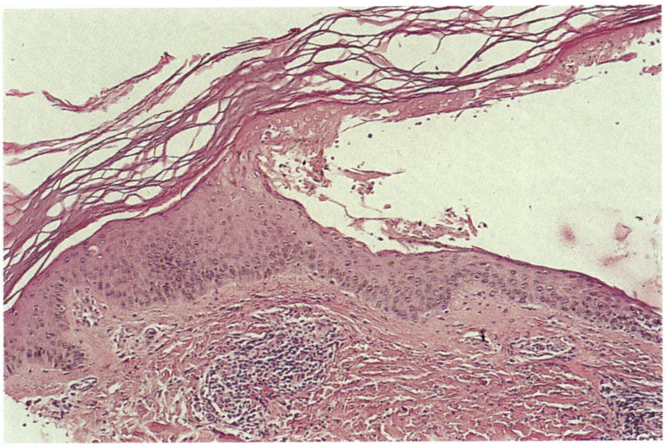

Figure 3–48. Although acute spongiotic dermatitis may progress to subacute and chronic stages, an alternative pathway is spontaneous or iatrogenic resolution. Lesions biopsied during resolution stages may not be recognized as representing a spongiotic process. This large intraepidermal vesicle has a necrotic roof; the base is formed by a regenerating epidermal layer devoid of spongiosis. The only clue to the inciting cause is the persistent angiocentric infiltrate of lymphocytes and eosinophils *(bottom left)* within the superficial dermis.

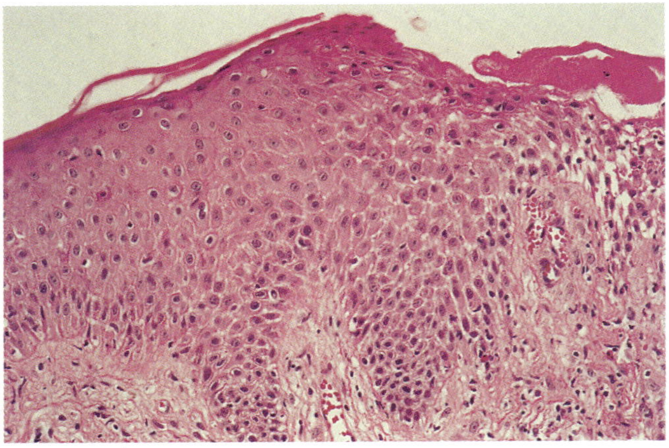

Figure 3–49. A lesion similar to that in Figure 3–48 in which the necrotic roof has been sloughed. At the edge of the previous blister *(right side of field)*, a small area of residual spongiosis is retained.

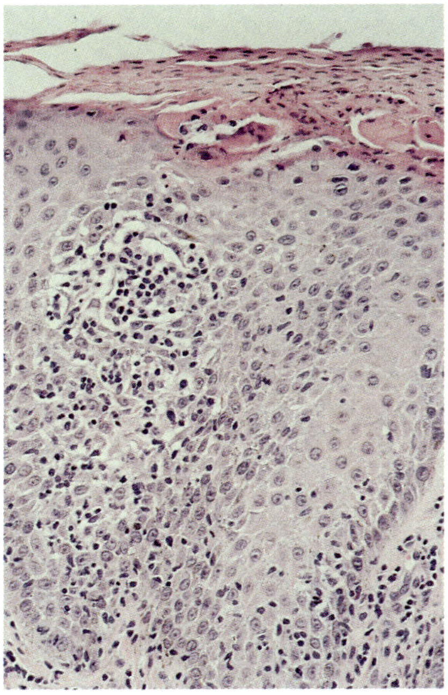

Figure 3–50. False-negative diagnosis of spongiotic dermatitis. In this chronic dermatitis, only acanthosis and inflammation persist. An important clue that this lesion was preceded by a spongiotic process is the presence of loculated serum that has not yet been shed within the stratum corneum.

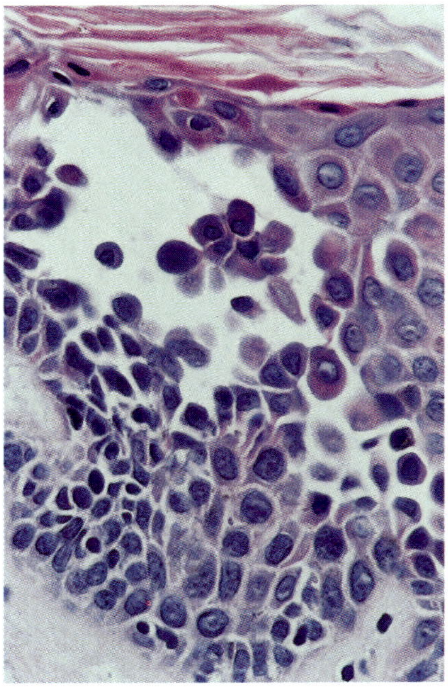

Figure 3–51. False-positive diagnosis of spongiotic dermatitis. Acantholysis must be differentiated from spongiosis and microvesicle formation. The former is characterized by rounded cells with hypereosinophilic (*i.e.,* dyskeratotic) cytoplasm. Prominent (*i.e.,* stretched) intercellular bridges, the hallmark of spongiosis, are not observed in acantholysis, even in the earliest stages, which here are appreciated as widened intercellular spaces.

4

Psoriasiform Dermatitis

Psoriasiform dermatitis is adapted from the New Latin word *psoriasis,* which derives from the Greek words for a condition *(-iasis)* of itching *(psor-).* Although the pathogenesis of pruritus is not understood, the term is appropriate because disorders that result in psoriasiform dermatitis may itch at some stages of their clinical evolution and because chronic scratching of pruritic skin invariably results in psoriasiform changes. True psoriasis is a disorder that can be clinically and histologically confused with other forms of psoriasiform dermatitis. Although psoriasis stands as the prototype for this family of epidermal reaction patterns, significant differences in gross appearance, clinical behavior, and histologic evolution exist among members of this group of different cutaneous diseases.

As illustrated in Chapter 1, epidermal hyperplasia consists of increased numbers of keratinocytes as a result of heightened proliferative rate, alteration in cell cycle, or decreased surface shedding. Preferential, albeit generally not exclusive, involvement of various epidermal layers has given rise to the terms *basaloid hyperplasia, acanthosis* (hyperplasia of the stratum spinosum), *hypergranulosis* (hyperplasia of the stratum granulosum), and *hyperkeratosis* and *parakeratosis* (a frequent but nonspecific concomitant feature of epidermal hyperplasia). In psoriasiform disorders, one or more layers may be diminished in prominence or entirely absent, as adjacent layers become markedly thickened. The prototype for a disorder characterized by epidermal hyperplasia is psoriasis, and considerable attention is devoted in daily practice to differentiation of true psoriasis from other disorders that may recapitulate some, but not all, of its clinical and histologic features.

Accurate diagnostic recognition of psoriasiform dermatitis is important because differentiation among psoriasis, chronic irritant dermatitis, and epidermal changes induced by underlying tumors or infection depends on histologic recognition of salient and reproducible features. The treatments for disorders that produce psoriasiform changes clinically and histologically may be quite different and, when specifically and appropriately targeted at accurately diagnosed diseases, often are quite effective.

Although the cellular and molecular biology of psoriasiform dermatitis is beyond the scope of this practical approach, it deserves brief mention. The inciting events that precipitate psoriasiform changes are frequently inflammatory and appear to involve dysregulation of cytokines and growth factors instrumental in the maintenance of normal epidermal proliferation. Aberrant molecular signals may be influenced by genetic factors, particularly in situations such as true psoriasis and its variants, and in the setting of chronic lesions of atopic dermatitis. Growing appreciation of the proinflammatory pathways and associated epidermal cytokine dysregulation that accompanies various forms of psoriasiform dermatitis should foster more complete understanding of the endogenous and environmental cues that govern keratinocyte proliferation.

The tinctorial characteristics of psoriasiform dermatitis may be remarkably helpful diagnostic features, along with assessment of lesion architecture and cytology. For example, although the normally dark-blue stratum granulosum is thickened in lichen simplex chronicus, it is thinned to absent in psoriasis. Small flecks of blue-purple stain in the stratum corneum may indicate mounds of parakeratosis seen in pityriasis rosea or guttate parapsoriasis or inflammatory cell infiltration of the stratum corneum, as observed in psoriatic Munro microabscesses in pustular psoriasis. Hints of blue-gray coloration in the dermis underlying a zone of psoriasiform epidermal hyperplasia may even indicate a subtle fibrohistiocytic proliferation responsible for inductive epithelial hyperplasia, as in early dermatofibroma. Cytoplasmic pallor within proliferating epidermal cells often correlates with glycogenation, as seen in pseudoepitheliomatous hyperplasia at the edge of a cutaneous ulcer. Such subtle alterations in hue provide an important diagnostic adjunct when initially viewing psoriasiform dermatitis at scanning magnification.

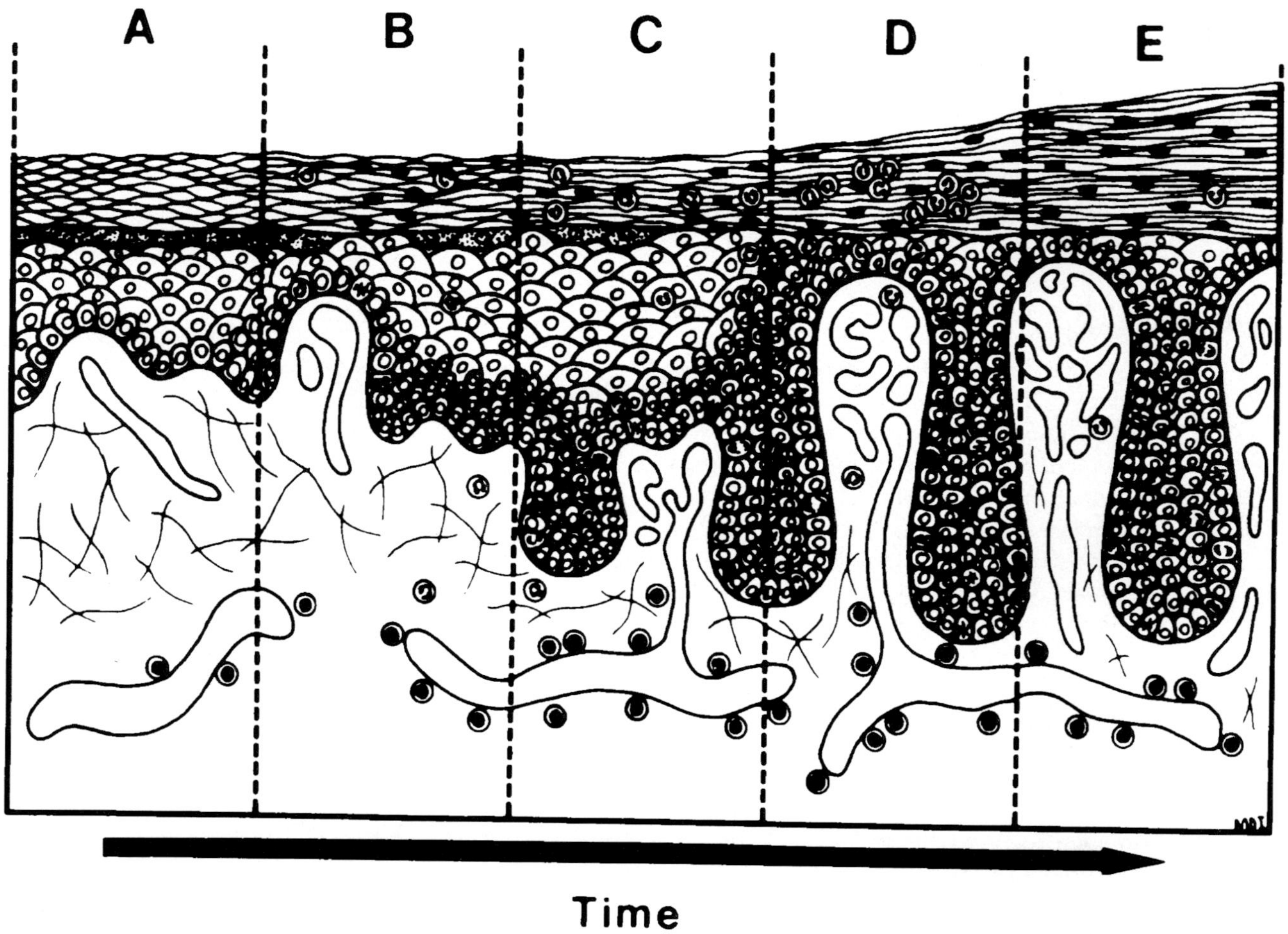

Figure 4–1. Temporal evolution of psoriasiform dermatitis: Psoriasis. *A* and *B,* The earliest manifestations of psoriasis involve subtle basal cell hyperplasia and focal parakeratosis, which evolve into *(C)* an initially irregular epidermal hyperplasia (*i.e.,* rete ridges extending unevenly into the underlying dermis) with parakeratosis containing occasional neutrophils and associated hypogranulosis. *B,* Even in early stages, capillary loops within dermal papillae may be ectatic and slightly tortuous, and there is a sparse-to-moderate mononuclear cell infiltrate about superficial venules. *D and E,* In established lesions, basaloid hyperplasia becomes regular (*i.e.,* even, downward extension of hyperplastic rete), and dermal papillae are edematous and extend upward to lie in close proximity to diffusely parakeratotic scale, often containing clustered neutrophils. Capillary loops within these hyperplastic papillae are markedly tortuous and ectatic at this juncture, and the stratum granulosum is generally absent.

Psoriasis

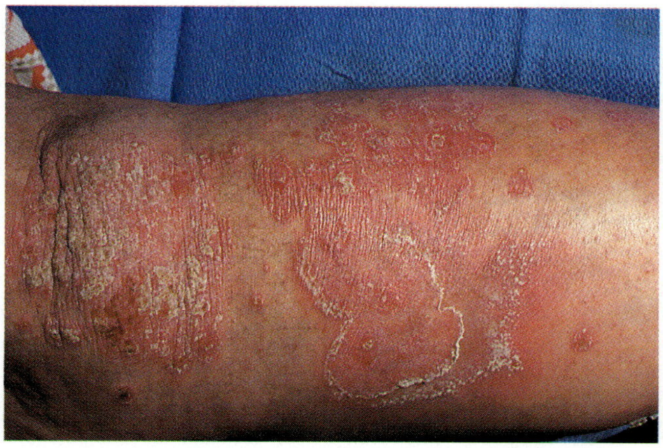

Figure 4–2. The clinical picture of psoriasis is predominated by arcuate and grouped pustules superimposed on boggy, erythematous plaques. Scale is not a predominant feature.

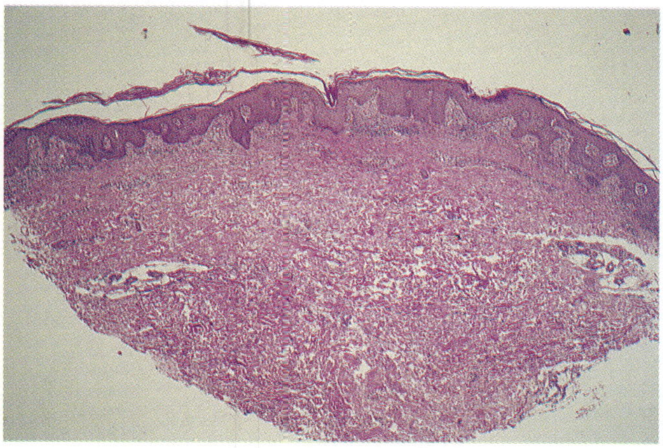

Figure 4–3. At scanning magnification, early psoriasis shows irregular acanthosis, the impression of a basophilic superficial perivascular infiltrate, and clear evidence of early scale abnormality characterized by compaction and exfoliation.

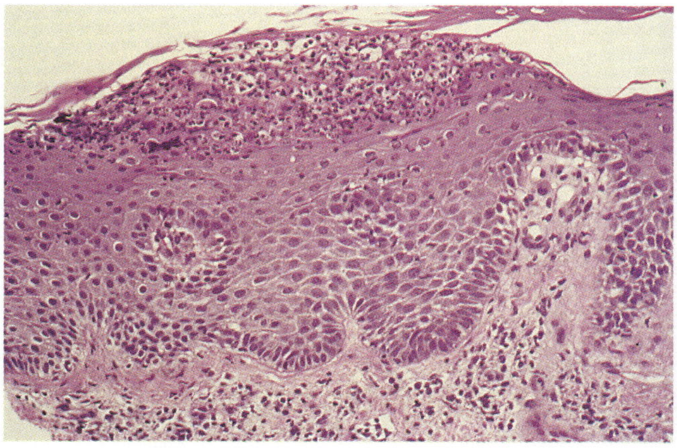

Figure 4–4. At higher magnification, subcorneal and intracorneal pustules formed by aggregated neutrophils are observed. The stratum granulosum is diminished, and the dermal papilla *(right)* contains a prominent, ectatic capillary loop.

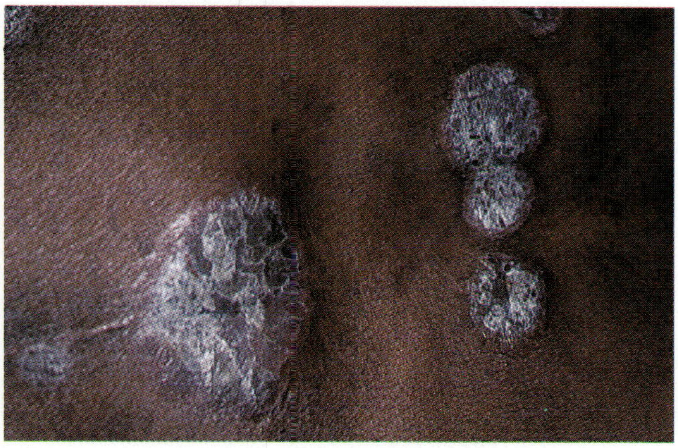

Figure 4–5. Psoriasis, established lesions. Well-demarcated plaques are typically covered by adherent, silvery scale.

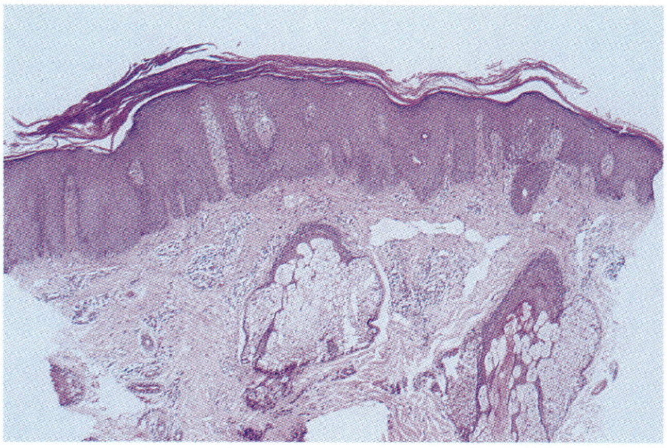

Figure 4–6. The biopsy specimen of established psoriasis is predominated by regular epidermal hyperplasia and compacted scale, which focally appears to lift off of the epidermal surface. The normal coalescence (*i.e.,* fusion) of rete ridges is accentuated in this biopsy with established basaloid hyperplasia.

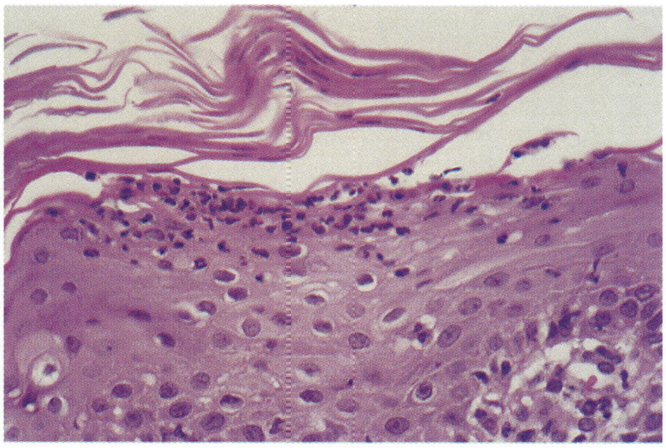

Figure 4–7. At higher magnification, the absence of stratum granulosum, the compacted parakeratotic scale, and the infiltration of the upper stratum spinosum by neutrophils (*i.e.,* spongiform pustule formation) are all apparent.

Reiter Syndrome

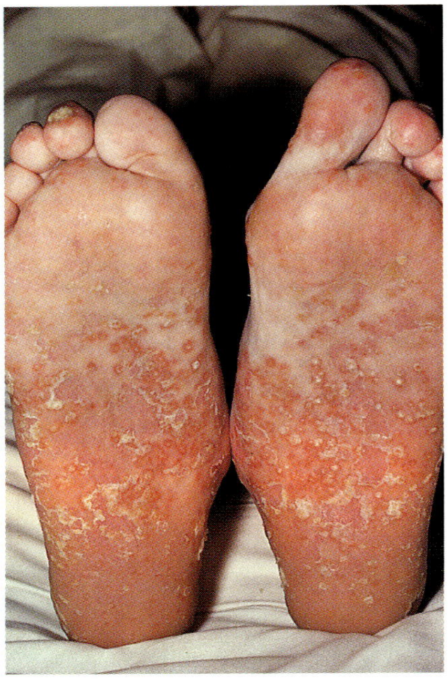

Figure 4–8. Clinically, lesions in Reiter syndrome include erythematous papules and plaques covered by scale and pustules on acral skin (*i.e.,* keratoderma blennorrhagicum), classic psoriasiform lesions elsewhere on the body surface, erythematous penile papules and plaques with central clearing (*i.e.,* balanitis circinata), and transient oral mucosal erosions or hyperkeratotic glossitis resembling geographic tongue.

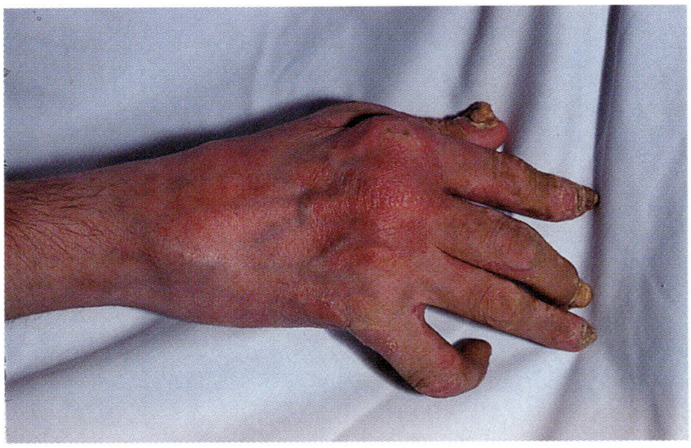

Figure 4–9. Associated arthritis is similar to psoriatic arthritis occurring in the absence of Reiter syndrome.

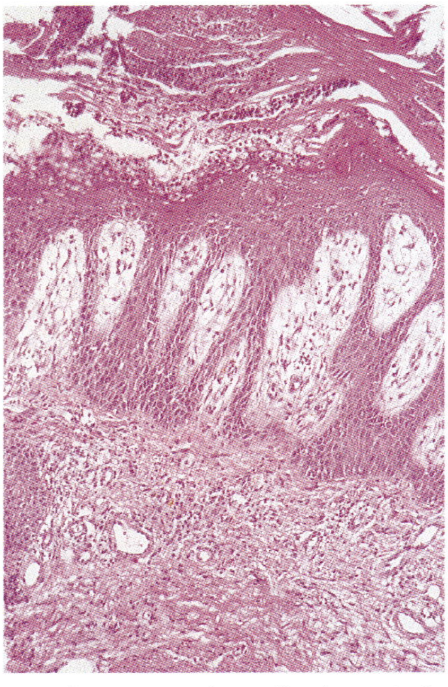

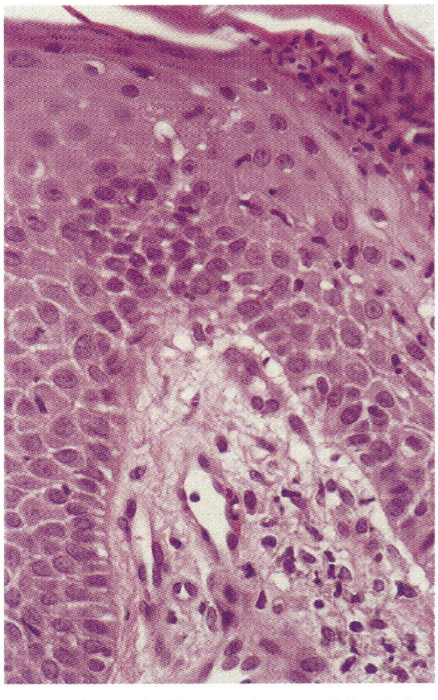

Figures 4–10 and 4–11. Histologically, the typical epidermal and dermal changes of psoriasis are observed in Reiter syndrome, although dermal edema and the neutrophilic inflammatory component may be more marked. Note the prominent intracorneal accumulations of neutrophils (Fig. 4–10) and the prominent, tortuous vessels within edematous dermal papillae (Fig. 4–11). The observation of large intracorneal pustules in the absence of a typical clinical history of eruptive or pustular psoriasis should raise the possibility of Reiter syndrome, particularly in young boys and in young to middle-aged men.

Lichen Simplex Chronicus/Prurigo Nodularis

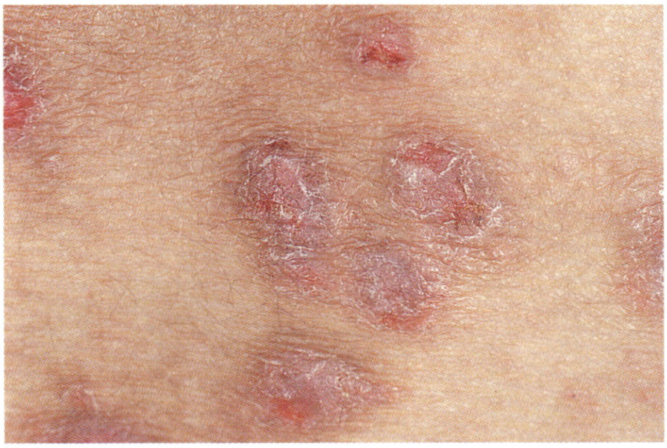

Figure 4–12. Lichen simplex chronicus and prurigo nodularis. Multiple nodules and plaques covered by scale also show evidence of hyperpigmentation and recent excoriation.

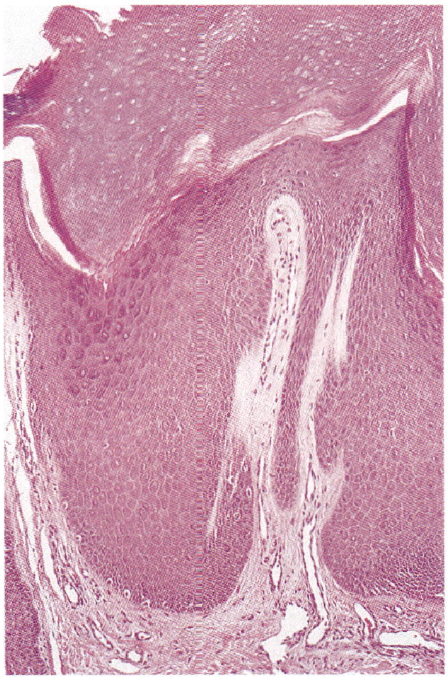

Figure 4–13. Histologically, in addition to irregular psoriasiform acanthosis and hyperkeratosis, there is a markedly *thickened* stratum granulosum and typical, vertically oriented fibrosis (*i.e.*, streaking) within dermal papillae.

Pseudoepitheliomatous Hyperplasia

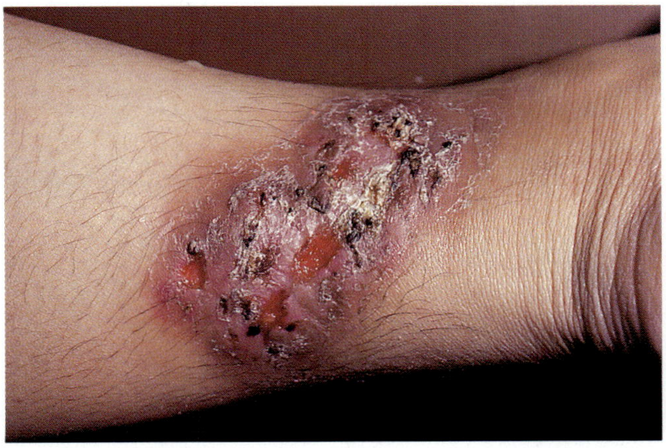

Figure 4–14. Pseudoepitheliomatous hyperplasia adjacent to chronic ulcer. A multifocal ulcer with zones of fibrosis and hyperkeratosis producing a tumor-like plaque. This lesion was self-induced.

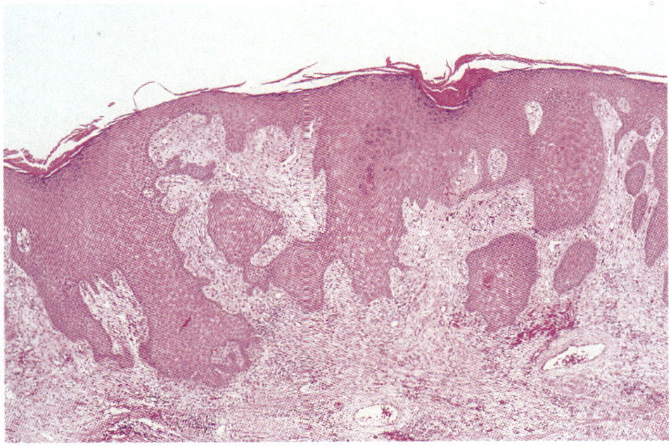

Figure 4–15. Reactive epidermal hyperplasia adjacent to one of the ulcerated foci. Note the jagged inferior border, which raises the possibility of superficially invasive squamous cell carcinoma.

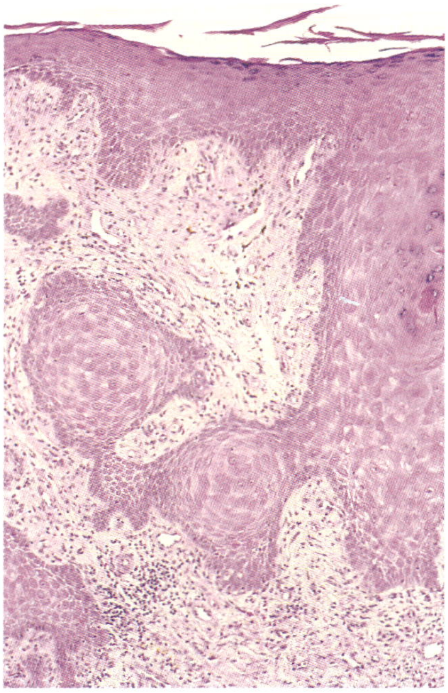

Figure 4–16. At higher magnification, the associated dermis is markedly fibrotic and inflamed. Significant dysplasia or single-cell invasion is not present in the epithelial elements.

Pityriasis Rubra Pilaris

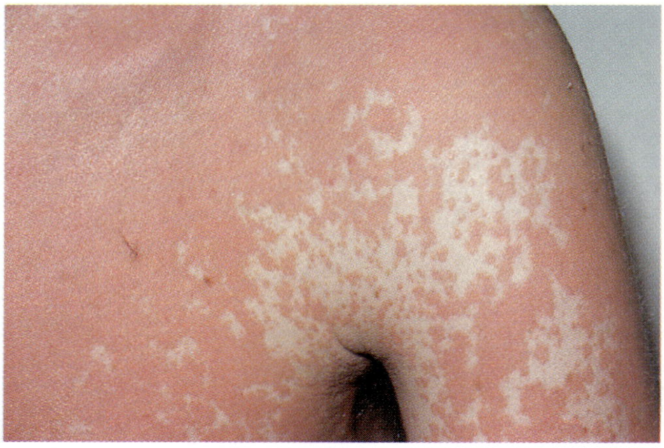

Figure 4–17. Pityriasis rubra pilaris. Interfollicular involvement, showing erythrodermic plaques with sharply defined islands of sparing.

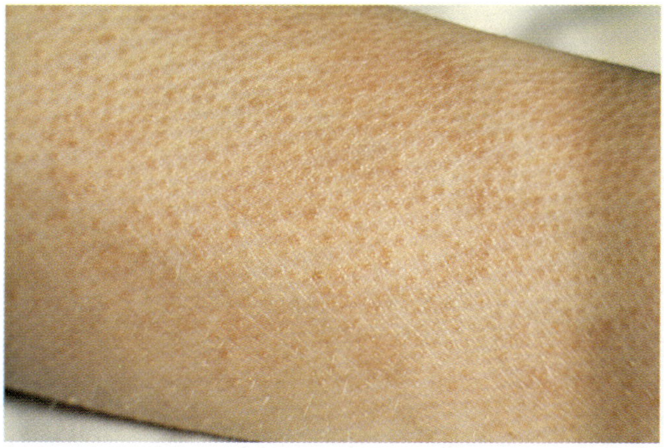

Figure 4–18. Pityriasis rubra pilaris with follicular involvement. Note the erythematous follicular papules with small central keratotic plugs.

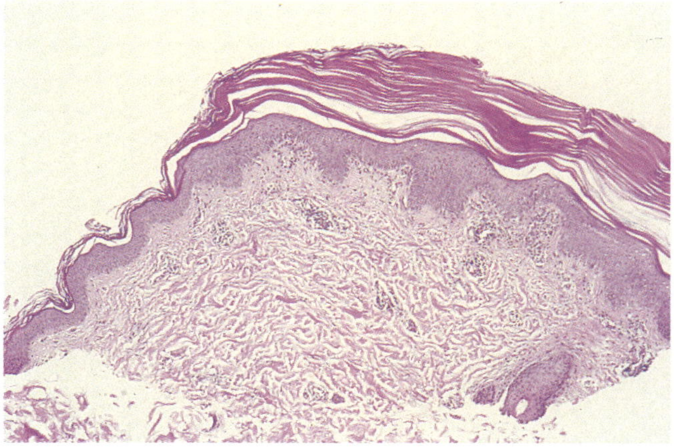

Figure 4–19. Biopsy of edge of interfollicular erythema demonstrates normal skin *(left one third)* juxtaposed with lesional skin *(right two thirds).* The lesion is characterized by slightly irregular psoriasiform epidermal hyperplasia and hyperkeratosis.

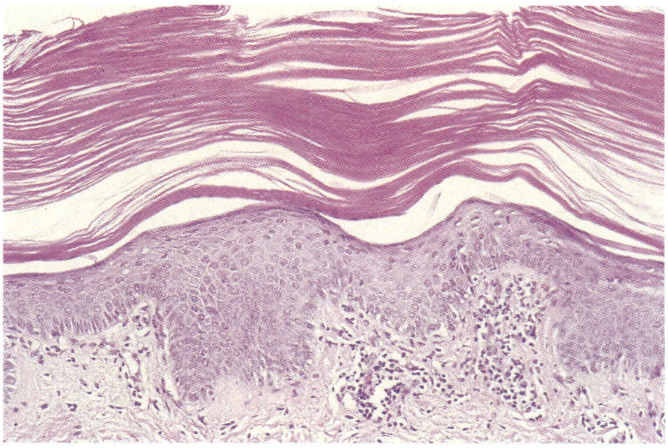

Figure 4–20. Scale devoid of neutrophilic infiltration (an important sign of psoriasis) and showing subtle zones of nuclear retention (parakeratosis), which alternate with orthokeratotic scale in both vertical and horizontal planes. The accentuation of parakeratosis at the orifice of a follicular infundibulum (*i.e.,* shoulder parakeratosis) is a typical feature of pityriasis rubra pilaris.

Pityriasis Rosea, Herald Patch

Figure 4–21. Pityriasis rosea, herald patch. Because this large eruptive plaque may precede the onset of typical lesions of pityriasis rosea, a biopsy may be performed to rule out psoriasis. In lightly pigmented individuals, the plaque is often salmon-colored; in darkly pigmented patients, it may be hyperpigmented, as depicted here.

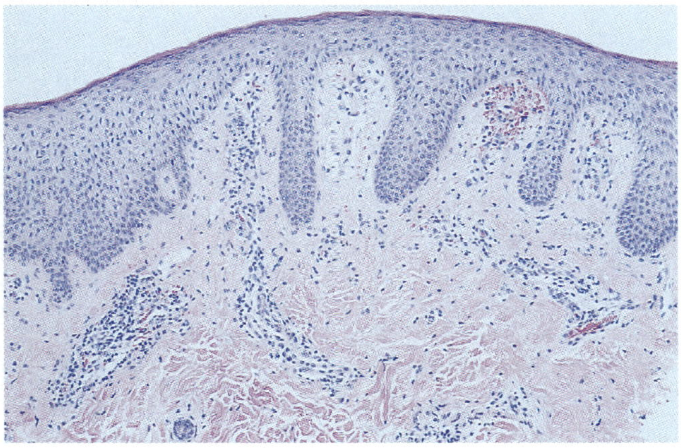

Figure 4–22. Biopsy specimen of the herald patch, which is really a plaque, shows psoriasiform epidermal hyperplasia without neutrophils in the stratum corneum (neutrophils would be typical of true psoriasis).

Psoriasiform Dermatitis Secondary to Stasis, Tumors, and Infection

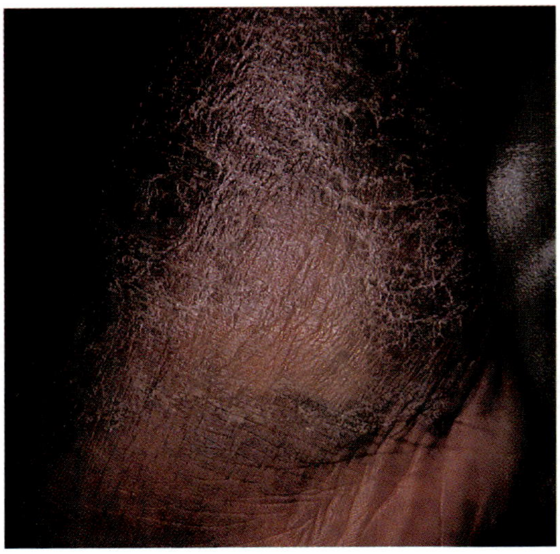

Figure 4–23. Stasis dermatitis with psoriasiform features. Clinical presentation of stasis dermatitis as scaling, hyperpigmented plaques on the lower extremity (see Figs. 17–18 to 17–20).

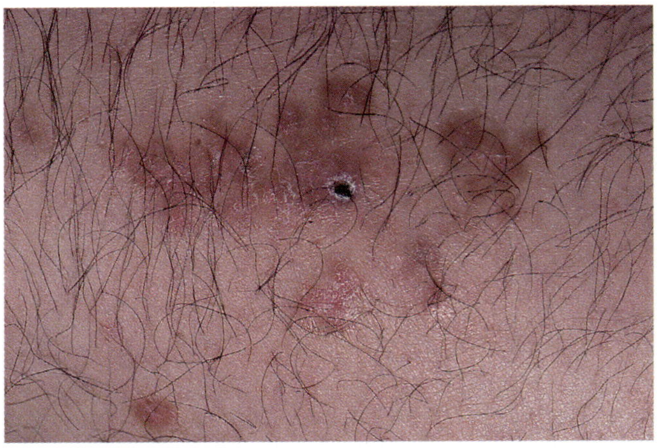

Figure 4–24. Psoriasiform epidermal hyperplasia overlying dermal tumors: Dermatofibroma. Multiple eruptive benign fibrous histiocytomas (*i.e.,* dermatofibromas) on the thigh producing a scale-covered plaque.

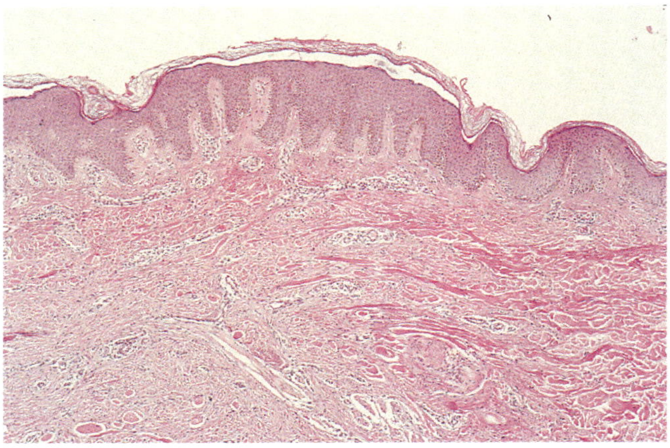

Figure 4–25. Psoriasis-like epidermal hyperplasia is obvious at scanning magnification; this lesion may be too subtle at this level of magnification to reveal itself initially as a dermatofibroma. Note, however, the hypercellular, altered dermis in the bottom left portion of this field.

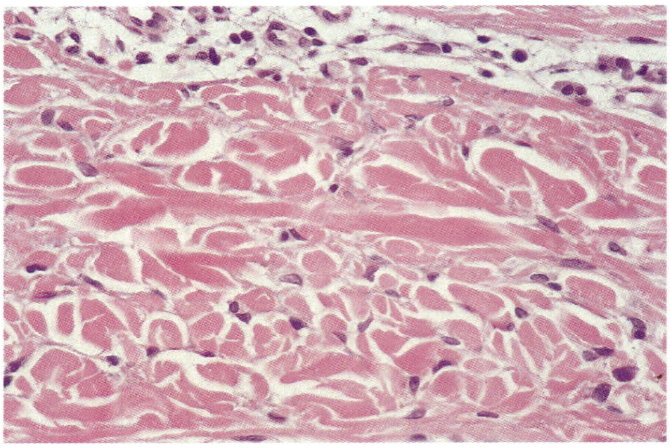

Figure 4–26. Inspection of the underlying dermis at a higher magnification of the lesion in Figure 4–25 shows proliferation of small fibroblasts within abnormal collagen bundles forming a symmetric dermal nodule.

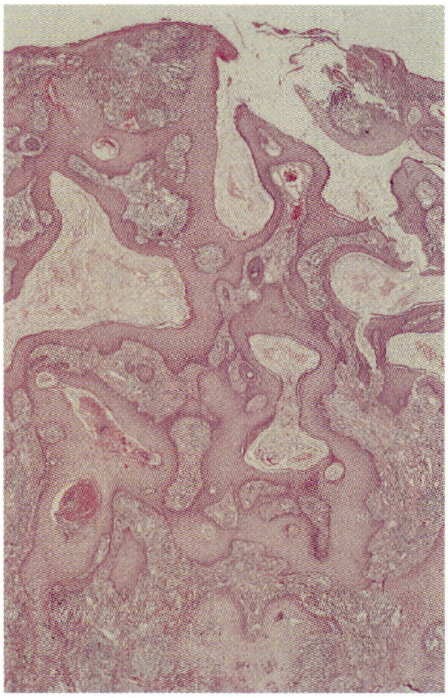

Figure 4–27. Epidermal hyperplasia associated with infection: Blastomycosis. On initial inspection, pseudoepitheliomatous epidermal hyperplasia predominates.

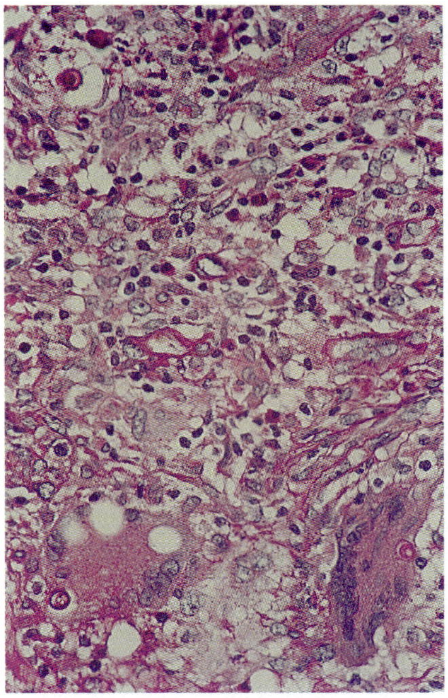

Figure 4–28. Epidermal hyperplasia associated with infection: Blastomycosis. The inflammatory infiltrate is composed of mononuclear cells, including multinucleated giant cells, and admixed neutrophils; with the periodic acid–Schiff stain, typical yeast forms are observed within giant cells.

5

Vesiculobullous Dermatitis

One of the most important and misunderstood areas of dermatopathology is vesiculobullous disease. This divergent group of disorders can be life threatening, and accurate diagnosis and implementation of correct therapy can have profound implications. The ability to make an accurate diagnosis, however, is often confounded by the histologic subtleties inherent in stage of lesion evolution, slight nuances in architecture, tinctorial characteristics, and inflammatory composition that distinguish certain disorders, and by the plethora of divergent stimuli that may eventuate in the common theme of an intraepidermal or a subepidermal blister (*e.g.,* antibody attack, cellular attack, ischemia, viral cytopathologic changes).

The nomenclature of blistering diseases is relatively simple. Vesicles (L. *vesicula,* meaning *small blister*) are lesions up to 1 cm in diameter. Bullae (L. *bulla,* meaning *bubble-like*) are larger blisters. Blisters may form from spongiosis, reticular degeneration, vacuolar degeneration, acantholysis, and lysis of dermal matrix *(dermolysis).*

We concentrate on disorders that commonly manifest as blisters at the most classic stage of their clinical and histologic evolution. Diseases that may form blisters but are better known for changes inherent in nonvesicular stages (*e.g.,* erythema multiforme) or disorders that occasionally, but not ordinarily, give rise to blisters and erosions (*e.g.,* lupus erythematosus, fixed drug eruption, lichen sclerosus) are not discussed.

One of the most useful applications of staining characteristics of cells and matrix is demonstrated in this category, in which the presence and localization of inflammatory cells can be detected at low-power magnification. Inflammatory cells generally appear as clusters of basophilia within the dermal or epidermal layers. Because some blistering disorders are relatively noninflammatory (porphyria, epidermolysis bullosa), detection of the presence or absence of inflammation based on tinctorial qualities at scanning magnification can be helpful in generation of the initial branch points of a diagnostic algorithm. Once identified, basophilic clusters of inflammatory cells can be categorized as to their location in the dermis and the type and level of blister (*e.g.,* subepidermal blister with alignment along dermal-epidermal interface [possible pemphigoid or linear IgA disease] or with aggregation within dermal papillae [probable dermatitis herpetiformis]).

Tinctorial pallor may also be useful in the diagnosis of vesiculobullous disorders according to hue. For example, keratinocytes showing a herpesvirus effect generally have a pale-pink cytoplasm as a result of ballooning degeneration. Pale, homogeneous eosinophilic matrix encasing superficial vessels may be seen in porphyria or in bullous lesions of diabetes, whereas normal vessels are usually surrounded by a fibrillar pink mantle.

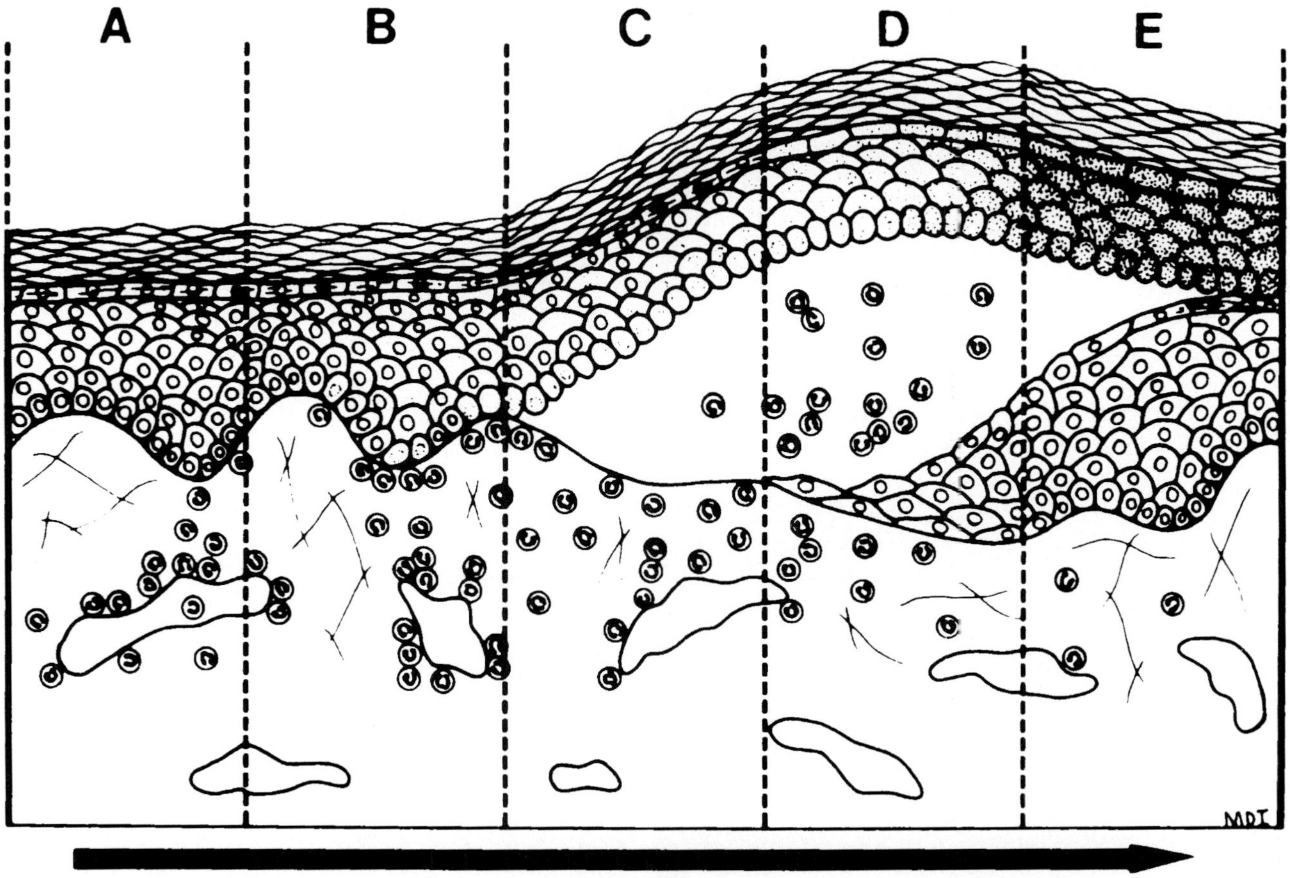

Figure 5–1. Temporal evolution of subepidermal inflammatory blister. *A,* The earliest phase of blister formation involves the local recruitment of inflammatory cells. Release of mediators by these cells, often in concert with concentration of these cells along with antibody and complement deposition along the dermal-epidermal junction *(B),* results in separation of the dermal and the epidermal layers *(C).* Initially, serum fills the forming cavity. *D,* Eventually, inflammatory cells infiltrate the cavity, and squamous epithelial cells begin to cover the blister base. *E,* On reaching confluence, these re-epithelializing cells begin to stratify, forming a new viable epidermal layer as the blister roof becomes progressively necrotic and eventually is sloughed. Biopsy of the edge of a blister may reveal several of these sequential steps and facilitate diagnosis. Biopsy of the center of the blister may confuse the diagnosis, because these sites frequently contain more chronic alterations.

Bullous Pemphigoid

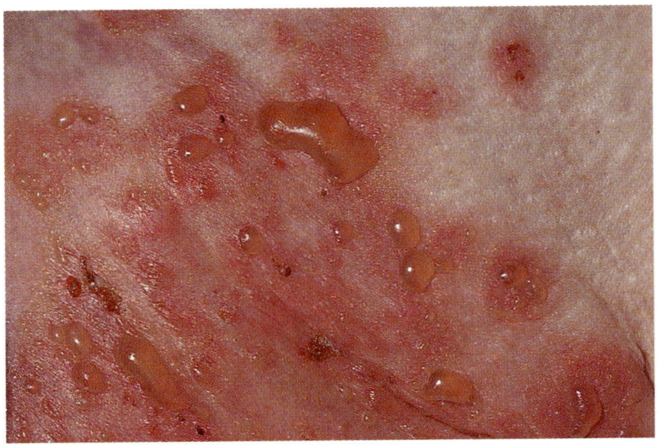

Figure 5–2. Bullous pemphigoid. Numerous tense bullae are present on erythematous bases. Occasionally, lesions begin and persist as pruritic, urticarial plaques. Erythematous, often urticarial plaques evolve into zones of microvesiculation and eventually form overt, fluid-filled bullae.

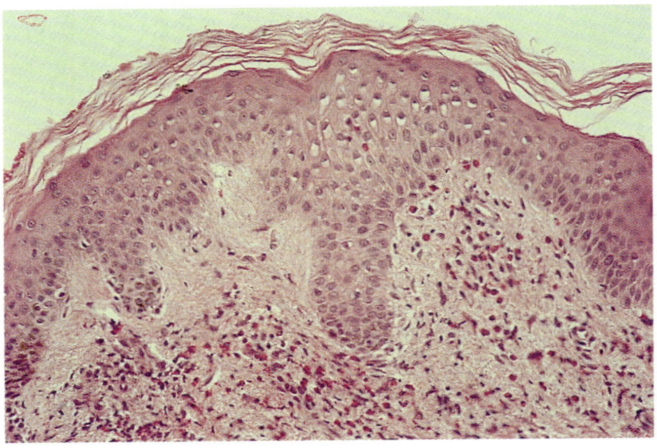

Figure 5–3. The earliest evolutionary phase of bullous pemphigoid consists of superficial perivascular infiltration by lymphocytes and eosinophils, with occasional eosinophils in close proximity to the dermal-epidermal junction. This pattern could represent a drug eruption or insect-bite reaction, but there is no spongiosis, and the presence of eosinophils along the basement membrane zone is unusual.

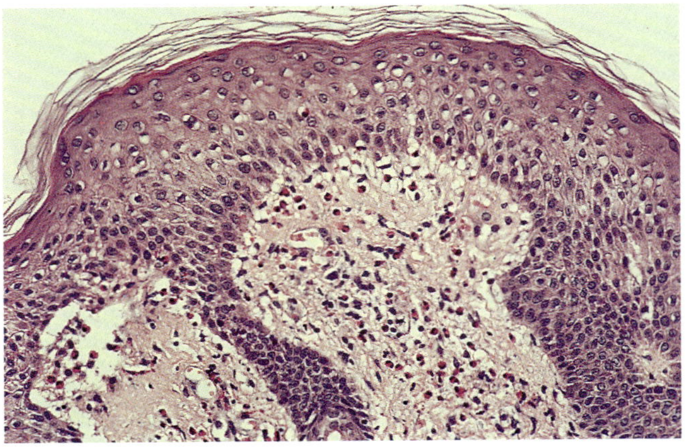

Figure 5–4. The apposition of degranulating eosinophils along the dermal-epidermal junction is followed by basal layer vacuolization and microvesicle formation *(bottom left).*

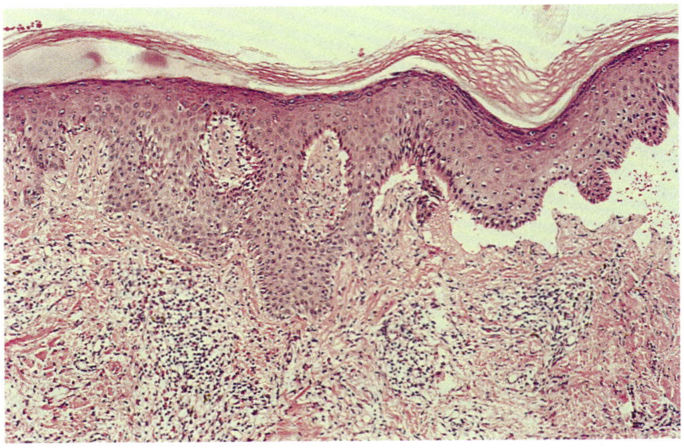

Figure 5–5. In time, a subepidermal blister forms, although at the edge *(left),* most of the changes seen in Figures 5–3 and 5–4 may be observed.

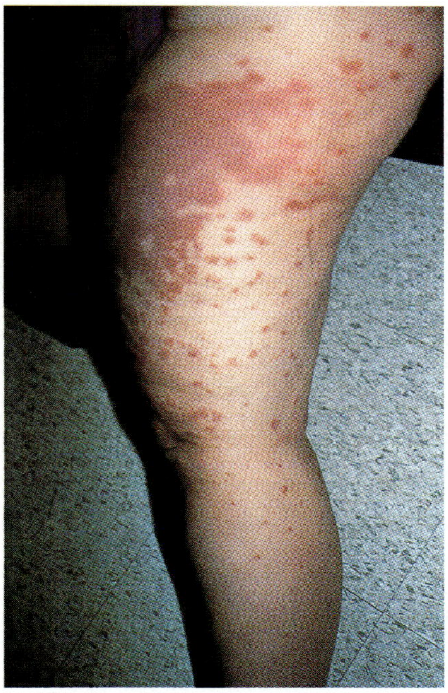

Figure 5–6. Herpes gestationis. Erythematous plaques with early vesiculation are present on the thigh of a pregnant woman. The histology of this disorder in indistinguishable from that of pemphigoid.

Dermatitis Herpetiformis

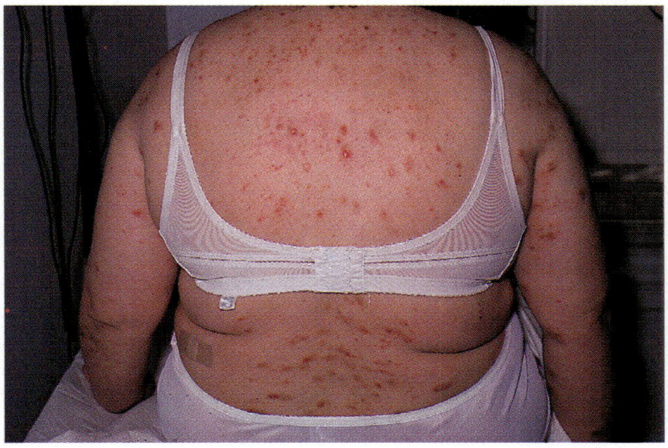

Figure 5–7. Clinical manifestations of dermatitis herpetiformis. Multiple erythematous vesicles and erosions are present on the back of a patient.

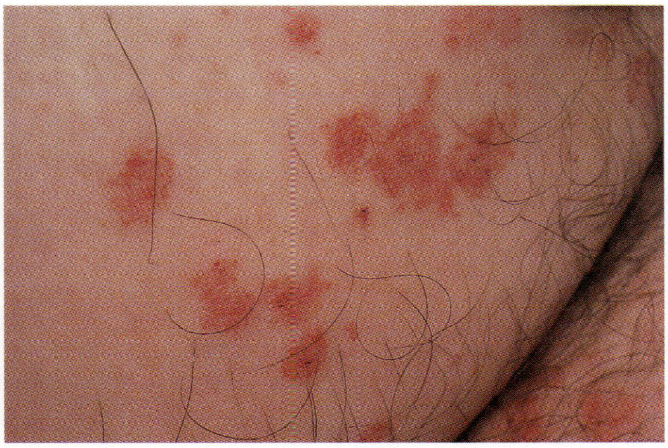

Figure 5–8. Closer inspection reveals their clustered, herpetiform arrangement. Often, vesicles have a predilection for the extensor surfaces of the extremities, and lesions are almost always intensely pruritic. The clinical differential diagnoses that accompany a biopsy specimen often include contact dermatitis and pruritic forms of pemphigoid.

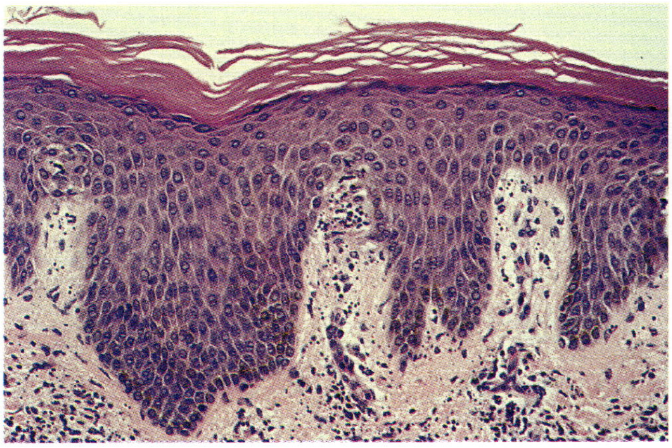

Figure 5–9. Histologic manifestations of dermatitis herpetiformis. An early lesion shows subtle accumulation of neutrophils, nuclear dust, and fibrin within the tips of dermal papillae. Because the epidermis in this biopsy specimen appears slightly hyperplastic and spongiotic, possibly owing to a primary irritant effect, the dermal changes could be overlooked in favor of an erroneous diagnosis of low-grade subacute spongiotic dermatitis.

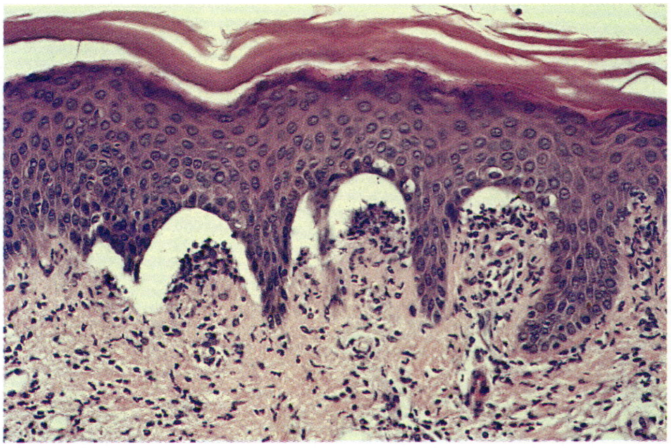

Figure 5–10. A better-developed lesion shows neutrophilic microabscesses at the tips of the dermal papillae, producing cleft-like zones of dermal-epidermal separation overlying each papilla. Eosinophils are notably absent.

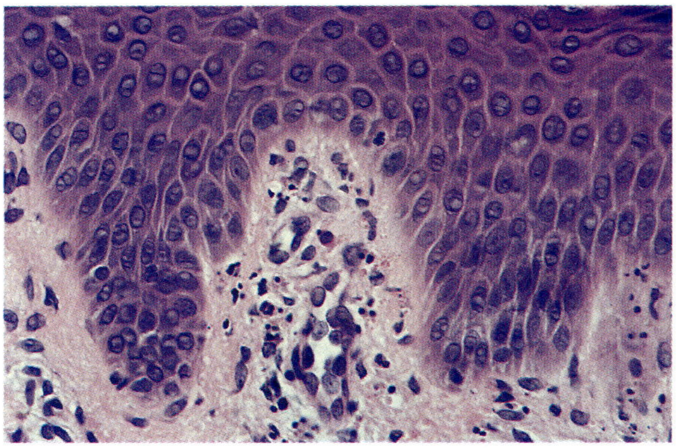

Figure 5–11. Sequential evolution of dermal papillary microabscess in dermatitis herpetiformis. Scant numbers of fragmented neutrophils and fibrin in dermal papillae lead to more overt aggregates of clumped fibrin and neutrophils associated with early microvesicle formation directly over the papilla.

Linear IgA Disease

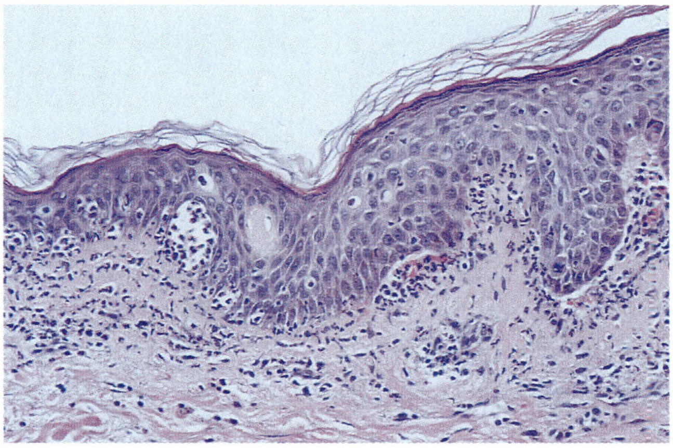

Figure 5–12. Linear IgA disease. In this biopsy specimen, neutrophils are both aggregated within dermal papillae and aligned along the entire dermal-epidermal junction, including rete tips *(bottom)*. Direct immunofluorescence reveals linear, not granular, deposits of IgA in a pattern that resembles C_3 and IgG deposition in pemphigoid. Linear IgA dermatosis is not a variant of dermatitis herpetiformis. Clinically, linear IgA dermatosis is characterized by a vesiculobullous eruption that may occur in childhood or after puberty. Lesions often form large bullae, may be annular in configuration, and occur randomly. In contrast to dermatitis herpetiformis, intestinal lesions and association with gluten-induced autoimmunity are the exception. Clinical presentation may mimic bullous pemphigoid.

Pemphigus

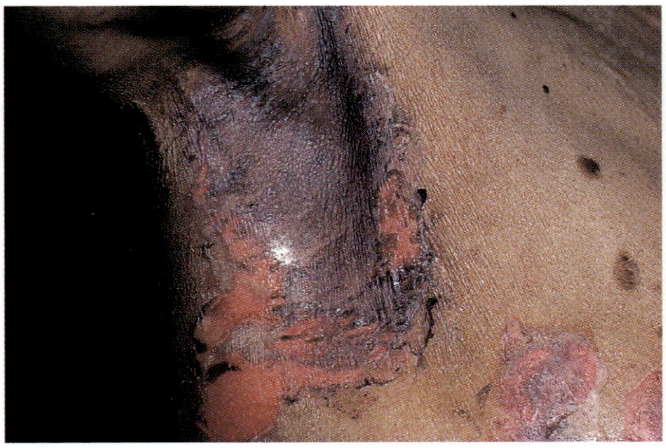

Figure 5–13. Pemphigus vulgaris. Eroded plaques are formed by confluent, thin-roofed bullae, here on intertriginous skin.

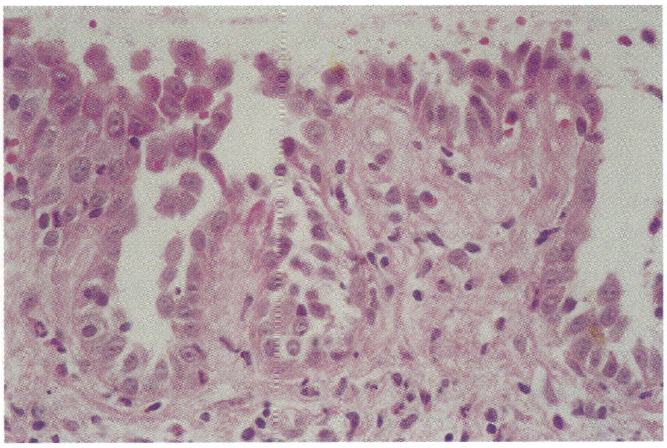

Figure 5–14. Rounded, acantholytic keratinocytes detached from neighboring cells are visible along the surface of the blister base in pemphigus vulgaris. The relatively rigid dermal papillae covered with a single row of adherent basal cells produce a characteristic tombstone pattern. The underlying inflammatory infiltrate is superficial, perivascular, and composed primarily of lymphocytes and eosinophils.

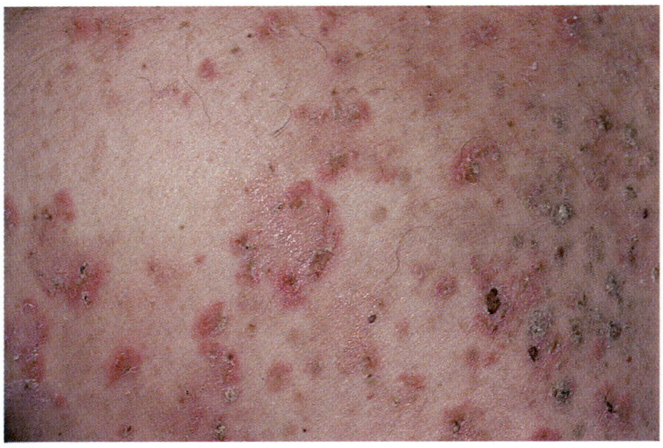

Figure 5–15. The clinical picture of pemphigus foliaceus (*i.e.*, superficial pemphigus) consists predominantly of superficial erosions with crust superimposed on erythematous plaques. Intact blisters may not be observed.

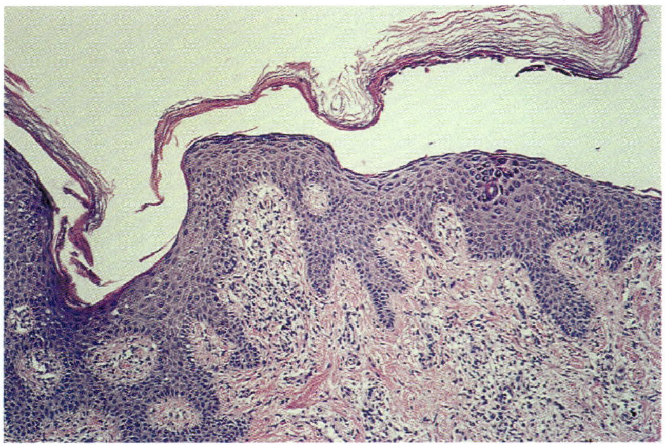

Figure 5–16. Biopsy specimens of the lesions in pemphigus foliaceus frequently reveal the base and a detached stratum corneum, which at scanning magnification may appear to represent normal skin.

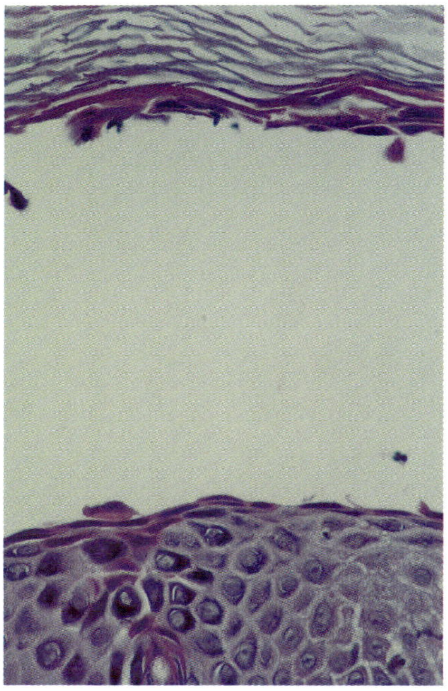

Figure 5–17. Closer inspection reveals that the stratum corneum and stratum granulosum have been sloughed as the roof of a very superficial acantholytic blister. Residual acantholytic cells are easily detected by their rounded, partially detached contours. The blister base in pemphigus foliaceus is therefore composed of an epidermal layer that is almost entirely intact.

Porphyria

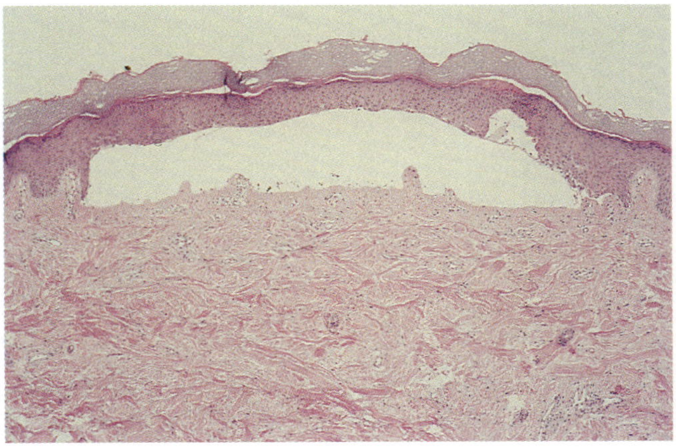

Figure 5–18. Porphyria cutanea tarda. At scanning magnification, there is a noninflammatory subepidermal blister. Forms of epidermolysis bullosa also produce noninflammatory blisters. Toxic epidermal necrolysis, a type of cytotoxic dermatitis (see Chapter 6 in textbook), is often described erroneously as another example of noninflammatory subepidermal blister formation.

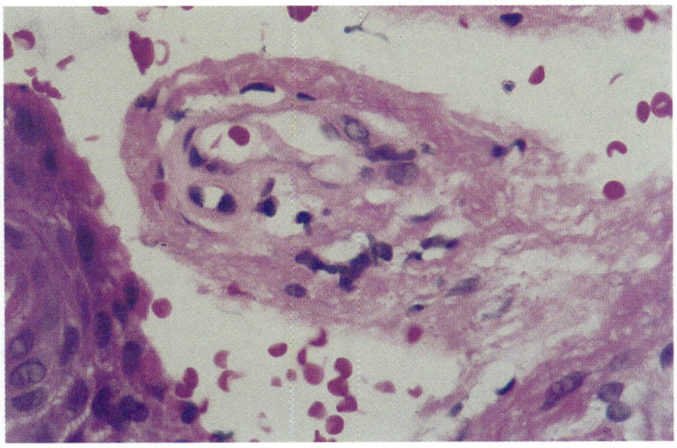

Figure 5–19. The vessels in each dermal papilla have thickened, hyalinized walls that are accentuated further by periodic acid–Schiff stain.

Bullous Vasculitis

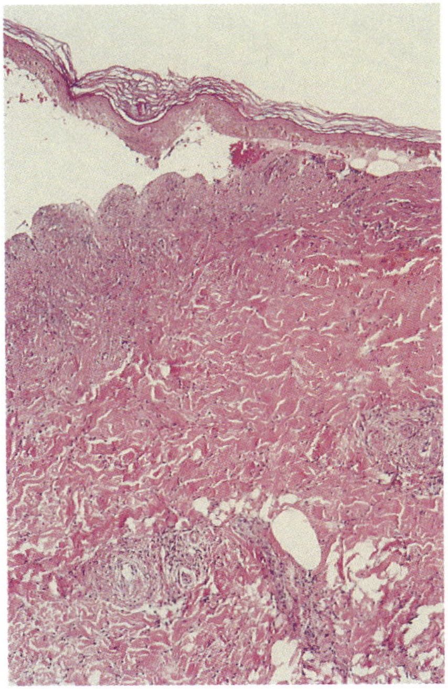

Figure 5–20. Edge of vasculitis blister revealing subepidermal separation, necrotic blister roof, and basophilic inflammatory cells aggregated around superficial and mid-dermal vessels.

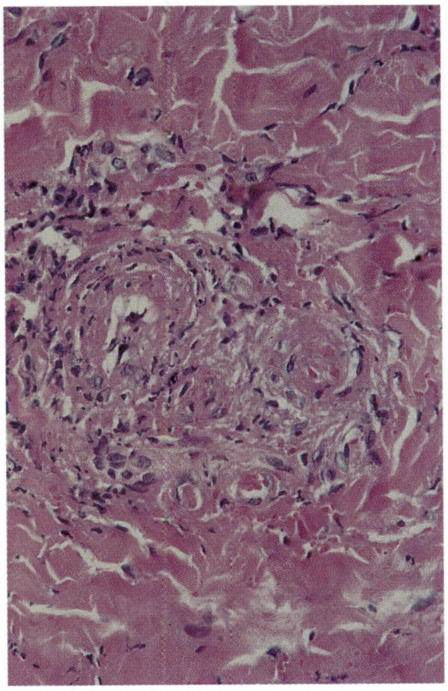

Figure 5–21. Higher magnification of involved dermal venules showing fibrinoid necrosis of vessel walls, nuclear dust, and luminal obliteration due to endothelial necrosis and microthrombus formation.

Viral Vesicles

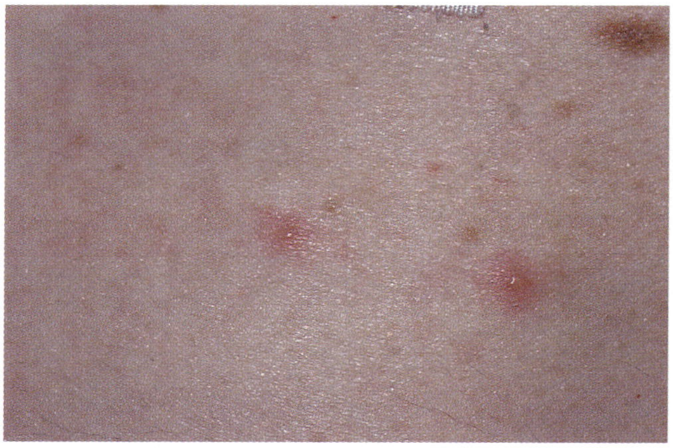

Figure 5–22. Varicella (chickenpox) showing drop-like vesicles on erythematous bases ("dew drops on rose petals").

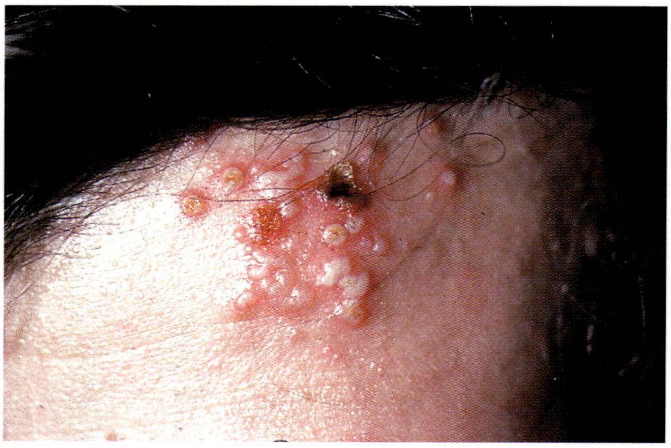

Figure 5–23. Herpes simplex, superinfected and presenting as grouped vesiculopustules.

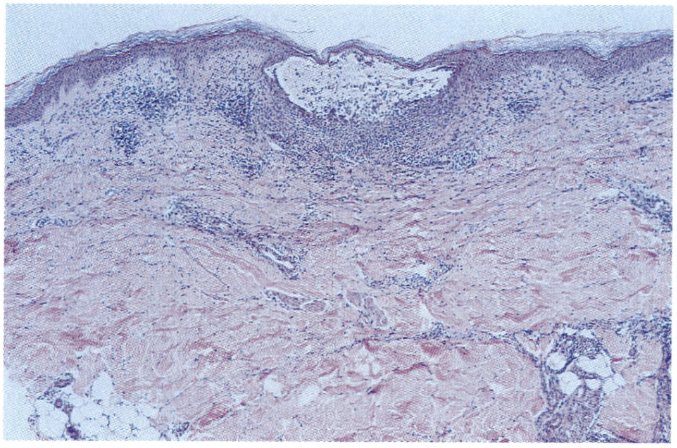

Figure 5–24. Herpes simplex: intraepidermal acantholytic vesicle with underlying dermal perivascular inflammatory infiltrate.

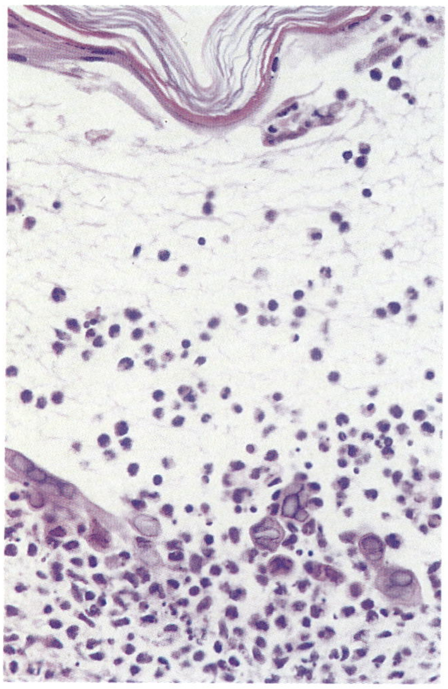

Figure 5–25. Vesicle cavity containing mixed inflammatory cells and rare, inconspicuous multinucleated giant cells exhibiting nuclear molding and characteristic pale-gray viral inclusions *(bottom)*.

Epidermolysis Bullosa

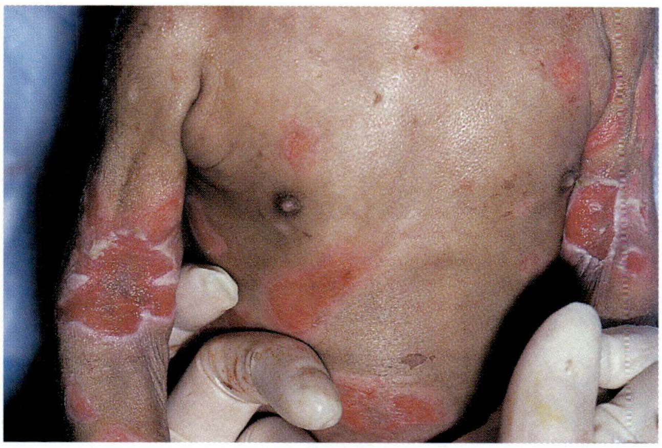

Figure 5–26. Epidermolysis bullosa. Junctional epidermolysis bullosa showing typical erosions in flexural creases.

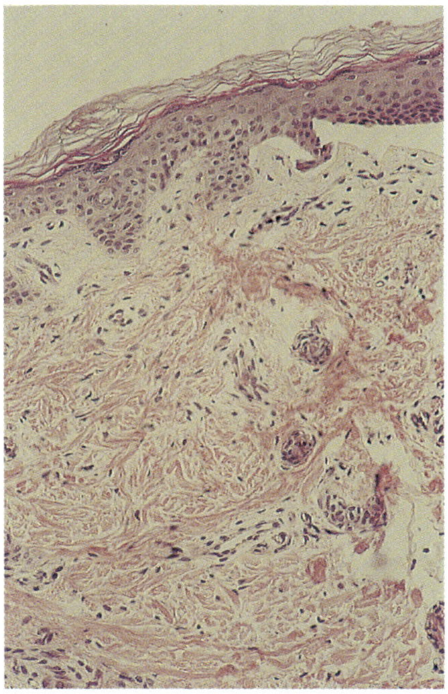

Figure 5–27. Dermal-epidermal blister cavity *(upper right)* in biopsy specimen; note relative absence of inflammation in underlying dermis.

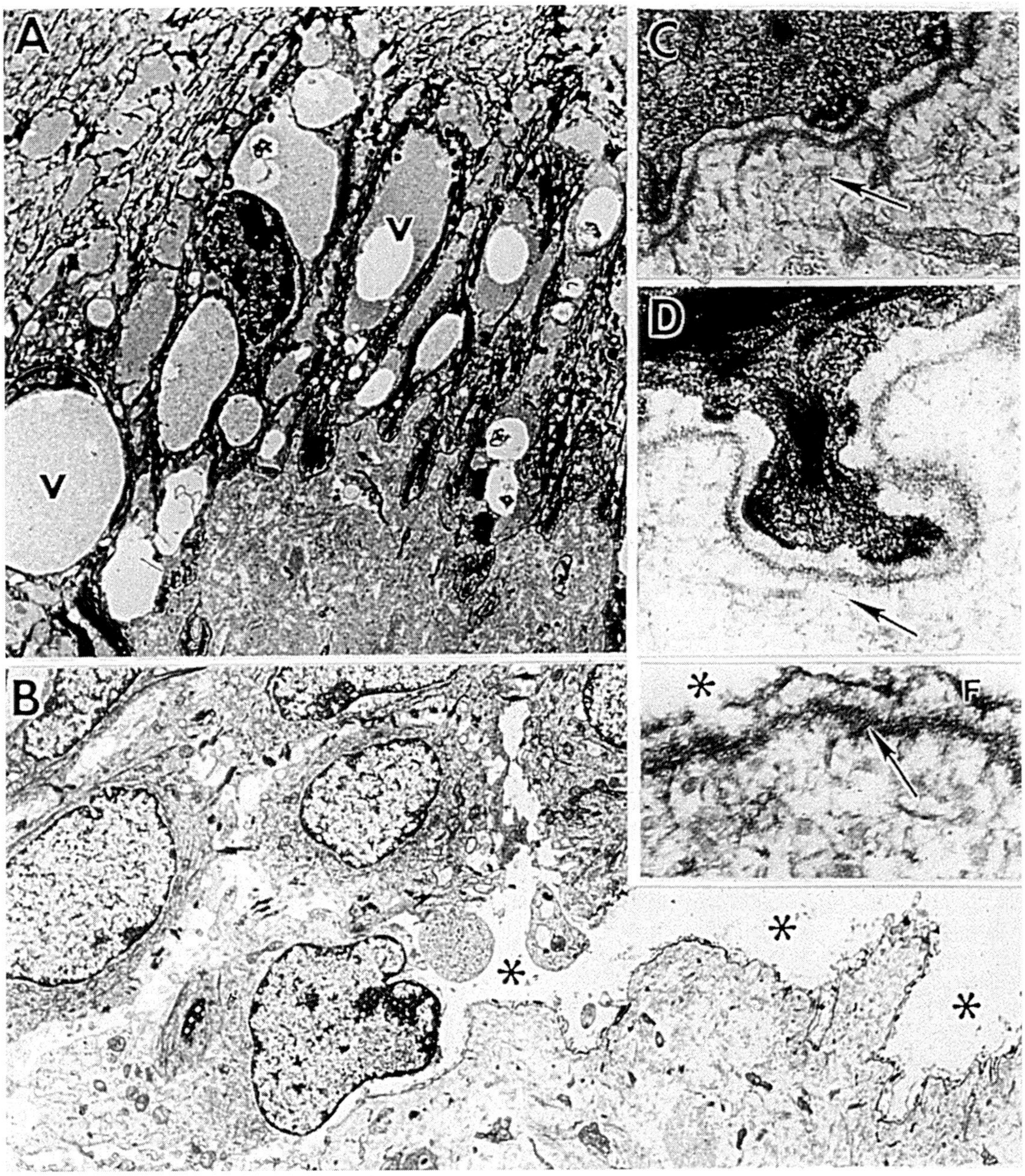

Figure 5–28. Diagnostic electron microscopy of types of epidermolysis bullosa. *A,* Vacuolated basal keratinocytes (V) in epidermolysis bullosa simplex. *B,* Lamina lucida split (*) in junctional epidermolysis bullosa (note *inset,* where lamina densa remains on blister base; F = fibrin coat on surface of base). *C,* Normal dermal-epidermal junction with full complement of anchoring fibrils *(arrow)* beneath the lamina densa. *D,* Markedly diminished anchoring fibrils in dystrophic (dermolytic) form of epidermolysis bullosa, at site where separation occurs beneath the lamina densa.

6

Cytotoxic Dermatitis

There are only a finite number of reaction patterns that may occur in human skin consequent to infiltration by reactive T lymphocytes. One pattern, depicted in Chapter 3, involves intercellular epidermal edema, or spongiosis. This occurs when antigen-specific T cells of the helper subtype infiltrate at sites of antigen challenge. Other subtypes of effector lymphocytes, however, may produce very different alterations within the epidermal layer. For example, experimentally, when autosensitized cytotoxic T cells enter the skin, the pattern consistently involves degeneration and death of keratinocytes *(cytotoxicity),* particularly those of the lower epidermal layers. Acute cytotoxicity may take the form of pale-pink to colorless basal cell layer vacuolization, an accelerated rate of programmed cell death (apoptosis), or direct cell-cell killing via effector-target cell apposition *(satellitosis).* Chronic cytotoxicity is manifested by abnormal keratinization *(dyskeratosis),* resulting in cells with dense eosinophilic cytoplasm, cell death with mummification of cytoplasmic contents (*colloid body* formation), or altered cellular maturation for a specific epidermal stratum (*squamatization* of the basal cell layer). These acute and chronic alterations, usually concentrated at the dermal-epidermal junction, coupled with lymphocyte infiltration along this interface, have earned for cytotoxic dermatitis the alternative designation of *interface dermatitis.*

At scanning magnification interface dermatitis is characterized by a variably dense, dark-blue band of inflammatory cells that obscures the normal pink epidermal and dermal strata. The underlying causes of most forms of cytotoxic dermatitis are protean, although it is generally assumed that autoantigens within the epidermal layer provoke an autoimmune reaction directed against keratinocytes. In connective tissue disorders, such as lupus erythematosus, the primary abnormality appears to reside in the effector pathway, with immune recognition and attack directed against epitopes, which are usually exempt from host surveillance. In other settings, such as erythema multiforme, infectious agents and ingested drugs are likely to alter epidermal antigens in a manner that provokes reactivity of an otherwise normal T-cell axis. Nevertheless, in conditions such as lichen planus, it remains unclear as to whether target or effector pathways are the primary stimulants for lesion formation.

The term *apoptosis* connotes *programmed cell death.* By *programmed,* it is implied that the cell is not simply starved as a result of nutrient depletion, or ripped apart, as in a traumatic wound. Rather, there are precise events determined at the genomic or receptor-mediated level that initiate nuclear degeneration involving chromosomal nicking by intrinsic endonucleases. Accordingly, apoptosis is an event that occurs normally in the epidermis as an essential component of follicular cycling, as well as pathologically as a result of cytotoxicity as a consequence of mediators, such as tumor necrosis factor (TNF) binding to the TNF receptor, which may stimulate an identical degenerative process.

Apoptotic cells show progressive nuclear pyknosis, eventual nuclear fragmentation, and cytoplasmic shrinkage such that intermediate filaments become increasingly prominent by routine histologic stains. Accordingly, such cells may appear to be *dyskeratotic.* Only refined stains that permit detection of chromosomal fragmentation within intact nuclei permit absolute distinction between early apoptotic cells and cells with an accelerated program for cytoplasmic keratinization.

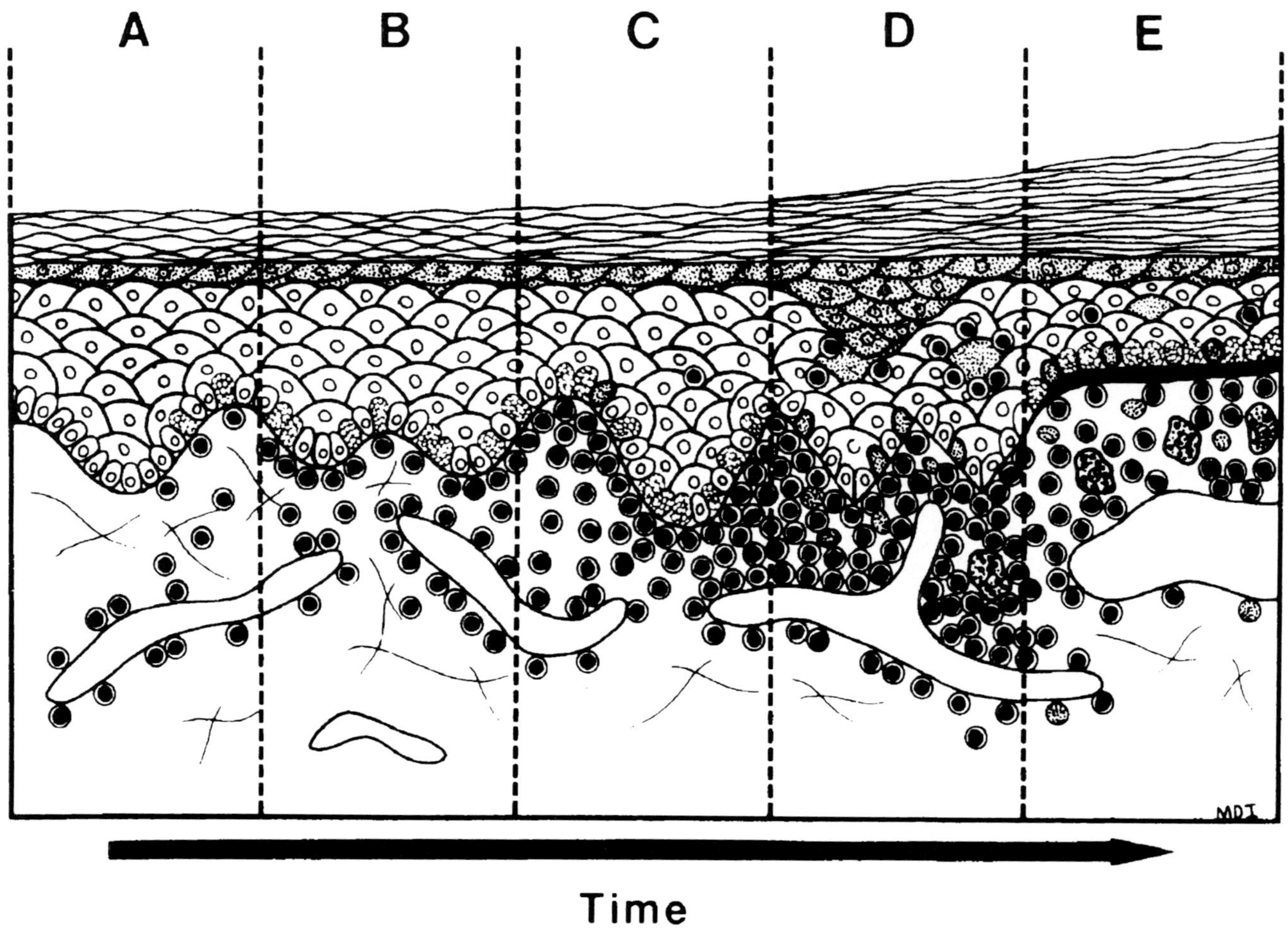

Figure 6–1. Temporal evolution of acute and chronic phases of cytotoxic dermatitis. *A through C,* The temporal evolution of prototypical cytotoxic dermatitis commences with a dermal angiocentric infiltrate with progressive alignment or tagging of lymphocytes along the dermal-epidermal interface. This is associated with degenerative alterations in basal keratinocytes. Note that by *C,* the infiltrate has begun to fill the papillary dermis, producing a band-like interstitial pattern as well as an angiocentric pattern. *D,* In certain disorders, such as lichen planus, chronicity takes the form of hyperkeratosis, hypergranulosis, and redefinition of the rete ridge pattern to form jagged "teeth." Note satellitosis of lymphocytes about midepidermal keratinocytes undergoing degenerative changes. *E,* In other conditions, such as discoid lupus erythematosus, chronicity produces hyperkeratosis and epidermal atrophy, with complete loss of the rete ridge pattern. Thickening of the basement membrane characteristically occurs in this disorder. Chronic destruction of basal cells containing melanin also results in accumulation of melanophages within the papillary dermis (*D and E,* melanophages = larger cells among lymphocytes).

Erythema Multiforme

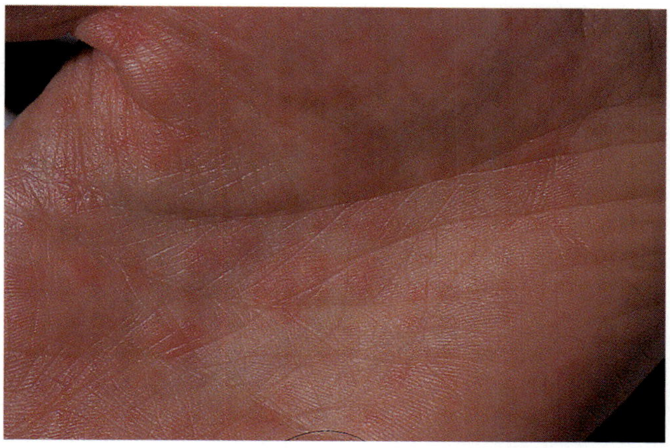

Figure 6–2. Erythema multiforme, early lesion. Erythematous macules and dermal plaques on the palm are the result of superficial perivascular lymphocytic infiltration with associated papillary dermal edema (see Fig. 6–3).

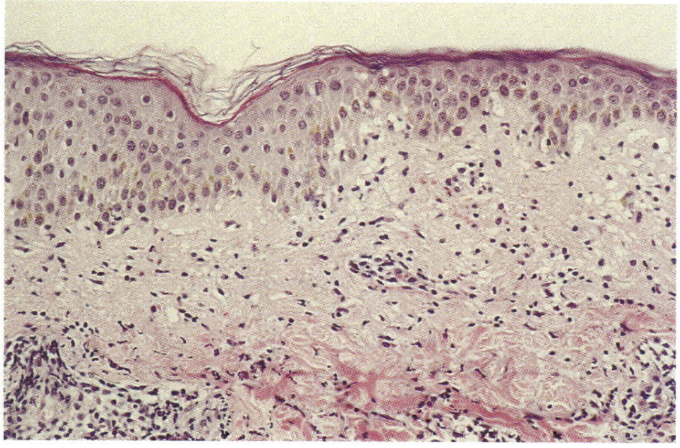

Figure 6–3. Superficial perivascular lymphocytic infiltration with associated papillary dermal edema.

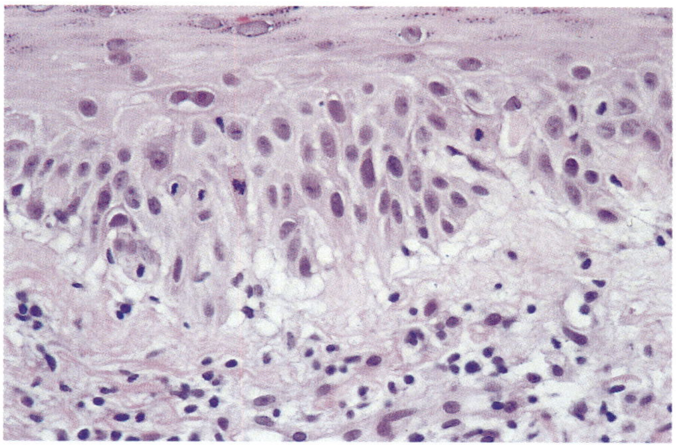

Figure 6–4. Higher magnification discloses characteristic early tagging of occasional lymphocytes along the dermal-epidermal interface, with early vacuolization of basal keratinocytes.

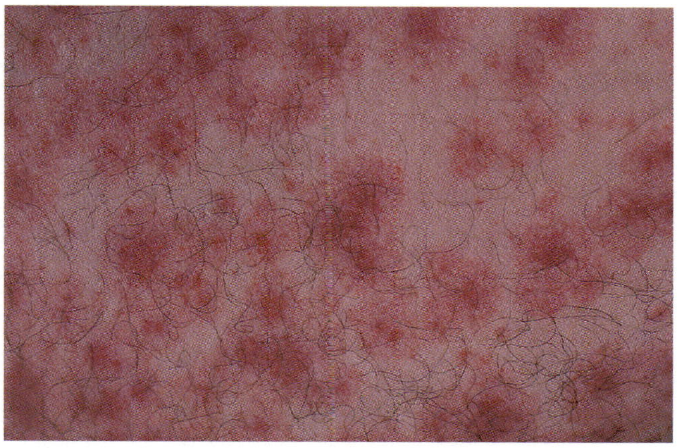

Figure 6–5. Erythema multiforme, advanced and healing lesions. Targetoid plaques are formed by central zones of epidermal necrosis and incipient vesiculation surrounded by a peripheral, advancing erythematous rim.

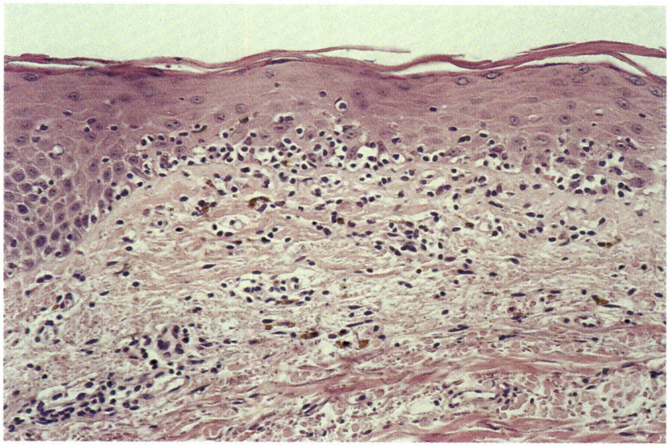

Figure 6–6. The rim shows well-developed alterations, which are depicted in earlier stages in Figures 6–3 and 6–4. Note the extensive lymphocyte tagging and basal cell layer vacuolization.

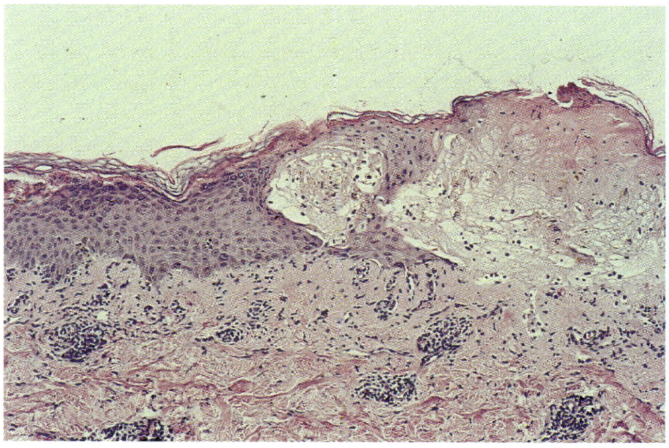

Figure 6–7. The center of the lesion *(right)* shows full-thickness epidermal necrosis with early detachment of the epidermal layer. The underlying dermis already has been partially recovered by re-epithelialization.

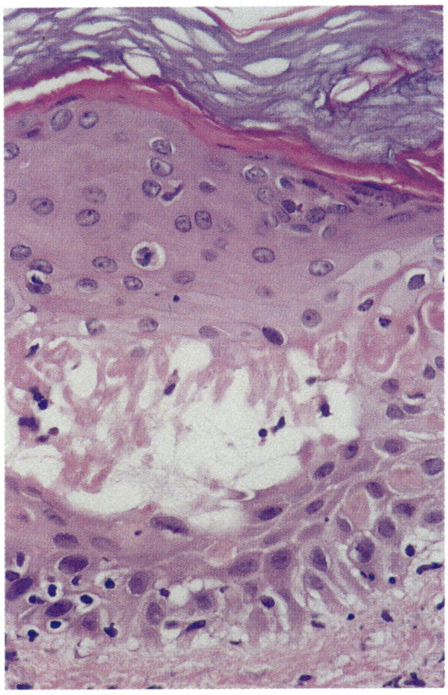

Figure 6–8. The basal cells of the former blister roof are ragged and necrotic. The basal cells of the re-epithelialized layer are infiltrated by lymphocytes, indicating that complete resolution of the inflammatory component has not yet occurred.

Acute and Chronic Graft-Versus-Host Disease

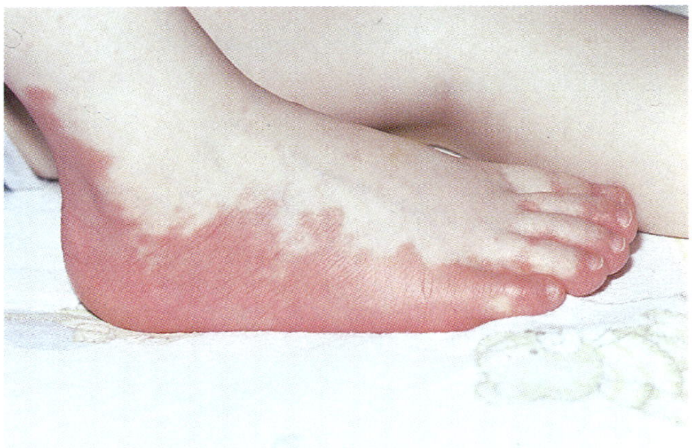

Figure 6–9. Acute graft-versus-host disease. There is confluent erythema of the palms and soles; elsewhere on the body surface, there may be a maculopapular exanthem.

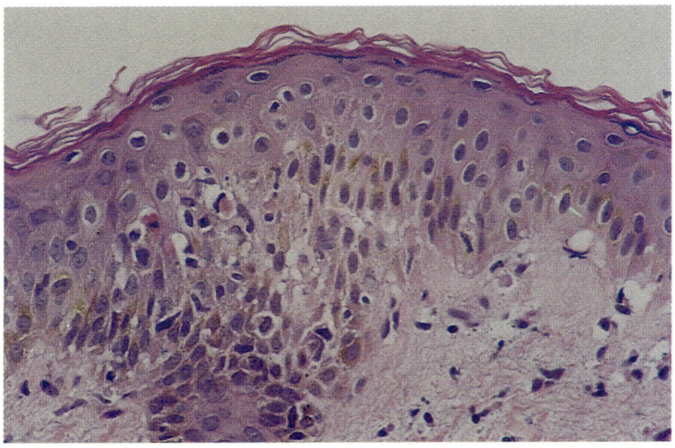

Figure 6–10. The histology is characterized by a relatively sparse infiltrate of lymphocytes within the papillary dermis, with migration of these cells into the overlying epidermal layer.

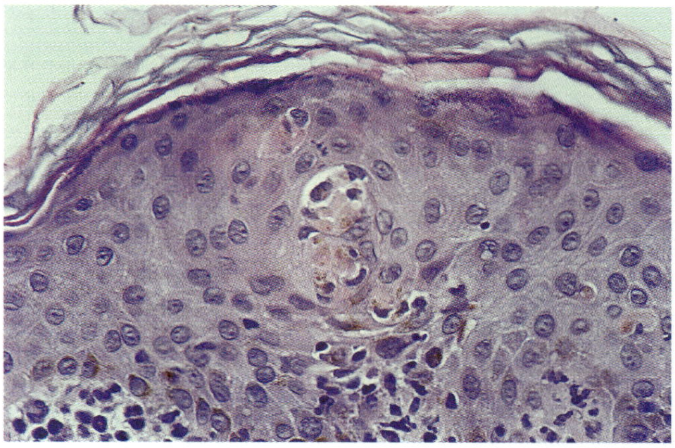

Figure 6–11. Both basal cell layer vacuolization and satellitosis may occur; the latter is characterized by aggregation of intraepidermal lymphocytes about a target keratinocyte undergoing necrosis *(center)*.

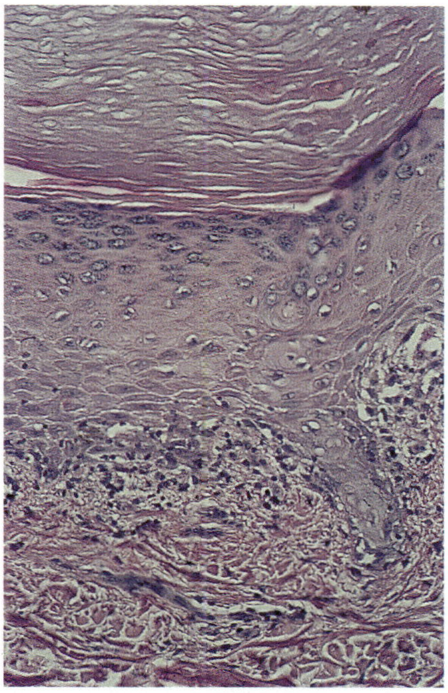

Figure 6–12. Lesions depicted in Figures 6–9 through 6–11 may become chronic, with progressive epidermal hyperplasia, hypergranulosis, and hyperkeratosis as well as development of a jagged dermal-epidermal interface infiltrated by lymphocytes in apposition to necrotic keratinocytes. These alterations resemble those of classic lichen planus, although the clinical setting in which they occur is very different. Acute graft-versus-host disease may also produce dermal sclerosis that is indistinguishable from scleroderma in certain individuals (*i.e.*, dermal sclerodermoid type).

Pityriasis Lichenoides et Varioliformis Acuta

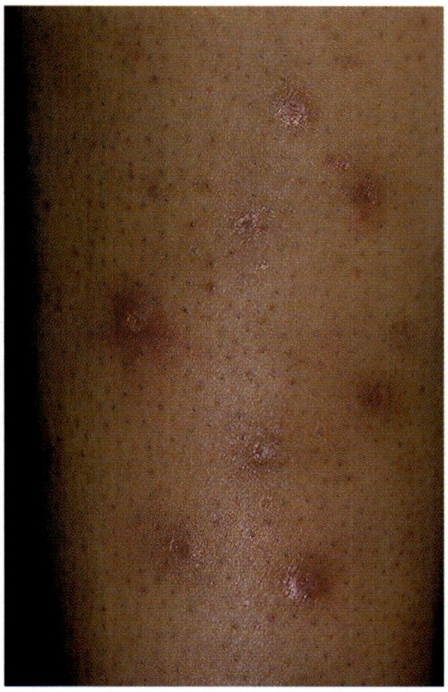

Figure 6–13. Pityriasis lichenoides et varioliformis acuta. Biopsy specimens of erythematous, indurated nodules generally reveal a superficial and deep angiocentric dermal infiltrate with an interface component at scanning magnification (see Fig. 6–14).

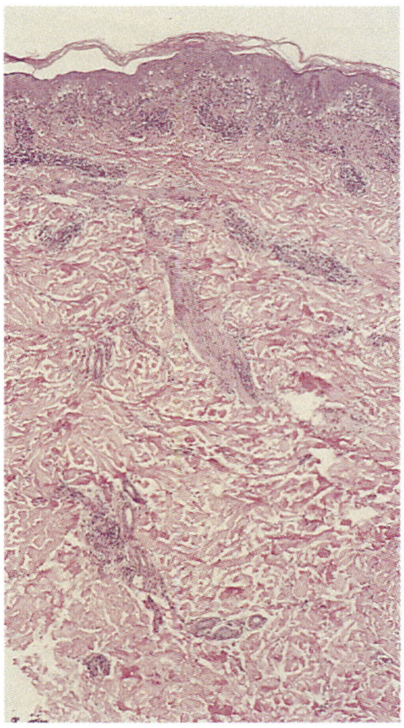

Figure 6–14. A superficial and deep angiocentric dermal infiltrate with an interface component is seen at scanning magnification.

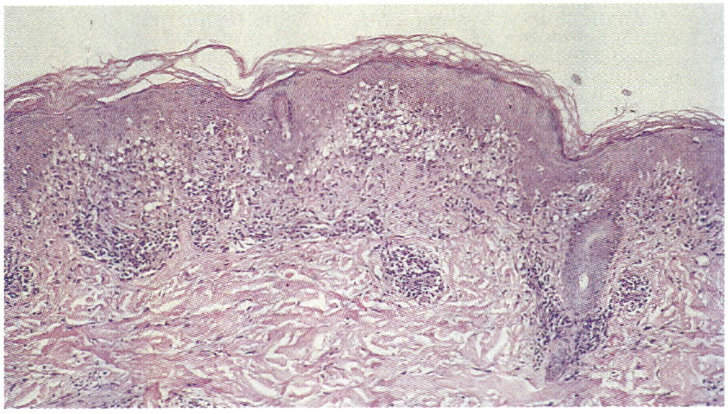

Figure 6–15. On closer inspection, early focal parakeratosis and basal cell layer vacuolization are observed.

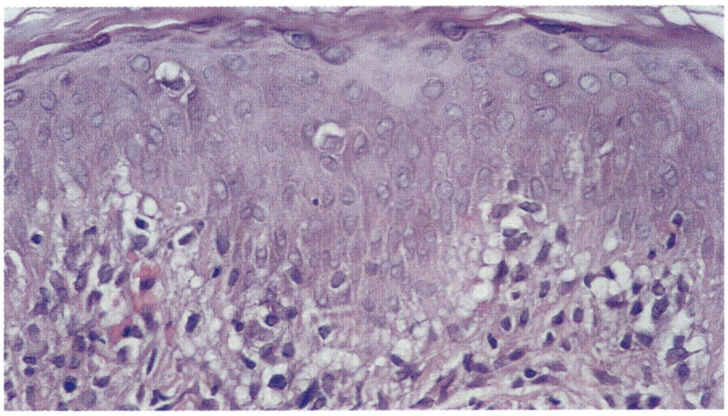

Figure 6–16. At even higher magnification, hemorrhage into the papillary dermis is observed *(left, center)*. In more advanced lesions, individual and zonal epidermal necrosis *(center)* and infiltration of parakeratotic scale by neutrophils are generally detected.

Lupus Erythematosus

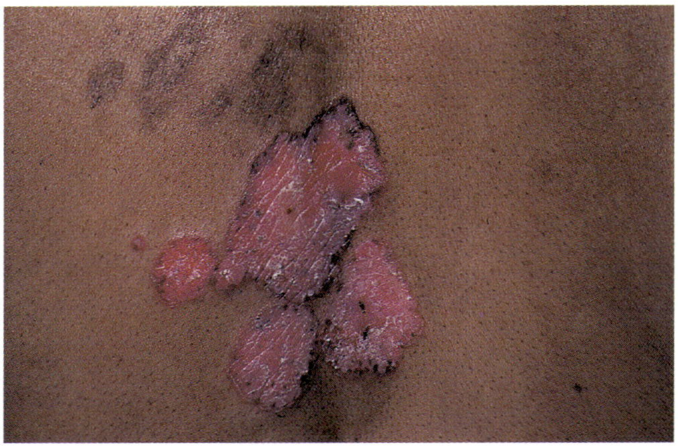

Figure 6–17. Discoid plaques of lupus erythematosus clinically show erythema, central atrophy and hyperkeratosis, and peripheral hyperpigmentation.

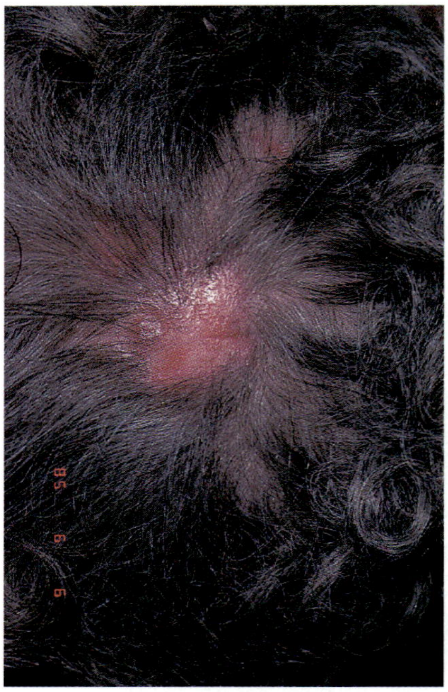

Figure 6–18. When hair-bearing surfaces are affected, hair loss often occurs.

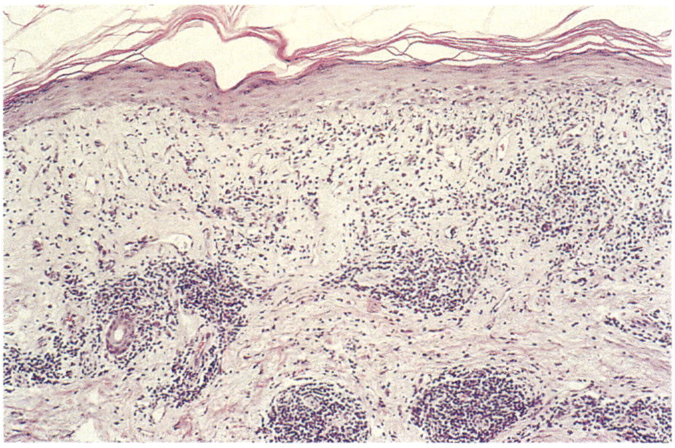

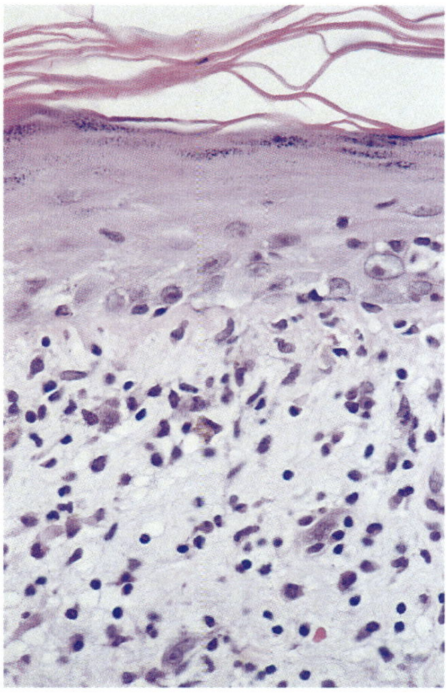

Figures 6–19 and 6–20. Histologically, there is a superficial and deep, perivascular and periadnexal infiltrate of lymphocytes; dermal pallor resulting from infiltration of pale-staining particulate mucin; and diffuse epidermal atrophy with associated basal cell layer vacuolization and hyperkeratosis. Note the association of subepidermal lymphocytes with degenerating basal cells in Figure 6–20.

Lichen Planus

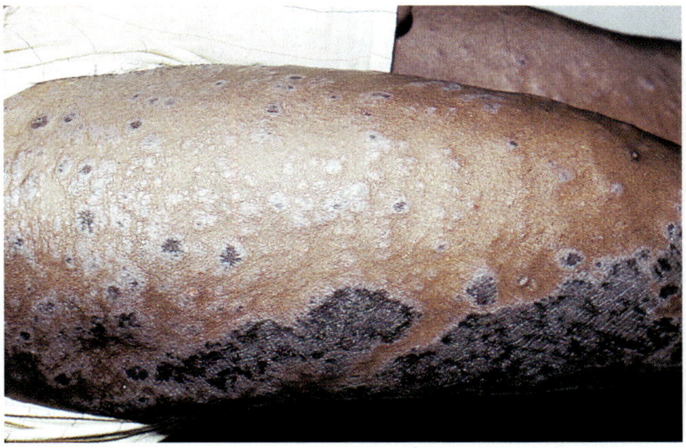

Figure 6–21. Clinically, lichen planus is characterized by numerous flat, pruritic papules that may coalesce to form hyperkeratotic plaques. Marked associated hyperpigmentation, resulting from chronic dermal pigment incontinence, is also present in this patient.

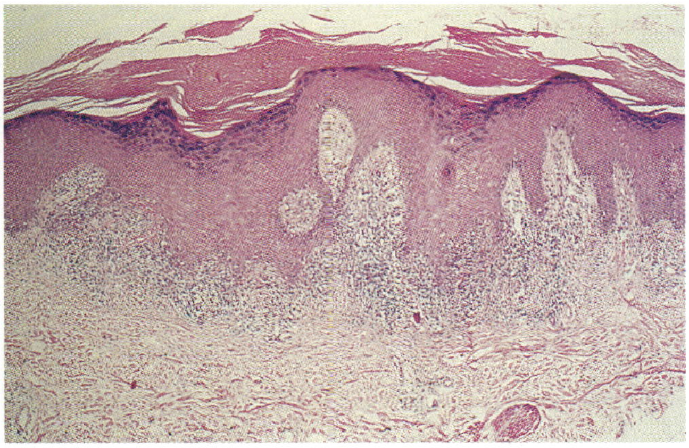

Figure 6–22. The characteristic histology of lichen planus at scanning magnification involves a band-like infiltrate of lymphocytes within the papillary dermis that is intimately associated with a jagged dermal-epidermal interface. The epidermal layer is hyperplastic, with hypergranulosis and hyperkeratosis.

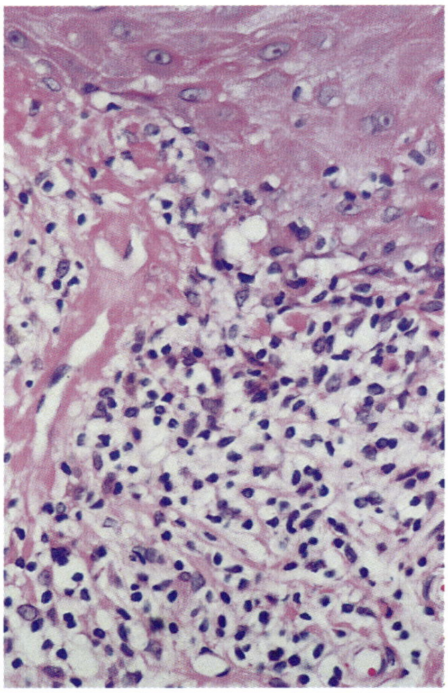

Figure 6–23. At higher magnification, lymphocytes infiltrating the dermal-epidermal interface are associated with basal cells with a polyhedral contour (*i.e.,* squamatized cells: *top right corner*) and small eosinophilic bodies (*i.e.,* colloid bodies) representing necrotic, anucleate epidermal cells.

Lichen Planopilaris

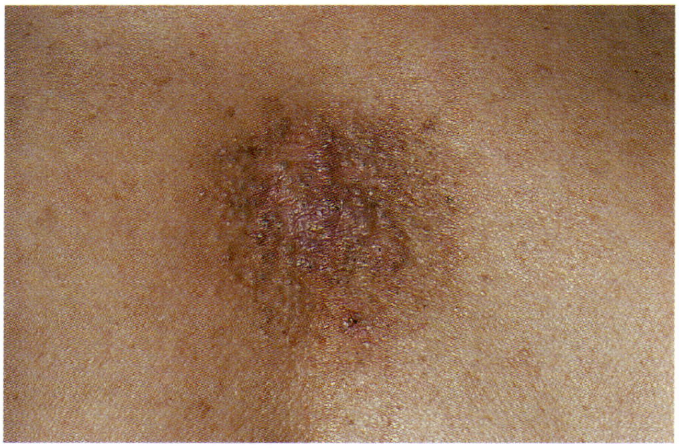

Figure 6–24. Lichen planus, follicular involvement (*i.e.,* lichen planopilaris). A cluster of follicular papules is associated with hyperpigmentation, indicative of chronic destruction of pigment-containing epithelial cells.

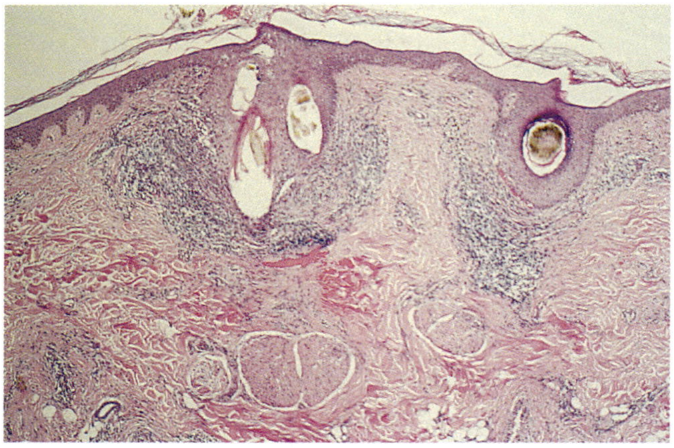

Figure 6–25. At scanning magnification, there is an interface infiltrate of lymphocytes about the dilated and plugged follicular infundibula.

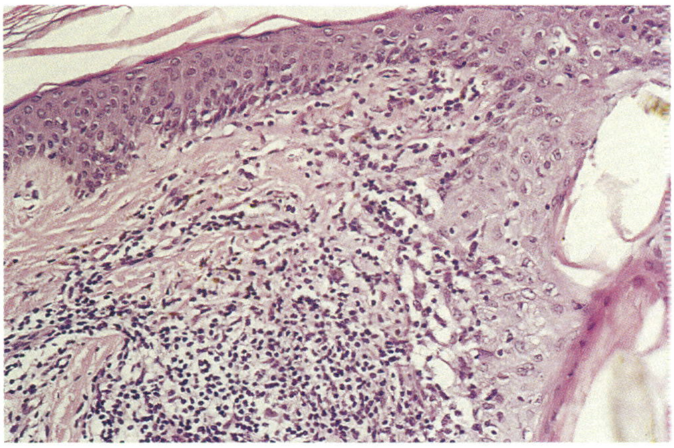

Figure 6–26. The infiltrate does not extend as deeply as in follicular lupus erythematosus, and the follicular epithelium is hyperplastic, not atrophic *(center right)*. As is the case in interfollicular lichen planus, the infundibular epithelium may also show hyperkeratosis and hypergranulosis, and the basal cells infiltrated by lymphocytes may demonstrate squamatization and colloid body formation.

Lichen Nitidus

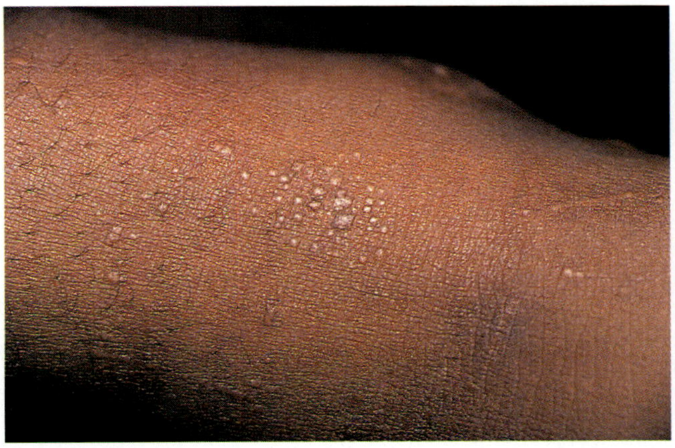

Figure 6–27. Lichen nitidus. Multiple nonfollicular papules, smaller than the flat-topped papules of lichen planus, are observed clinically.

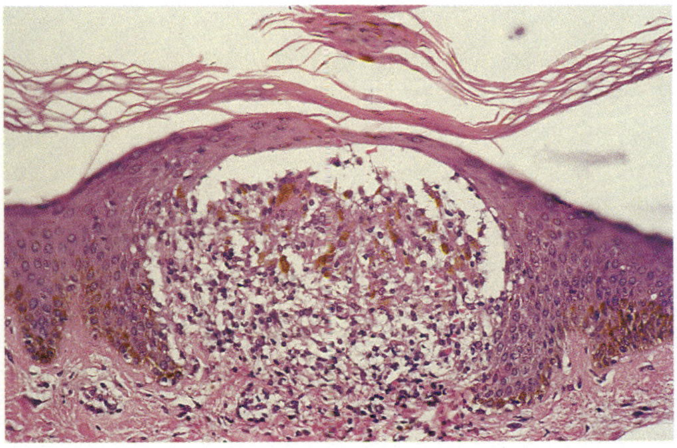

Figure 6–28. Histologically, there is a micronodule of inflammatory cells (*i.e.,* histiocytes and lymphocytes) embraced by an epidermal collarette. Interface changes similar to those observed in lichen planus are observed in the basal cell layer of the overlying epidermis.

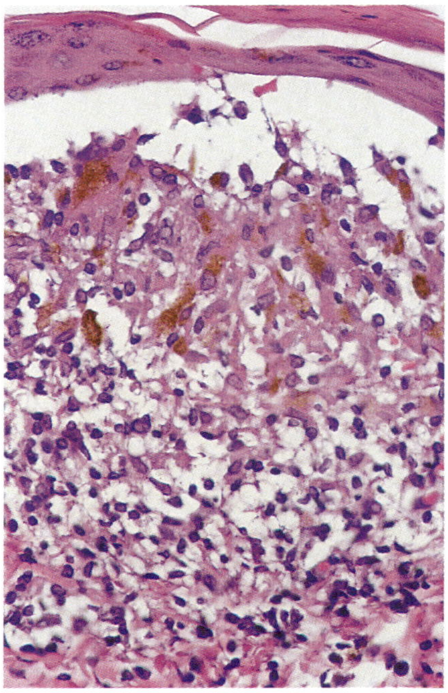

Figure 6–29. At high magnification, the majority of inflammatory cells are histiocytic. The overlying epidermis is separated from the infiltrate by a cleft-like space resulting from destruction of basal cells and associated dermal-epidermal integrity.

Lichenoid Drug Eruption

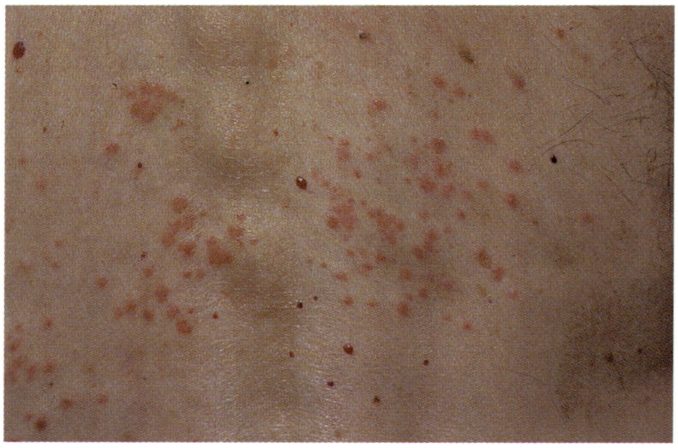

Figure 6–30. Lichenoid drug eruption. Multiple flat, erythematous papules are observed clinically (smaller, darker papules are incidental hemangiomas).

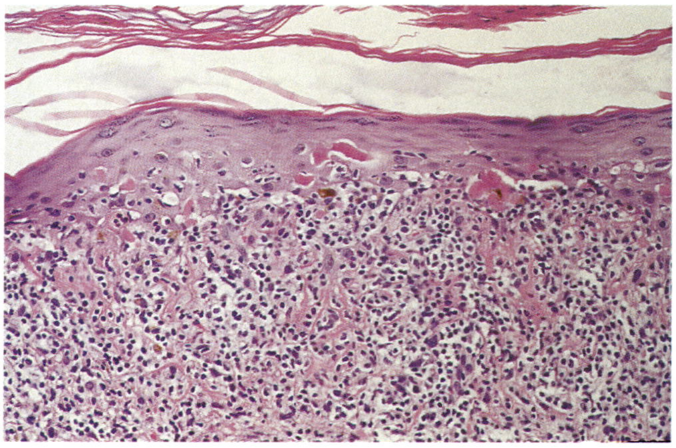

Figure 6–31. At medium magnification, there is a band-like inflammatory infiltrate associated with chronic interface changes, which include prominent single-cell epidermal necrosis with colloid body formation. The scale shows focal compact hyperorthokeratosis *(extreme top right)* and parakeratosis.

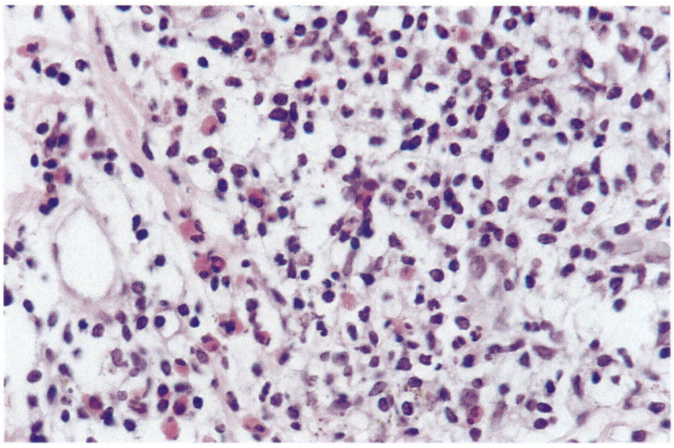

Figure 6–32. Eosinophils *(center)* and lymphocytes are observed in the infiltrate, in contrast to true lichen planus, which contains only lymphocytes.

Fixed Drug Eruption

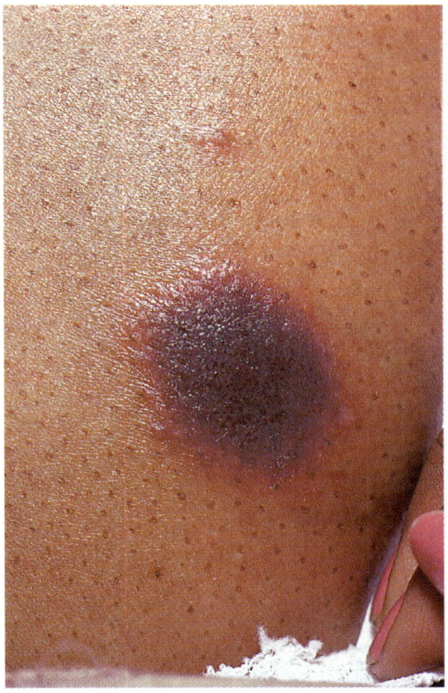

Figure 6–33. Fixed drug eruption. A chronic zone of macular hyperpigmentation has become indurated and peripherally erythematous. This is indicative of recrudescence of this fixed form of cytotoxic dermatitis.

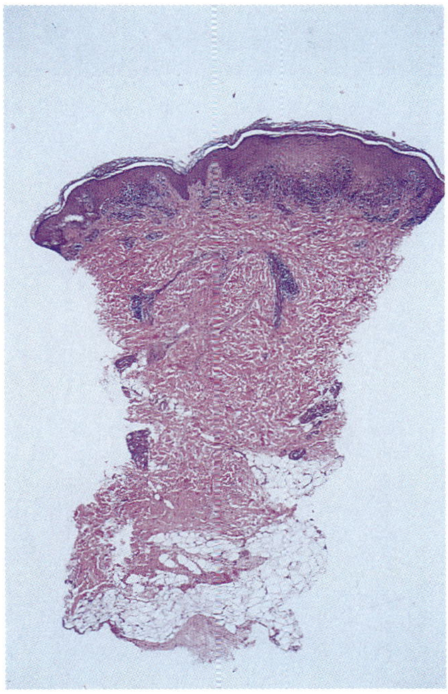

Figure 6–34. Histologically, there is a superficial and mid-dermal angiocentric infiltrate, as well as a prominent lichenoid component within the papillary dermis. Zonal necrosis of keratinocytes may also be observed.

Lichenoid Secondary Syphilis

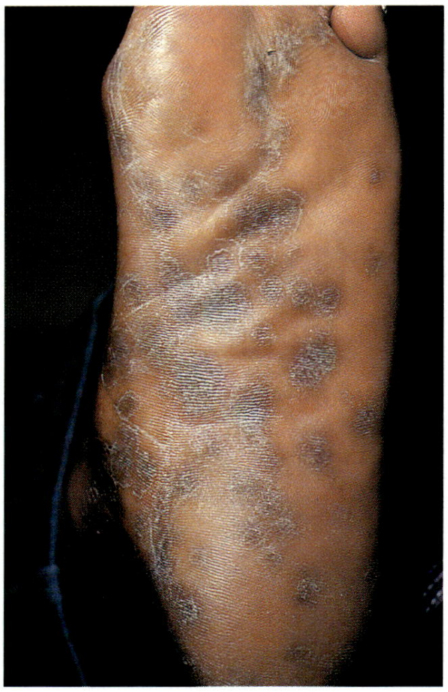

Figure 6–35. Lichenoid secondary syphilis. Hyperpigmented, scaling plaques on the palms and soles are frequently observed.

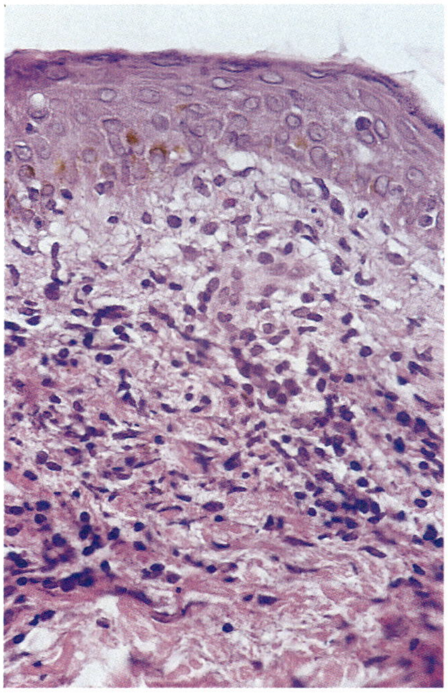

Figure 6–36. A biopsy specimen reveals a band-like interstitial infiltrate of mononuclear cells within the papillary dermis associated with variable basal cell layer vacuolization. Granulomatous foci also are often observed (note the vague collection of pale histiocytes centrally beneath the epidermal layer).

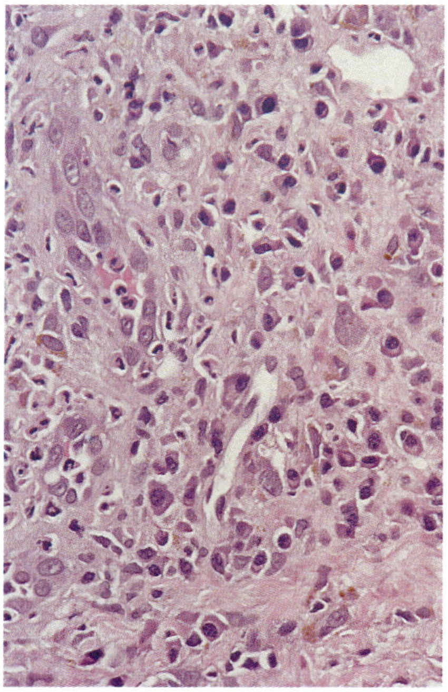

Figure 6–37. Plasma cells *(top and center)* and enlarged endothelial cells that focally occlude microvascular lumens are usually detected.

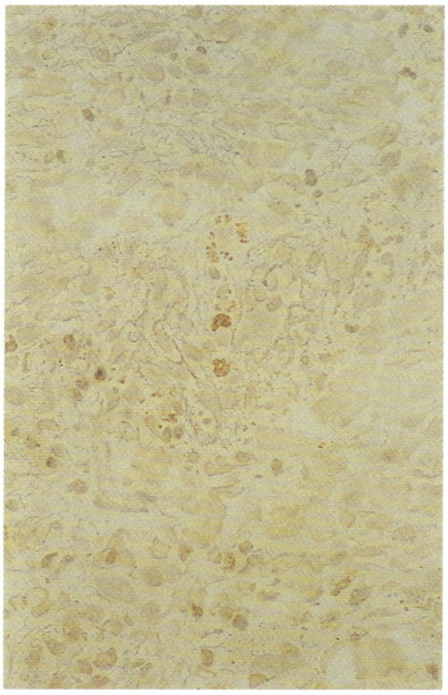

Figure 6–38. Dieterle stain may reveal slender, spiraling organisms within perivascular connective tissue or within the epidermal layer *(center)*, although serologic confirmation often is more sensitive than tissue stains in establishing a definitive diagnosis.

Lichenoid Eruption of AIDS

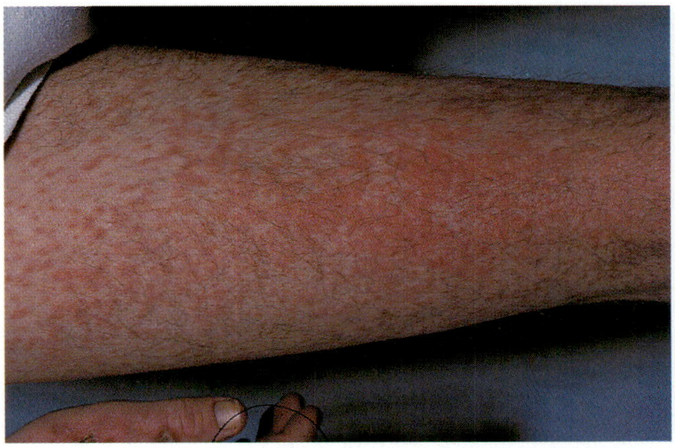

Figure 6–39. Lichenoid eruption in a patient with acquired immunodeficiency syndrome (AIDS). Clinically, there may be a maculopapular exanthem, raising the possibility of viral rash or drug eruption.

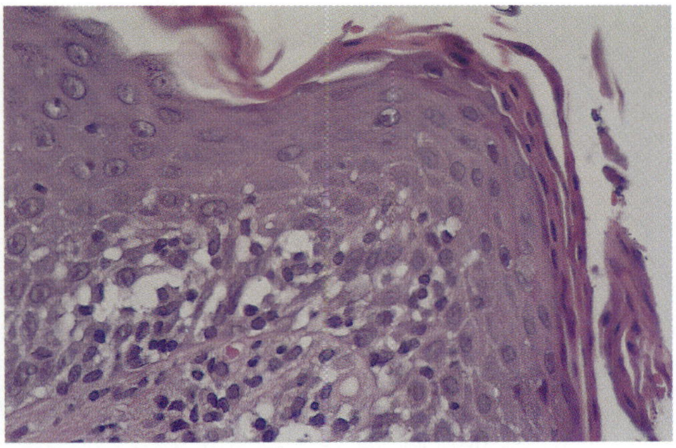

Figure 6–40. Interface change may resemble that seen in acute graft-versus-host disease, although epidermal alterations, such as parakeratosis and hyperplasia, may also be present.

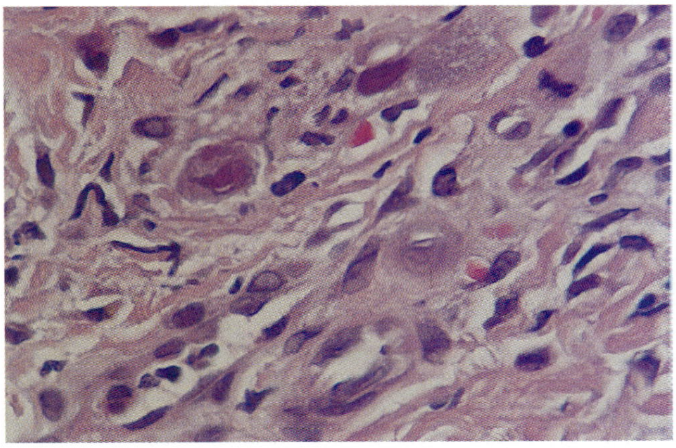

Figure 6–41. The inflammatory component should be inspected closely for evidence of associated pathology or infection; in this case, inclusions of cytomegalovirus were observed in some cells *(left center).*

7

Angiocentric Dermatitis

The term *angiocentric dermatitis* is used here to define disorders characterized throughout their course primarily by perivascular inflammatory infiltrates, with or without vasculitis. Although all forms of dermatitis are angiocentric from the outset, some are eventually predominated by subsequent localization of immune cells into nonangiocentric tissue compartments (*e.g.,* the epidermis in the case of spongiotic and cytotoxic dermatitis and the subcutaneous fat in the case of panniculitis). Because the epidermis is relatively unaltered in angiocentric dermatitis, these conditions are often diagnosed at scanning magnification once the normal overlying epidermal layer is appreciated. *Vasculitis,* an unfortunate term merely implying inflammation of the vessel, is used to describe vessel injury manifested by varying degrees of endothelial degeneration and necrosis. Accordingly, "vasculitis" is present when endothelial cells exhibit little more than degenerative cytoplasmic vacuolization and hypereosinophilia. Classic fibrinoid necrosis defines a condition in which injury has so progressed as to render the vessel wall permissive to the leakage of blood cells and serum components, including fibrin.

The term *lymphocytic vasculitis* deserves special attention. It implies damage to the vessel wall provoked primarily by lymphocytes and is generally recognized by a perivascular angiocentric pattern with associated hemorrhage but without classic fibrinoid necrosis of the vessel wall. Lymphocytic vasculitis is a reaction pattern that may be seen in a diverse array of conditions, including erythema multiforme, pityriasis lichenoides et varioliformis acuta, and pigmentary purpura, and in dysplastic and malignant cutaneous lymphocytic infiltrates. The setting of pure angiocentric dermatitis without evidence of epidermal alteration or chronicity may suggest the exanthem of systemic viral infection.

The hues that characterize angiocentric dermatitis are often of great assistance in generating and following an algorithm in the direction of a correct diagnosis. Urticaria, for example, may be first perceived as a superficial zone of pale pink-white pallor within an otherwise pink-red dermis. Gyrate erythemas (*e.g.,* erythema annulare centrifugum) are frequently recognized by virtue of dark-blue aggregates of inflammatory cells that are tightly applied to the walls of dermal vessels, producing a "coat-sleeve" effect. Necrotizing vasculitis, on the other hand, is characterized by granular aggregates of vessel-associated fibrin, which typically is pink-purple. This quality is also helpful in differentiating fibrin thrombi from thrombi resulting from cryoglobulins, which have a characteristic pale-pink, homogeneous appearance.

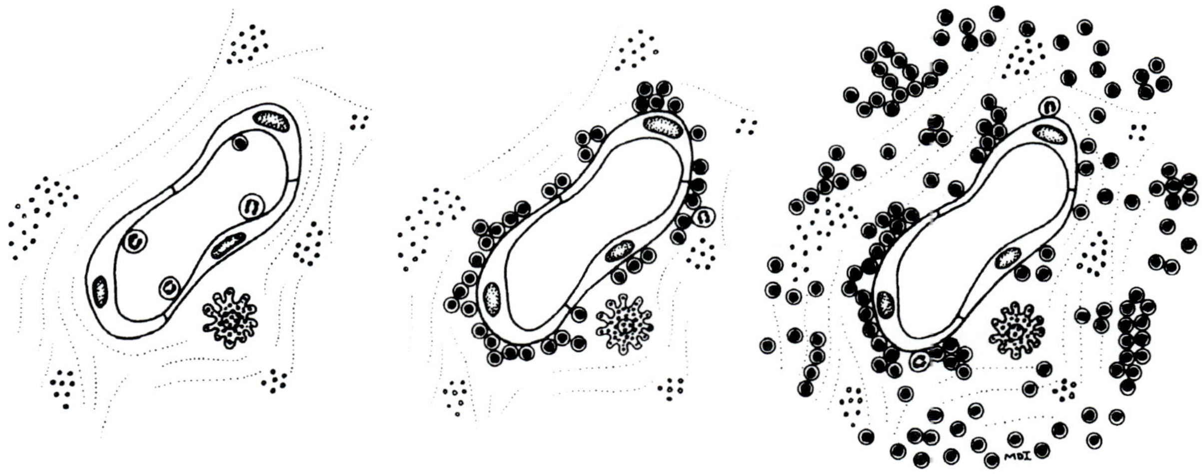

Figure 7–1. Temporal evolution of angiocentric dermatitis. The earliest phases of angiocentric dermatitis *(left)* are often characterized by little more than margination of leukocytes along the endothelial lumen. In time, transmural diapedesis results in accumulation of leukocytes in the immediate perivascular space *(center).* Depending on the nature of the provocative agent or antigen and the adhesion pathways that are set into motion, leukocytes may migrate away from the vessel wall, producing an interstitial pattern as well as an angiocentric pattern *(right).* The latter phenomenon often occurs in insect-bite reactions to injected antigen.

Urticaria

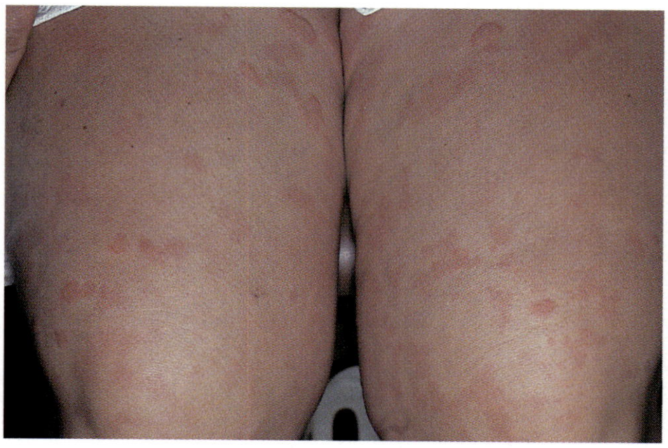

Figure 7–2. Urticaria. Clinically, there are erythematous, edematous, often circinate or polycyclic plaques covered by a normal epidermal surface. Individual lesions generally last for less than 24 hours.

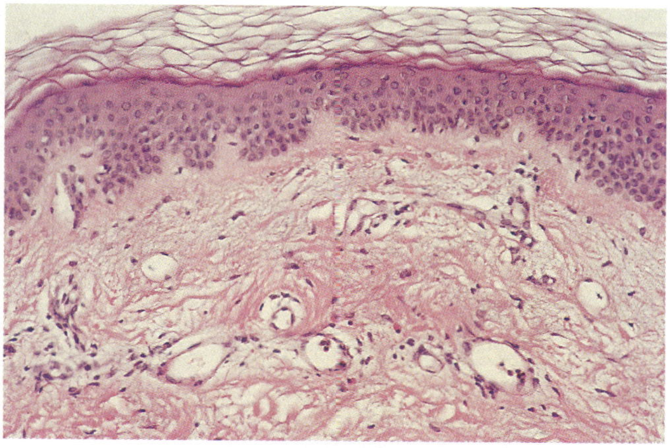

Figure 7–3. At scanning magnif cation, there is superficial dermal edema and dilated lymphatic and blood vascular channels. The edema is manifested as a widening of spaces that separate adjacent collagen bundles.

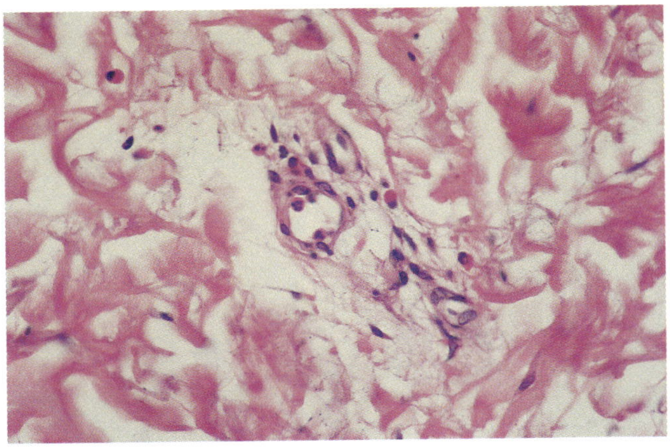

Figure 7–4. At higher magnification, there is a scant inflammatory infiltrate composed of lymphocytes and occasional neutrophils and eosinophils within an edematous perivascular space. The finding of intraluminal neutrophils *(center)* adherent to the endothelial luminal membrane is characteristic.

Figure 7–5. Dermatographism, or urtication, at sites of trauma or stroking is a form of physically induced urticaria.

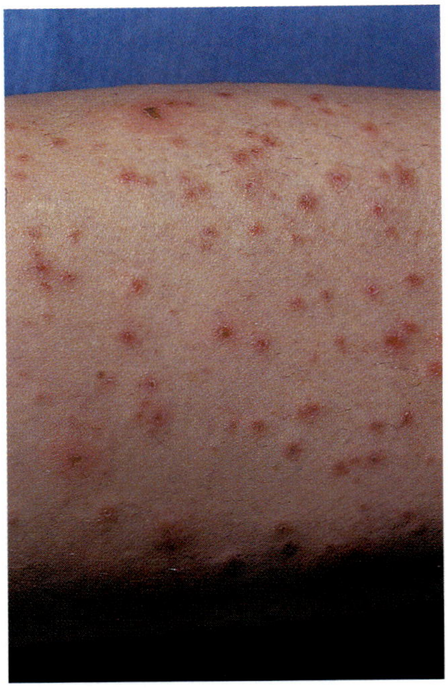

Figure 7–6. The condition known as *pruritic urticarial papules and plaques of pregnancy* (PUPPP) is characterized by often excoriated, discrete, erythematous papules.

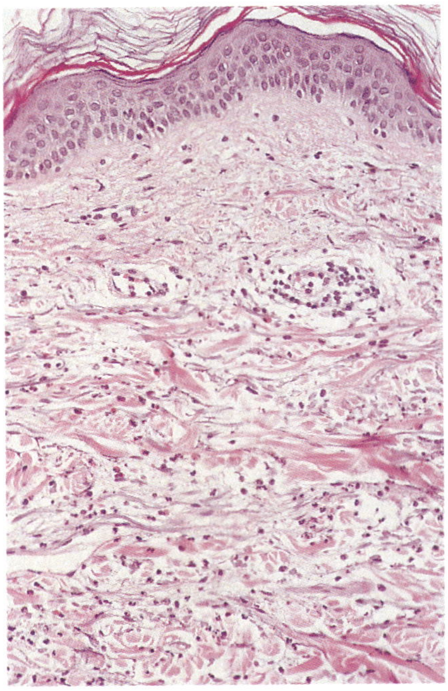

Figure 7–7. Neutrophil-rich urticaria. Note the interstitial and angiocentric pattern of neutrophil infiltration within an edematous superficial dermis.

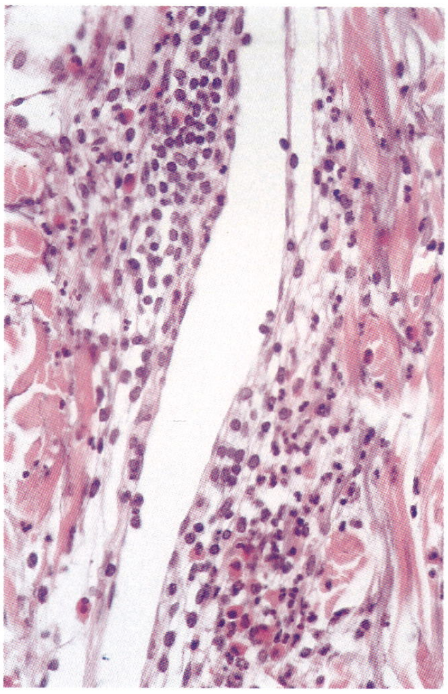

Figure 7–8. Higher magnification of an involved vessel from Figure 7–7 demonstrates an angiocentric infiltrate of lymphocytes and neutrophils with adherent neutrophils within the vessel lumen *(center)*.

Erythema Marginatum

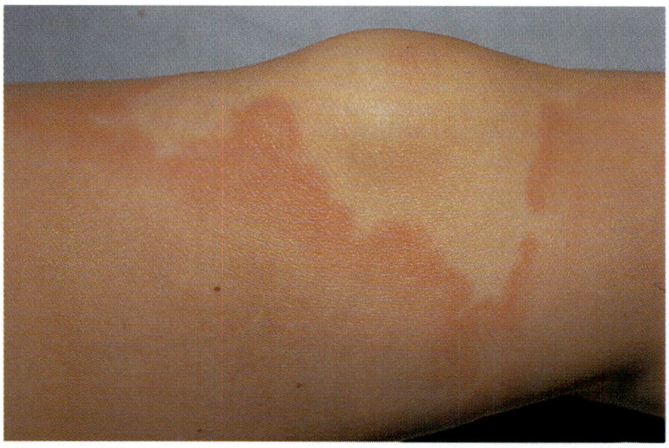

Figure 7–9. Erythema marginatum. Clinically, there are confluent zones of erythema and edema with a characteristic sharply demarcated advancing border.

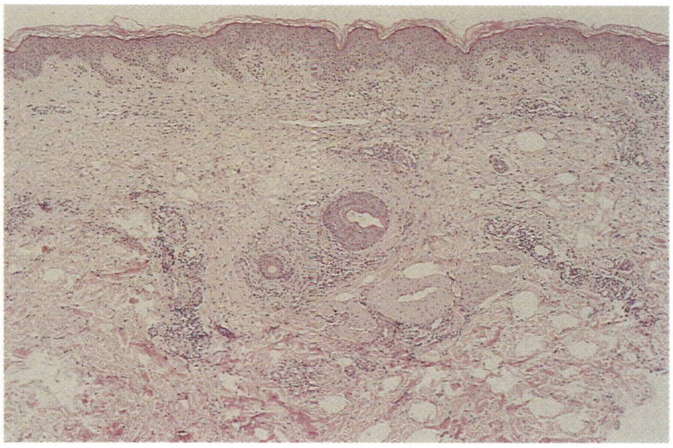

Figure 7–10. At scanning magnification, there is an angiocentric and interstitial inflammatory infiltrate within the superficial and mid-dermis, beneath a normal overlying epidermal layer.

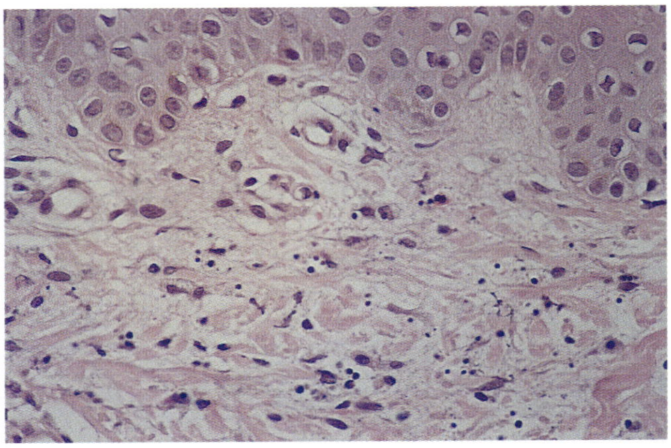

Figure 7–11. The urticarial quality of erythema marginatum is appreciated in this field, showing superficial dermal edema and an interstitial infiltrate of neutrophils, similar to the histologic picture of neutrophil-rich urticaria. In both, however, lymphocytes also participate, and accordingly, these lesions are not considered primarily to be in the category of granulocytic dermatitis.

Erythema Annulare Centrifugum

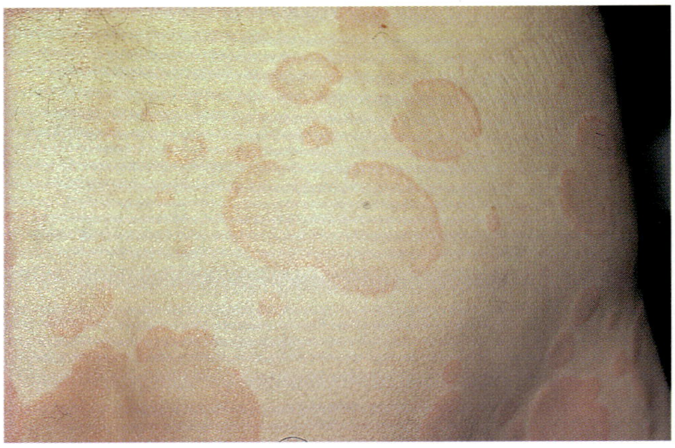

Figure 7–12. The gross pathology of erythema annulare centrifugum is characterized by annular, erythematous plaques, often with a fine, adherent collarette of scale that trails just behind the advancing edge of each lesion.

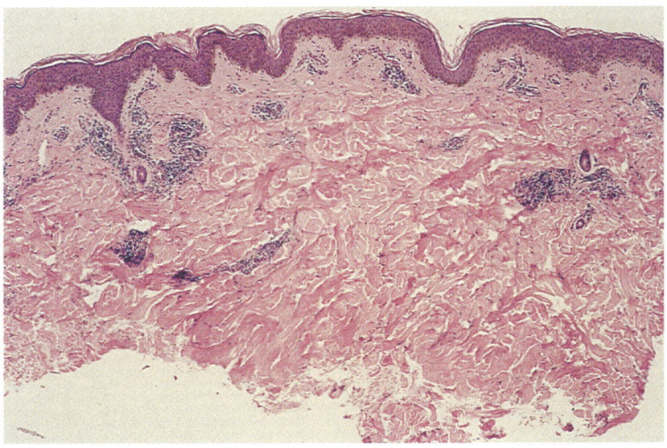

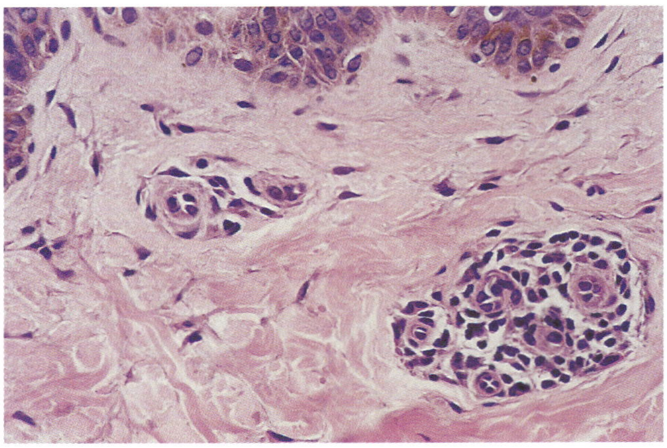

Figures 7–13 and 7–14. Histologically, there is a superficial and sometimes mid-dermal angiocentric infiltrate of lymphocytes, which are tightly aggregated in the perivascular space (*i.e.*, coat-sleeve pattern). When the biopsy specimen includes the edge of a lesion, foci of mild epidermal hyperplasia and parakeratosis may be detected in the overlying epidermal layer.

Erythema Chronicum Migrans

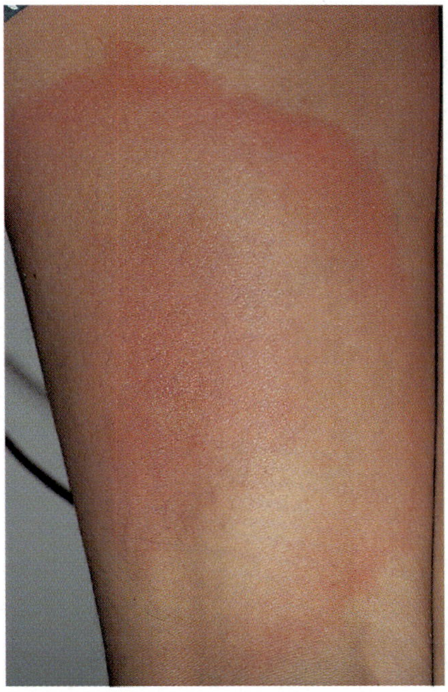

Figure 7–15. Erythema chronicum migrans. An expanding, indurated, erythematous plaque developed at the site of a previous tick bite. There is no epidermal change at the advancing border of this annular lesion, in contrast to erythema annulare centrifugum.

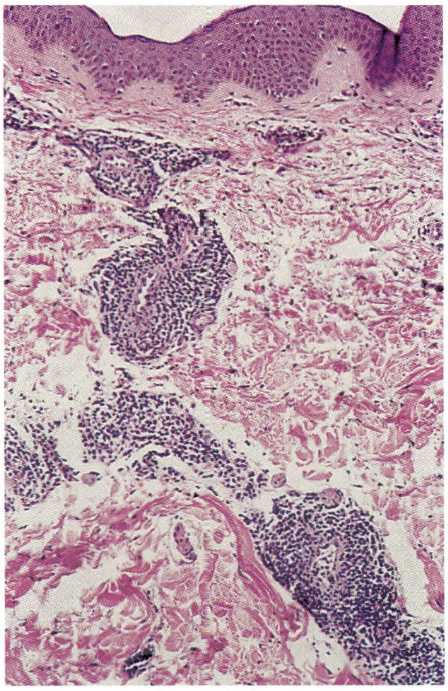

Figure 7–16. The tight, perivascular lymphocytic infiltrate appreciated in erythema annulare centrifugum is even more prominent and extends more deeply into the dermis in erythema chronicum migrans.

Polymorphous Light Eruption

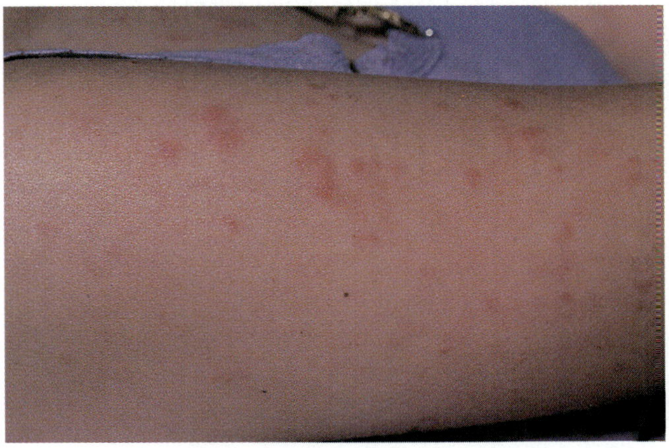

Figure 7–17. Polymorphous light eruption. Clinical lesions vary from papules to plaques to vesicles at sites of sun exposure.

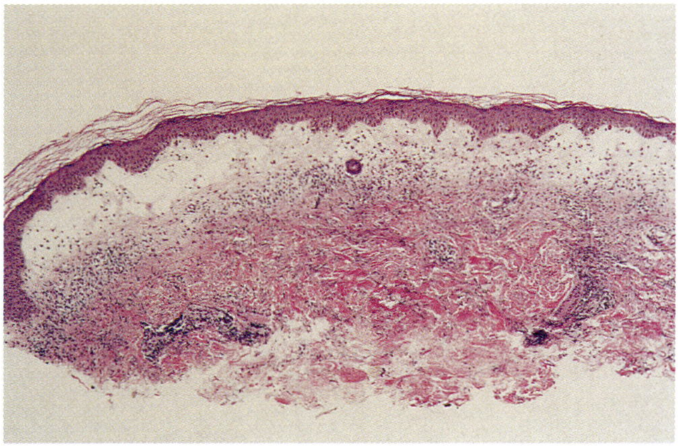

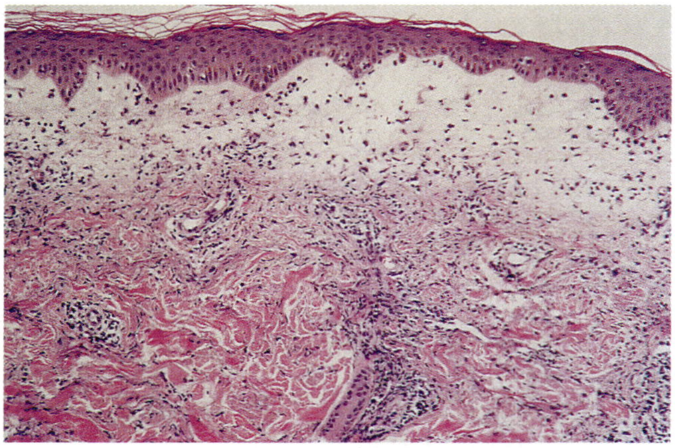

Figures 7–18 and 7–19. Scanning (Fig. 7–18) and medium (Fig. 7–19) magnification of a representative biopsy specimen of an early lesion reveals a brisk, superficial and mid-dermal, angiocentric, lymphocytic infiltrate associated with marked papillary dermal edema. Unlike phototoxic and photoeczematous eruptions, where epidermal dyskeratosis and spongiosis, respectively, occur, the epidermal layer is relatively unaffected in a polymorphous light eruption.

Jessner Lymphocytic Infiltrate

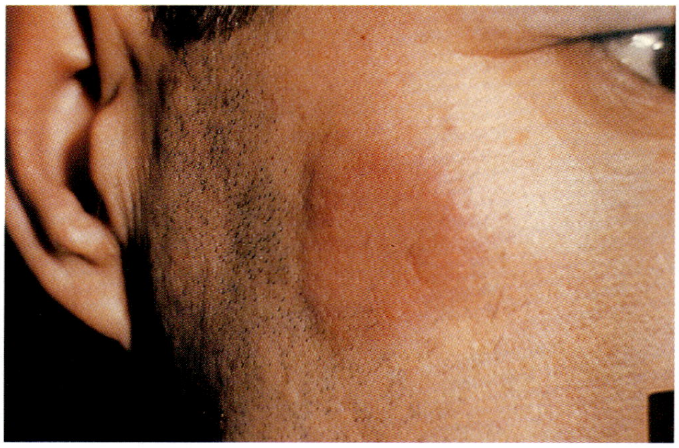

Figure 7–20. Jessner lymphocytic infiltrate. A well-formed, boggy, erythematous plaque on the face with little or no evidence of epidermal or follicular involvement.

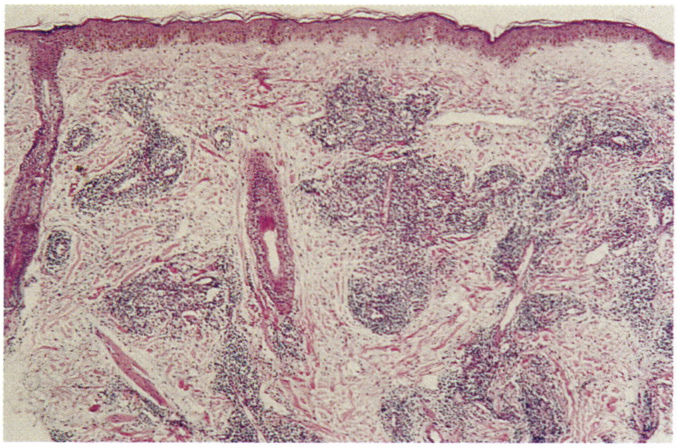

Figure 7–21. Low magnification of a biopsy specimen reveals a brisk angiocentric mononuclear cell infiltrate in the superficial and deep dermis. Although this clinical picture may raise the possibility of a predominantly dermal form of lupus erythematosus, note that hair follicles and other adnexal structures are not affected by the inflammatory infiltrate.

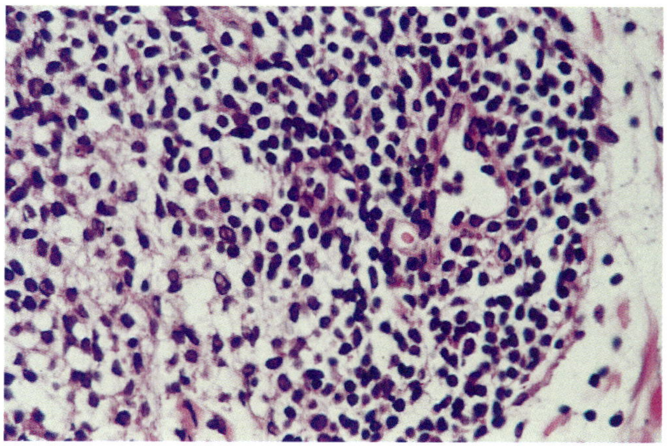

Figure 7–22. The mononuclear cells are composed of small lymphocytes admixed with larger, pale-staining histiocytes; foci of associated extracellular mucin may also be observed.

Dermal Delayed Hypersensitivity Reaction

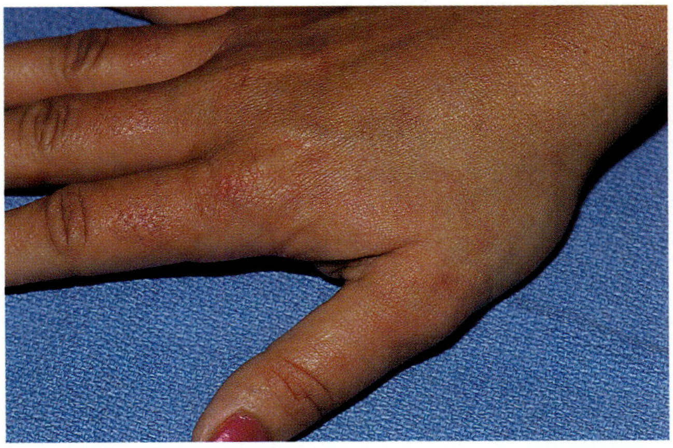

Figure 7–23. Clinical lesions in dermal delayed hypersensitivity may vary from vague zones of erythema to urticarial plaques; pruritus is common.

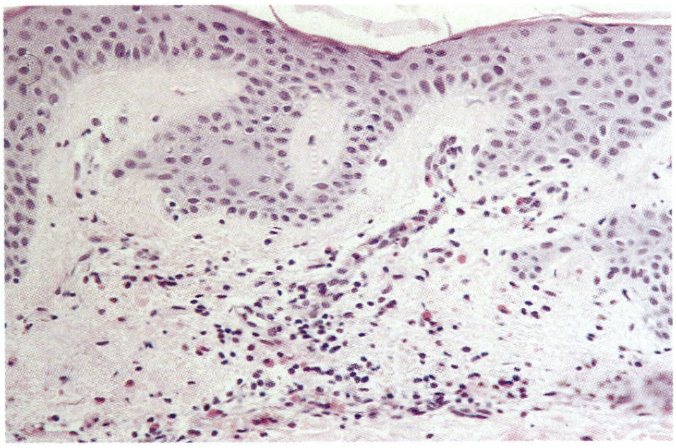

Figure 7–24. Biopsy specimens reveal superficial and sometimes deep perivascular lymphocytic infiltrate without significant epidermal alterations. Admixed eosinophils are often encountered.

Necrotizing Neutrophilic Venulitis

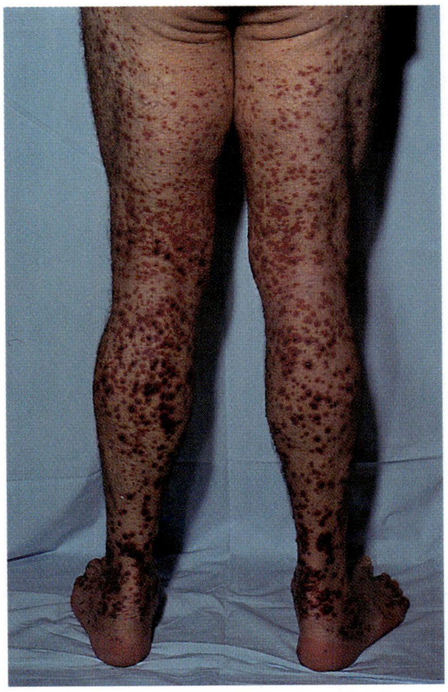

Figure 7–25. Necrotizing neutrophilic venulitis. These palpable purpura lesions characteristically involve the lower extremities.

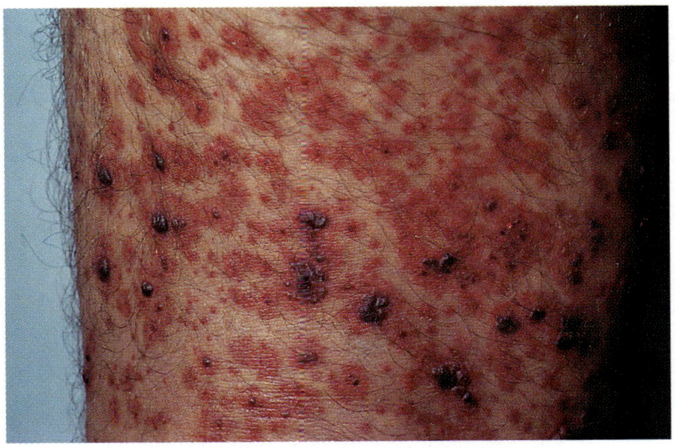

Figure 7–26. Some lesions show early blister formation, the result of extensive epidermal necrosis (see Fig. 7–29).

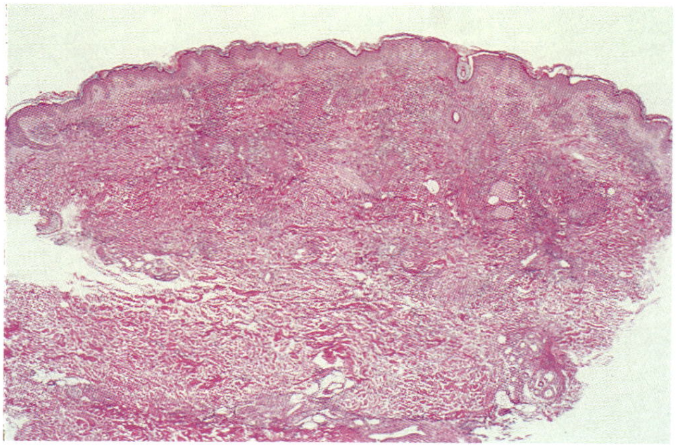

Figure 7–27. On scanning magnification, there is a superficial angiocentric infiltrate, often with a red-purple hue due to associated hemorrhage and fibrin deposition.

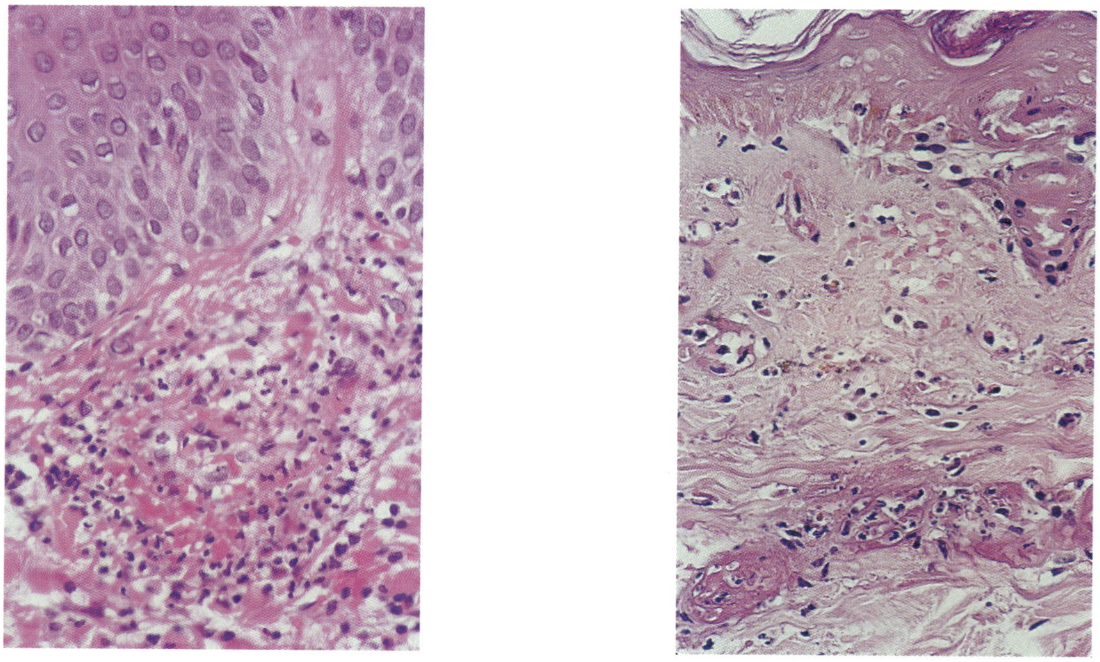

Figures 7–28 and 7–29. Individual venules within the superficial vascular plexus show fibrinoid necrosis, fibrin thrombus formation, and an angiocentric cuff of fragmented neutrophils (*i.e.*, nuclear dust) and lymphocytes. The epidermis in Figure 7–29 shows ischemic necrosis, with loss of nuclear basophilia.

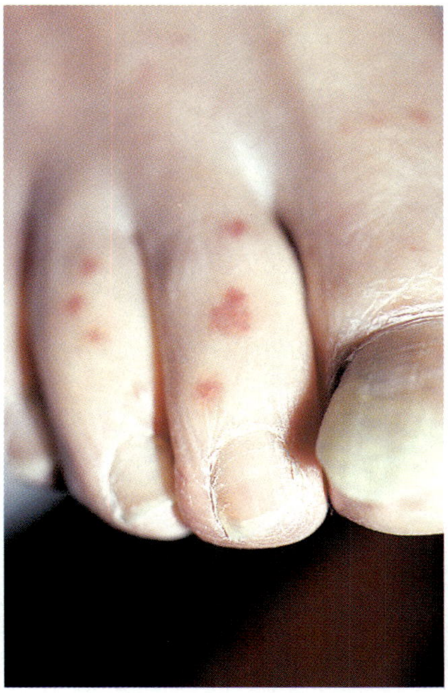

Figure 7–30. Necrotizing vasculitis: Cryoglobulinemia. These purpuric lesions occur on distal extremities and digits, which are prone to lower temperatures and thromboembolic events.

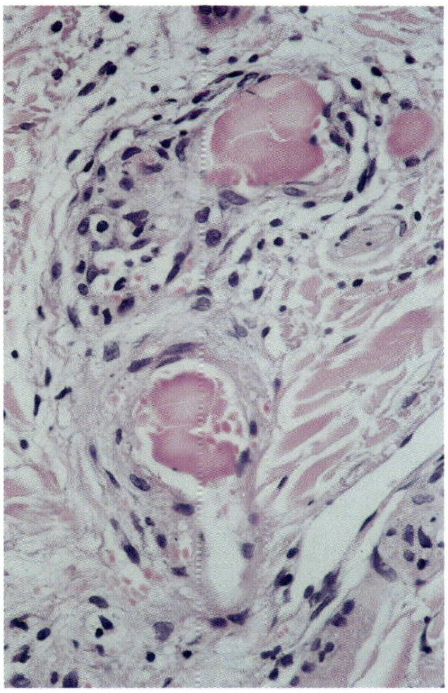

Figure 7–31. Cryoglobulins appear histologically as pale pink, homogeneous thrombi within vessels.

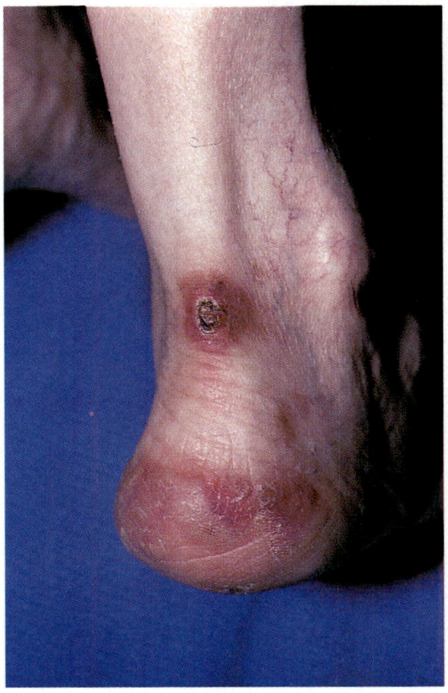

Figure 7–32. Erythema elevatum diutinum. More chronic necrotizing vasculitis is manifested by long-standing hemorrhagic nodules with ulceration, typically on distal extremities.

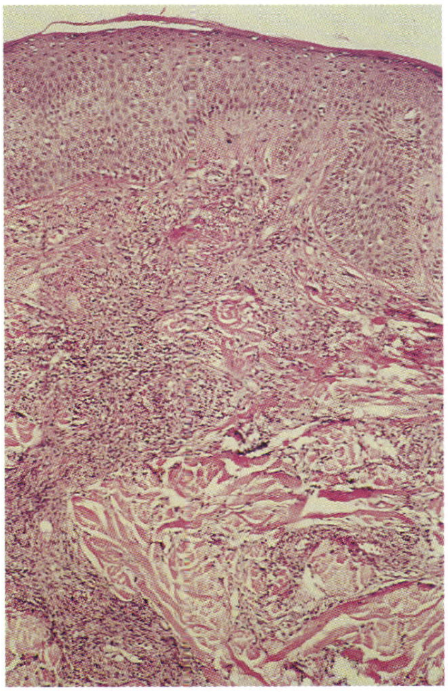

Figure 7–33. Histologically, there is a brisk, superficial and mid-dermal mixed inflammatory infiltrate composed of lymphocytes and neutrophils associated with necrotizing vascular injury (see also Fig. 7–34).

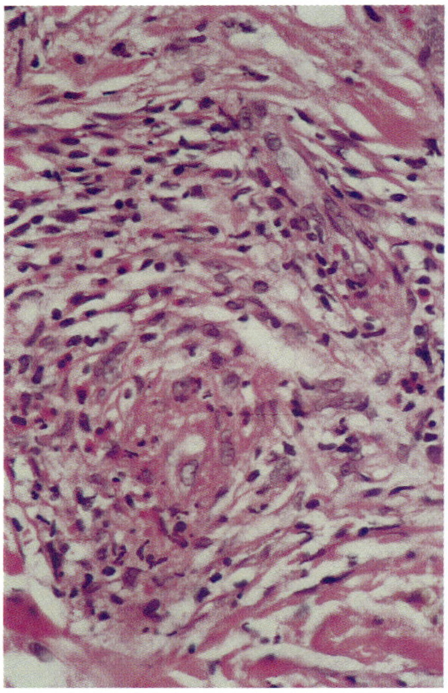

Figure 7–34. There is superficial dermal and perivascular fibrosis *(top),* a manifestation of chronic, repeated vascular insult.

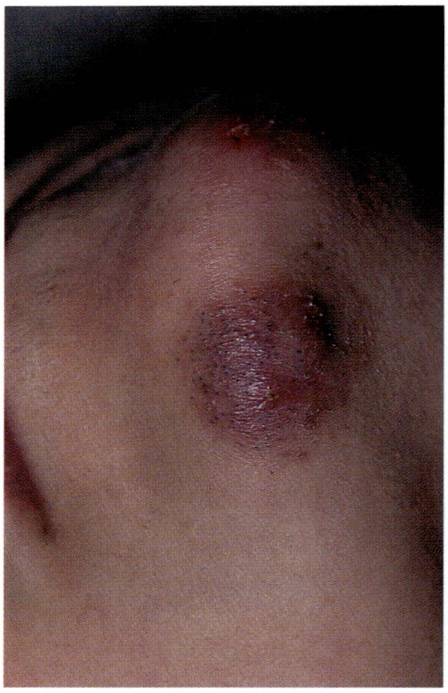

Figure 7–35. Granuloma faciale, a form of localized necrotizing neutrophilic vasculitis that occurs most often on the face. A typical, erythematous, brown-purple facial plaque with patulous follicular openings.

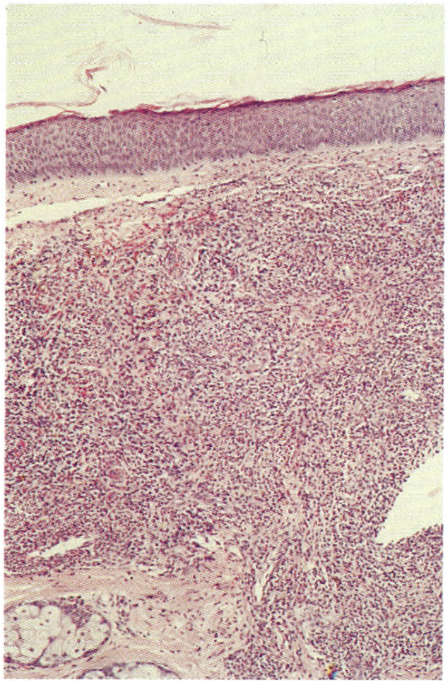

Figure 7–36. Scanning magnification reveals coalescent aggregates of inflammatory cells within the superficial and deep dermis; these begin as angiocentric foci, although many vessels are now obliterated. Note the characteristic sparing of the dermis directly beneath the epidermal layer and around hair follicles (not shown); this area is known as the Grenz zone.

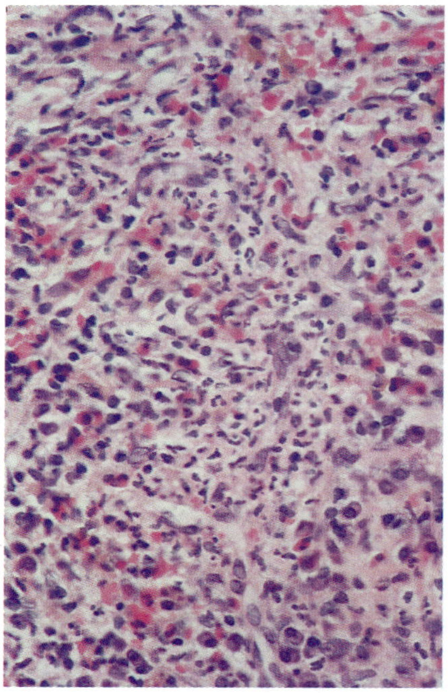

Figure 7–37. At higher magnification, foci of fragmented neutrophils demarcate sites of preexisting vessels that have been nearly totally obliterated. Note surrounding plasma cells, eosinophils, and lymphocytes.

Lymphocytic Vasculitis

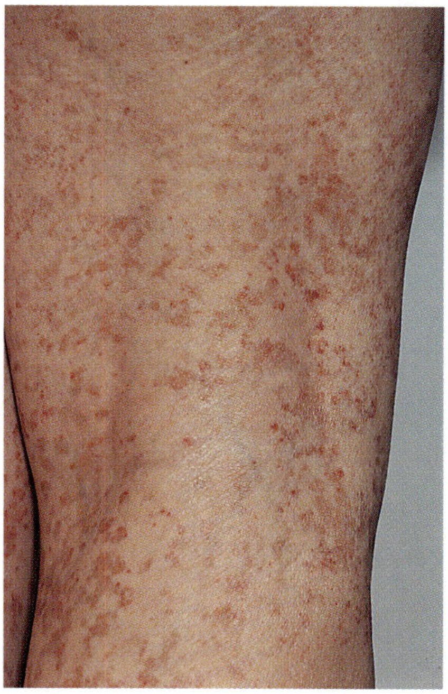

Figure 7–38. Lymphocytic vasculitis, pigmentary purpura type. Multiple asymptomatic, red-brown macules and shallow plaques are evident.

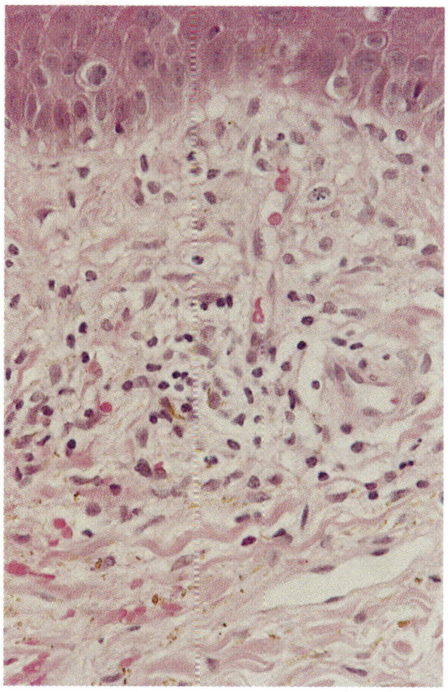

Figure 7–39. Angiocentric lymphocytic inflammation in progressive pigmentary purpura is distinctively centered about capillary loops within the most superficial regions of the papillary dermis. Recent perivascular hemorrhage and hemosiderin deposits are testimony to this subtle form of vascular injury.

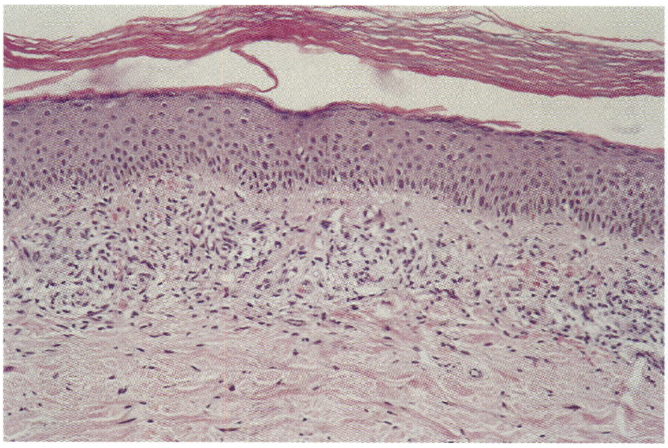

Figure 7–40. The angiocentric inflammatory component in some lesions is brisk, leading to a lichenoid pattern via confluence (*i.e.*, lichenoid purpura).

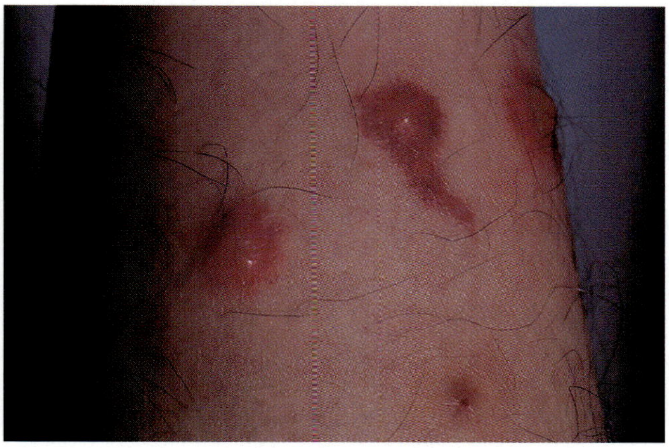

Figure 7–41. Insect-bite reaction with lymphocytic vasculitis. Purpuric nodules occur at sites of arthropod stings.

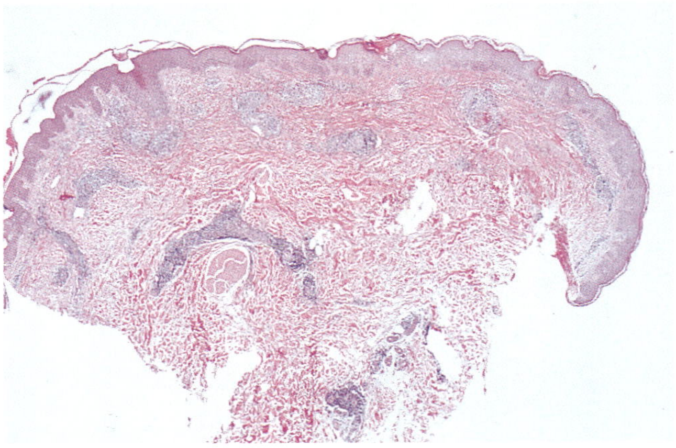

Figure 7–42. Scanning magnification reveals a superficial and deep angiocentric inflammatory infiltrate beneath an essentially normal epidermal layer.

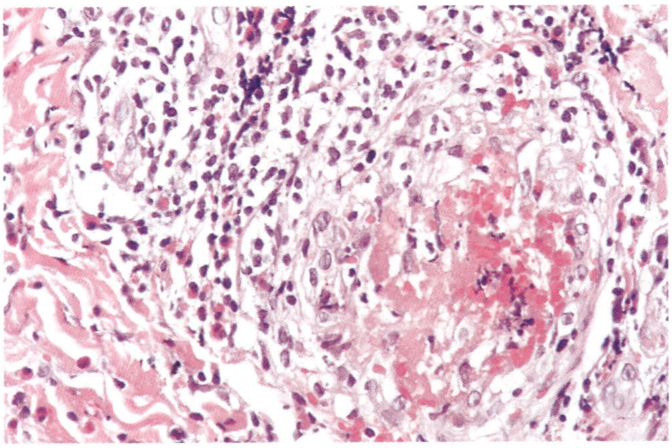

Figure 7–43. Extensive vascular injury and necrosis, with luminal obliteration by coagulated fibrin, are associated with a perivascular lymphocytic infiltrate containing occasional eosinophils.

Cutaneous Polyarteritis Nodosa

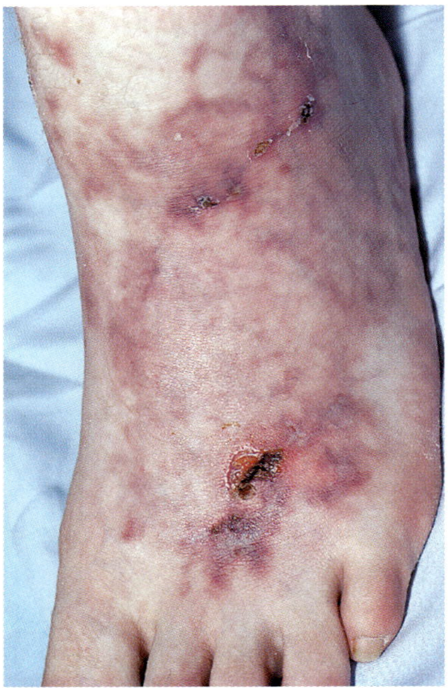

Figure 7–44. Cutaneous polyarteritis nodosa. Painful, nodular lesions are located along the line of arteries underlying the skin of the dorsum of the foot. Note the livedo pattern of mottled erythema that accompanies the vascular insult.

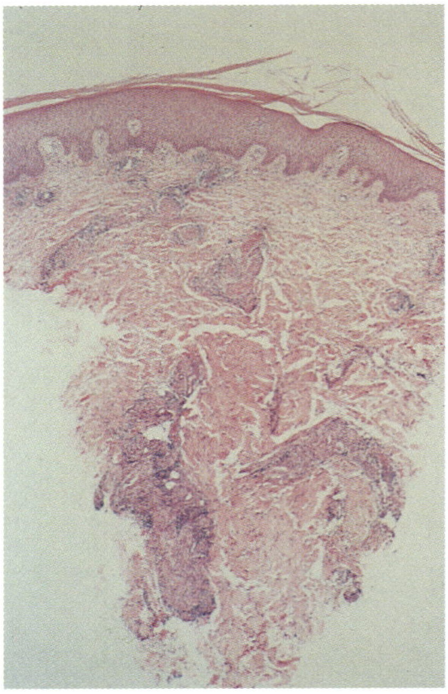

Figure 7–45. A deep biopsy specimen that includes a medium-sized cutaneous artery infiltrated by inflammatory cells.

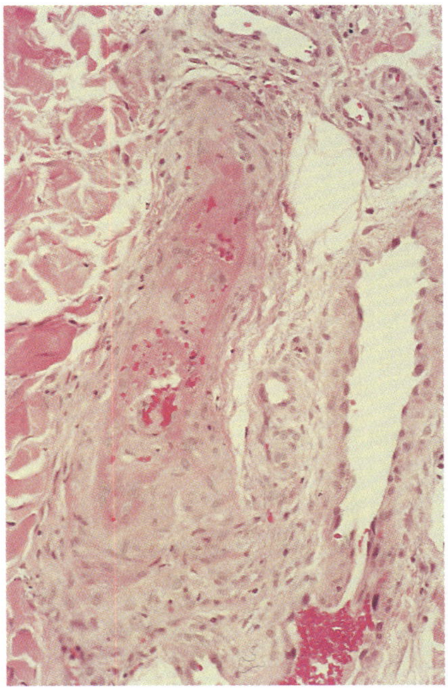

Figure 7–46. Higher magnification of affected arteries *(left center)* reveals mixed inflammatory cells within the vessel wall.

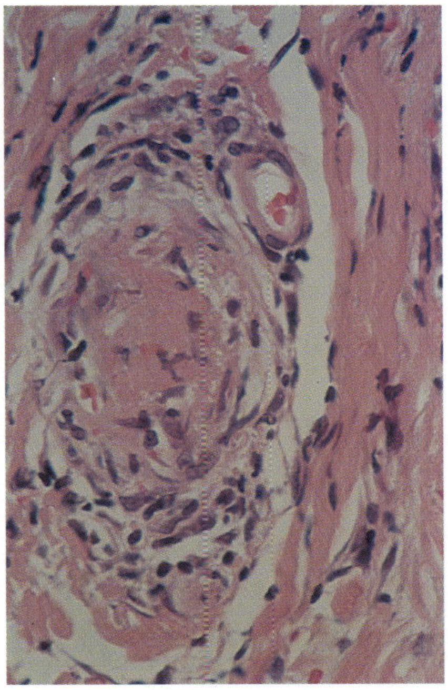

Figure 7–47. Luminal obliteration by fibrin and cellular debris. Obsolescent lesions demonstrate marked intimal fibrosis and luminal recanalization.

Migratory Thrombophlebitis

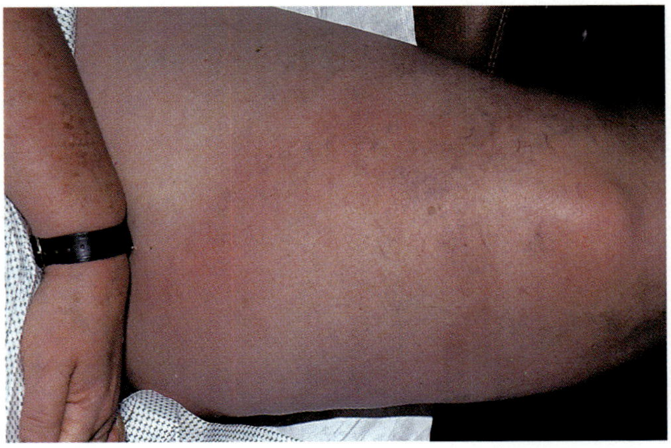

Figure 7–48. Superficial migratory thrombophlebitis. Coalescent nodules form linear plaques that are exquisitely tender.

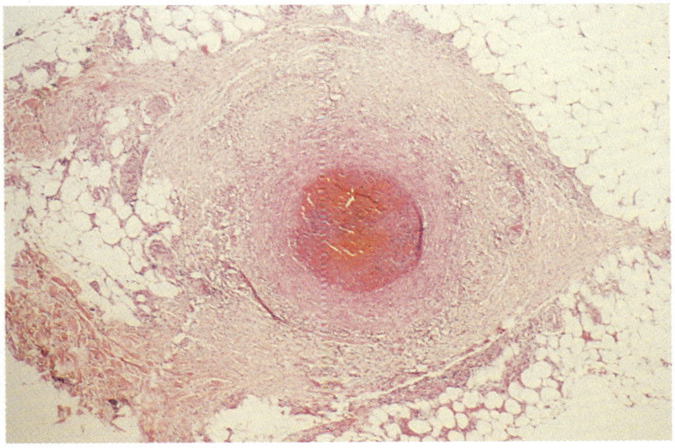

Figure 7–49. A subcutaneous vein is occluded by a thrombus and shows thickening of its wall due to edema and inflammatory infiltration.

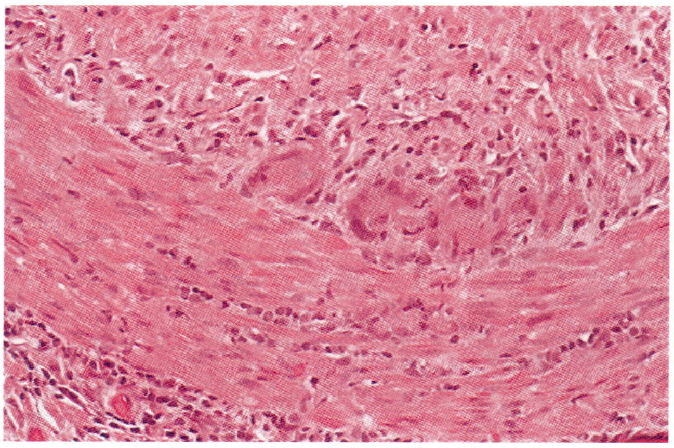

Figure 7–50. The wall of the affected vein is infiltrated by mononuclear cells and occasional multinucleated giant cells.

Malignant Atrophic Papulosis

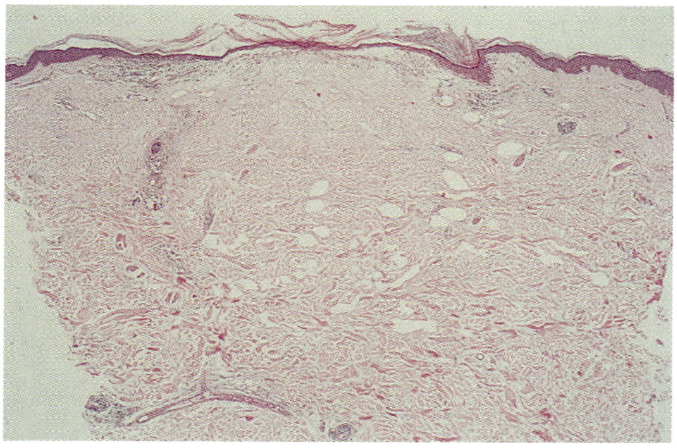

Figure 7–51. Rare form of angiocentric dermatitis: Malignant atrophic papulosis. At scanning magnification, there is a wedge-shaped dermal infarct *(top center)* bordered by an angiocentric lymphocytic infiltrate and surmounted by epidermal atrophy and hyperkeratosis.

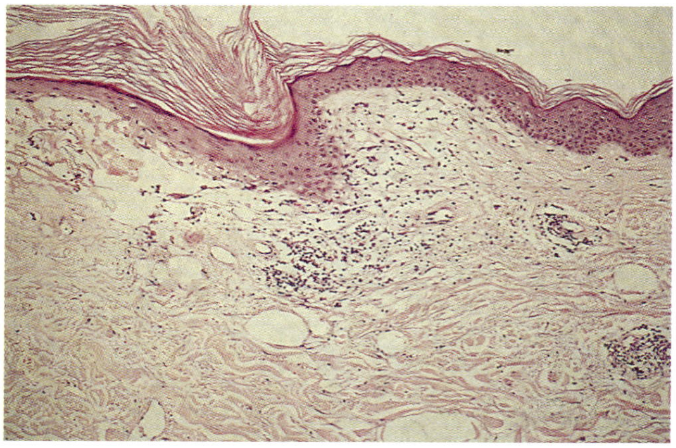

Figure 7–52. Higher magnification reveals cuffs of lymphocytes about small venules; occasionally, necrotizing injury is documented at the base of the zone of infarcted dermis *(left center)*.

8

Granulocytic Dermatitis

Granulocytes are defined here as mature hematopoietic cells that display cytoplasmic granules visible by high-power light microscopy. Accordingly, granulocytes are segregated in the categories listed in Table 8–1.

There are only a finite number of dermatoses that are predominated by granulocytes. The prototypic cause of granulocytic infiltration of skin is bacterial infection. Neutrophils within scale crust associated with superficial forms of bacterial infection (impetigo) produce a clinical and histologic picture often referred to as *impetiginization*. Clinical pustules are generally associated with microabscesses, which consist of small, tumor-like aggregates of granulocytes. Microabscesses may occur within or beneath the stratum corneum, within the epidermis or follicular epithelium, or within the dermis. *Pyoderma* is a term used to refer to diffuse, extensive, and permeative infiltration of the dermis by granulocytes.

Neutrophilic aggregates are often pink-purple due to the admixture of granular eosinophilic cytoplasm, nuclear fragmentation, and fibrin frequently encountered at acutely inflamed tissue sites. Impetiginization of stratum corneum manifests as discrete regions of basophilia that may initially be confused with densely compacted parakeratosis. At higher magnification, associated bacterial colonies are seen as particulate deep-blue regions clustered within the inflammatory debris. Infiltrates of eosinophils, as would be expected, stain more intensely red than neutrophils and, in the setting of Wells syndrome, are associated with granular, brightly eosinophilic zones of altered collagen ("flame figures"). The tinctorial characteristics of granulocytic infiltrates are subtle yet characteristic and, once recognized, contribute to the ability to recognize aggregates of these cells, even at scanning magnification.

Table 8–1. Types of Granulocytes in Human Dermatitis

Granulocyte Type	Characteristic Feature	Prototypic Disorder
Neutrophil	Multilobed nucleus	Impetigo
Eosinophil	Bilobed nucleus, densely eosinophilic cytoplasmic granules	Wells syndrome
Basophil	Bilobed nucleus, vague amphophilic cytoplasmic granules	Rarely* encountered in human skin

*Characteristic of experimental dermatitis in guinea pig skin.

Impetigo

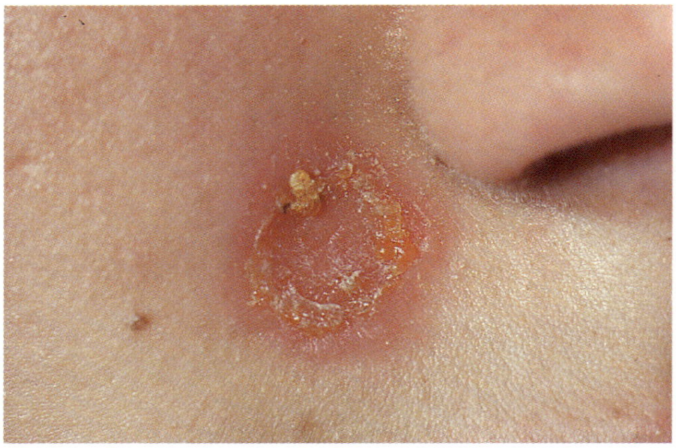

Figure 8–1. Bacterial superinfection results in characteristic honey-colored crust surmounting this shallow facial erosion of impetigo.

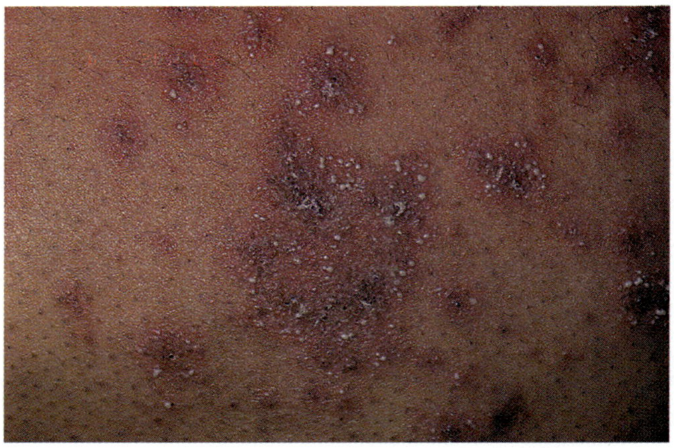

Figure 8–2. Impetigo herpetiformis, showing multiple grouped pustules covering an erythematous and focally eroded zone of intensive bacterial colonization.

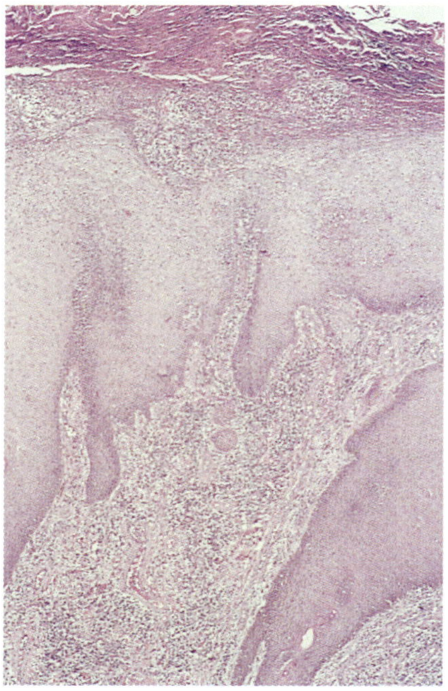

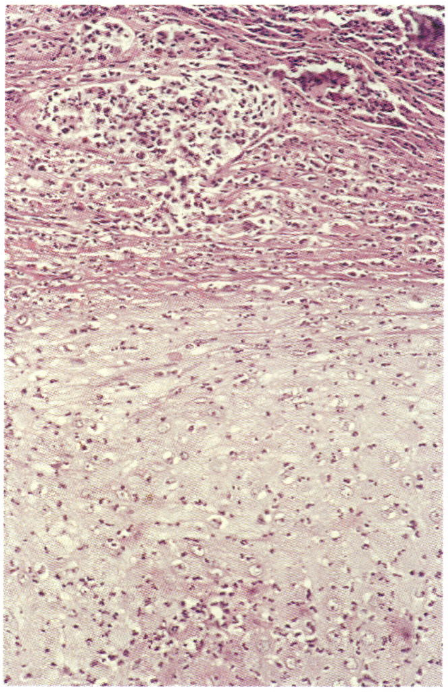

Figures 8–3 and 8–4. The edge of an impetiginized ulcer shows pseudoepitheliomatous hyperplasia surmounted by scale crust heavily infiltrated by neutrophils and colonized by bacteria.

Subcorneal Pustular Dermatosis

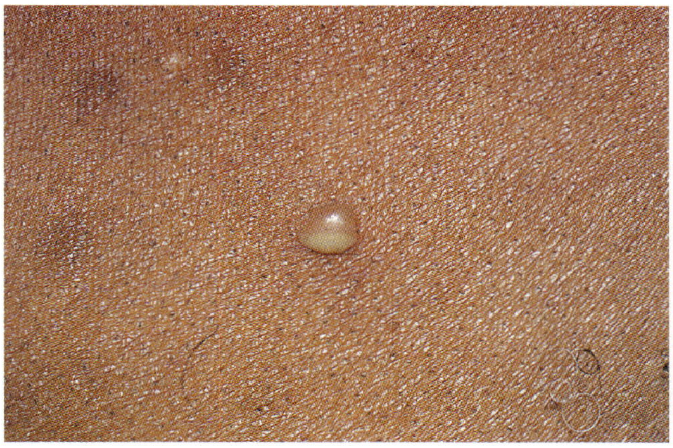

Figure 8–5. Subcorneal pustular dermatosis. A solitary subcorneal vesiculopustule shows an interface between serum exudate *(top half)* and purulent exudate *(bottom half)*.

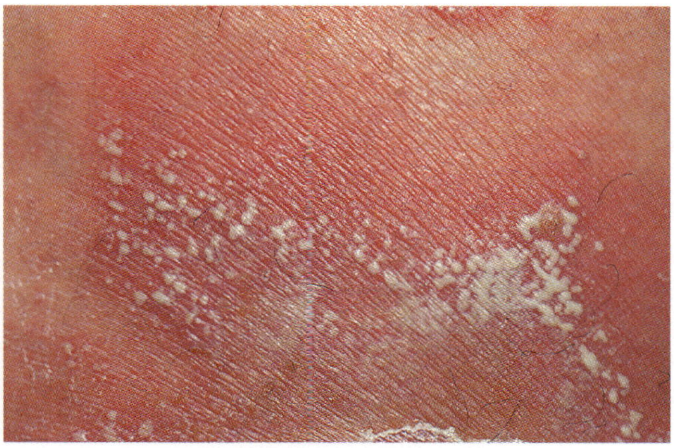

Figure 8–6. An established plaque of subcorneal pustular dermatosis shows multiple coa escent pustules on an erythematous base.

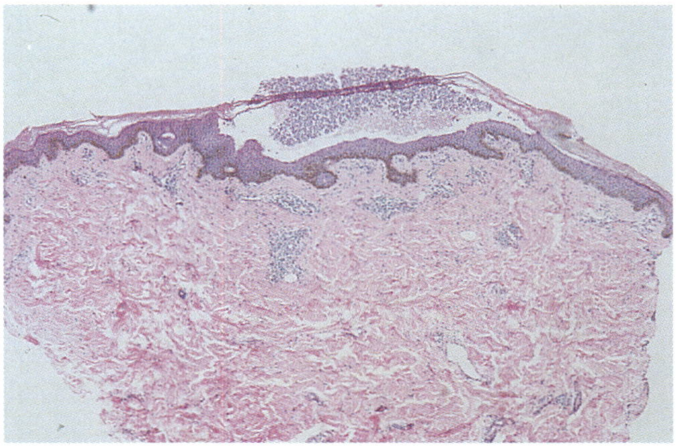

Figure 8–7. Scanning magnification discloses a pure accumulation of neutrophils directly beneath the stratum corneum *(top center)*.

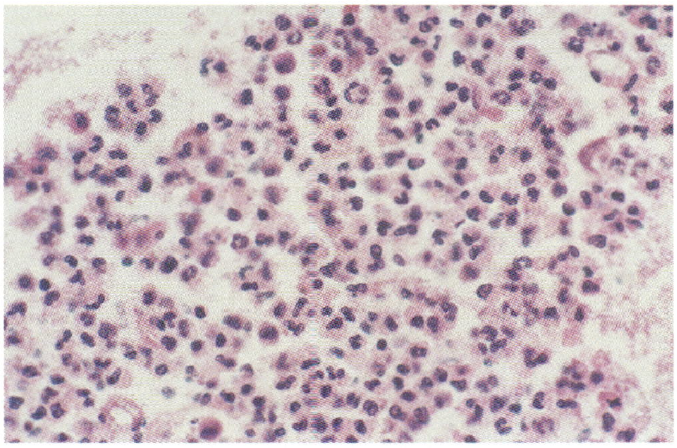

Figure 8–8. Higher magnification to show detail of neutrophils within subcorneal pustule. In contrast to pustular psoriasis, changes of psoriasiform ep dermal hyperplasia do not predominate, and neutrophils do not significantly accumulate in the epidermal layers (*e.g.,* as in spongiform pustules).

Pustular Candidiasis

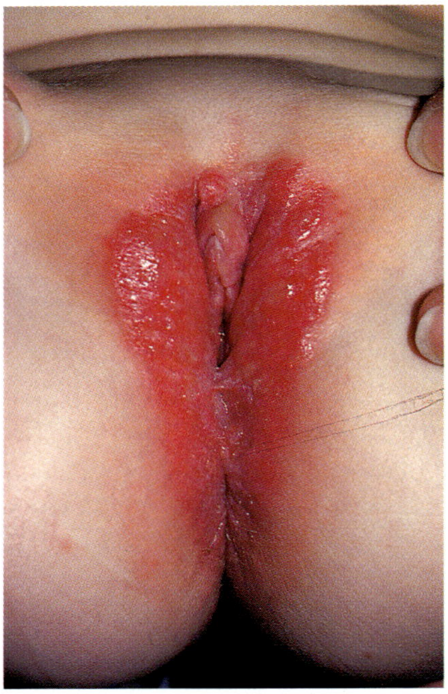

Figure 8–9. Pustular candidiasis. Beefy red pustular eruption affecting genital skin in the diaper region of an infant.

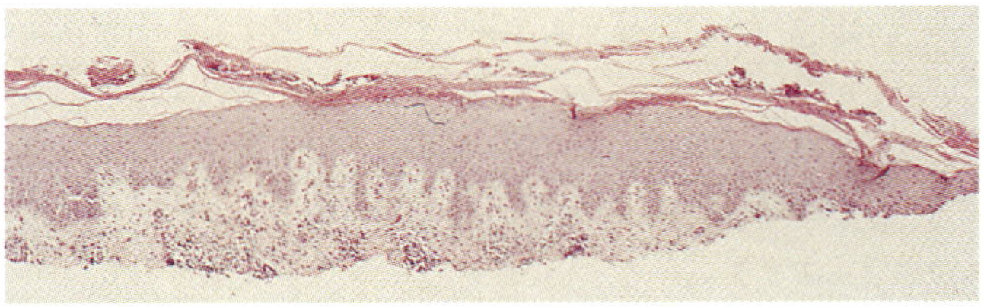

Figure 8–10. Scanning magnification reveals dense aggregates of neutrophils within a stratum corneum overlying a diffusely hyperplastic epidermal layer.

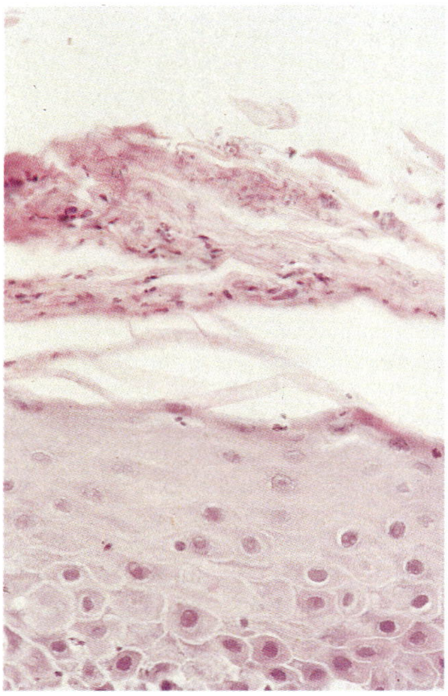

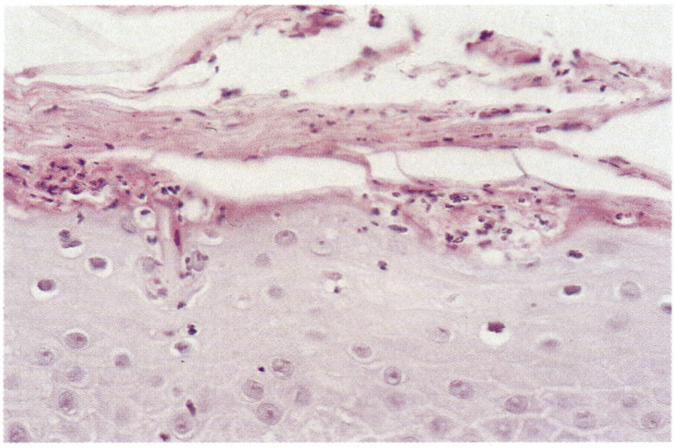

Figures 8–11 and 8–12. Higher magnification of budding yeast forms (Fig. 8–11), stained by periodic acid–Schiff, within the affected stratum corneum. In Figure 8–12, the yeast are admixed with early subcorneal pustules.

Erythema Toxicum Neonatorum

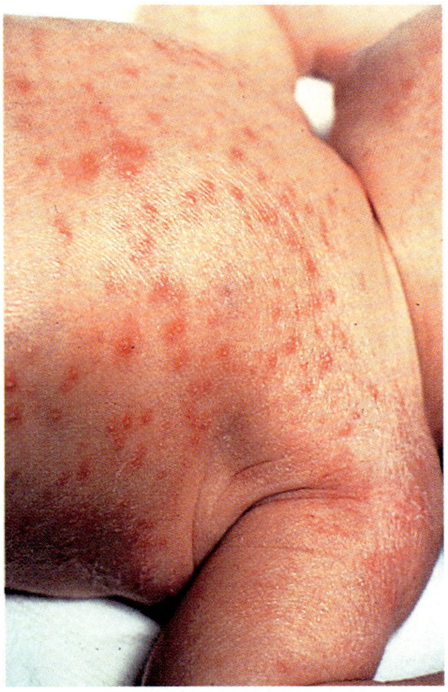

Figure 8–13. Erythema toxicum neonatorum. Multiple erythematous pustules are present on the truncal skin of a newborn.

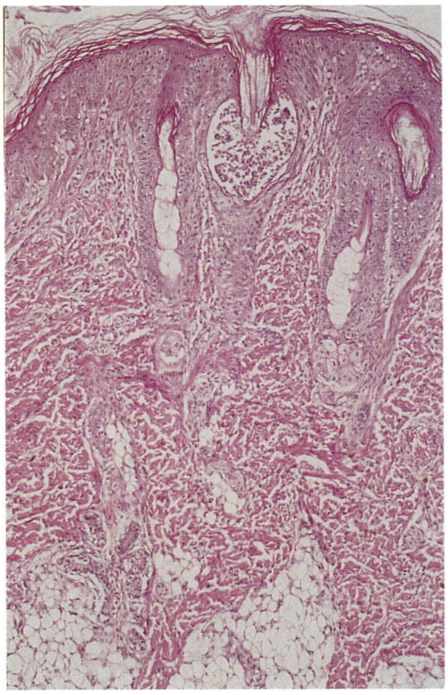

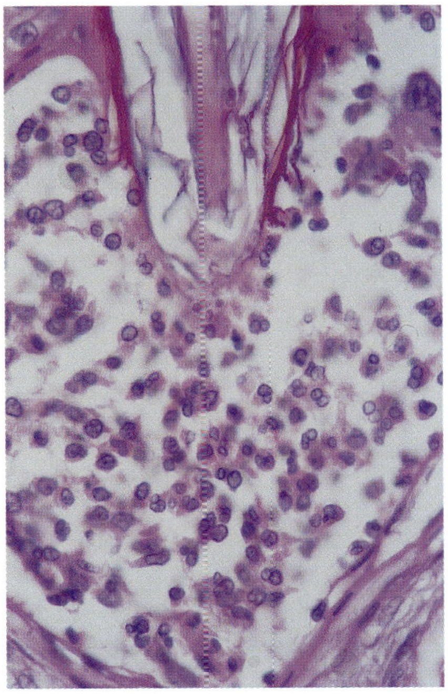

Figures 8–14 and 8–15. Histologically, there are follicular infundibular pustules composed almost exclusively of eosinophils containing characteristically bilobed nuclei.

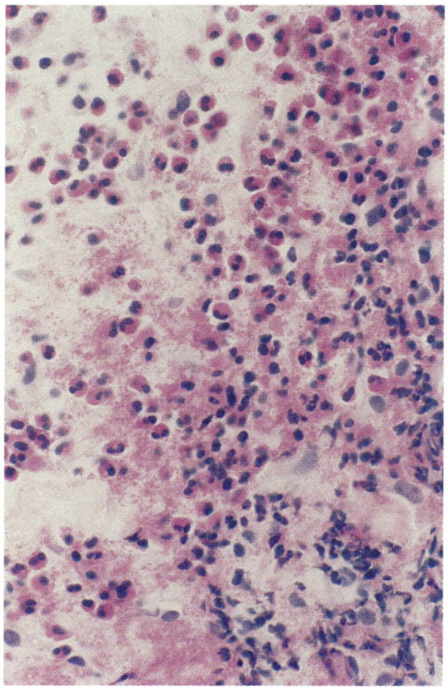

Figure 8–16. Scraping of superficial pustules permits examination of the inflammatory component as a smear. When eosinophils predominate in this clinical setting, this approach will obviate a skin biopsy.

Pustular Folliculitis

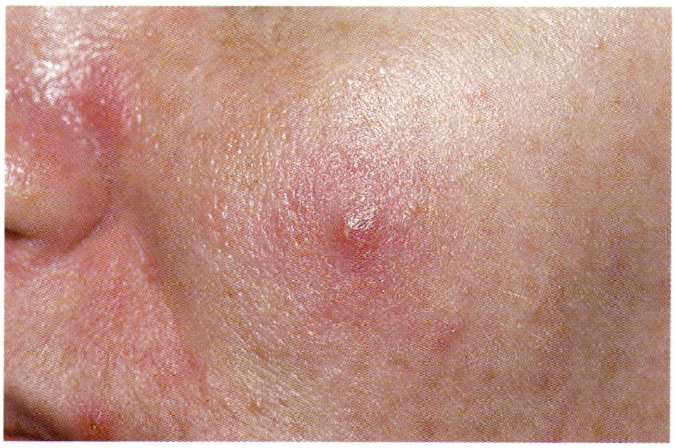

Figure 8–17. The clinical appearance of pustular folliculitis is that of erythematous papules that develop central pustules.

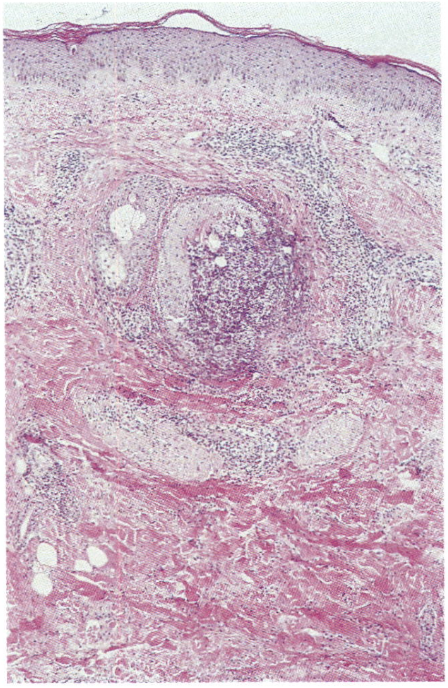

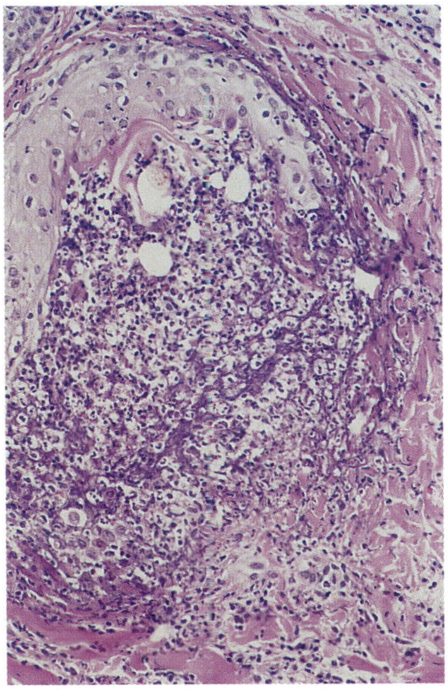

Figures 8–18 and 8–19. Biopsy specimen reveals destructive follicular infundibular pustules composed of neutrophils. Follicular perforation *(center)* may result in inflammation secondary to follicular contents extruded into the dermis.

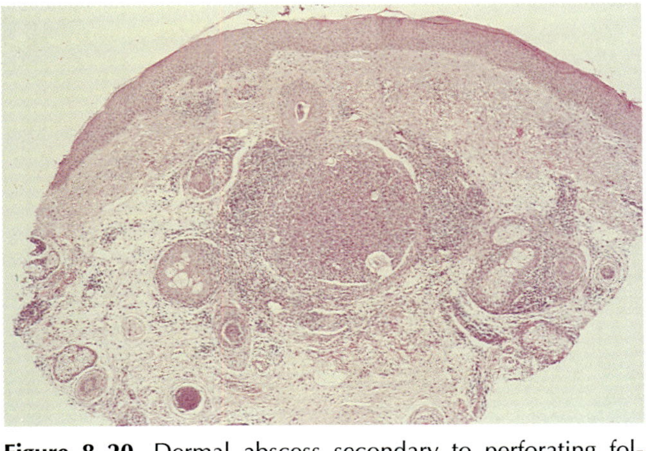

Figure 8–20. Dermal abscess secondary to perforating folliculitis. A mid-dermal abscess composed of neutrophils contains a free *Demodex* mite *(bottom center),* evidence that follicular perforation was the cause of this lesion.

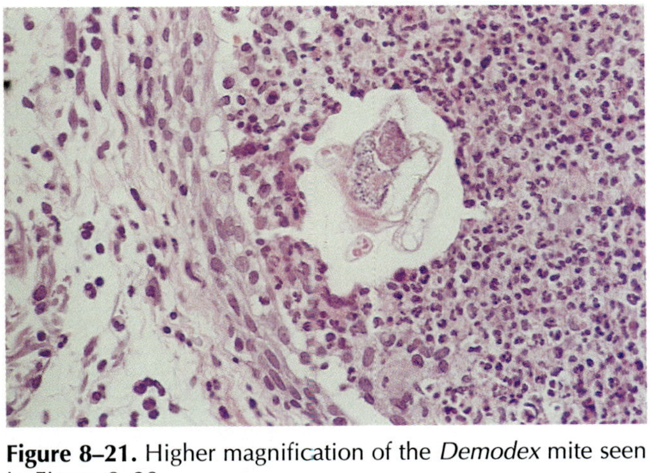

Figure 8–21. Higher magnification of the *Demodex* mite seen in Figure 8–20.

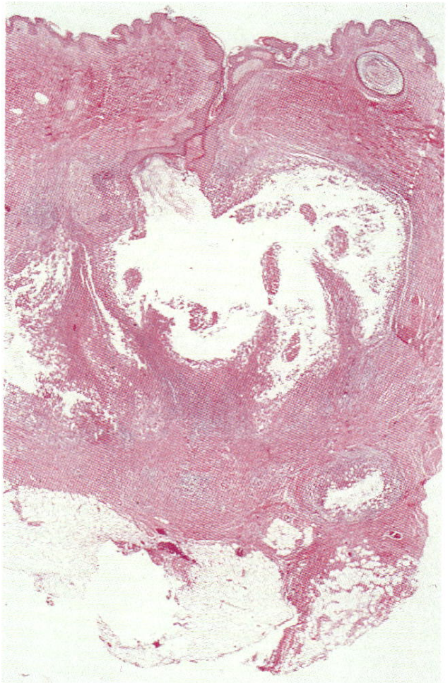

Figure 8–22. A large dermal abscess is secondary to rupture of a follicular cyst.

Acute Febrile Neutrophilic Dermatosis

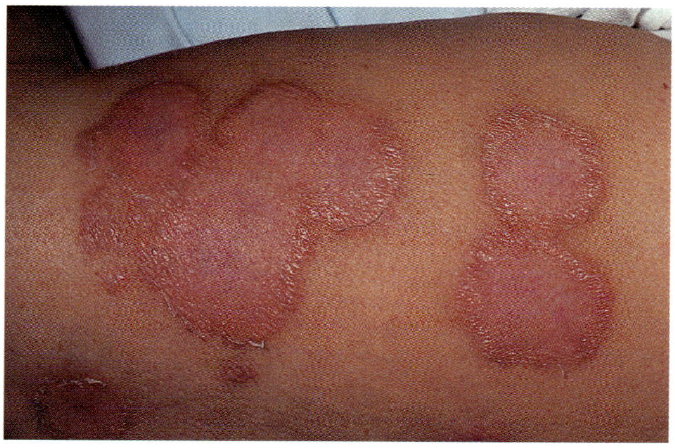

Figure 8–23. Acute febrile neutrophilic dermatosis (*i.e.,* Sweet syndrome). The clinical appearance is characterized by raised, tender erythematous plaques.

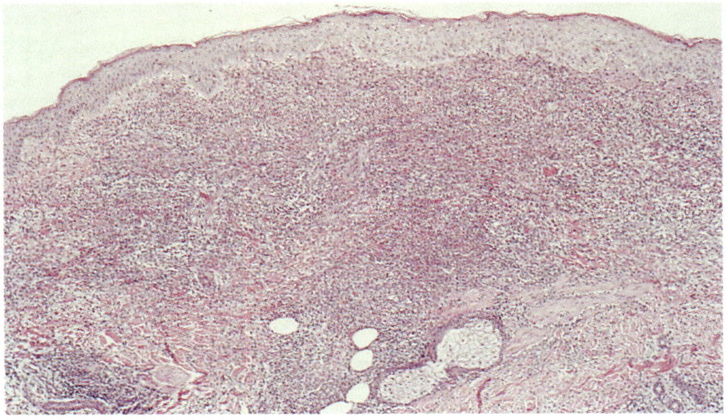

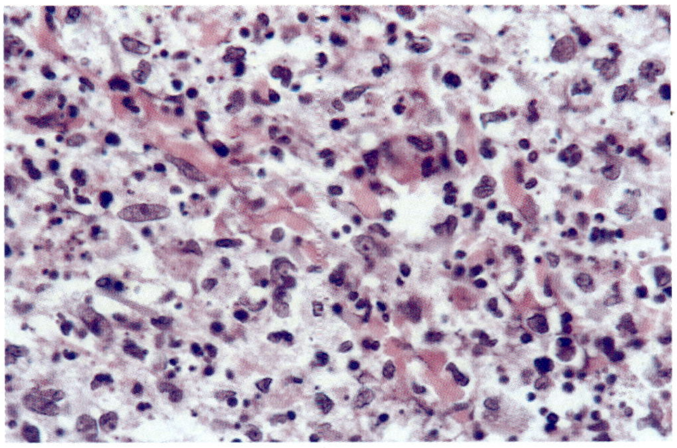

Figures 8–24 and 8–25. Comparison between acute febrile neutrophilic dermatosis (Figs. 8–24 and 8–25) and eosinophilic cellulitis (Figs. 8–26 and 8–27). The former is composed primarily of neutrophils and fibrin within the superficial and deep dermis. Pronounced lesions may be indistinguishable from early pyoderma gangrenosum. Primary vasculitis is not observed, although secondary injury to entrapped vessels may be documented.

Eosinophilic Cellulitis

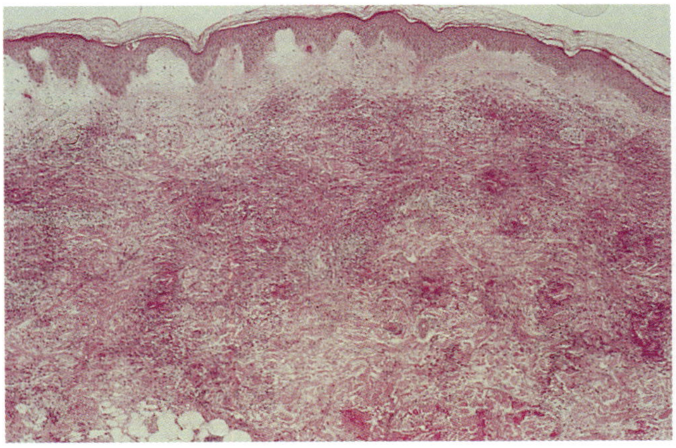

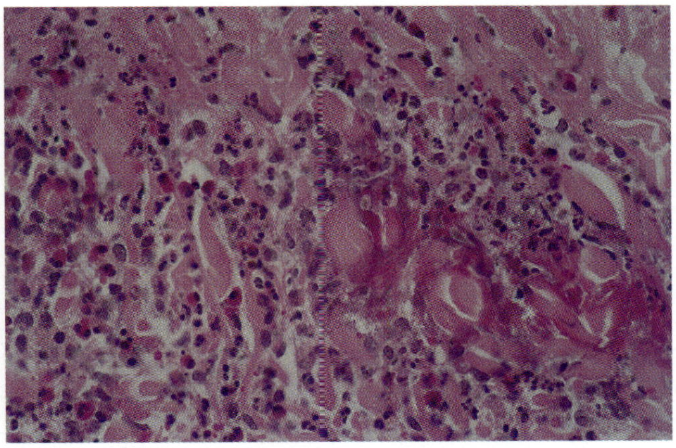

Figures 8–26 and 8–27. Wells syndrome (eosinophilic cellulitis) is characterized by patchy superficial and deep infiltrates composed predominantly of eosinophils. Eosinophilic degeneration of collagen bundles associated with degranulating eosinophils (Fig. 8–27) is typical, and such zones are termed flame figures.

Pyoderma Gangrenosum

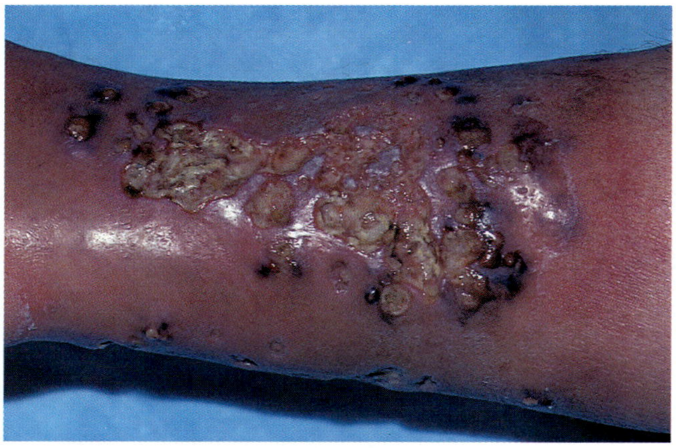

Figure 8–28. The typical clinical appearance of pyoderma gangrenosum shows well-demarcated ulcers with undermined, red-purple borders.

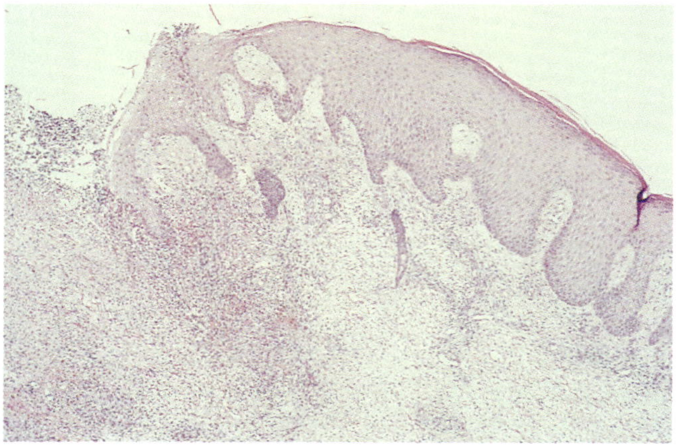

Figure 8–29. A biopsy specimen of the edge of an ulcer *(top left)* shows early pseudoepitheliomatous hyperplasia and a marked dermal inflammatory infiltrate.

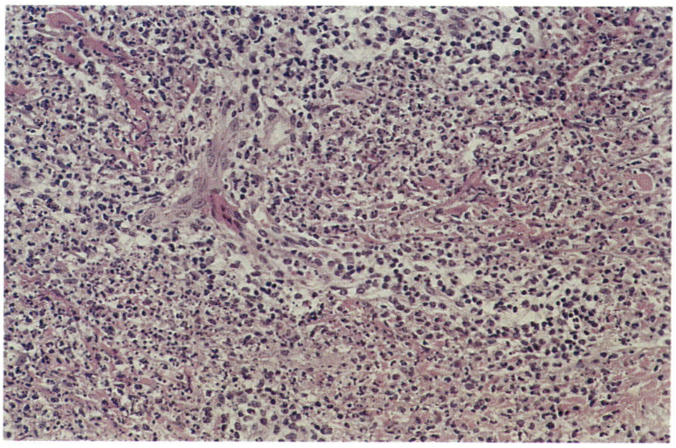

Figure 8–30. Beneath the ulcer base, the dermis is entirely replaced by sheets of neutrophils.

Infectious Pyodermas

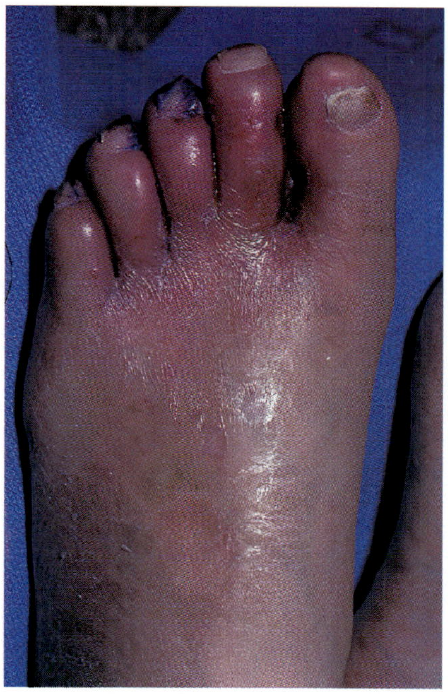

Figure 8–31. Bacterial pyoderma. The ischemic foot of this diabetic patient has become superinfected by bacteria, producing increased erythema, edema, and local pain.

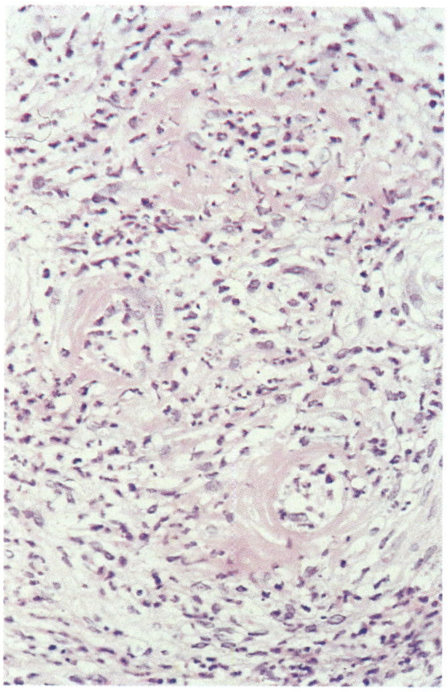

Figure 8–32. Biopsy specimens and culture reveal a mixed inflammatory infiltrate composed predominantly of neutrophils; Gram stain revealed intracellular bacteria. Certain pyodermas may be characterized by marked epidermal hyperplasia (*e.g.*, blastomycosis-like pyoderma).

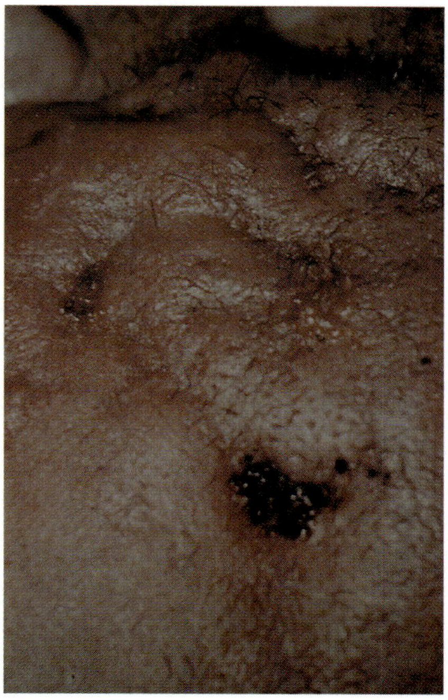

Figure 8–33. Actinomycosis. Boggy, indurated facial skin contains several draining sinus tracts.

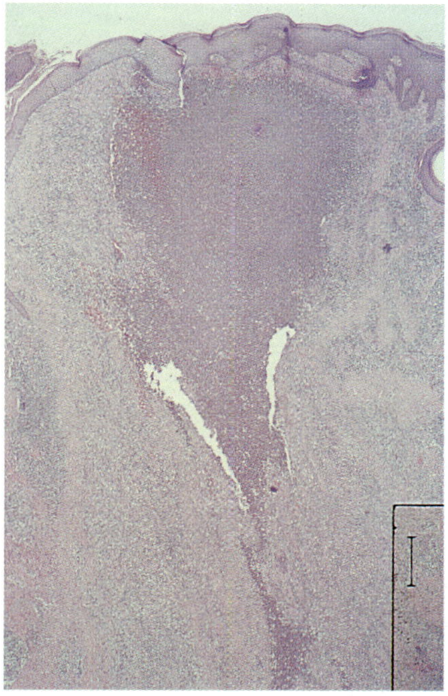

Figure 8–34. Scanning view of a sinus tract that extends from the epidermal layer into deep subcutaneous tissue. The central portion is filled with abscess-like aggregates of neutrophils; the borders of the tract are composed of granulation tissue.

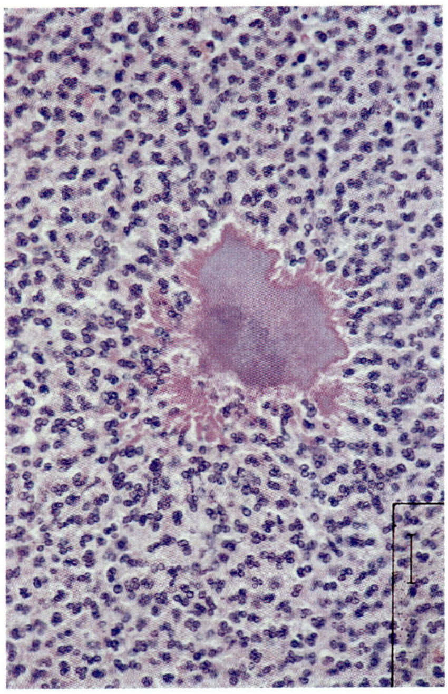

Figure 8–35. Closer inspection of the abscess-like zone reveals characteristic sulfur granules of *Actinomyces* (bar = 100 μm).

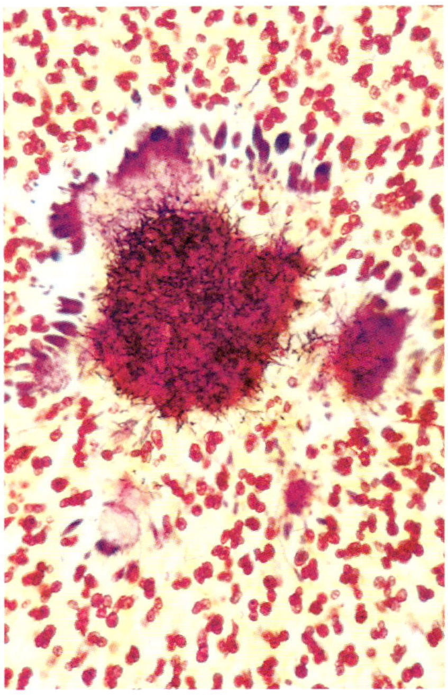

Figure 8–36. Slender filaments extend from the perimeter of the basophilic granule and stain intensely with Gram stain.

9

Granulomatous Dermatitis

Granulomatous dermatitis designates the diverse array of cutaneous inflammatory disorders characterized by dermal and sometimes subcutaneous granulomas. A granuloma is a localized collection of activated histiocytes that may or may not be rimmed by lymphocytes and/or show central necrosis. Activated histiocytes are macrophage-derived cells that ingest either foreign particulates or protein antigens, resulting in attempted lysosomal degradation or antigen processing and presentation. Such histiocytes often become enlarged, sometimes exhibit multinucleation, and generally show conspicuous pale eosinophilic cytoplasm resembling epithelial cell cytoplasm. Thus, such cells are often referred to as *epithelioid histiocytes.* On aggregation, these histiocytes may form syncytial masses of cells that mimic the coalescent growth of true epithelium.

Particulate material ingested by histiocytes is often basophilic or may be birefrigent and detectable by polarization microscopy within cytoplasmic granules. Other putative stimuli of epithelioid cell transformation may not be detected, although arrays of lysosomes presumably activated by these provocative agents may be visible, as in the case of the eosinophilic, star-shaped cytoplasmic "asteroid body" often seen in sarcoidosis. Multinucleation within granulomas may be of diagnostic significance, as in cutaneous tuberculosis, where such cells often have deep-blue wreath-like configurations of nuclei about the cell perimeter (Langhans giant cells). Foreign body giant cells, on the other hand, tend to have more centrally clustered nuclei without a well-defined wreath-like configuration. The presence or absence of central eosinophilic necrosis within granulomas is of limited diagnostic assistance, although the *prototypic* lesion of sarcoidosis is often described as composed of predominantly noncaseating, "naked" (free of surrounding lymphocytes) granulomas. Granulomas with extensive necrosis, on the other hand, often suggest the presence of causative organisms, as is the case in mycobacterial and deep mycotic infections.

Some granulomas form aggregates about altered or *necrobiotic* collagen. Necrobiosis may be associated with pale blue-gray mucin deposition, as in granuloma annulare; deeply eosinophilic fibrinoid degeneration of collagen, as in rheumatoid nodule; or pale-pink sclerosis and homogenization of collagen bundles, as is typical of necrobiosis lipoidica. In all of these disorders, well-formed granulomas are characterized by an array of histiocytes radially arranged about the perimeter of the necrobiotic zone, with the long axes of each cell in parallel *(palisaded granulomas).*

The pattern formed by granulomatous inflammation in the skin may at times be of diagnostic assistance. For example, although in sarcoidosis granulomas may be randomly scattered throughout the superficial and deep dermis, in leprosy they tend to wind around neuromuscular bundles in a serpiginous manner. Granulomas in secondary syphilis are poorly formed and tend to be concentrated within the papillary dermis in association with cytotoxic alteration of the basal cell layer. In the case of granulomatous inflammation that accompanies follicular perforation, the histiocytic aggregates are centered about the offending pilar epithelium.

Infectious Granulomas

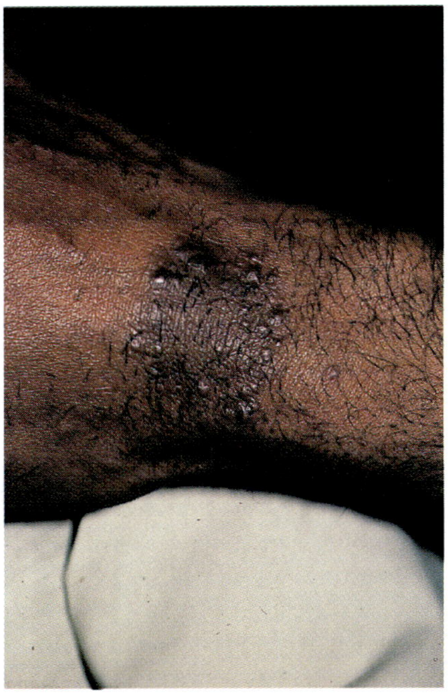

Figure 9–1. Infectious granulomas: Cryptococcosis (also see Figs. 9–2 and 9–3). The skin of a renal transplant patient shows a hyperpigmented plaque studded by small, firm papules.

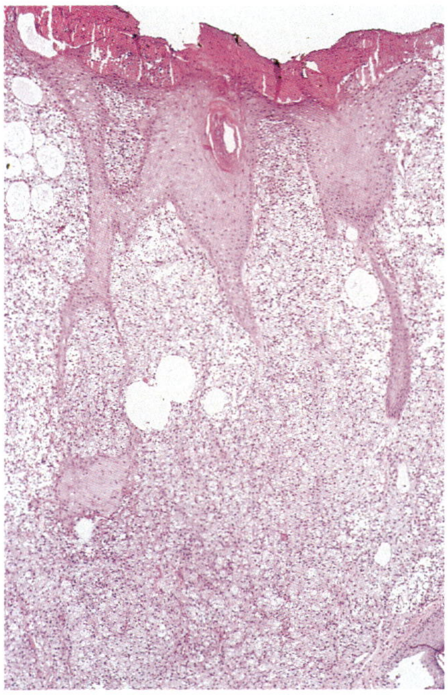

Figure 9–2. A diffusely granulomatous response is present in the dermis, underlying reactive epidermal hyperplasia.

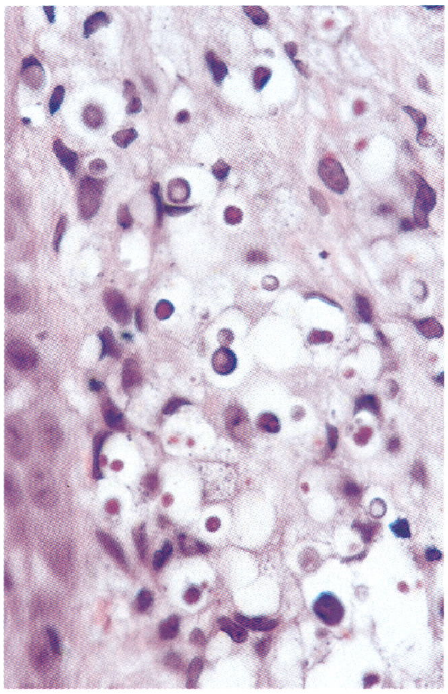

Figure 9–3. Periodic acid–Schiff stain reveals a narrow-necked, budding spore *(center)* surrounded by a clear halo, representing a mucinous capsule.

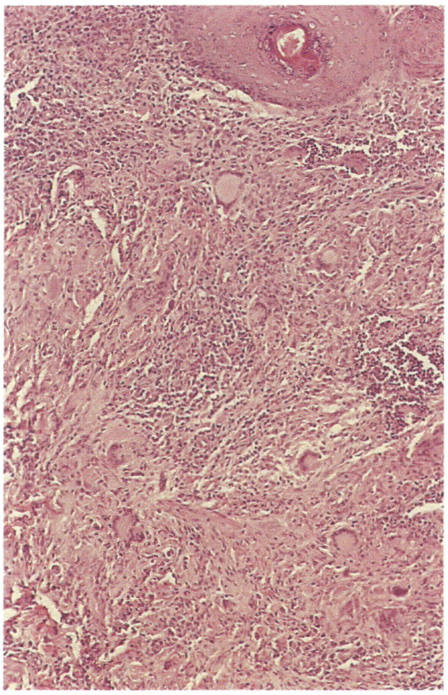

Figure 9–4. Infectious granulomas: Histoplasmosis (also see Figs. 9–4 through 9–6). This lesion is characterized by diffuse granulomatous inflammation of the superficial and deep dermis.

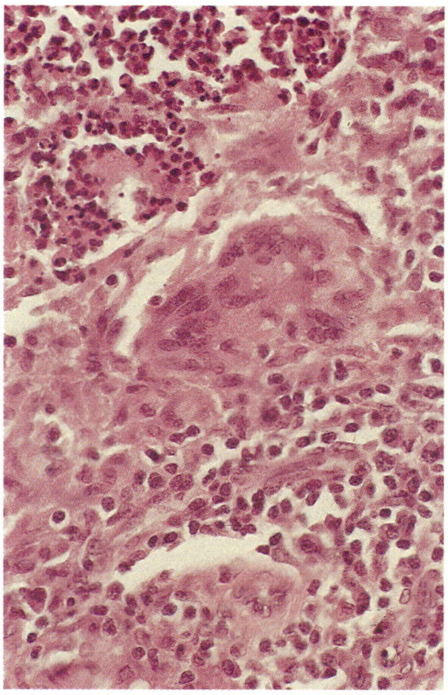

Figure 9–5. Note the prominent multinucleated giant cells, in which rounded clear zones *(center)* are detected. These zones represent cytoplasmic lacunae where spores reside.

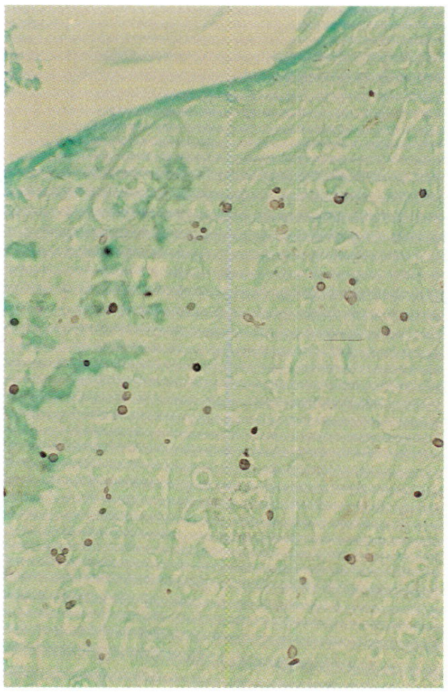

Figure 9–6. Silver stain reveals numerous spores 2 to 4 μm in diameter.

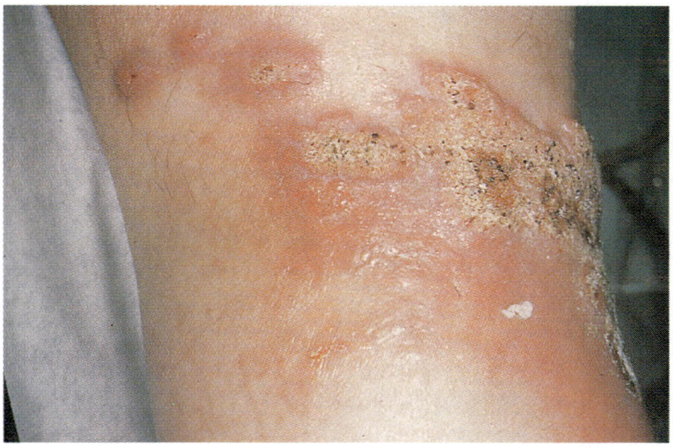

Figure 9–7. Infectious granulomas: Chromomycosis (also see Figs. 9–8 and 9–9). The clinical picture of verrucous nodules and plaques on the lower extremity is typical.

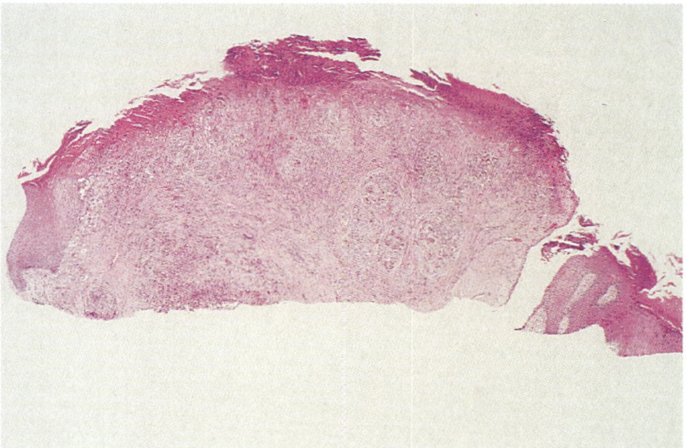

Figure 9–8. A biopsy specimen reveals epidermal ulceration bordered by hyperplasia and a dense dermal inflammatory infiltrate composed of noncaseating granulomas as well as aggregates of neutrophils.

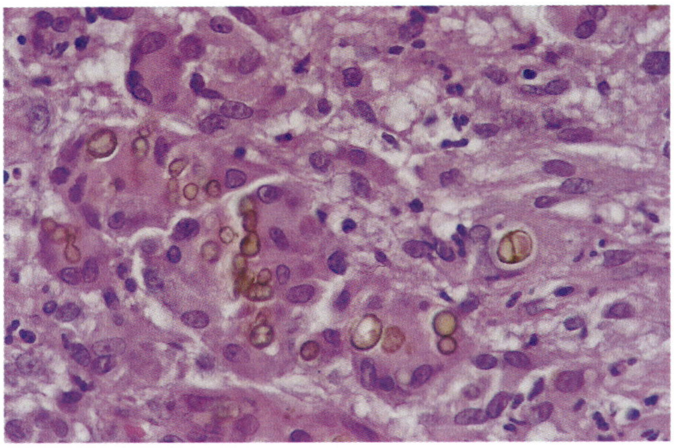

Figure 9–9. Organisms are endogenously pigmented, copper-colored spores within multinucleated giant cells. They do not reproduce by budding but rather by formation of septa within individual spores *(center right).*

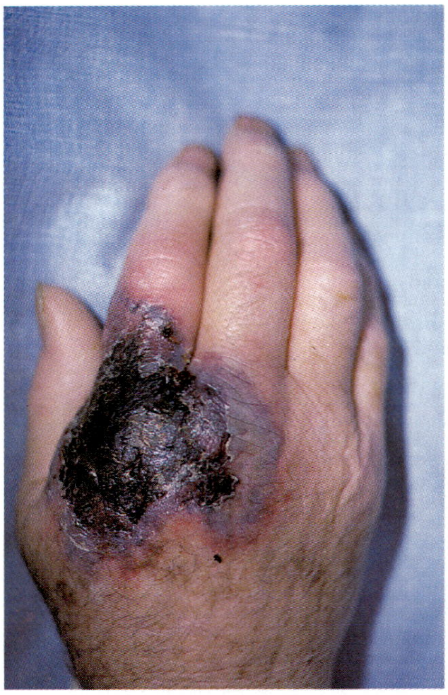

Figure 9–10. Infectious granulomas: Mucormycosis (also see Figs. 9–11 through 9–13). Necrotic and ulcerated plaque on the dorsum of the hand of an immunosuppressed patient.

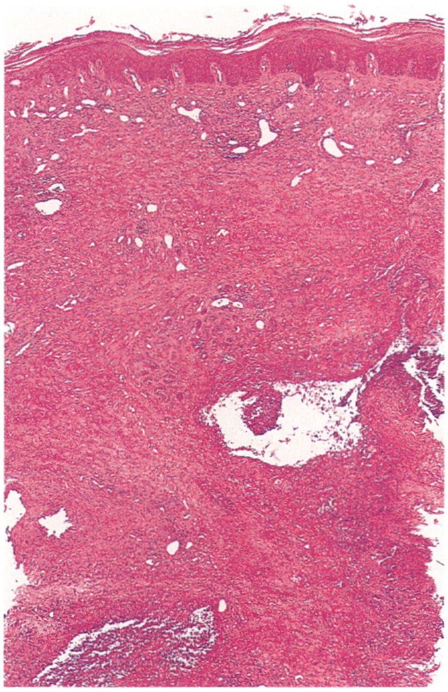

Figure 9–11. Diffuse, vague, granulomatous inflammation, granulation tissue, and cystic necrosis are present in the dermis.

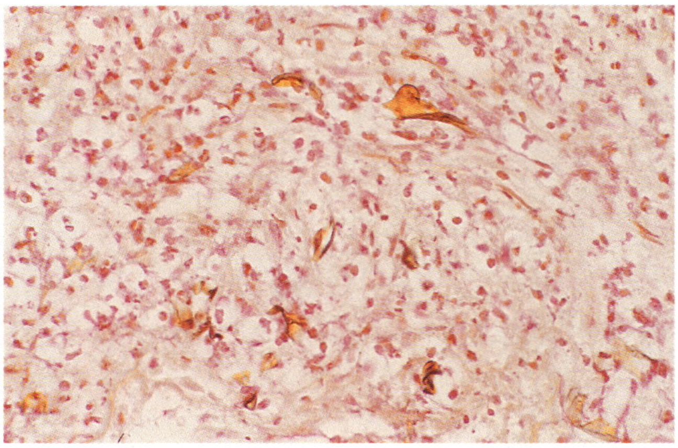

Figure 9–12. Silver stain reveals twisted, ribbon-like hyphae in the deep dermis.

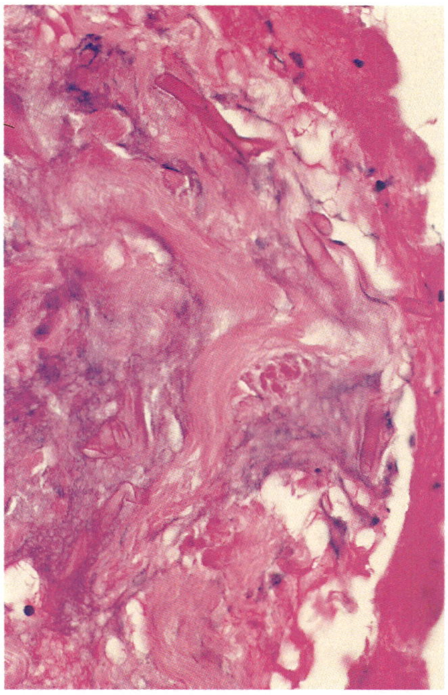

Figure 9–13. In a necrotic region, pleomorphic, nonseptate hyphae are also observed *(center top)* with periodic acid–Schiff stain.

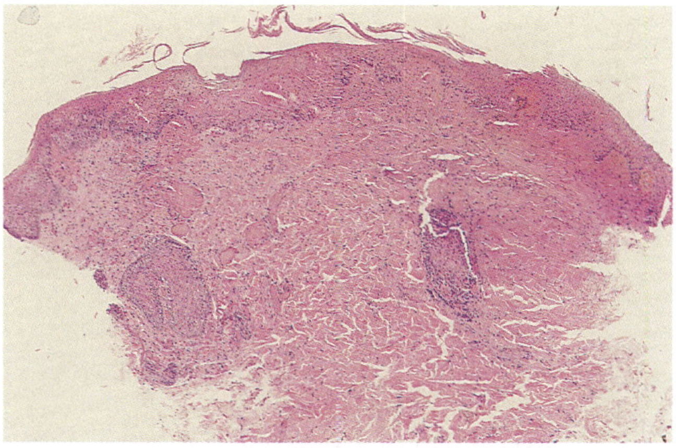

Figure 9–14. Infectious granulomas: Aspergillosis (also see Figs. 9–15 and 9–16). At scanning magnification, there is a patchy, vague granulomatous infiltrate within the superficial and deep dermis.

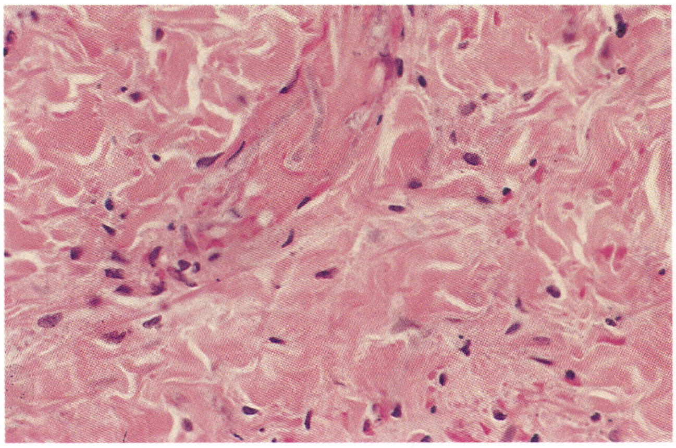

Figure 9–15. Closer inspection of a region *(center left)* in Figure 9–14 reveals pale blue-gray hyphae within small vessels, indicative in this case of thromboembolic dissemination to the skin.

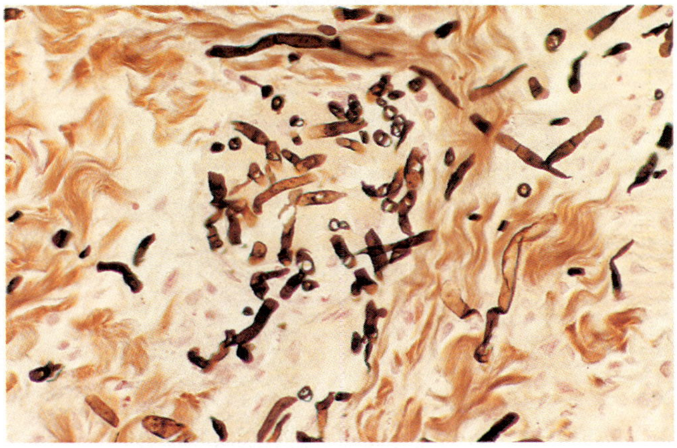

Figure 9–16. Silver stain reveals numerous septate hyphae that branch at acute angles.

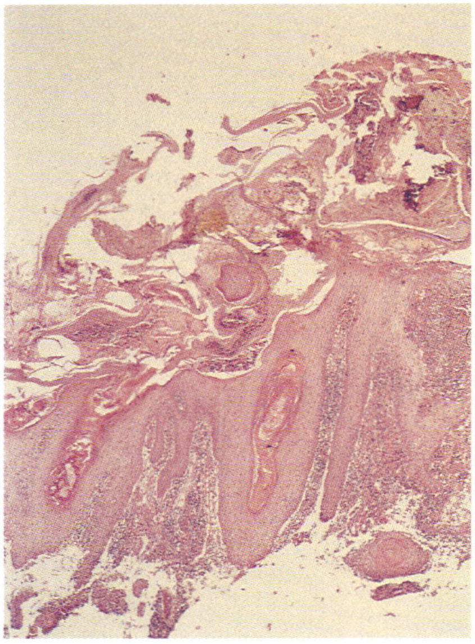

Figure 9–17. Infectious granulomas: Coccidioidomycosis. A biopsy specimen of a tender, ulcerated, verrucous nodule in a patient with systemic coccidioidomycosis. The inflammatory infiltrate in the dermis is mixed and focally granulomatous with focal caseous necrosis; the epidermis shows reactive hyperplasia similar to that seen in early blastomycosis.

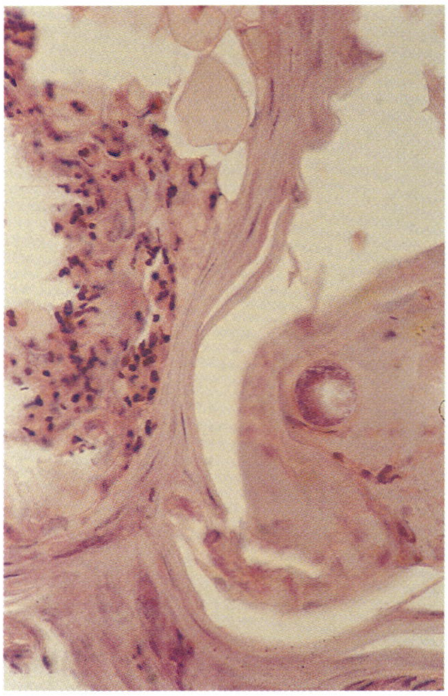

Figure 9–18. Within the stratum corneum, a sporangium containing endospores *(center right)* is identified in this case of coccidioidomycosis.

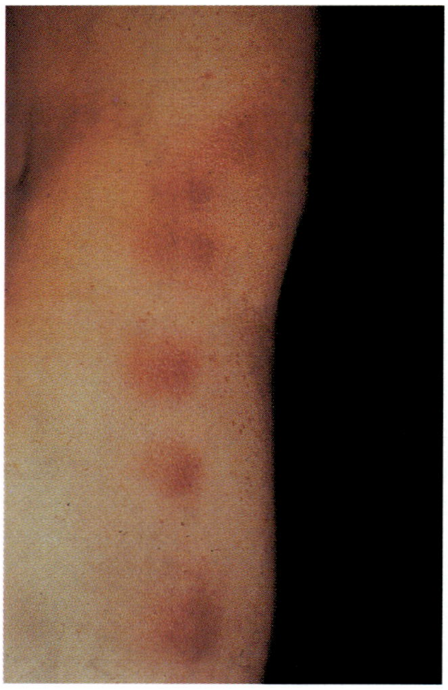

Figure 9–19. Infectious granulomas: Sporotrichosis (also see Figs. 9–20 through 9–23). A linear array of erythematous nodules drains a primary site of infection in a patient with lymphocutaneous sporotrichosis.

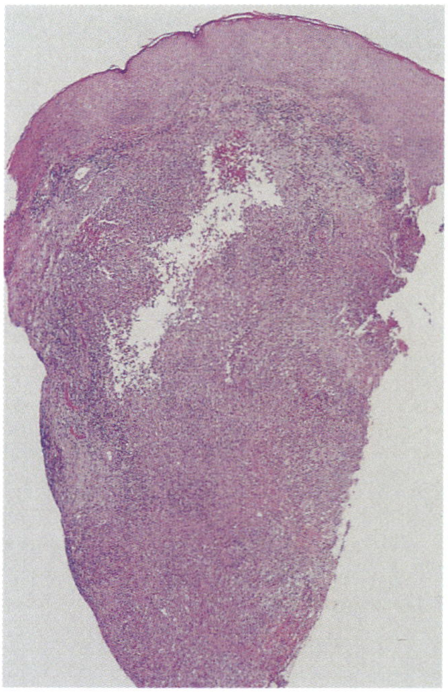

Figure 9–20. At scanning magnification, the inflammatory infiltrate is composed of lymphocytes, neutrophils, plasma cells, and monocytes, with foci of granuloma formation.

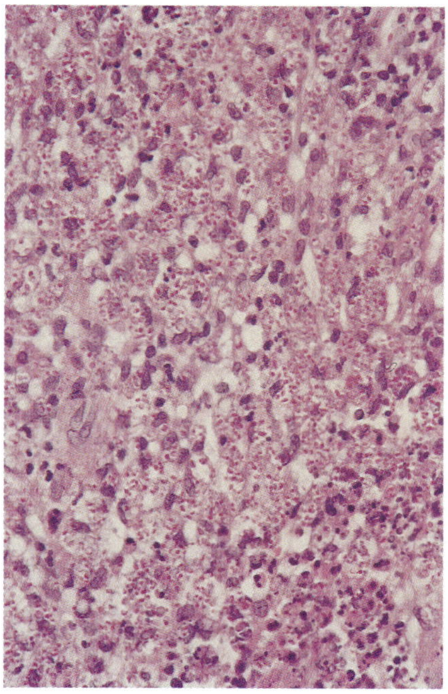

Figure 9–21. The histiocytic component of the inflammatory infiltrate contains numerous spores, which stain positive with periodic acid–Schiff.

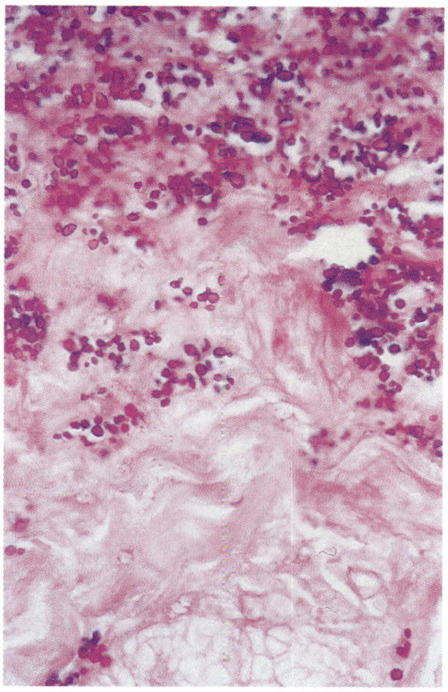

Figure 9–22. Positive periodic acid–Schiff stain of numerous spores.

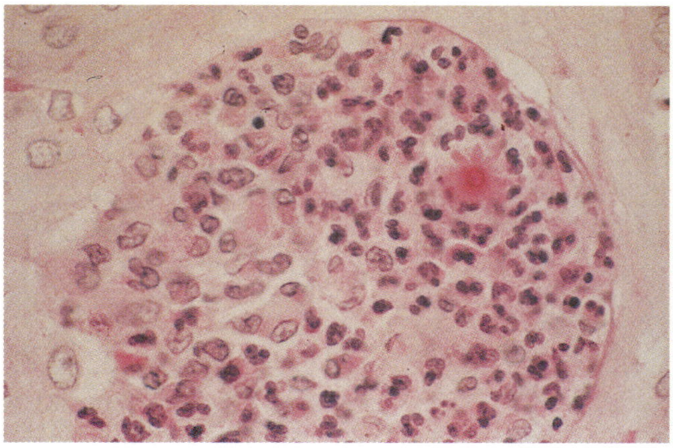

Figure 9–23. Asteroid bodies *(center right),* which here represent central spores with homogeneous eosinophilic radiations, are occasionally observed.

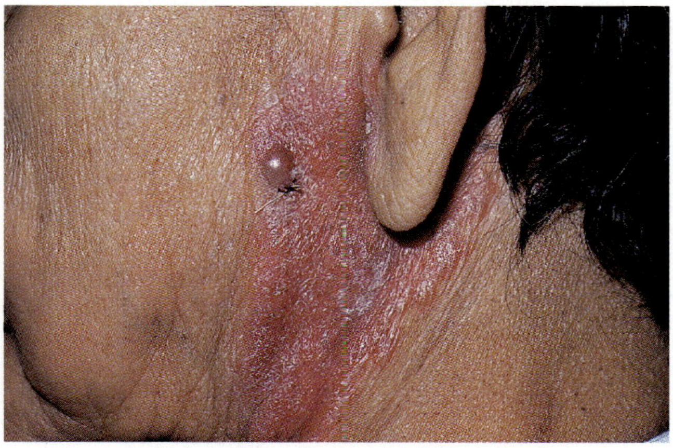

Figure 9–24. Infectious granulomas: Atypical mycobacteria (also see Figs. 9–25 through 9–27). Primary inoculation sites may be manifest as solitary nodules, sometimes in linear array, mimicking sporotrichosis.

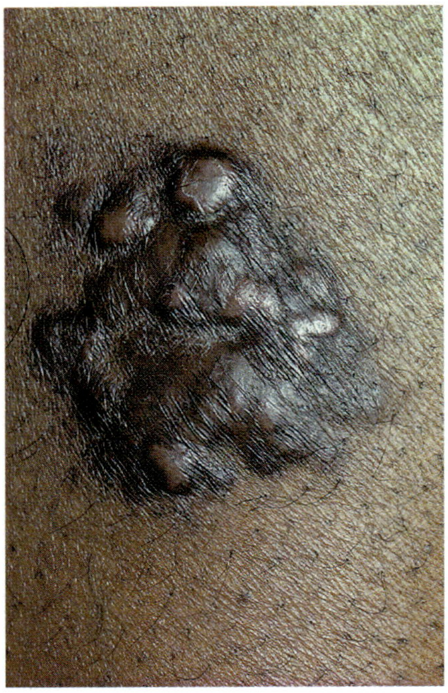

Figure 9–25. Primary inoculation sites may also be manifest as multiple nodules, here associated with hyperpigmentation.

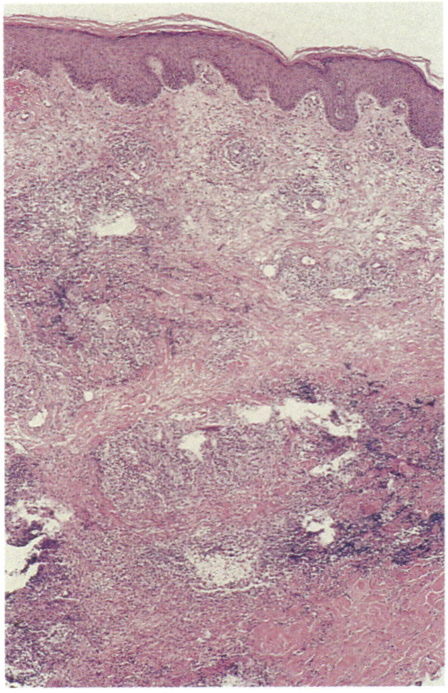

Figure 9–26. Histologically, there is a mixed inflammatory infiltrate within the superficial and deep dermis, which may contain vaguely granulomatous foci and necrosis.

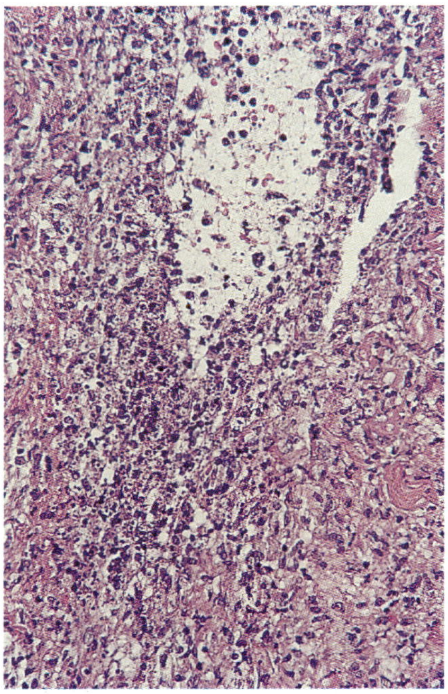

Figure 9–27. Vaguely granulomatous foci and necrosis. With time, classic epithelioid granulomas may supervene.

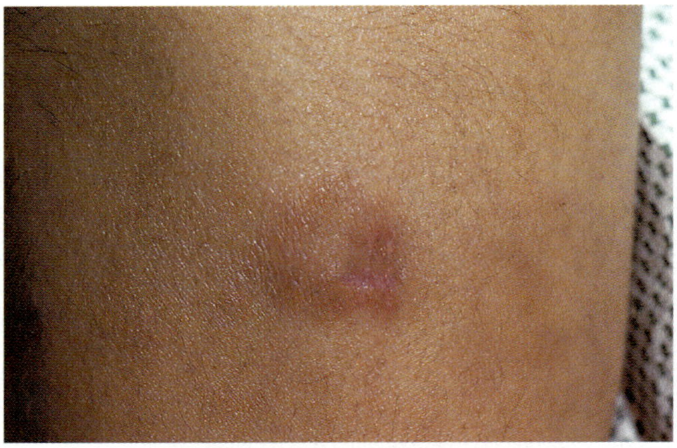

Figure 9–28. Cutaneous tuberculosis. Erythematous papules and small nodules may be present (also see Figs. 9–29 through 9–31).

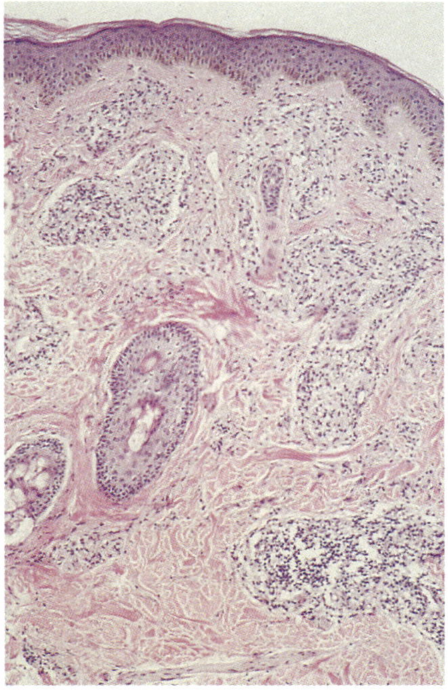

Figure 9–29. A biopsy specimen demonstrates a superficial and deep dermal mononuclear cell infiltrate.

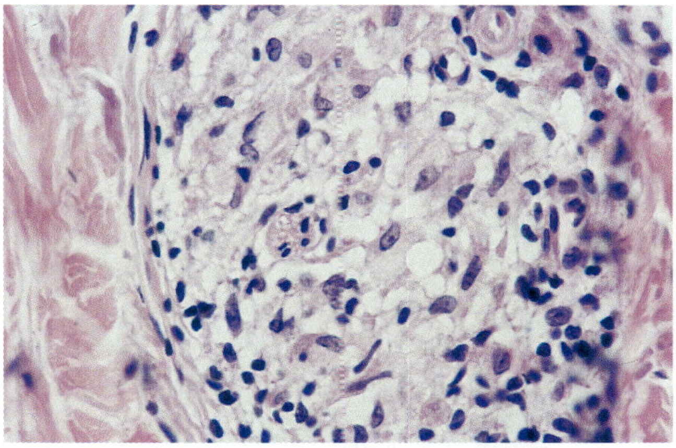

Figure 9–30. On higher magnification, these foci are predominantly epithelioid histiocytes and lymphocytes. In contrast to tuberculoid leprosy, dermal nerves are not damaged.

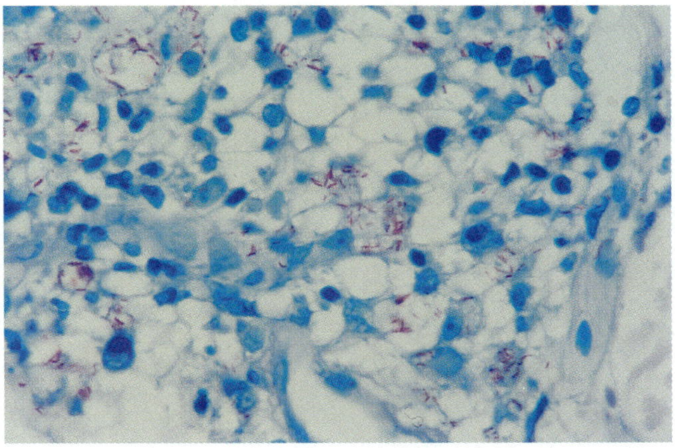

Figure 9–31. Acid-fast stain reveals characteristic mycobacteria within dermal histiocytes.

Foreign Body Granulomas

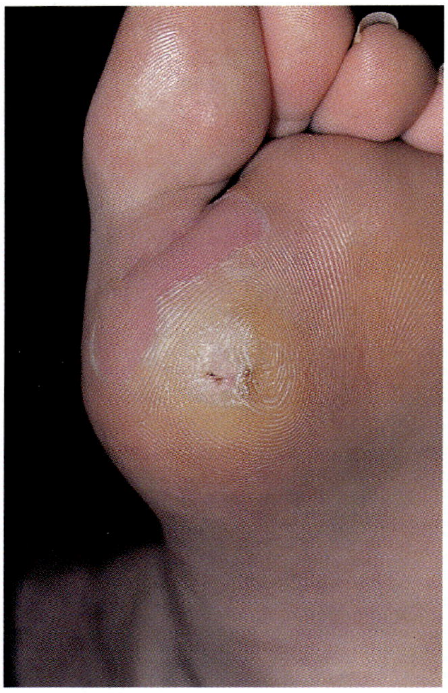

Figure 9–32. A foreign-body granuloma at the site of previous surgical removal of a plantar wart.

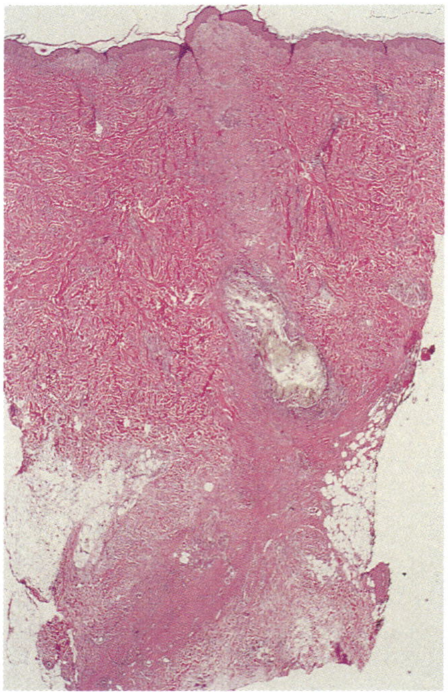

Figure 9–33. This foreign body granuloma reveals scar formation associated with granulomatous inflammation to foreign material.

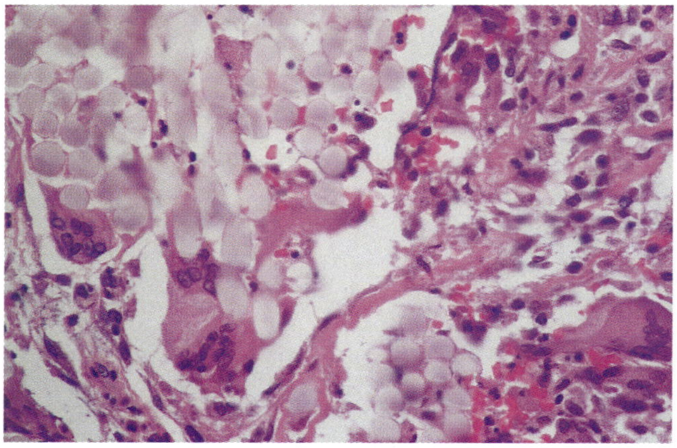

Figure 9–34. Retained suture material *(top and center left)* is present within foci of fibrosis and granulomatous inflammation.

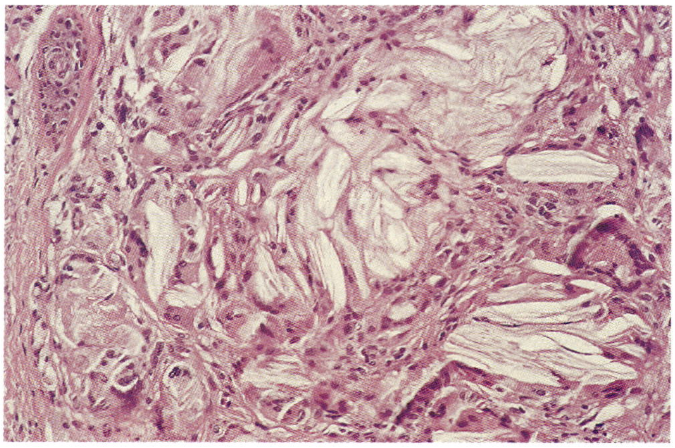

Figure 9–35. Foreign-body giant cell response to site of cyst rupture demonstrates cleft-like spaces formed by cholesterol from membranous cyst contents.

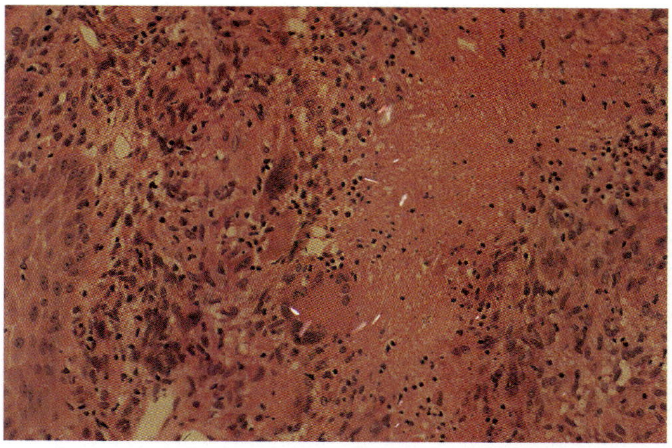

Figure 9–36. Polarization microscopy of foreign-body reaction at the site of traumatically introduced foreign material reveals birefringent material as clear clefts within multinucleated histiocytes.

Granulomas Due to Mineral Particulates

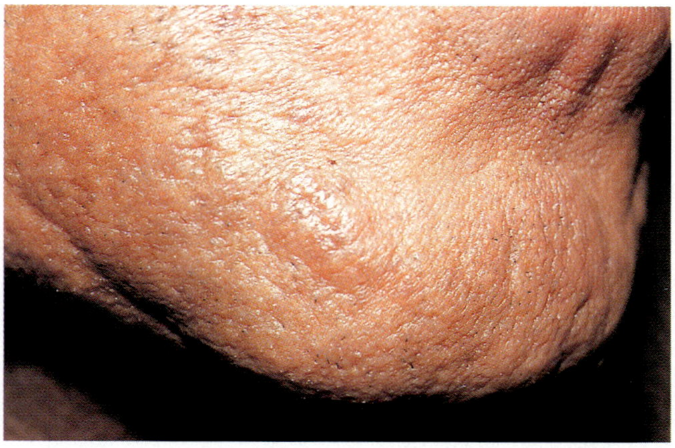

Figure 9–37. Granulomatous response to silica occurred many years after its local introduction into the dermis.

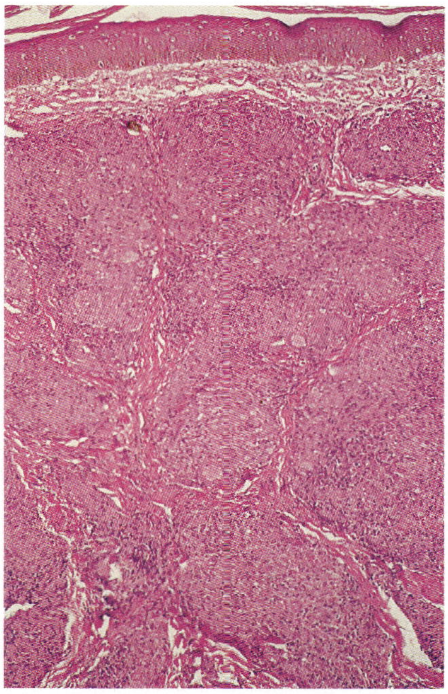

Figure 9–38. Well-formed granulomas within the superficial and mid-dermis mimic sarcoidosis.

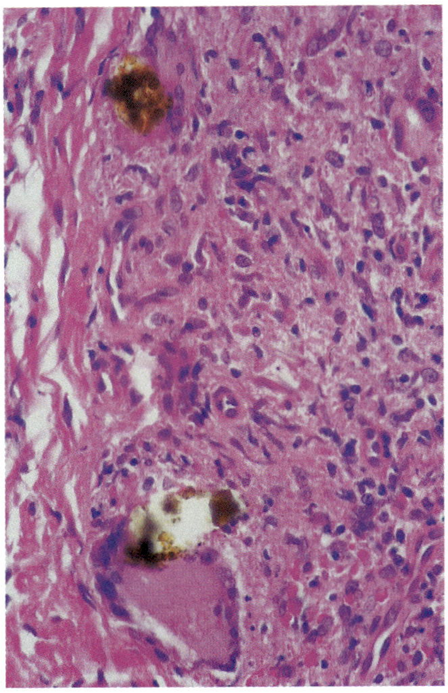

Figure 9–39. Sites of deposition of refractile silica crystals associated with brown hemosiderin are visible even by routine microscopy. Polaroscopy, clinical history, and, occasionally, x-ray–dispersive electron microscopy for elemental analysis may facilitate accurate diagnosis.

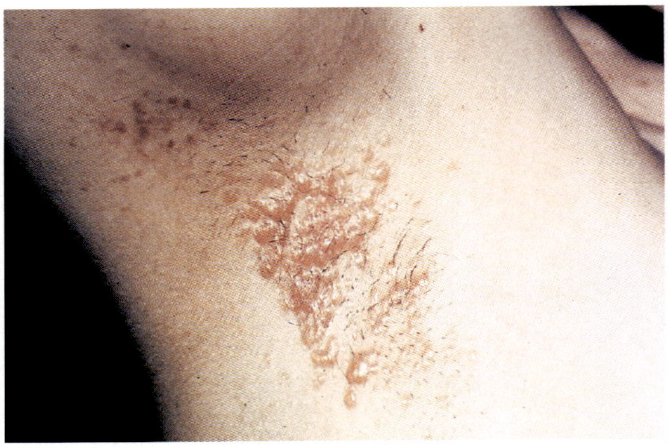

Figure 9–40. Zirconium granulomas. Boggy red-brown papules are present at the site of application of zirconium-containing antiperspirant.

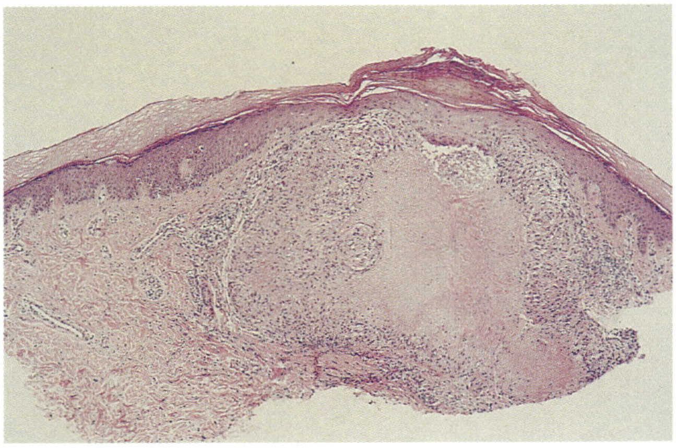

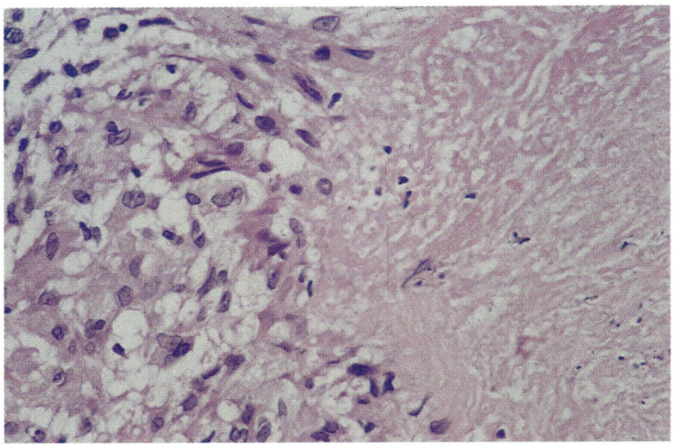

Figures 9–41 and 9–42. Epithelioid granulomas have foci of central caseous necrosis. Although zirconium and beryllium usually do not cause necrosis, this case of zirconium-induced granulomatous dermatitis demonstrated prominent zones of necrosis *(right).*

Sarcoidosis

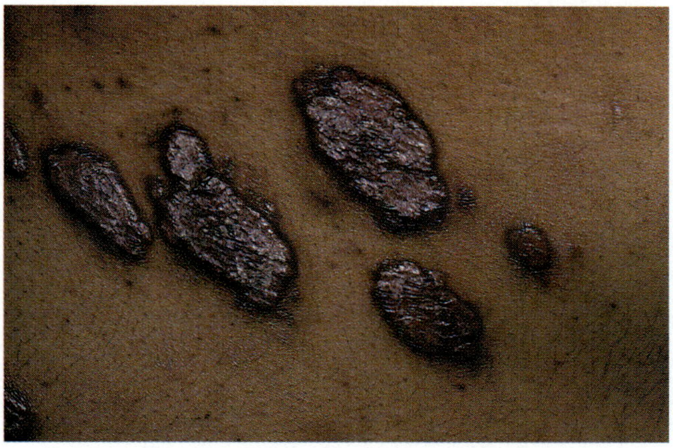

Figure 9–43. Sarcoidosis. Erythematous plaques raise the clinical differential of lupus erythematosus, sarcoidosis, or infection.

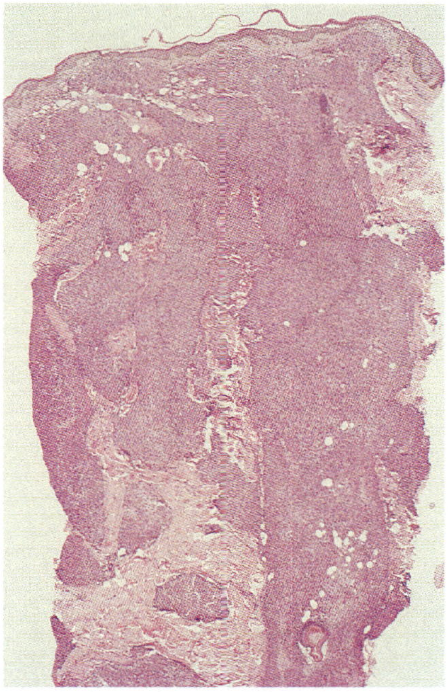

Figure 9–44. Scanning magnification reveals numerous confluent granulomas within the superficial and deep dermis.

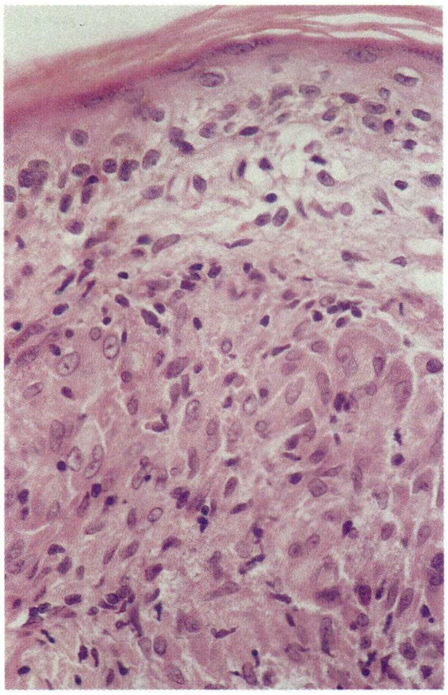

Figure 9–45. High magnification demonstrates epithelioid granulomas devoid of both significant central necrosis (noncaseating granulomas) and a substantial peripheral rim of lymphocytes (naked granulomas). Special stains and culture of fresh tissue in sarcoidosis are invariably negative for organisms.

Granuloma Annulare

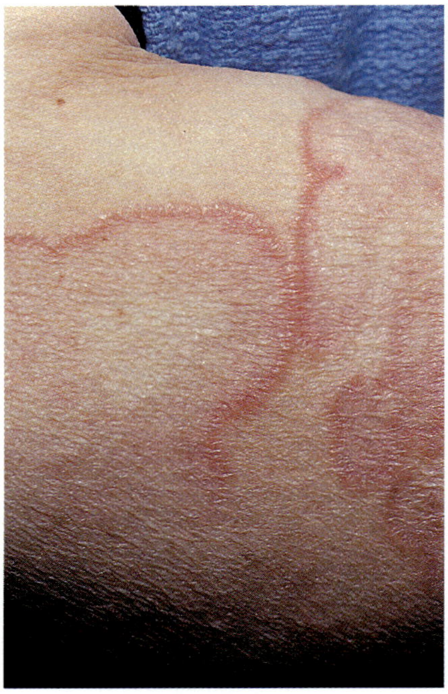

Figure 9–46. Granuloma annulare. Clinical lesions consist of annular, dermal plaques with central clearing and raised, erythematous borders.

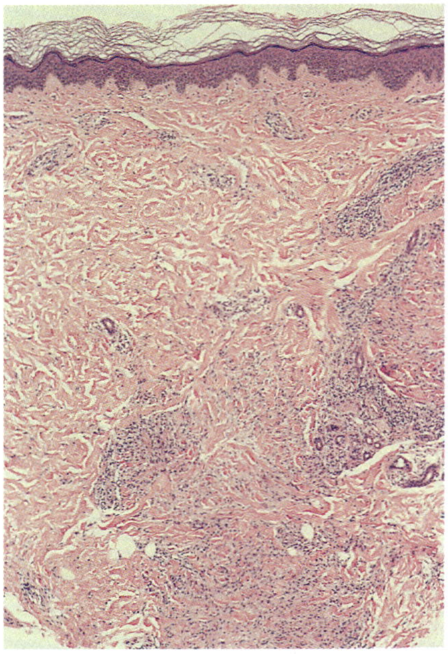

Figure 9–47. Early lesions typically show an interstitial pattern of infiltration by inflammatory cells (see also Fig. 9–48).

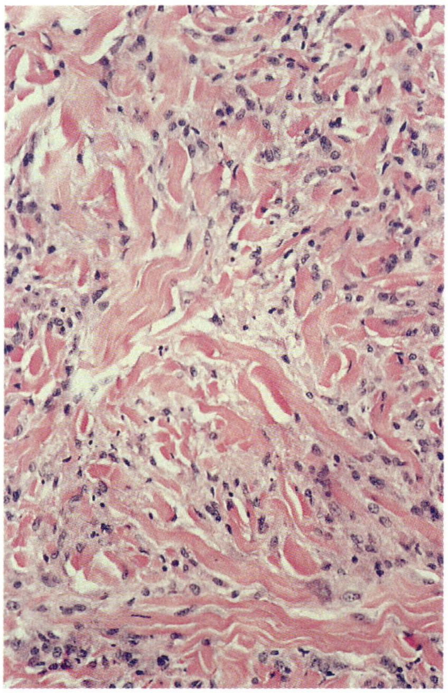

Figure 9–48. Mononuclear cells are present among collagen bundles in association with variable mucin deposition.

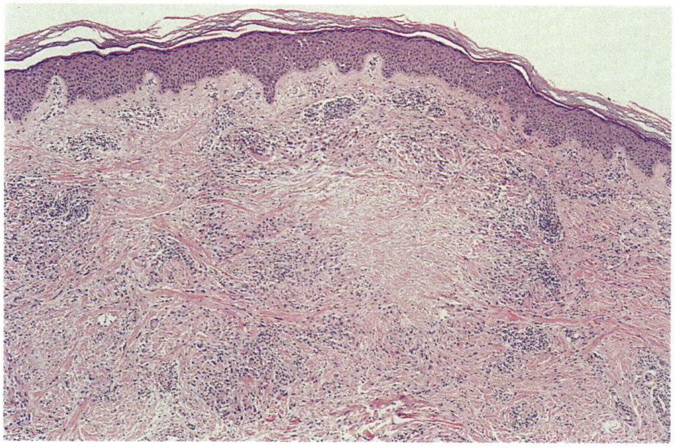

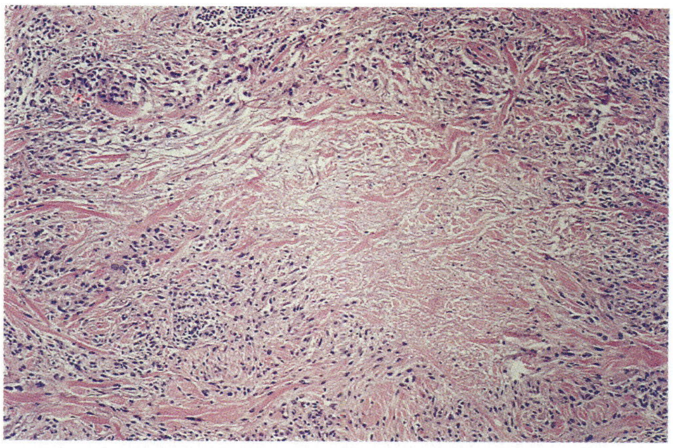

Figures 9–49 and 9–50. Well-developed lesions of granuloma annulare show zones of mucinous necrobiosis of collagen, surrounded by mononuclear cells with an infiltrative pattern similar to that described in Figures 9–47 and 9–48. Around the perimeters of zones of necrobiotic collagen are palisades of monocytes, forming a vaguely granulomatous pattern of inflammation.

Rheumatoid Nodule

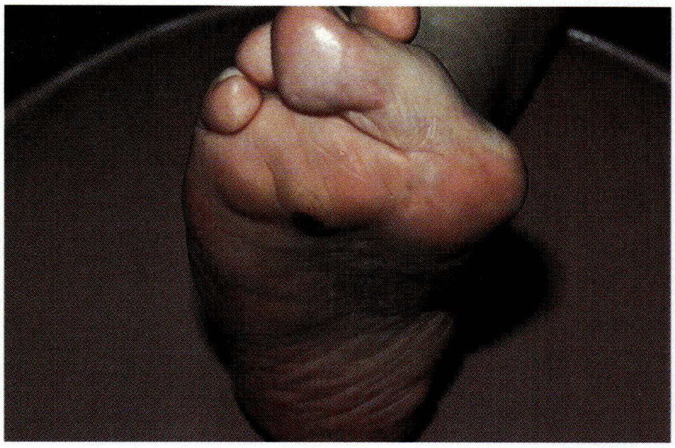

Figure 9–51. Rheumatoid nodule. Firm nodules are associated with the joints on the plantar aspect of the foot of this patient.

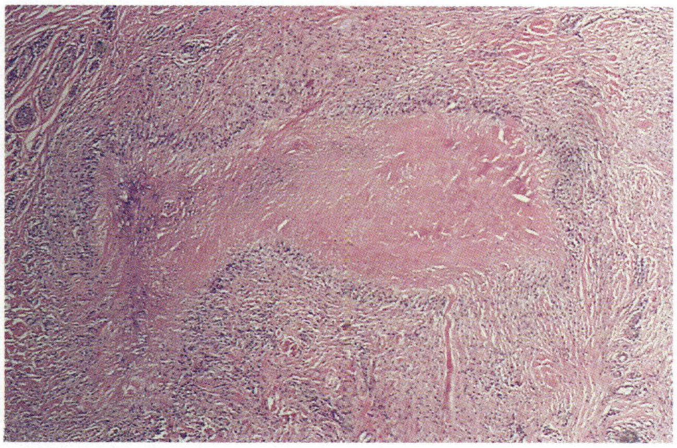

Figure 9–52. The pathology of Figure 9–54 consists of zones of fibrinoid necrobiosis, surrounded by palisades of histiocytes and a fibrotic stroma.

Necrobiosis Lipoidica

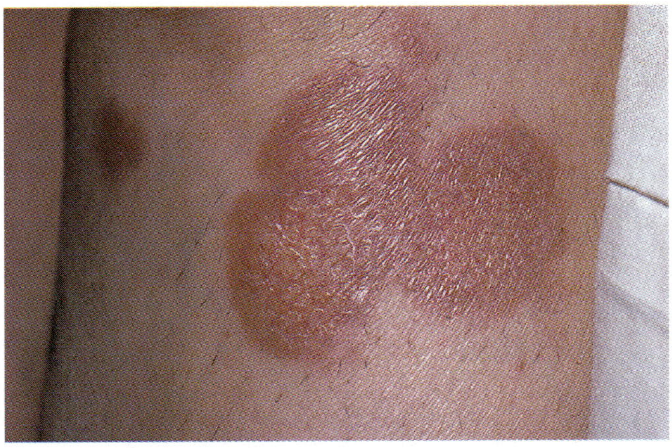

Figure 9–53. The gross pathology of necrobiosis lipoidica consists of pale, erythematous to waxy yellow plaques with telangiectasia and an atrophic, overlying epidermal layer. Lesions often affect the anterior aspects of the lower extremities.

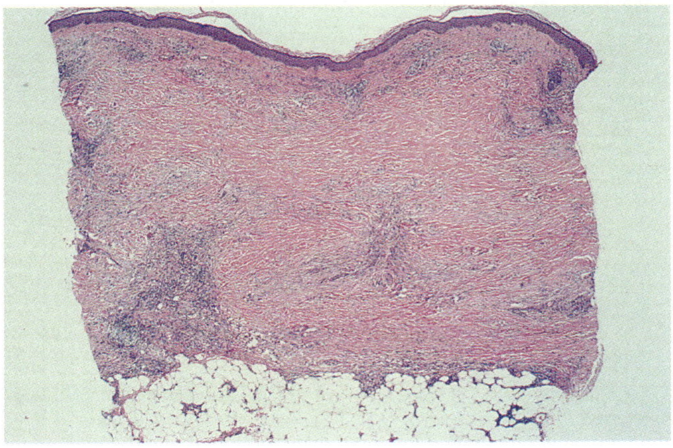

Figure 9–54. Histologically, layers of inflammation alternate with broad zones of fibrosis in the horizontal plane.

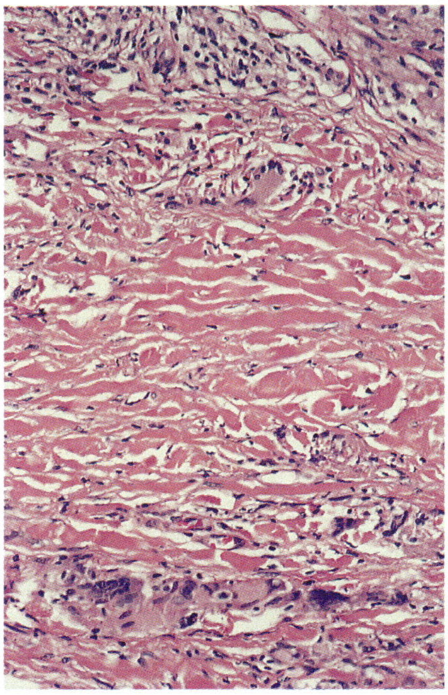

Figure 9–55. Higher magnification of Figure 9–54 demonstrates a central zone of fibrotic dermis sandwiched between two bands of inflammatory infiltrate composed of lymphocytes and histiocytes, some of which are multinucleated.

Elastolytic Granuloma

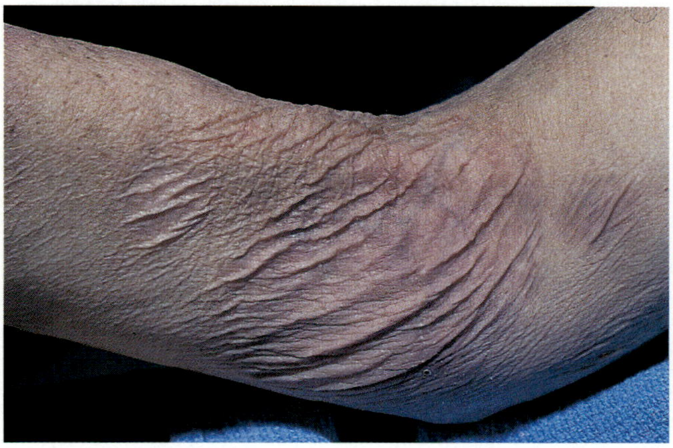

Figure 9–56. The clinical appearance of elastolytic granuloma demonstrates the consequence of loss of dermal elastic recoil; the lesion is more wrinkled and redundant than the surrounding, unaffected skin.

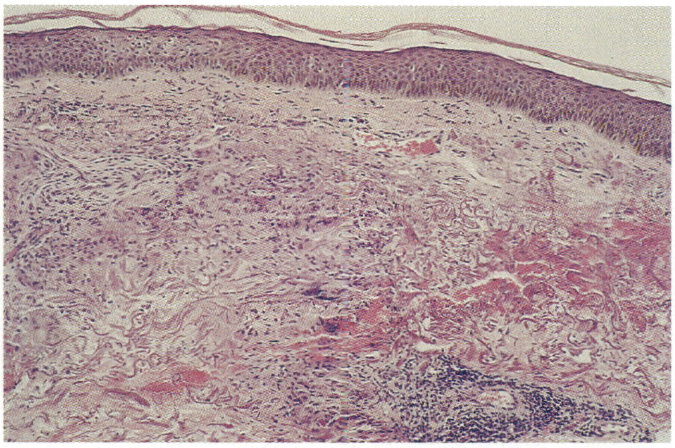

Figure 9–57. A biopsy specimen reveals a patchy granulomatous infiltrate within the dermis.

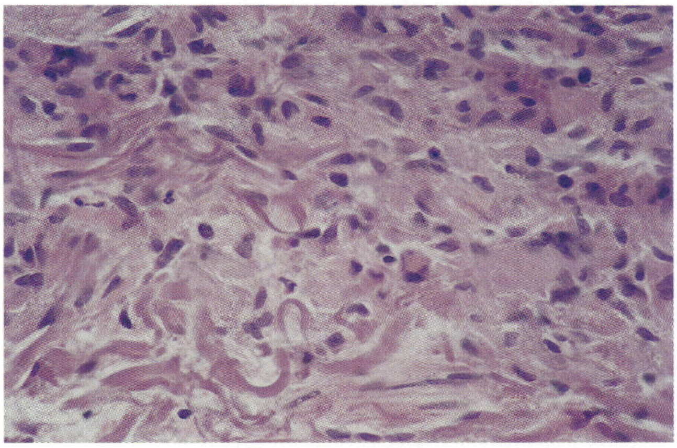

Figure 9–58. On higher magnification, this demonstrates phagocytosis of altered and fragmented elastic fibers by histiocytes within the granulomas.

Granulomatous Cheilitis

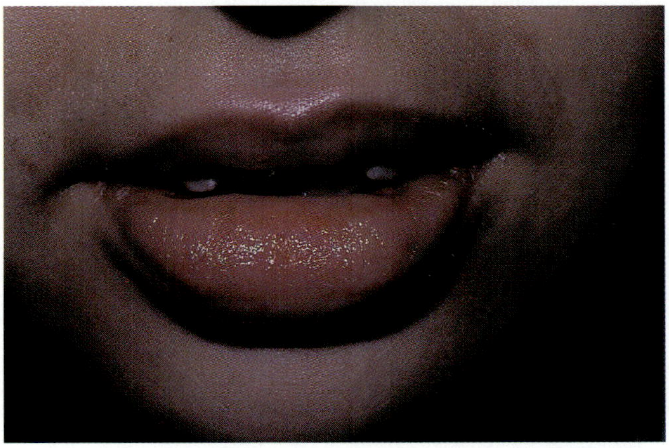

Figure 9–59. Clinical manifestations of granulomatous cheilitis include development of permanent swelling and induration of the lips.

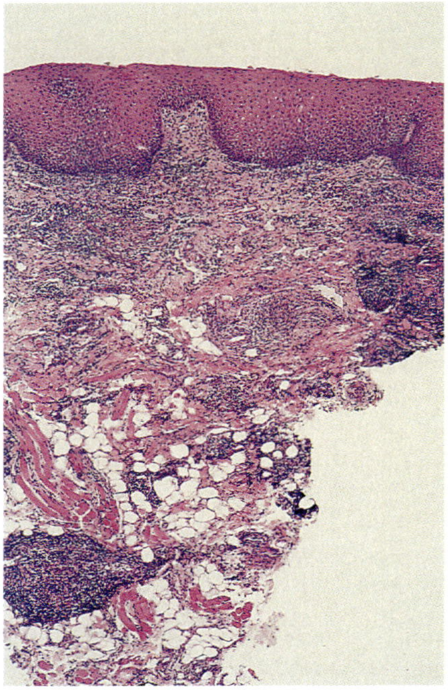

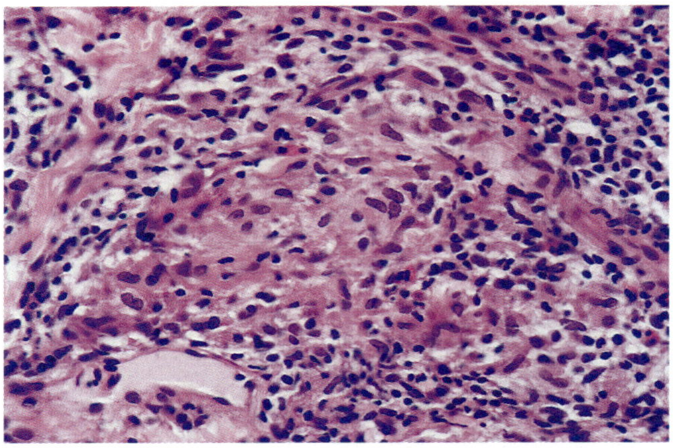

Figures 9–60 and 9–61. Biopsy specimens reveal multiple sarcoidal granulomas within submucosal connective tissue. Extension into fat or underlying muscle may occur.

Wegener Granulomatosis

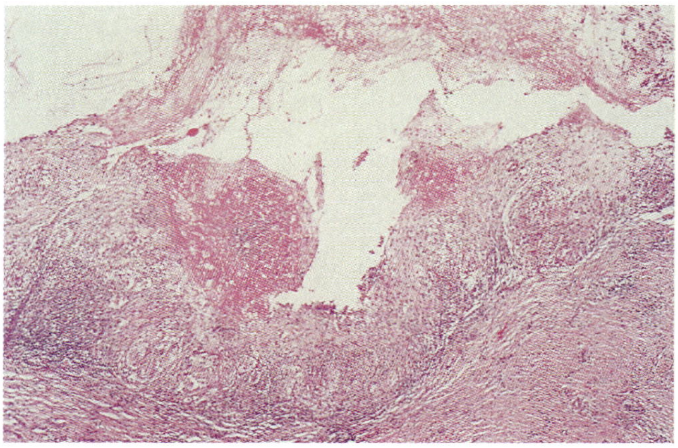

Figure 9–62. Wegener granulomatosis. At scanning magnification, there is epidermal and dermal ulceration associated with a brisk, underlying, inflammatory infiltrate.

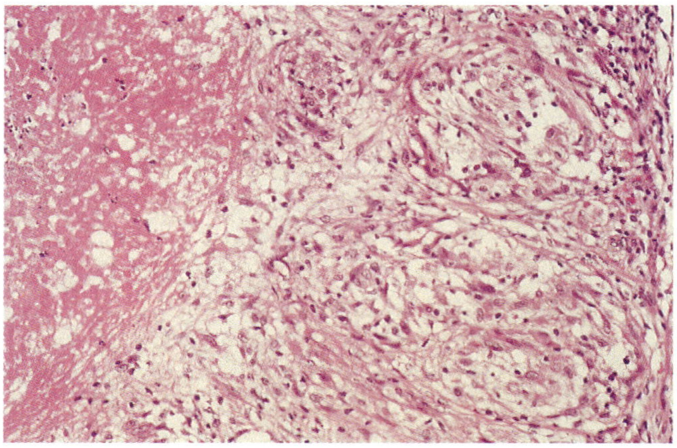

Figure 9–63. Characteristic features at higher magnification include geographic zones of fibrinoid necrosis *(top left)* bordered by a loosely aggregated granulomatous response.

10

Cutaneous Panniculitis

The word *panniculitis* implies a primary inflammatory process involving the subcutaneous fat. Panniculitis may arise as an immunologic disorder in which antigenic targets specifically located in characteristic regions of the subcutis (*e.g.,* septa or lobules) are attacked by host inflammatory cells. Alternatively, panniculitis may be the result of ischemia to the subcutis, with secondary invasion of inflammatory cells. In addition, panniculitis may arise when endogenous enzymes (*e.g.,* as in pancreatitis or pancreatic carcinoma) or exogenous toxic substances gain access to subcutaneous tissue. Finally, infectious processes centered predominantly within the fat or infiltrative processes involving the hematopoietic system can result in secondary inflammatory changes in subcutaneous fat that may closely mimic primarily immunologic insults.

Unlike the epidermis and dermis, the subcutaneous fat reacts to inflammation and trauma in a limited number of ways. Fat becomes neither hyperplastic nor hypertrophied in response to trauma, and extracellular fluid within the fat is usually localized to the adventitial connective tissue that courses through the thin septa that separate lobules composed of confluent aggregates of adipocytes. Fat undergoing necrosis frequently provokes a histiocytic inflammatory response in which lipid is engulfed by macrophages to form foamy cells similar to xanthoma cells. Zones of fat necrosis frequently resolve with fibrosis, although microcysts may form in regions of fat necrosis before infiltration by fibroblasts and vessels. Dissolution of the cell membranes of adipocytes produces pooled regions of lipid frequently referred to as *liquefactive fat necrosis.* Such zones may have a pale-blue hue. Accumulation of pale-pink material between intact adipocytes often signifies atrophy and a peculiar associated form of fibrosis referred to as *hyalinization,* which is typically encountered in lupus panniculitis. Degenerating and necrotic adipocytes also may undergo *saponification,* in which calcium salts are deposited in zones of fat necrosis. Occasionally, the lipid within the degenerating adipocytes may form needle-shaped clefts, as seen in the rare disorder subcutaneous fat necrosis of the newborn and in *sclerosing lipogranuloma* (an iatrogenic disorder representing a response to injected oils or paraffin).

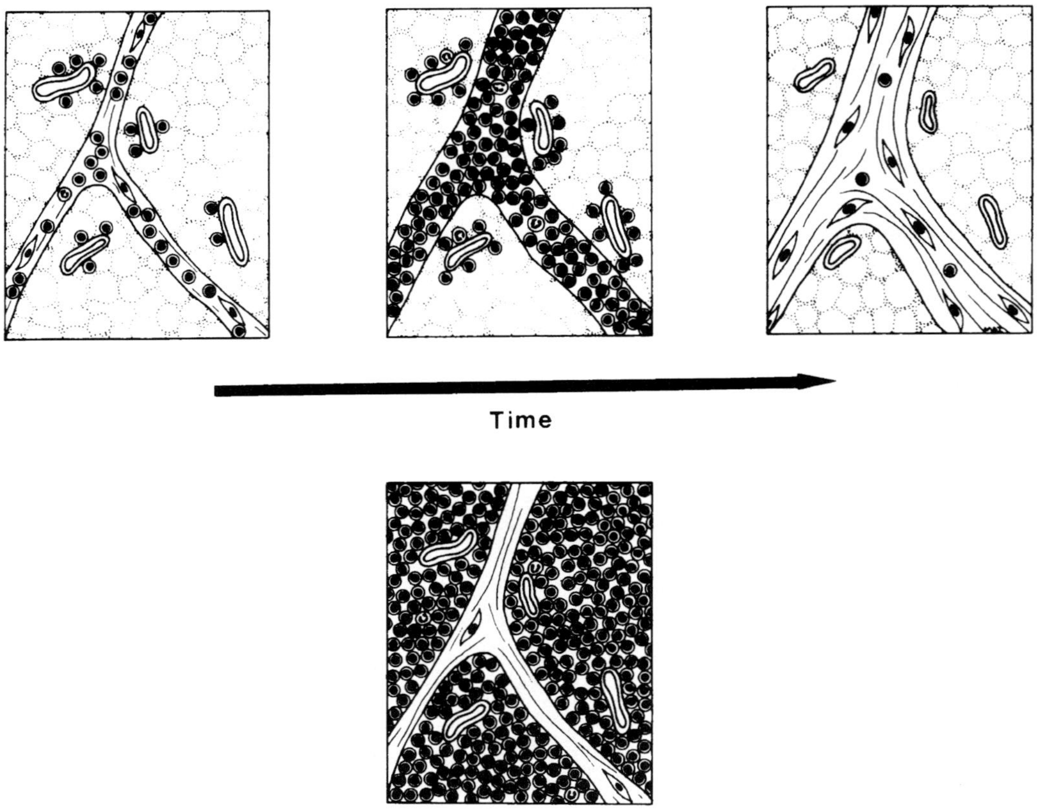

Figure 10–1. Schematic representation of the temporal evolution of septal panniculitis. The earliest inflammatory events involve small venules within septa and in paraseptal adipose tissue *(top left).* This inflammation results in gradual widening of the septum as it becomes filled with mononuclear cells *(top middle).* At this point, perivenular inflammation in paraseptal adipose tissue may also be prominent, but this limited involvement of the lobule should not be confused with true lobular panniculitis *(bottom middle),* in which lobules are diffusely involved by inflammation and septa are relatively spared. With chronicity, the septum may become permanently thickened by scar tissue *(top right).*

Erythema Nodosum

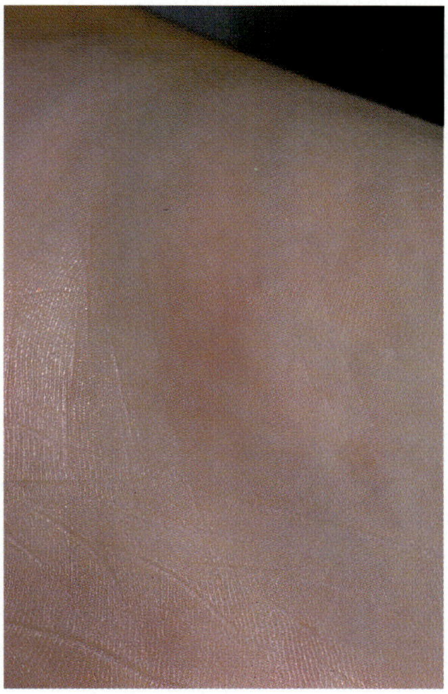

Figure 10–2. A poorly defined, erythematous, painful, deep-seated nodule is typical of early erythema nodosum.

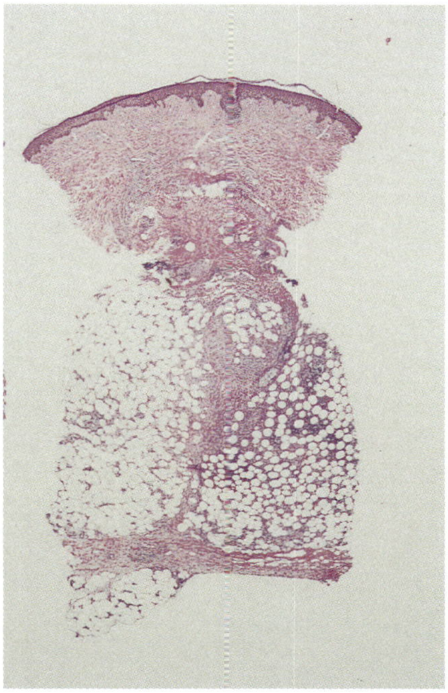

Figure 10–3. Scanning magnification reveals inflammation and expansion of a septum *(center)* within the subcutis. There also is some degree of paraseptal lobular involvement, perhaps accentuated by a tangential plane of section.

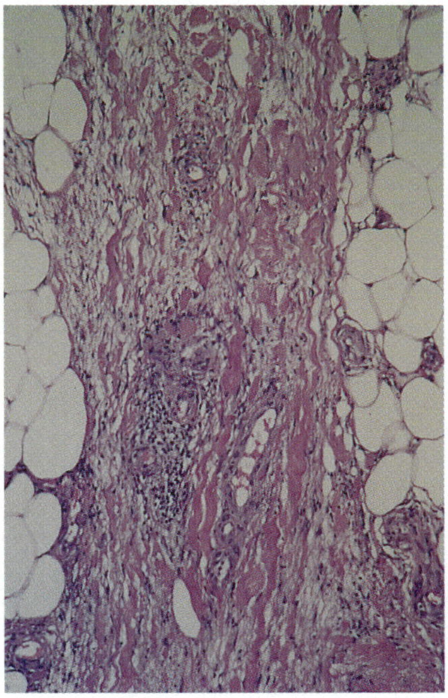

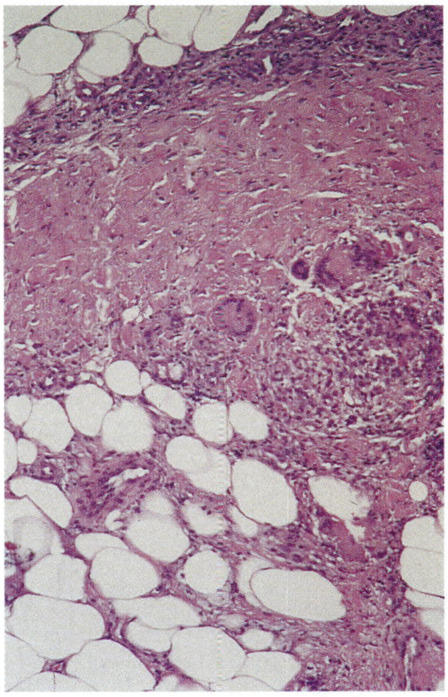

Figures 10–4 and 10–5. Inspection at higher magnification reveals granulomatous aggregates within edematous septa, perivenular lymphocytic infiltrates, variable numbers of eosinophils, and occasional giant cells. Vasculitis is not present.

Erythema Induratum

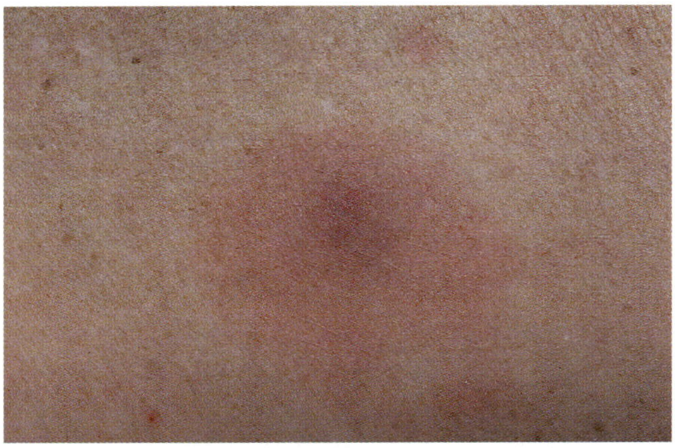

Figure 10–6. Erythema induratum. The gross pathology consists of indurated, erythematous, painful lesions. There is a dusky purple center surrounded by a pale-pink rim of erythema.

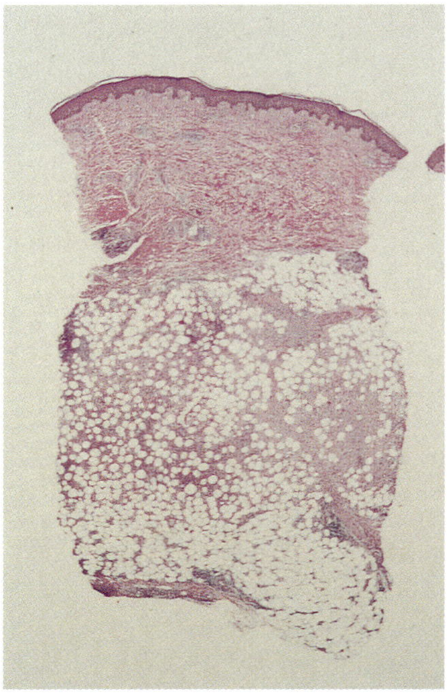

Figure 10–7. Biopsy specimens reveal diffuse inflammation within the lobule *(center).*

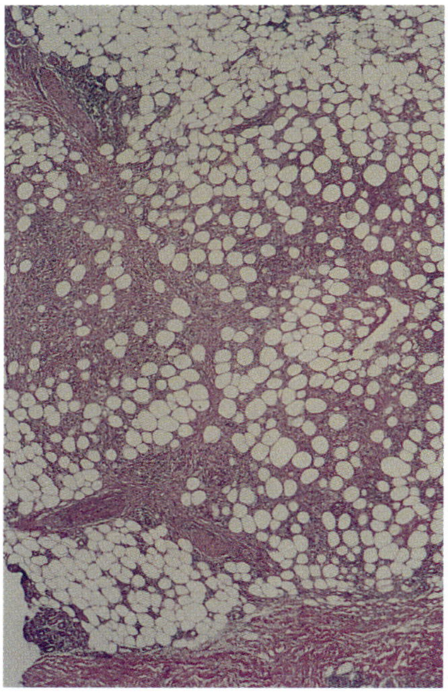

Figure 10–8. In contrast to erythema nodosum, vascular injury is focally observed *(bottom left).*

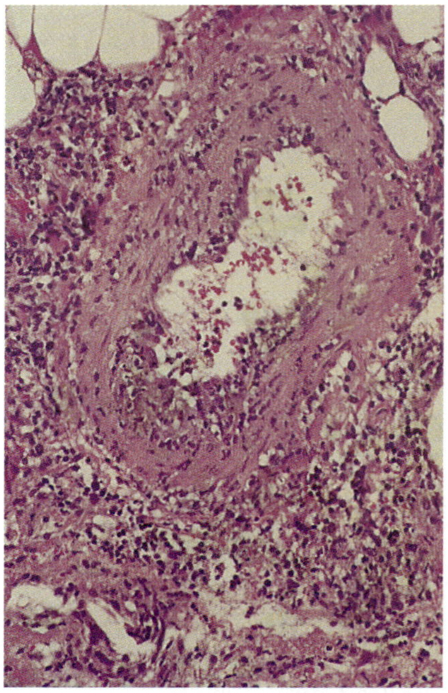

Figure 10–9. Erythema induratum. Higher magnification of the inflammatory infiltrate reveals foci of vasculitis.

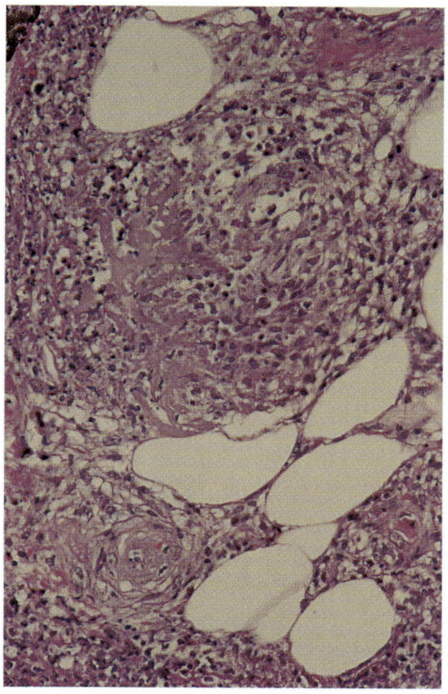

Figure 10–10. Higher magnification of the inflammatory infiltrate also reveals necrosis within granulomatous foci *(center)*.

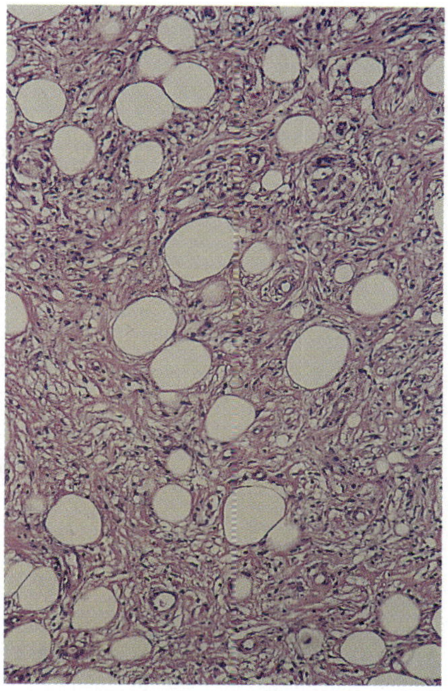

Figure 10–11. Older lesions may show diffuse fibrosis within the lobule.

Polyarteritis Nodosa with Panniculitis

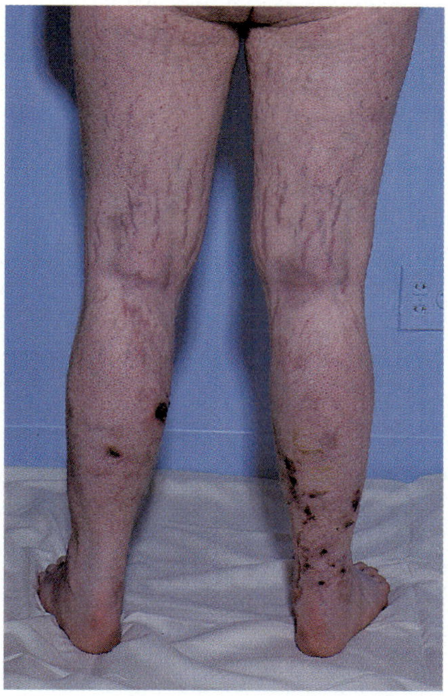

Figure 10–12. Panniculitis associated with polyarteritis nodosa. The lower extremities of this transplant patient are enlarged and indurated due to diffuse panniculitis. Focally, overlying skin has broken down, suggesting associated ischemia. The striae on the posterior thighs are a result of chronic treatment with corticosteroids.

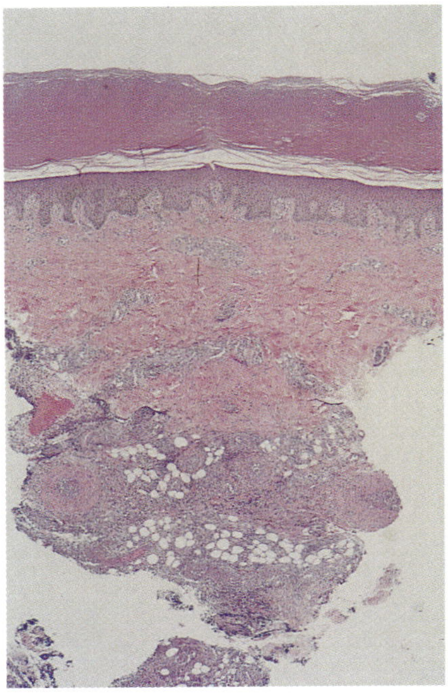

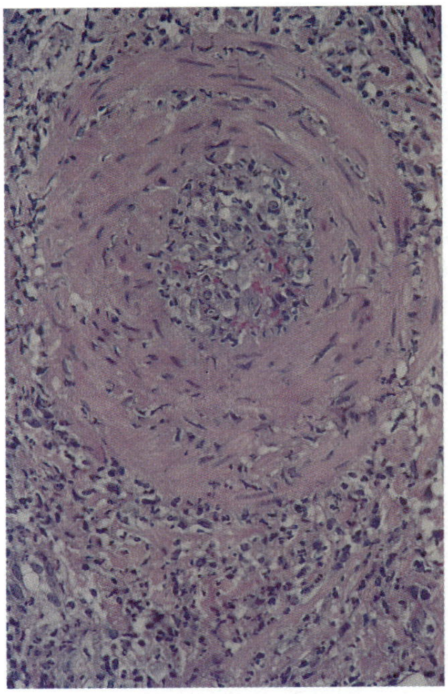

Figures 10–13 and 10–14. Biopsy specimens from the foot reveal vasculitis, characterized by neutrophils and mononuclear cells. The affected vessels were confirmed to be medium-sized arteries by elastic tissue staining, which allowed detection of residual, albeit fragmented, internal elastic laminae.

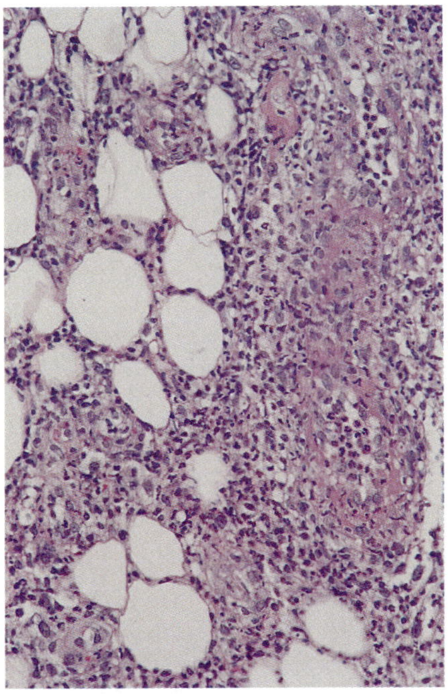

Figure 10–15. Biopsy specimens from the foot also reveal secondary lobular panniculitis, involving neutrophils and mononuclear cells. Although erythema induratum also may show vasculitis and panniculitis, both arteries and veins are involved, and the primary lobular panniculitis is granulomatous, often resembling infection with tubercle bacilli.

Lupus Panniculitis

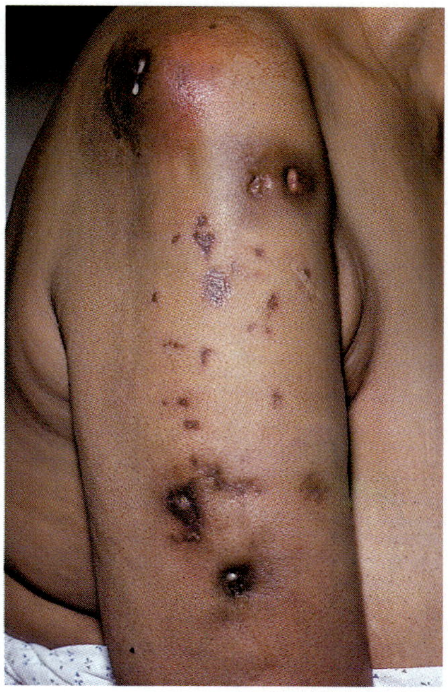

Figure 10–16. Panniculitis of lupus erythematosus. Multiple erythematous nodules are present, many with central ulceration.

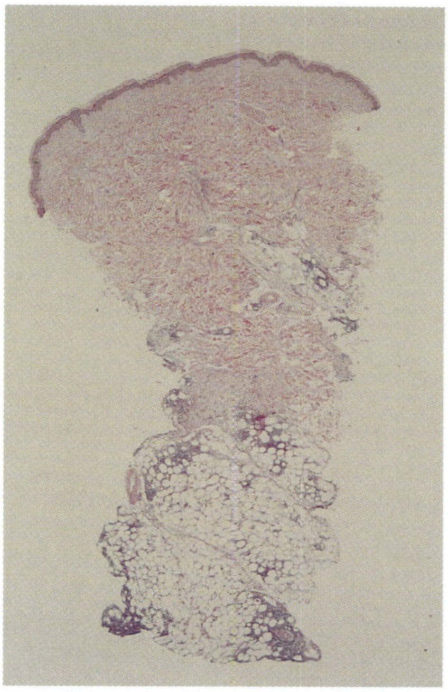

Figure 10–17. Scanning magnification of an early lesion shows deep dermal and subcutaneous aggregates of mononuclear cells. Eccrine coils, when present, are also frequently involved by the inflammatory infiltrate.

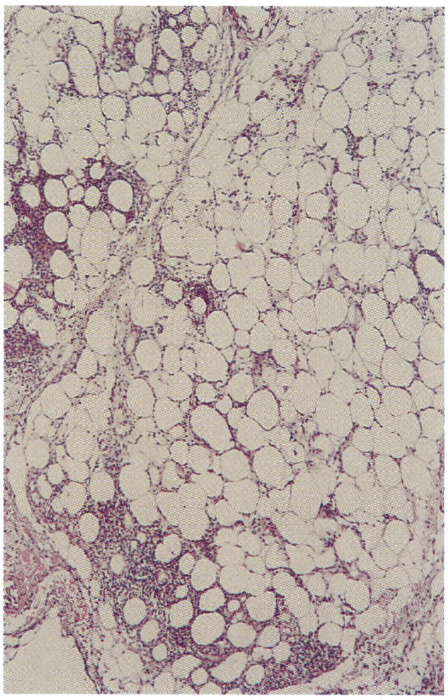

Figure 10–18. Lymphocytes and plasma cells predominate in this focus; adipocytes within the lobule are variably atrophic and separated by characteristic, pale, hyalinized matrix *(top right)*.

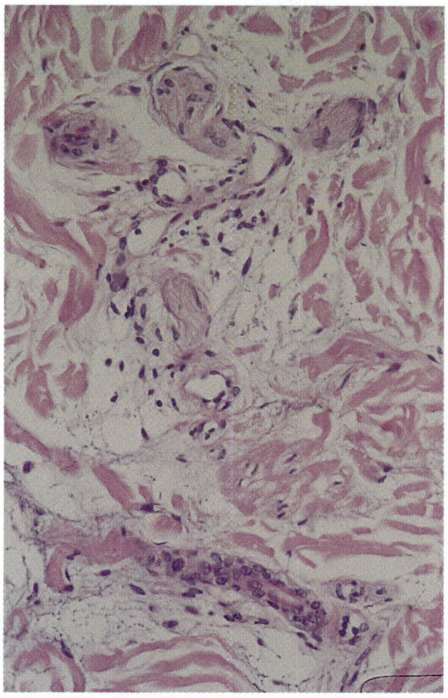

Figure 10–19. Thin, beady strands of pale blue mucin are conspicuous about neurovascular bundles and eccrine epithelium.

Miscellaneous Forms of Panniculitis

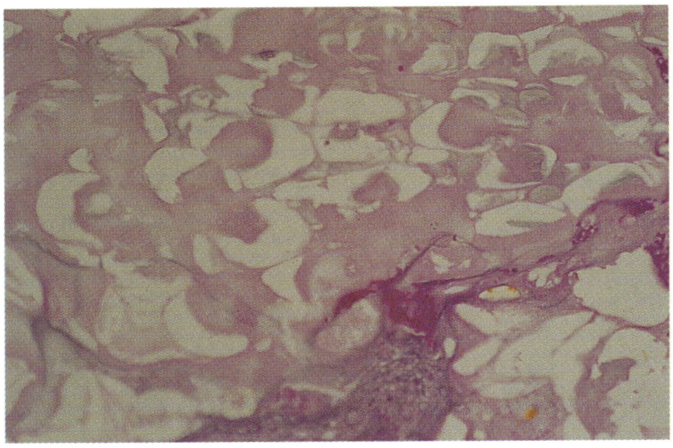

Figure 10–20. Panniculitis of pancreatitis and pancreatic carcinoma is characterized by hyalinized, coagulative necrosis of adipocytes within the lobule and associated saponification with calcification *(bottom center).*

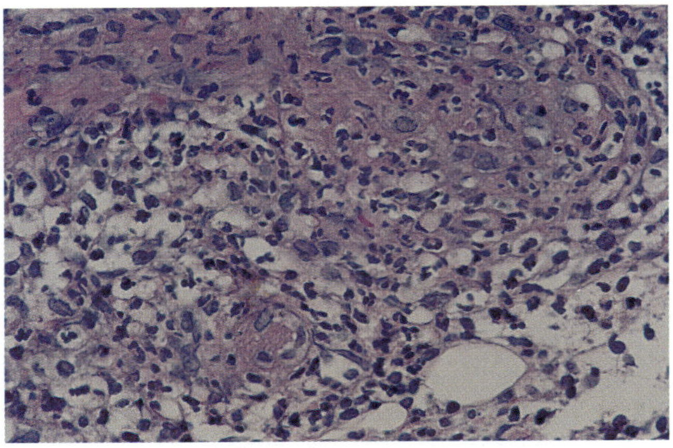

Figure 10–21. Mixed inflammation in a fat lobule without a specific pattern of primary panniculitis prompted special stains for fungi and mycobacteria in this case of infectious panniculitis.

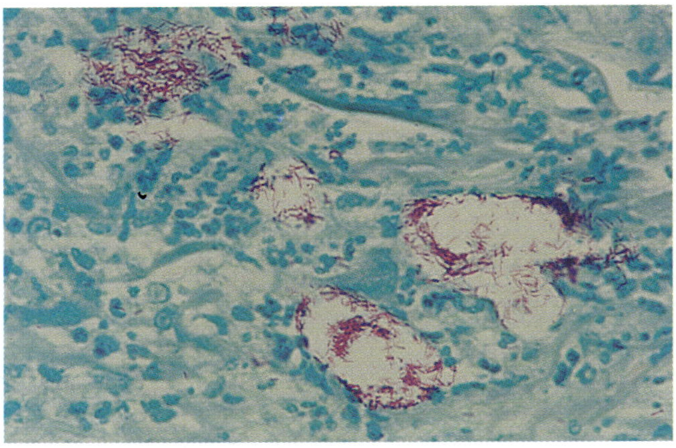

Figure 10–22. In this case (see Fig. 10–21), atypical mycobacteria were detected in large numbers.

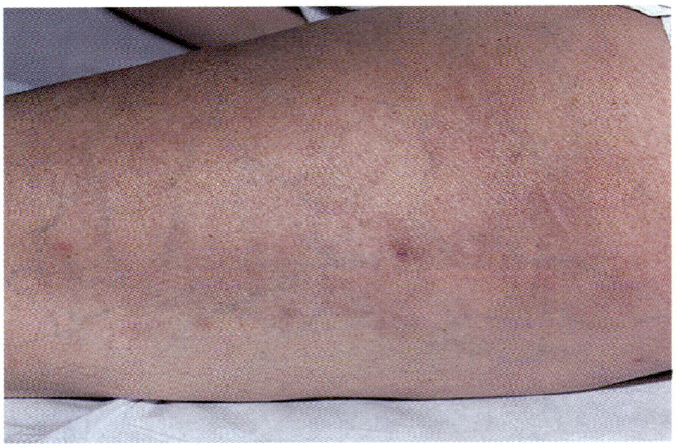

Figure 10–23. Factitial panniculitis. Indurated, erythematous skin with residual small papules and pinpoint scabs representing injection sites.

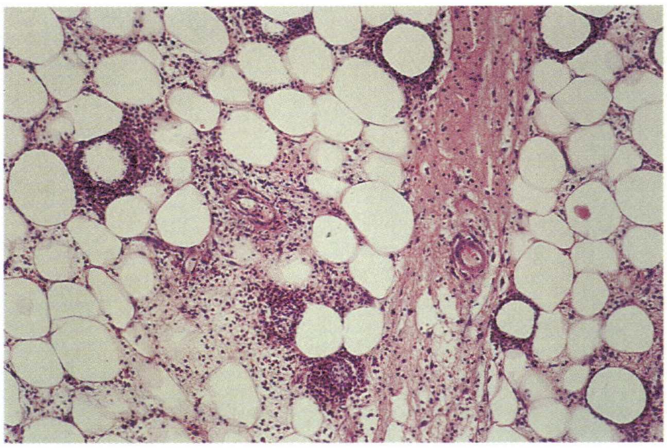

Figure 10–24. Factitial panniculitis may be both septal and lobular, and inflammatory cells are focally tightly clustered about individual cells, potentially indicating uneven distribution of the injected toxic material.

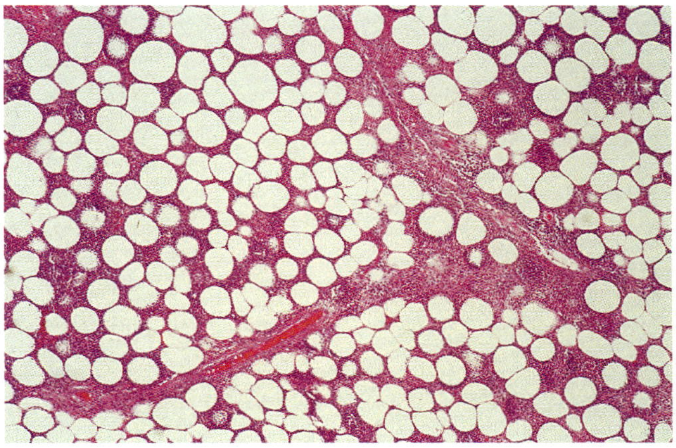

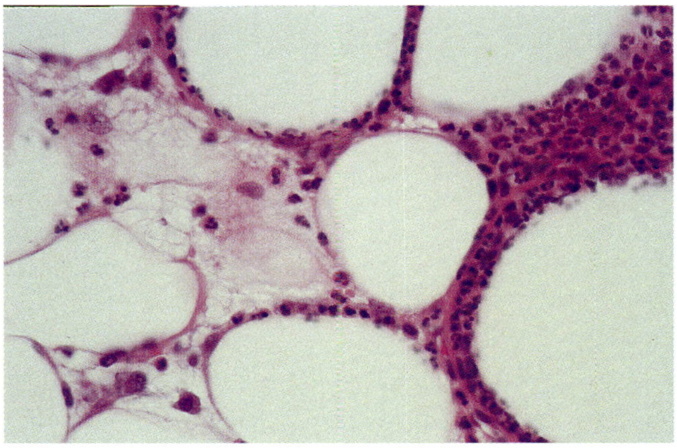

Figures 10–25 and 10–26. Relapsing febrile nodular nonsuppurative panniculitis (Weber-Christian disease). In the earliest stages, characteristic histologic changes include diffuse lobular infiltration by inflammatory cells, predominantly neutrophils (Fig. 10–25) and foci of degenerating adipocytes (Fig. 10–26, *left of field*). In contrast to infectious panniculitus, discrete microabscesses do not occur.

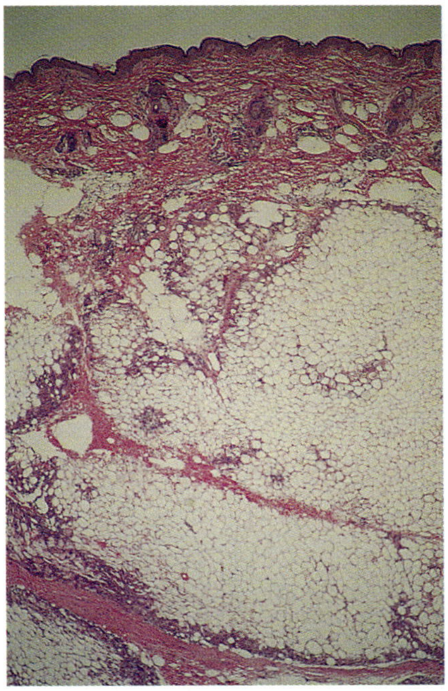

Figure 10–27. Subcutaneous fat necrosis of the newborn. Mixed inflammatory cells are centered about lobular aggregates of degenerating subcutaneous fat.

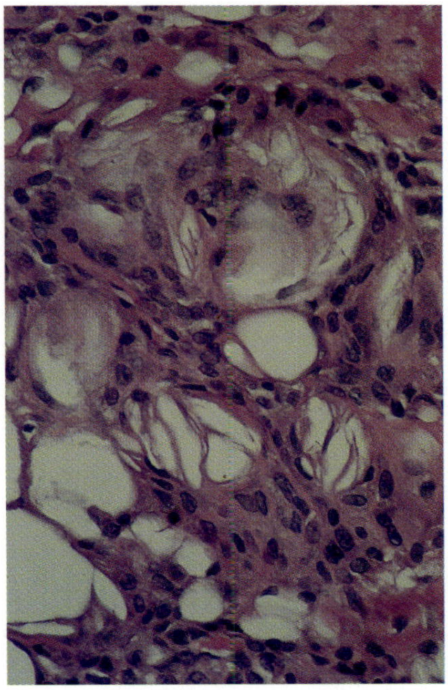

Figure 10–28. Individual adipocytes (see Fig. 10–27) contain characteristic clefts within their cytoplasm, which on polarization of frozen sections represent birefringent crystals.

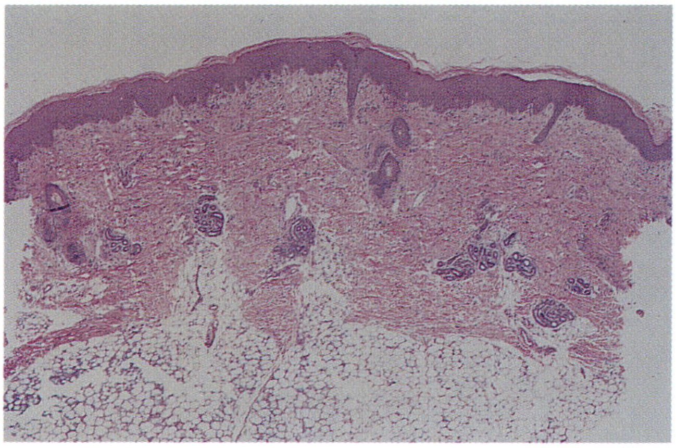

Figure 10–29. Sclerema neonatorum. In contrast to subcutaneous fat necrosis of the newborn, inflammation is inconspicuous to absent; therefore, it does not represent a true panniculitis.

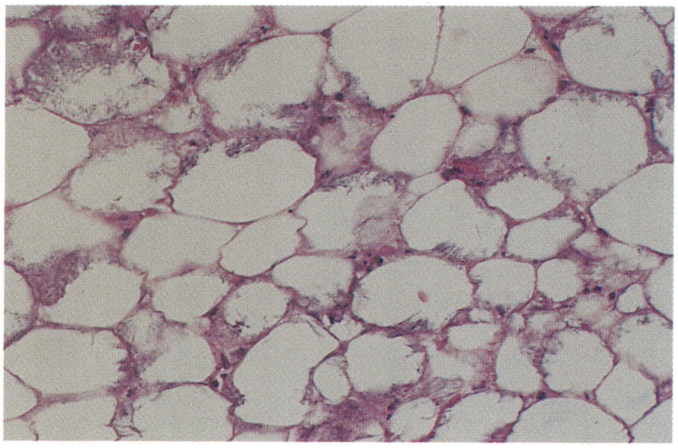

Figure 10–30. Individual adipocytes (see Fig. 10–29) contain fine, needle-shaped clefts at the cell perimeter.

III

Neoplasms

11

Epidermal Tumors

Tumors of the surface epidermis can be one of the most diagnostically problematic areas in dermatopathology. Major issues, such as the difference between benign and malignant, arise routinely. Moreover, many of the neoplasms have ambiguous or vague architectural or cytologic features that defy accurate classification. A major problem is that chronically inflamed keratoses acquire a degree of reactive atypia that may superficially mimic carcinoma. Specific examples of this potential pitfall are demonstrated, and histologic features are portrayed for differentiation of reactive nuclear alterations from true dysplasia and anaplasia within keratinocytes.

In describing cutaneous epidermal neoplasms, it is important to understand the meanings of the words *dysplasia, anaplasia,* and *atypia.* The same issues, of course, are related to tumors of adnexal epithelium and melanocytes, which are illustrated later. For this discussion, the word *dysplasia* (*dys-* means abnormal or faulty, and the Greek word *plasis* means development or, literally, molding) refers to cytologic and architectural characteristics with some but not all of the characteristics of malignancy. *Anaplasia,* on the other hand, connotes the prototypic malignant cell, devoid of significant differentiation. *Atypia,* perhaps the most problematic of the terms, simply means not typical or normal. In a sense, therefore, dysplastic cellular processes are atypical. However, atypia encompasses much more than dysplasia. There are, for example, the reactive atypia of an inflamed epithelial neoplasm or a re-epithelializing ulcer base and the degenerative atypia of virally infected or metabolically poisoned cells. Understanding and correctly using these terms are critical to an algorithmic approach to differential diagnosis of cutaneous epithelial tumors.

The tinctorial characteristics of epidermal tumors are an important adjunct to accurate diagnosis. Although benign basaloid tumors (*e.g.,* seborrheic keratoses) tend to be symmetric basophilic nodules or plaques at scanning magnification, squamoid tumors (*e.g.,* keratoacanthomas) are considerably more eosinophilic. The same is true for basal and squamous cell carcinoma, with the former often presenting as discrete blue nests and nodules in the dermis and the latter presenting as infiltrative pink cords and fascicles. At a cytologic level, the degree of nuclear basophilia may correlate with dysplasia, as dark-blue heterochromatin becomes coarsely aggregated within affected nuclei. Virally infected nuclei of ordinary warts, on the other hand, characteristically are recognized by their steel-gray pallor. Cytoplasmic inclusions in molluscum contagiosum *(molluscum bodies)* are differentiated from condensed cytokeratin aggregates of ordinary warts by virtue of the tendency of the former to be more "red in the blue layer" (stratum granulosum) and more "blue in the red layer" (stratum corneum), a phenomenon related to alterations in viral structure as the particles pass from lower to higher epidermal strata.

Epidermal Nevus

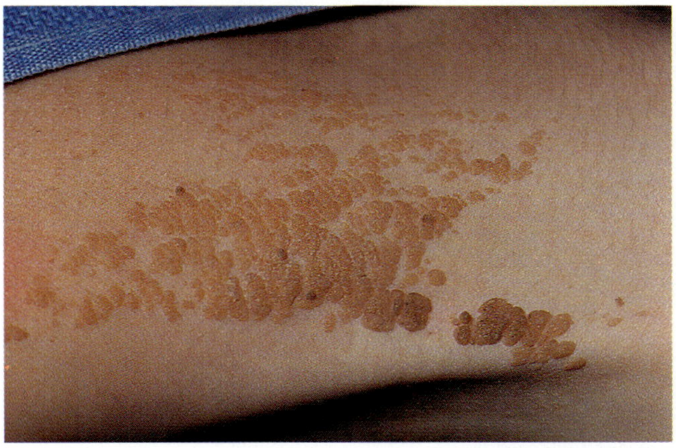

Figure 11–1. Clinical appearance of epidermal nevus. Typical lesions are grouped, with keratosis-like plaques arranged in linear array.

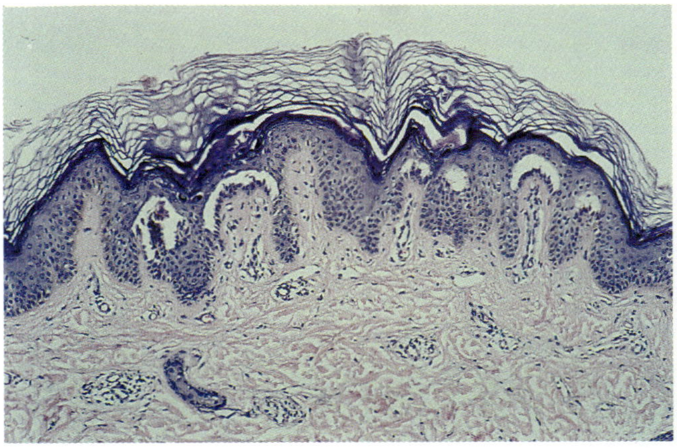

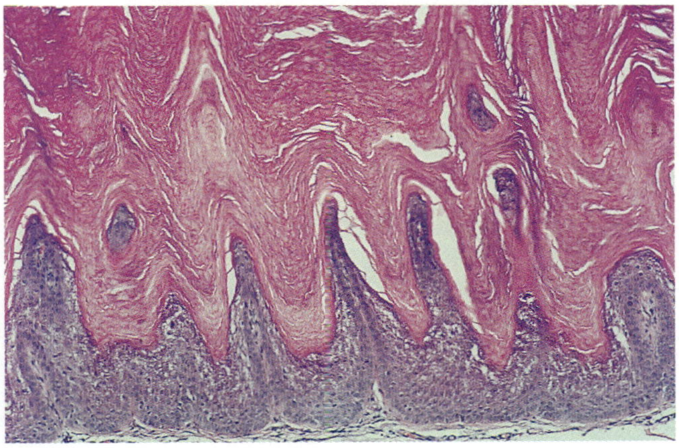

Figures 11–2 and 11–3. Histologically, verrucous acanthosis begins abruptly and is accompanied by various degrees of hyperkeratosis. Lesions may closely resemble those of seborrheic keratosis, and correlation with clinical parameters is generally required in formulating a correct diagnosis. Note that the lesions also show secondary focal acantholytic dyskeratosis (Fig. 11–2) and epidermolytic hyperkeratosis (Fig. 11–3).

Acanthosis Nigricans

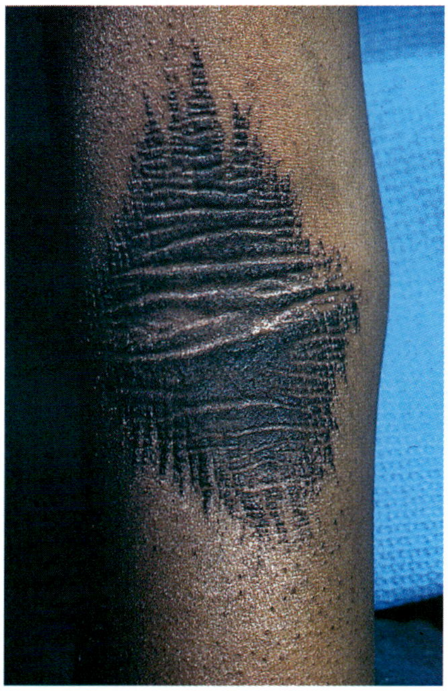

Figure 11–4. Acanthosis nigricans. This hyperpigmented plaque is characteristically located in a flexural crease or an intertriginous region.

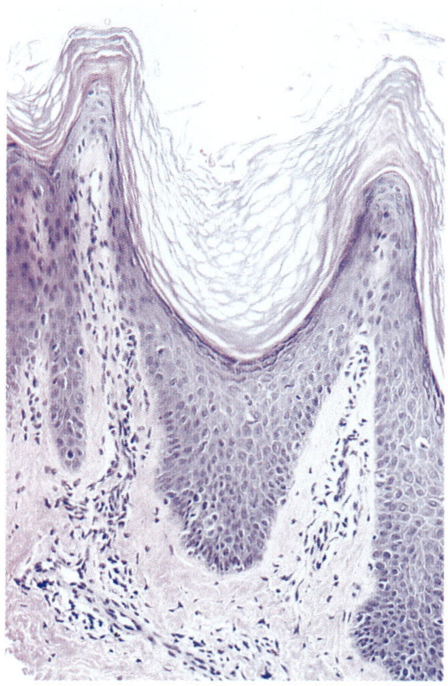

Figure 11–5. Histologically, there is papillomatosis and mild epidermal hyperplasia with hyperkeratosis. Findings may be subtle, appear nonspecific, or be mistaken for an epidermal nevus or seborrheic keratosis.

Seborrheic Keratosis

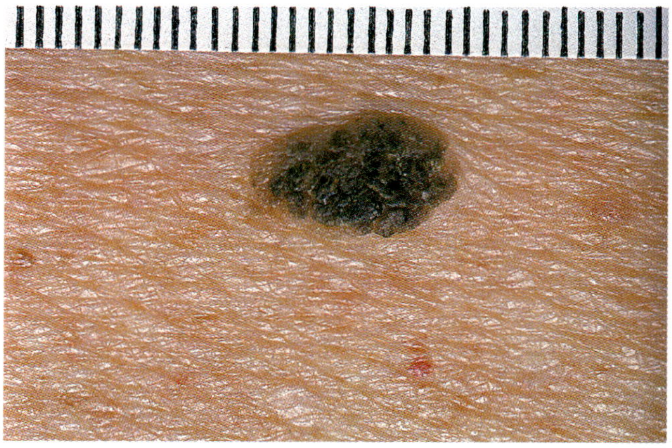

Figure 11–6. Gross pathology of seborrheic keratosis is a well-defined, hyperkeratotic, pigmented plaque that appears to be stuck onto the epidermal surface. Keratotic plugs may be helpful in distinguishing these lesions from those of melanocytic origin.

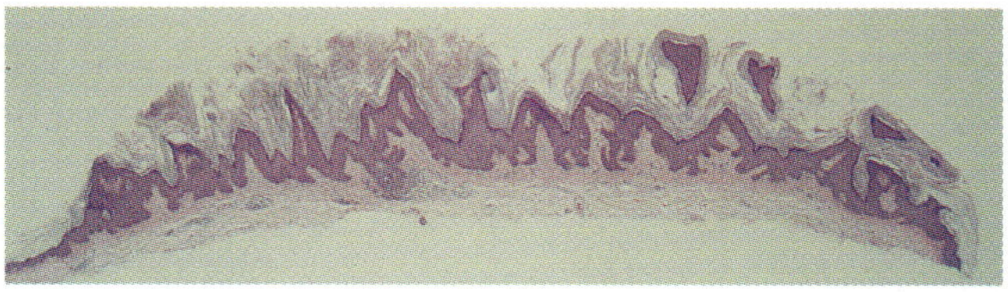

Figure 11–7. At scanning magnification, seborrheic keratoses may have an exophytic verrucous surface.

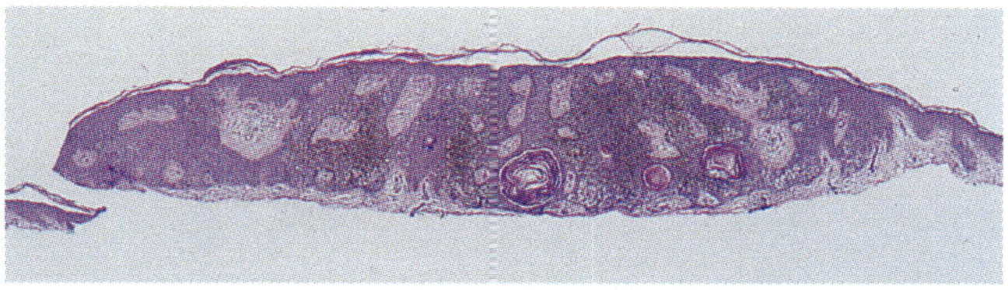

Figure 11–8. At scanning magnification, seborrheic keratoses also may show endophytic growth.

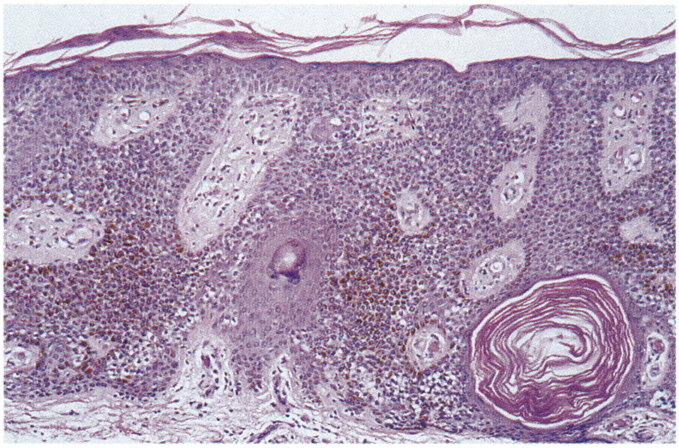

Figure 11–9. Common to all lesions is proliferation of benign basaloid epithelial cells, which resemble normal stratum basalis. The associated dermis is thickened and hyalinized just below the dermal-epidermal junction of the tumor. This is an important diagnostic clue when dealing with curetted, tangentially oriented fragments.

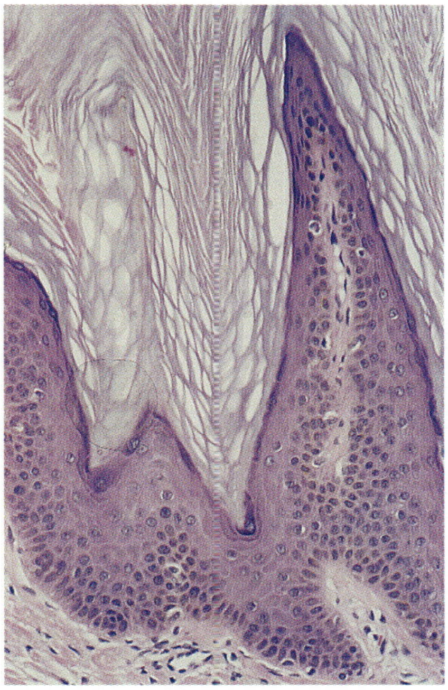

Figure 11–10. The scale of seborrheic keratosis is generally hyperkeratotic, with a prominent, basket-weave appearance.

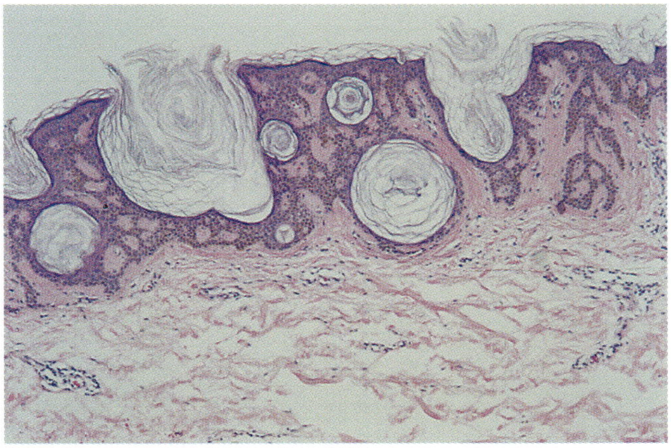

Figure 11–11. Prominent keratin-filled horn cysts are present within the tumor *(center)* or communicate with the epidermal surface (*i.e.,* pseudohorn cysts).

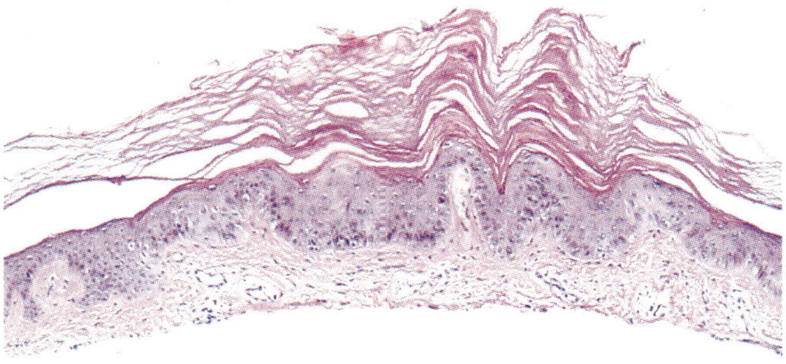

Figure 11–12. Large cell acanthoma variant is composed of squamoid cells that are several times the diameter of normal keratinocytes within the adjacent stratum spinosum.

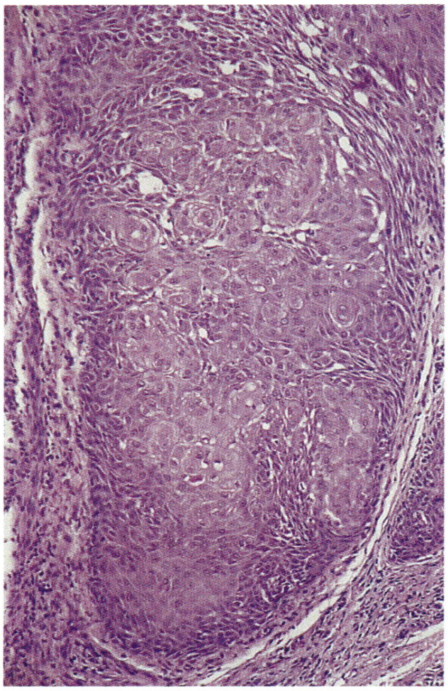

Figure 11–13. Irritated seborrheic keratosis is characterized by prominent squamatization and eddy formation.

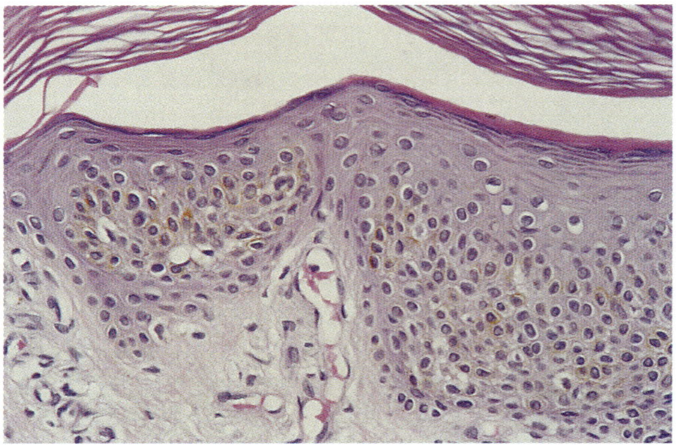

Figure 11–14. In intraepidermal epithelioma pattern, basaloid elements are nested within an otherwise normal epidermal layer.

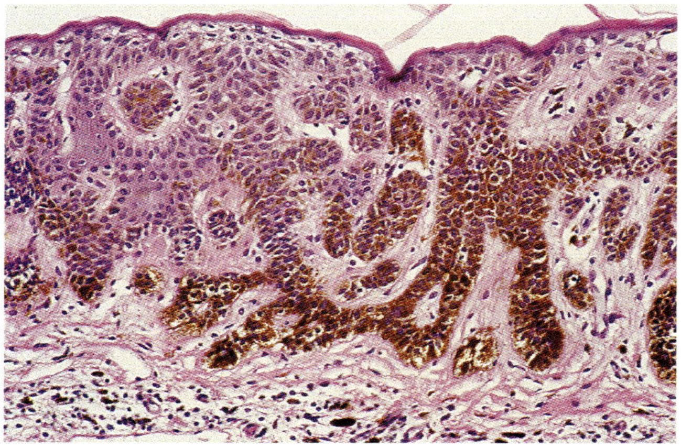

Figure 11–15. In the adenoidal variant of seborrheic keratosis, there are heavily melanized endophytic cords of pigmented neoplastic epithelium within the superficial dermis.

Clear Cell Acanthoma

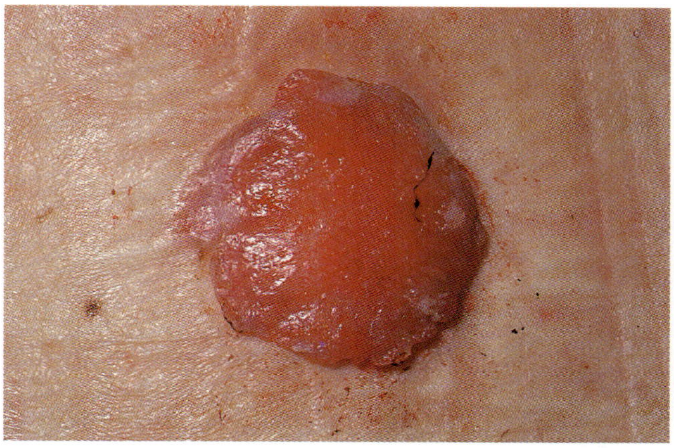

Figure 11–16. Clear cell acanthoma. This lesion from the lower extremity demonstrates a typical oozing surface; the clinical impression was basal cell carcinoma.

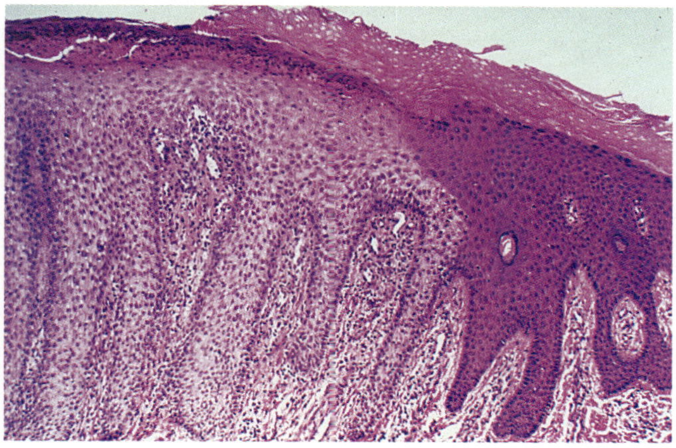

Figure 11–17. The biopsy specimen reveals a well-demarcated endophytic neoplasm sharply juxtaposed with the adjacent epidermis because of the clear, highly glycogenated cytoplasm of the tumor cells.

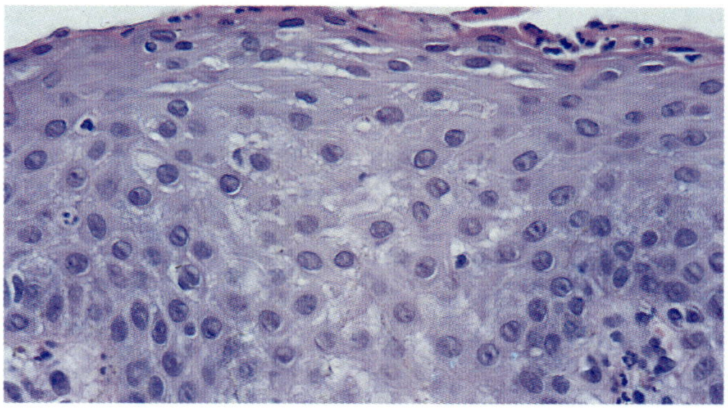

Figure 11–18. An additional diagnostic feature is the presence of neutrophils that percolate within the epithelial elements of this neoplasm.

Keratoacanthoma

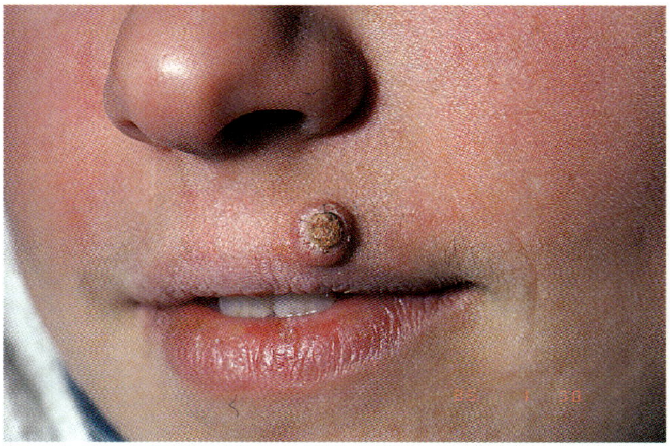

Figure 11–19. Keratoacanthoma. This crater-like nodule has a prominent central keratin plug, which, on histologic examination, forms much of the tumor mass.

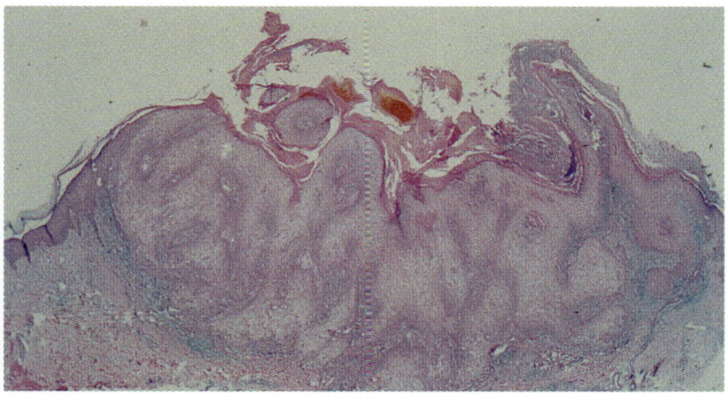

Figure 11–20. The first stage of the histologic sequential evolution of this neoplasm is proliferative, in which epithelial elements predominate.

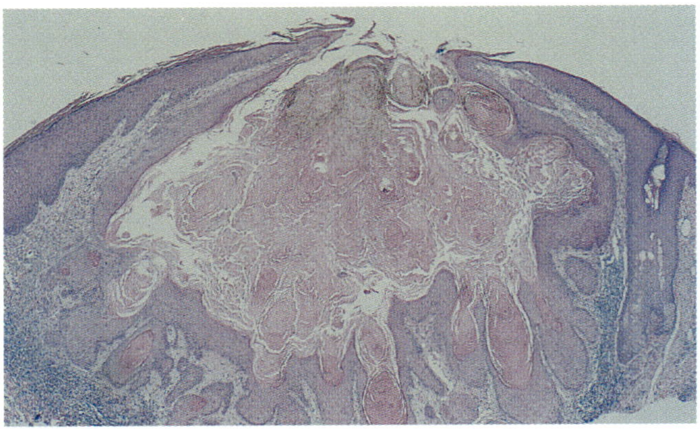

Figure 11–21. In the middle stage, the well-formed keratotic crater is surrounded by endophytic lobules of proliferating epithelium.

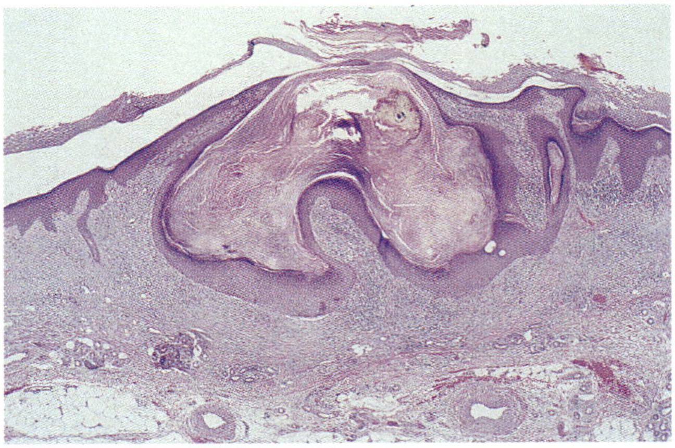

Figure 11–22. In the regressing later phase, there is fibrosis at the base of the lesion, attenuated epithelial elements, and incipient extrusion of the central keratotic plug.

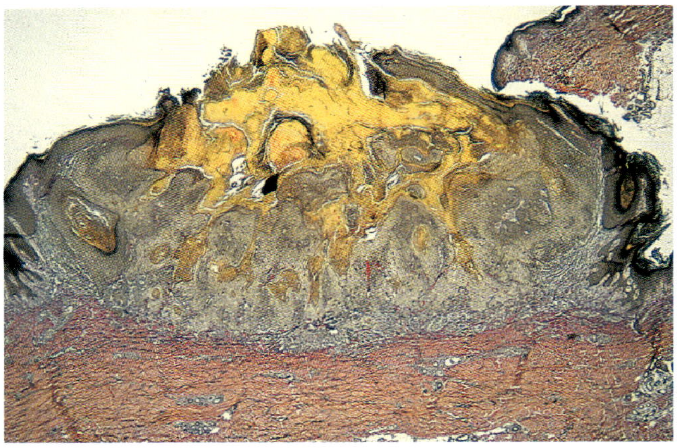

Figure 11–23. Keratoacanthoma: Distinguishing characteristics. Lesions are bilaterally symmetric. (Elastic tissue stain.)

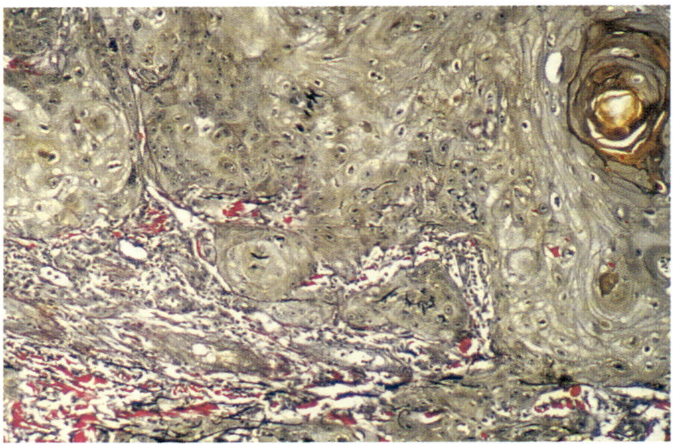

Figure 11–24. The lesions also often contain elastic fibers, which have penetrated into the epithelial elements.

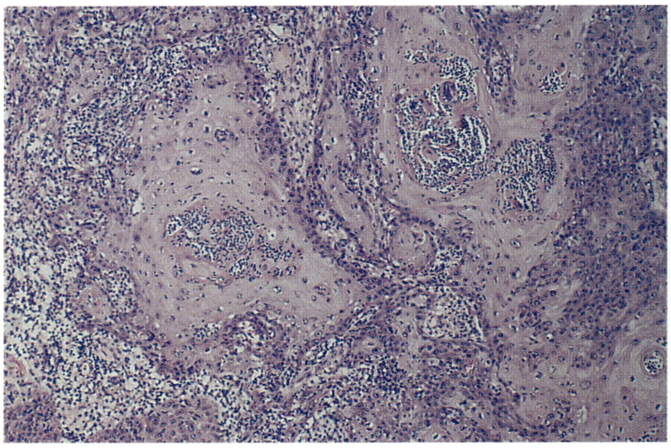

Figure 11–25. Neutrophilic microabscesses are often seen within their epithelial elements; they retain a more basaloid layer at the perimeter of endophytic, pseudoinvasive epithelial lobules.

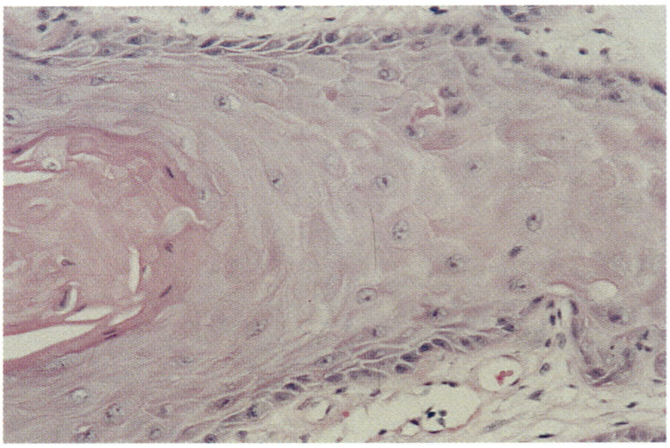

Figure 11–26. The lesions also exhibit glassy, homogeneous cytoplasm with abrupt keratinization devoid of an intervening granular layer (*i.e.,* trichilemmal keratinization).

Warty Dyskeratoma

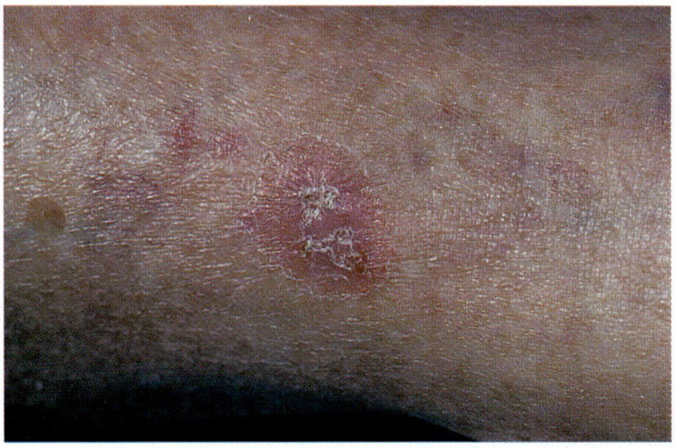

Figure 11–27. Warty dyskeratoma. An erythematous papule with central hyperkeratosis raises the possibility of proliferative actinic keratosis or squamous cell carcinoma.

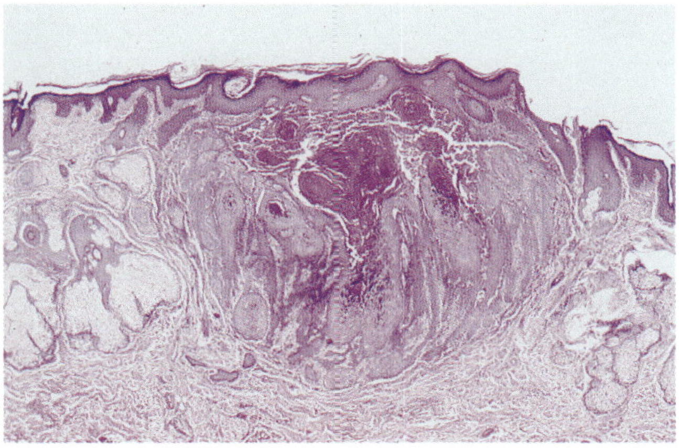

Figure 11–28. A biopsy specimen reveals a verrucous lesion with both exophytic and downward growth into an inflamed dermis. Numerous suprabasal clefts resulting from acantholysis are present.

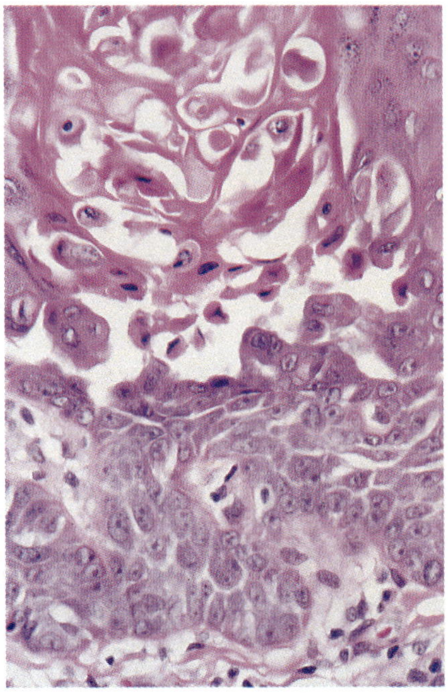

Figure 11–29. Closer examination of the acantholytic tumor cells reveals large, eosinophilic rounded cells with perinuclear halos and small, dense cells with pyknotic nuclei arising in association with parakeratotic scale (*i.e.,* corps ronds and corps grains, respectively).

Verrucae

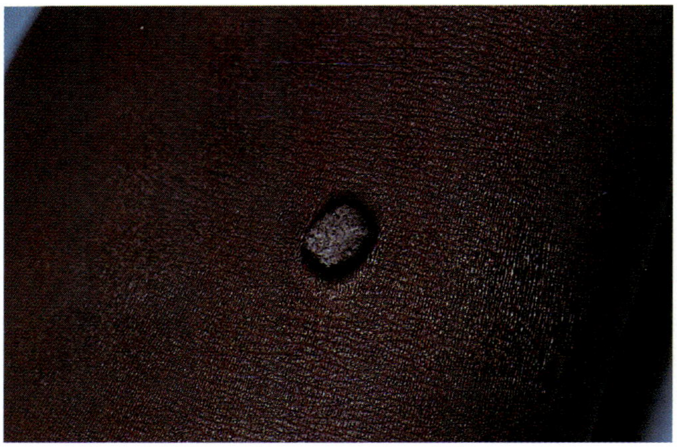

Figure 11–30. The clinical lesion of verruca vulgaris consists of a raised, flat-topped papule with a rough, hyperkeratotic surface.

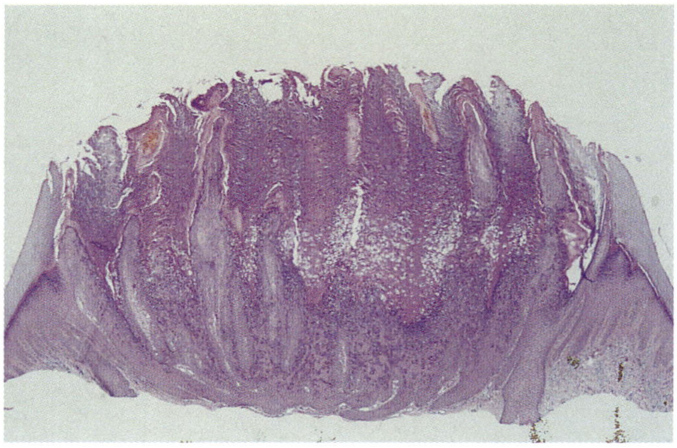

Figure 11–31. Architecturally, lesions are symmetric verrucous keratoses with prominent exophytic as well as endophytic components.

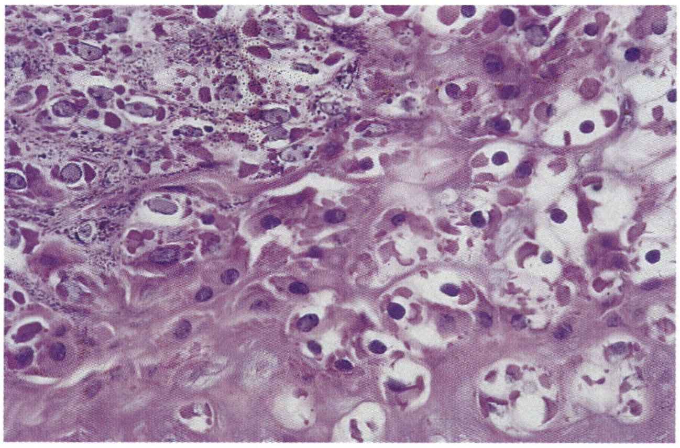

Figure 11–32. Viral cytopathic change is manifested by clearing and pallor of nuclear chromatin, cytoplasmic swelling and vacuolization, and condensation of cytokeratin to form densely eosinophilic intracellular aggregates.

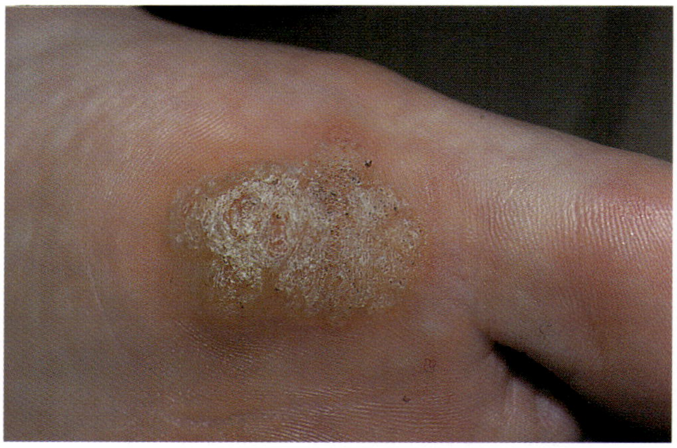

Figure 11–33. Verruca plantaris. A slightly raised, hyperkeratotic plaque characteristically affects the ball of the foot; note punctate zones of hemorrhage from superficial wart vessels.

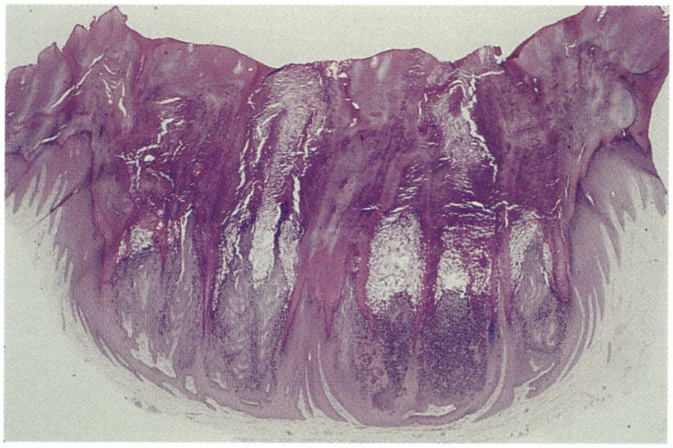

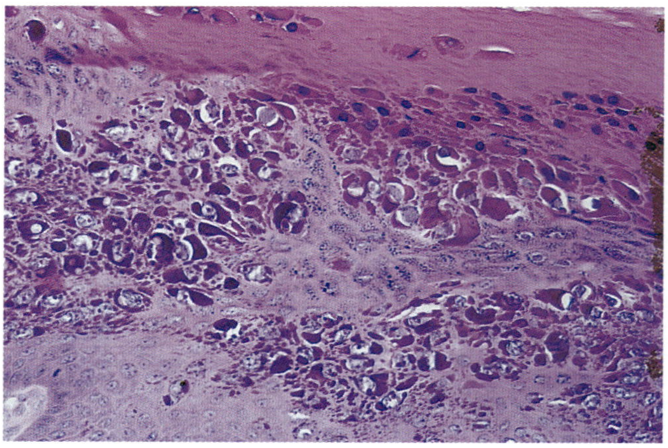

Figures 11–34 and 11–35. Histologically, these lesions differ from verruca vulgaris in their mainly endophytic architecture (Fig. 11–34) and the prominence of condensed cytokeratin, which sometimes is mistaken for the more rounded molluscum bodies (Fig. 11–35).

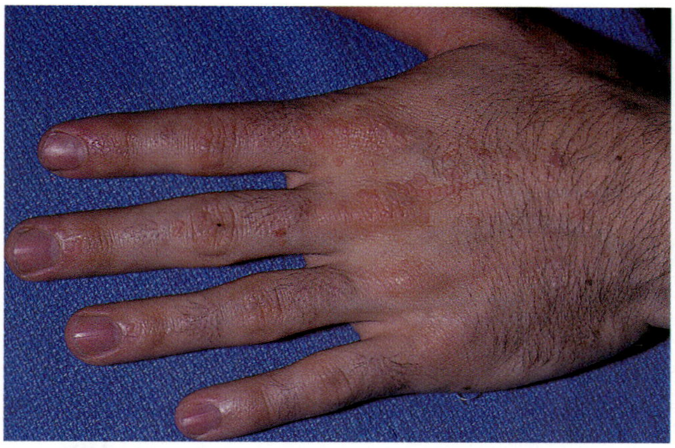

Figure 11–36. Verruca plana. Coalescent, raised, flesh-colored papules are arranged in linear distribution, indicating the path of inoculation.

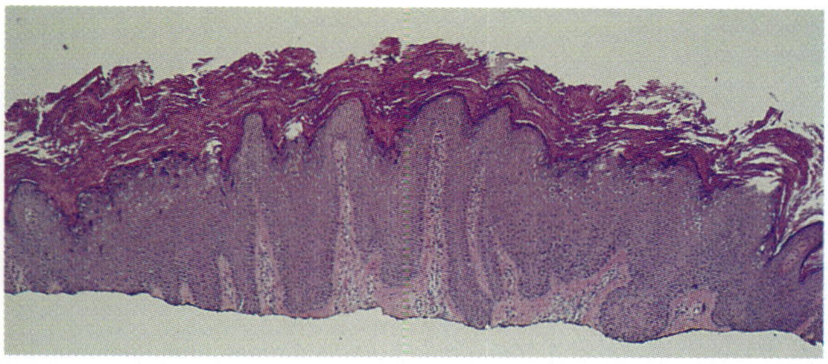

Figure 11–37. The histologic appearance of verruca plana is more subtle than that of verruca vulgaris or palmar or plantar verrucae, with only mild exophytic and endophytic verrucous hyperplasia and associated hyperorthokeratosis and parakeratosis.

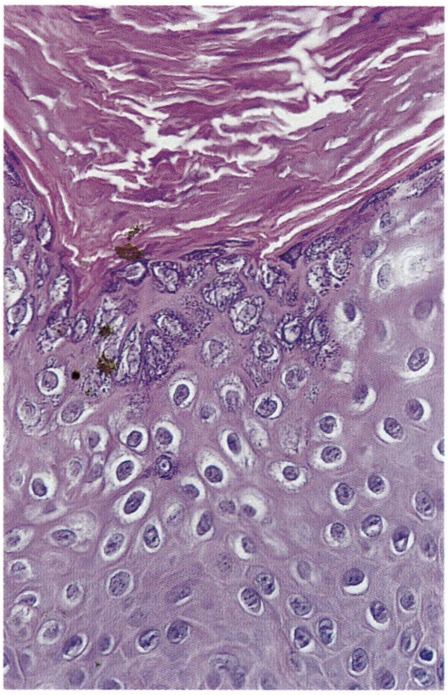

Figure 11–38. Cytoplasmic swelling and vacuolization (*i.e.,* koilocytosis) and nuclear pallor within the uppermost epidermal layers are evidence of an active viral cytopathic effect. These cytologic alterations are more subtle than those encountered in most other types of verrucae.

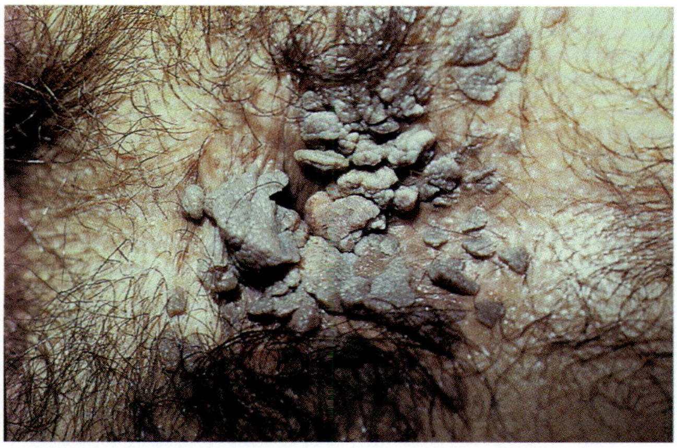

Figure 11–39. The clinical appearance of condyloma acuminatum is characterized by numerous cauliflower-like excrescences affecting anogenital skin.

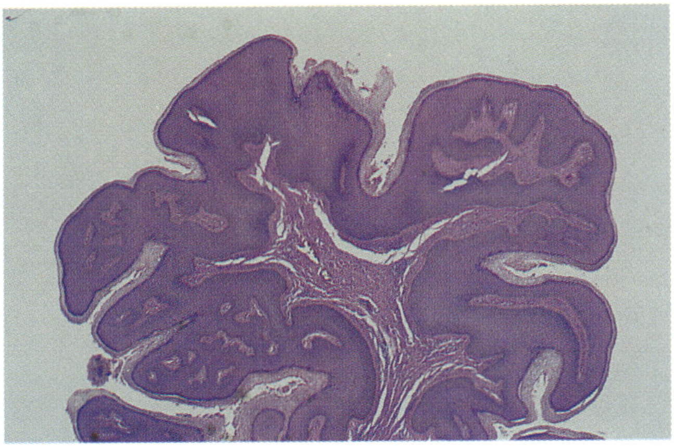

Figure 11–40. Lesional architecture of condyloma acuminatum at scanning magnification is that of a fibroepithelial polyp with an elaborate epidermal surface.

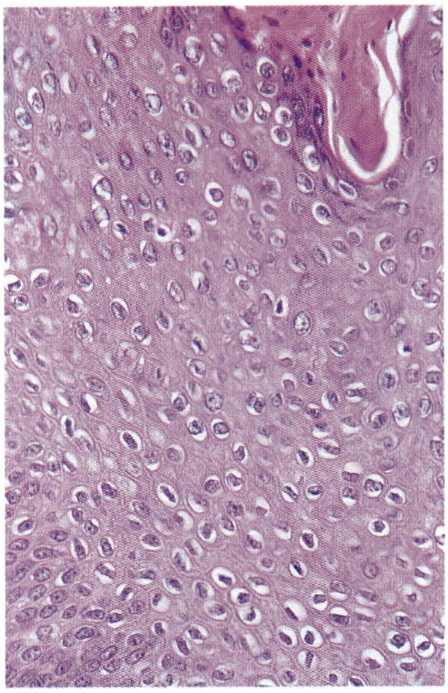

Figure 11–41. At higher magnification, perinuclear vacuolization, nuclear angulation, and occasional binucleated cells, which collectively indicate koilocytosis, are observed near the surface of the epithelial layer.

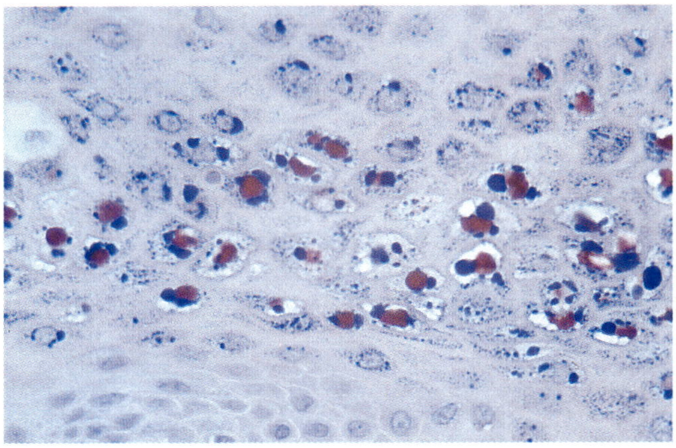

Figure 11–42. Immunohistochemical detection of human papillomavirus protein within tumor nuclei confirms the diagnostic impression of condyloma in difficult cases.

Molluscum Contagiosum

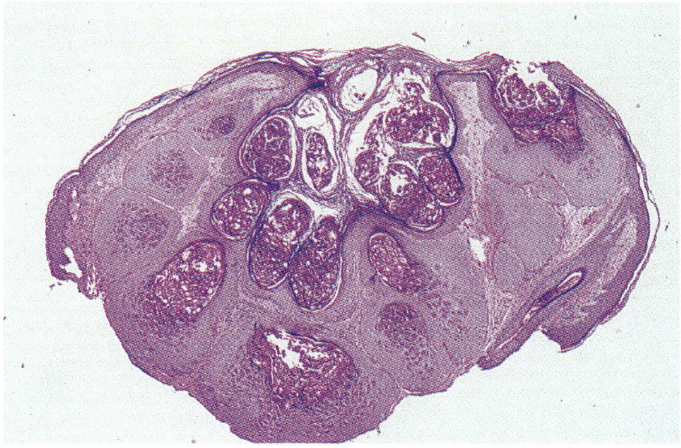

Figure 11–43. Molluscum contagiosum. The lesion shows a symmetric downgrowth of epithelium and a central cornified plug.

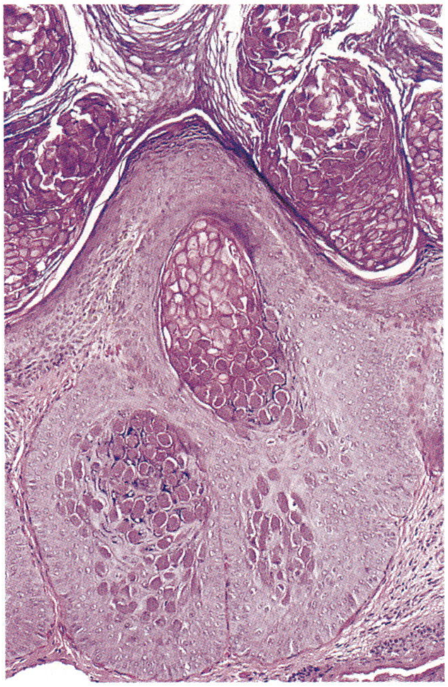

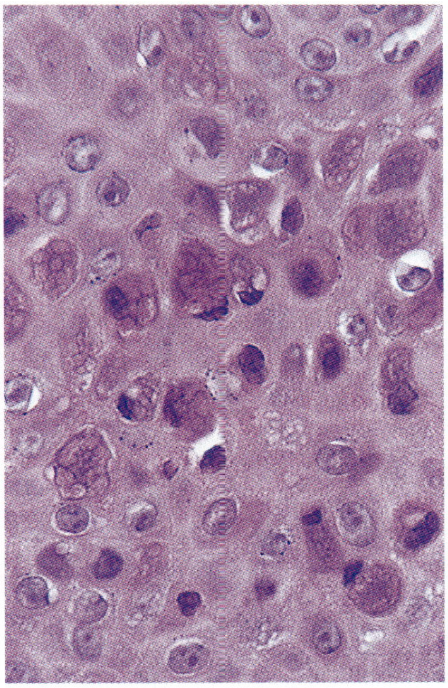

Figures 11–44 and 11–45. The central cornified plug contains numerous molluscum bodies. These bodies are eosinophilic, rounded cytoplasmic inclusions with a bubbly quality.

Actinic Keratosis

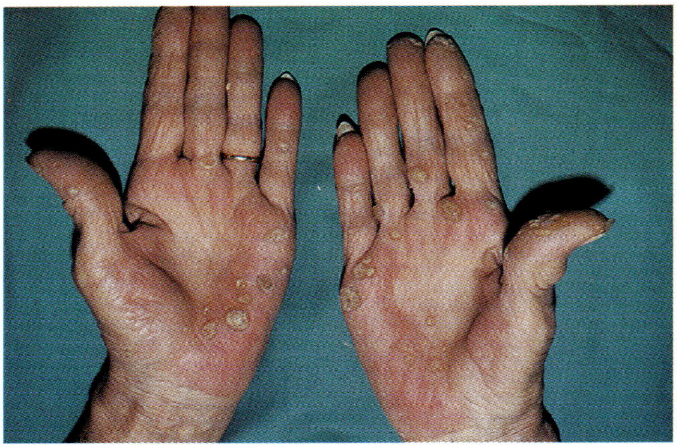

Figure 11–46. Dysplastic keratoses. Arsenical keratoses typically involve the palmar surfaces, although they otherwise resemble active keratoses.

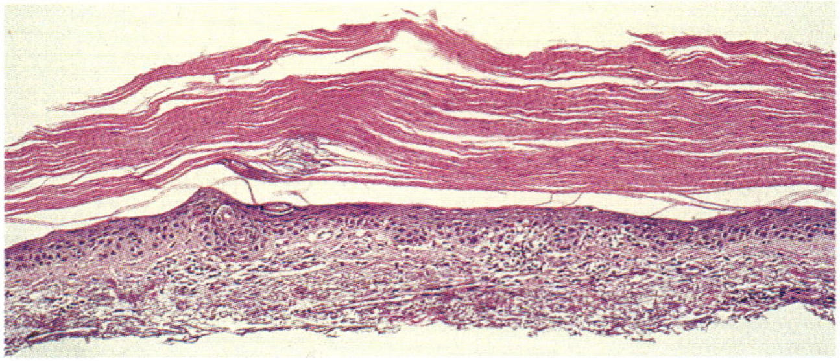

Figure 11–47. Actinic keratosis. Lesions may be atrophic, with loss of epidermal rete ridges and diffuse thinning of the epidermal layer.

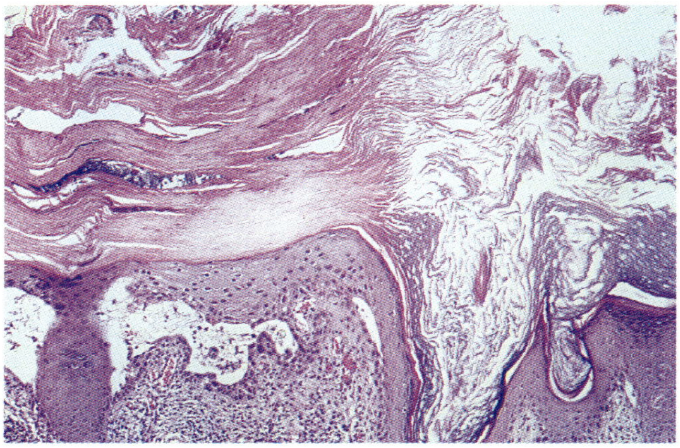

Figure 11–48. Alternatively, lesions may be proliferative, with endophytic budding of atypical basaloid cells. This lesion also shows suprabasal acantholysis, a frequent finding in actinic keratoses. Note the diffuse parakeratotic scale overlying lesions depicted here and in Figure 11–47.

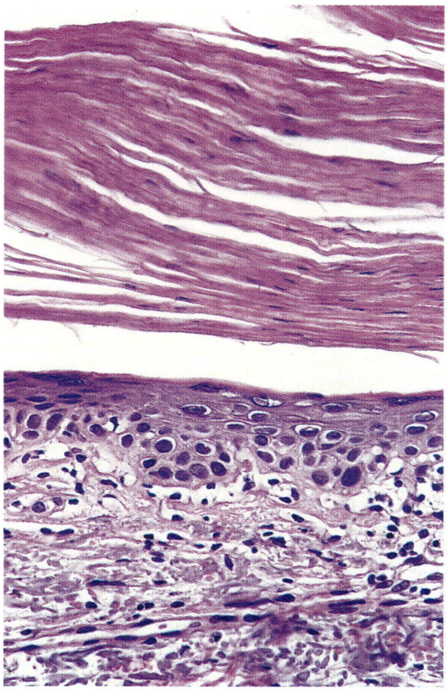

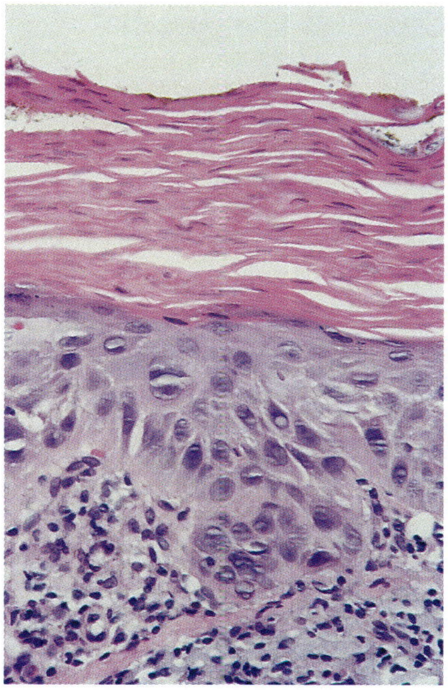

Figures 11–49 and 11–50. A hallmark of actinic keratoses is dysplasia affecting the lower epidermal layers. This is evidenced by nuclear enlargement, contour angulation, and hyperchromasia. Note that plump, atypical nuclei are also retained in the overlying parakeratotic scale, a diagnostic clue when superficial curettings disclose only stratum corneum and fail to demonstrate full-thickness epidermis. The lesion in Figure 11–50 shows severe dysplasia, indicating transitional areas to carcinoma in situ.

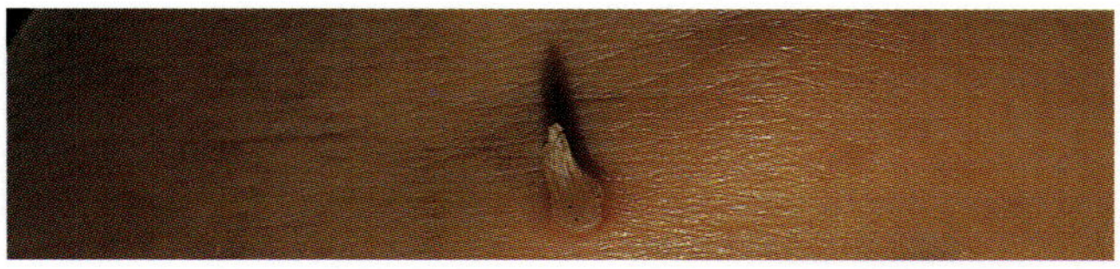

Figure 11–51. Proliferative actinic keratosis with horn formation. A cutaneous horn represents a tower of compacted scale and is not entirely dissimilar to a true animal horn.

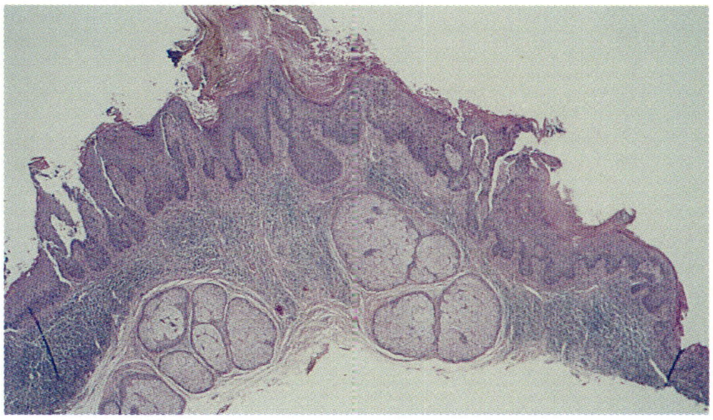

Figure 11–52. Early horn formation is evidenced by a spire of compacted parakeratotic scale emanating from the center of this proliferative actinic keratosis.

Squamous Cell Carcinoma

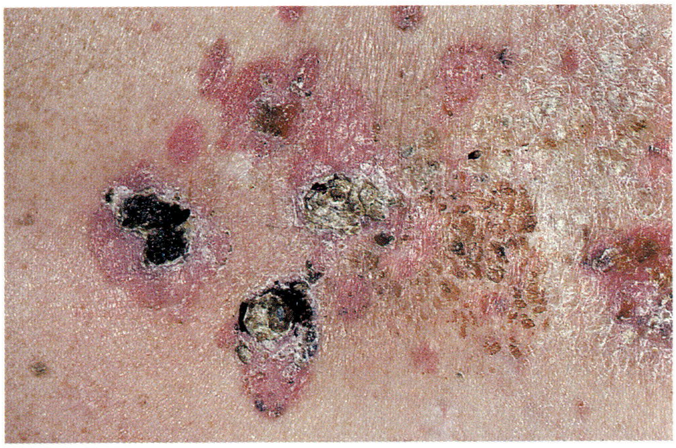

Figure 11–53. Squamous cell carcinoma in situ. Clinically, scaling erythematous plaques may be confused with subacute to chronic inflammatory dermatitis.

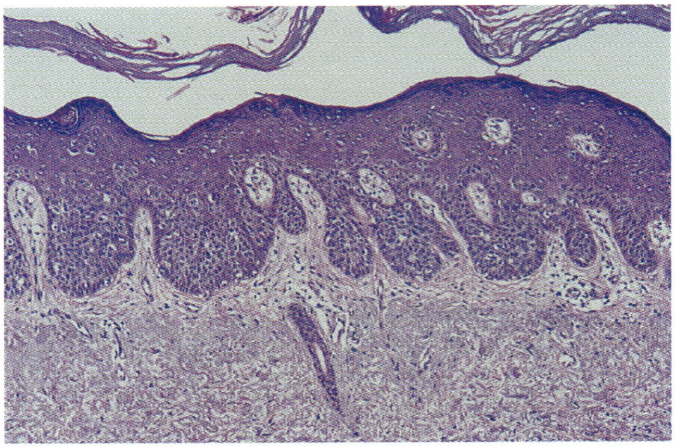

Figure 11–54. Nests of anaplastic keratinocytes are present in an intraepidermal epithelioma pattern within this expanded epidermal layer.

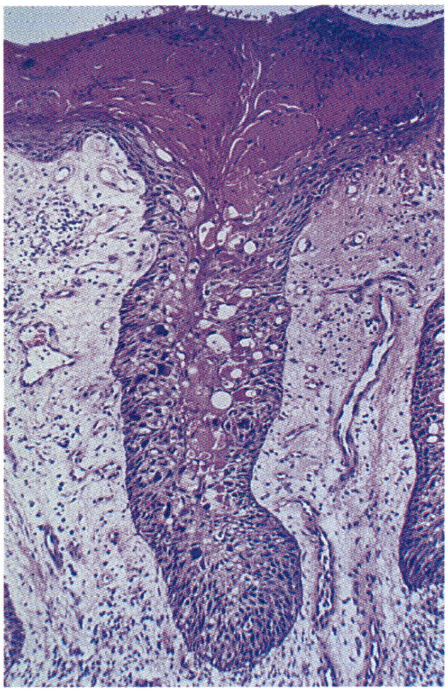

Figure 11–55. Growth within the acrosyringium and superficial dermal portion of the eccrine duct also may occur.

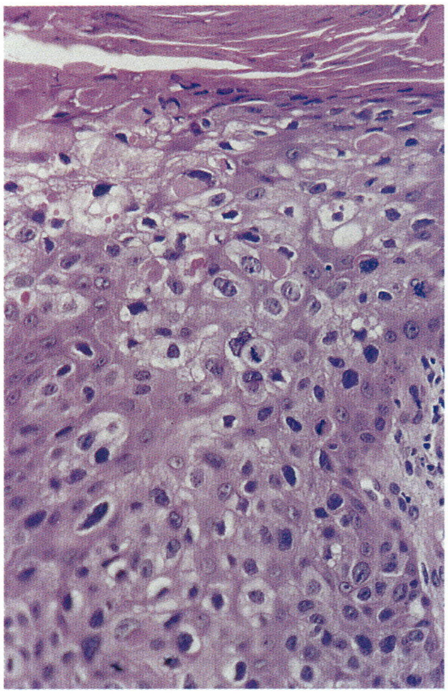

Figure 11–56. Closer inspection reveals that anaplastic tumor cells are confined to the epidermal layer. These cells are often glycogenated, imparting a relatively clear cytoplasm. Note the absence of a stratum granulosum, with an abrupt transition to atypical, compacted parakeratotic scale.

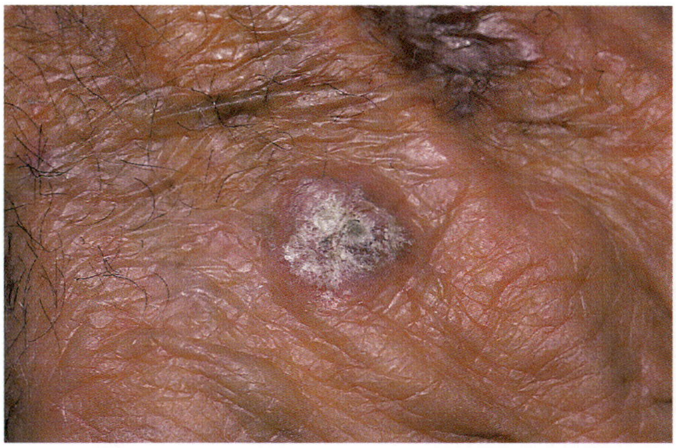

Figure 11–57. Invasive squamous cell carcinoma. A raised and asymmetric facial nodule has a cornified and focally ulcerated center.

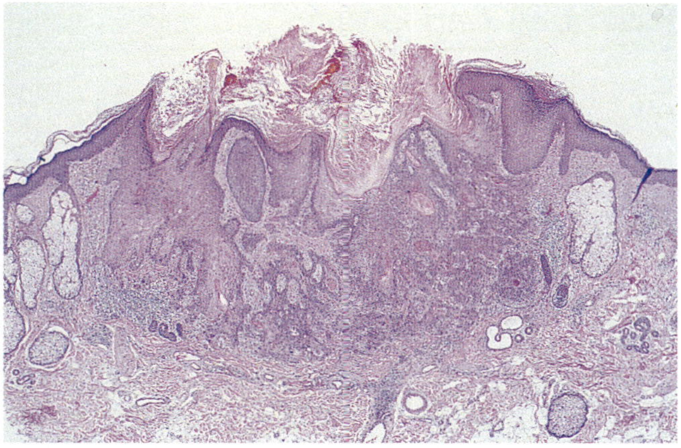

Figure 11–58. A biopsy specimen reveals endophytic tongues of atypical epithelium within a fibrotic, inflamed dermis. Note the central zone of hyperkeratosis and parakeratosis.

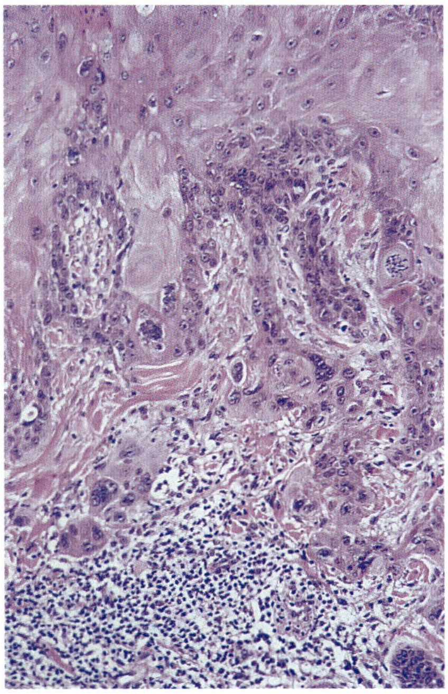

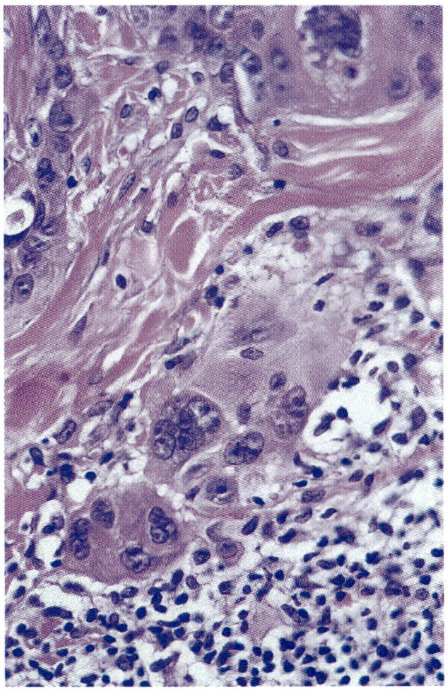

Figures 11–59 and 11–60. In contrast to keratoacanthoma, true stromal invasion by malignant cells is easily documented in invasive squamous cell carcinoma.

Basal Cell Carcinoma

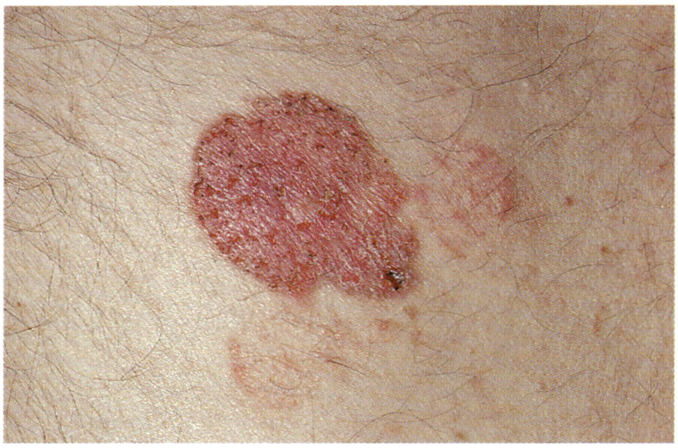

Figure 11–61. A plaque-like, focally pigmented superficial multicentric basal cell carcinoma. Like some forms of squamous cell carcinoma in situ, such lesions may be confused with dermatitis.

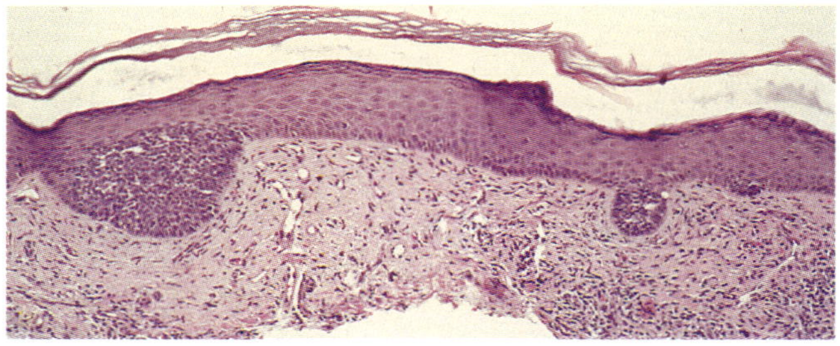

Figure 11–62. A biopsy specimen reveals seemingly discontinuous buds of basal cell carcinoma of the superficial multicentric type arising from the epidermal layer.

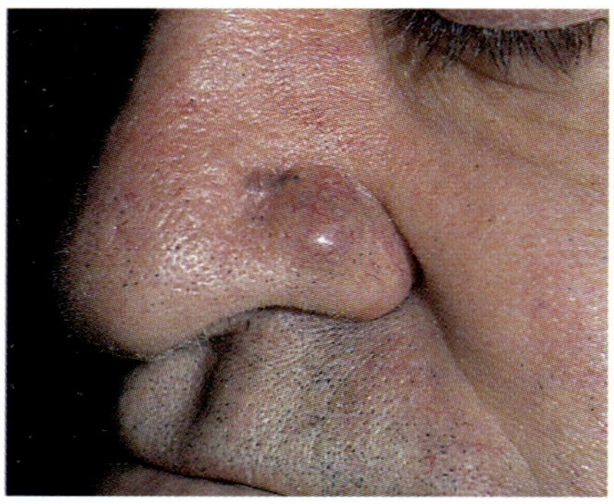

Figure 11–63. A nodular basal cell carcinoma on the nose presents as a pearly lesion with prominent telangiectasia.

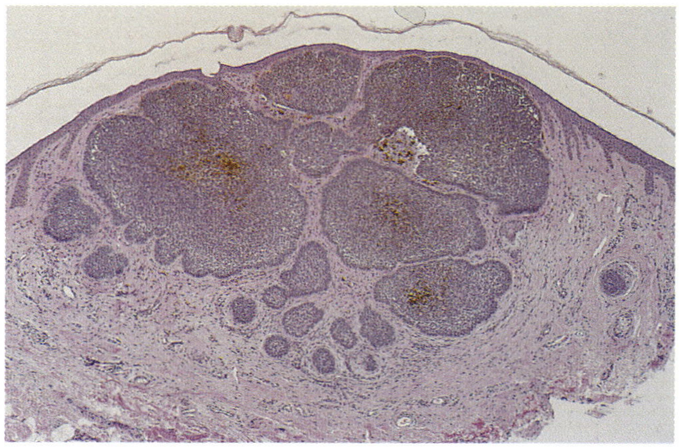

Figure 11–64. A biopsy specimen reveals strands and nests of basal cells invading a mucinous stroma, which focally separates from the epithelial elements to form clefts (*i.e.*, separation artifact). The tumor islands are characterized by peripheral palisading; focal, single-cell necrosis; and occasional mitotic figures.

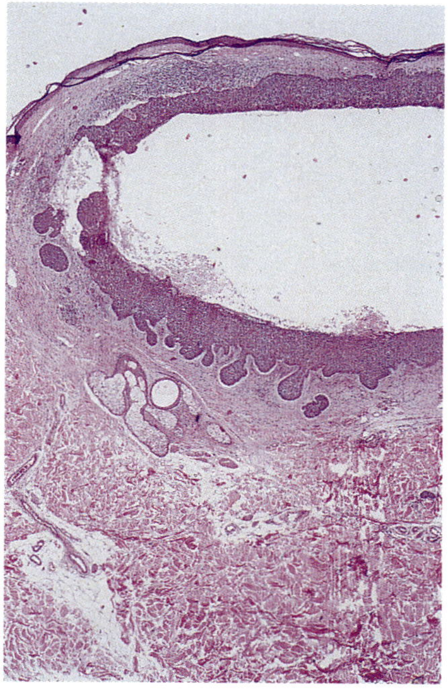

Figure 11–65. Cystic basal cell carcinoma.

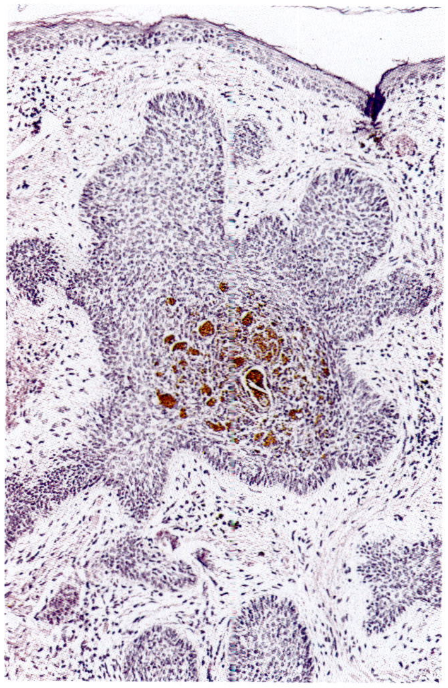

Figure 11–66. Pigmented basal cell carcinoma.

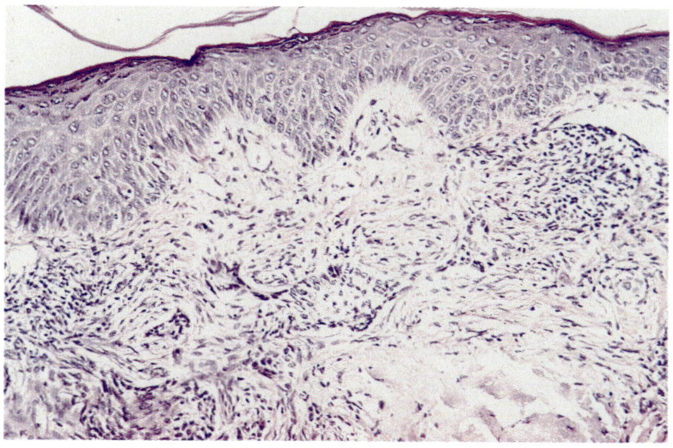

Figure 11–67. Sclerosing basal cell carcinoma. This lesion is composed of thin cords of fusiform tumor cells that grow insidiously within a cellular, desmoplastic stroma.

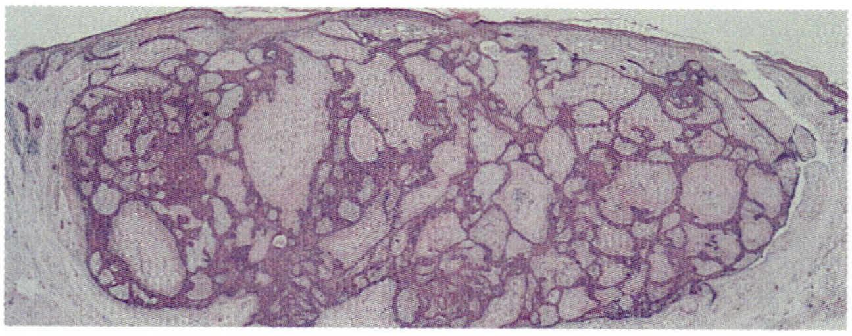

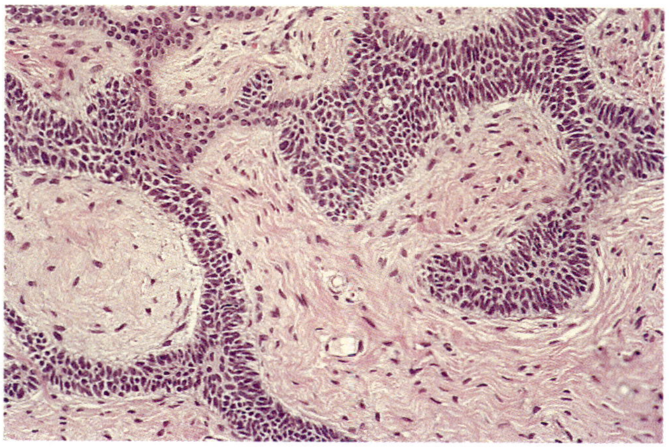

Figures 11–68 and 11–69. Fibroepithelioma of Pinkus. This well-differentiated form of basal cell carcinoma is characterized by a symmetric proliferation of anastomosing thin epithelial strands (Fig. 11–68) within a well-developed fibrotic stroma (Fig. 11–69).

12

Adnexal Tumors

As with epidermal tumors, adnexal neoplasia is one of the most challenging topics in dermatopathology. This is in part because of the enormous number of individual tumors and variant forms and the complicated nomenclature. In addition, many systems of classification have relied on presumed histodifferentiation and histogenesis—an approach with clear-cut limitations in light of recent evidence indicating ambiguous and multiple differentiation pathways for many lesions. In general, adnexal tumors of skin do not derive directly from mature appendageal epithelium. Rather, they originate from totipotential stem cells and differentiate along adnexal pathways. This explains why many adnexal tumors bear little resemblance to their mature counterparts and how multiple differentiation pathways may be followed simultaneously in single tumors.

In this atlas, cutaneous adnexal neoplasms are classified according to the following patterns, without regard to histodifferentiation: partially and fully cystic tumors; tumors forming small nests, cords, and ducts; tumors forming sheets or large nodules; and infiltrative, malignant tumors. This approach permits elimination of a large number of adnexal neoplasms at a glance and limits the diagnostic algorithm to a manageable number of possibilities. Although only the more common tumors are displayed, approximately more than 95% of the adnexal neoplasms encountered in routine practice are illustrated.

It also should be emphasized that when an adnexal neoplasm is encountered that does not conform completely to the diagnostic features portrayed in this atlas, it does not necessarily represent a new or rare entity. More likely is the possibility that such a neoplasm is a variant of a more common tumor form. Adnexal tumors often show "hybrid" features, such as coincident spiradenoma and cylindroma in one tumor or a cyst with mixed infundibular and trichilemmal differentiation. Such lesions should be described as exhibiting mixed features, and their diagnoses therefore appropriately combine more than one entity. A more critical issue, however, is deciding whether an adnexal tumor is benign or malignant. In general, the presence of mitotic activity and individual cell necrosis favors is a malignant process, although exceptions do exist (*e.g.,* numerous mitoses in early pilomatricomas, necrosis in proliferating variants of trichilemmal cysts).

Accurate identification of adnexal neoplasms is important, despite the frequent comment that once it has been decided whether such a tumor is benign or malignant, precise classification does not matter. First, it is requisite that adnexal tumors be differentiated from tumors with different biologic behaviors (*e.g.,* trichoepithelioma versus basal cell carcinoma, proliferating trichilemmal cyst versus squamous cell carcinoma). Second, certain adnexal tumors occur in the setting of well-recognized syndromes associated with internal disease (*e.g.,* trichilemmomas and sebaceous epitheliomas in the setting of breast and gastrointestinal carcinoma, respectively). Certain adnexal tumors (*e.g.,* cylindroma) may be inherited and occur as multiple lesions that require clinical monitoring, follow-up, and, often, repeated surgical intervention. Finally, some adnexal tumors arise in the setting of lesions potentially programmed for malignant degeneration (*e.g.,* a syringocystadenoma arising in a nevus sebaceus, the latter being a tumor that even more frequently gives rise to basal cell carcinoma).

Staining characteristics of adnexal tumors are often helpful in directing the dermatopathologist along defined diagnostic pathways and branch points. At scanning magnification, for example, outer root sheath differentiation in tumors often presents as pale-pink regions (*e.g.*, trichilemmoma), whereas neoplasms with hair matrix elements may be dark blue (basaloid areas of pilomatricoma). Highly glycogenated neoplasms recapitulating embryonic acrosyringium may contain pale to clear cells (nodular hidradenoma), whereas those differentiating along apocrine lines are often composed of cells that are deep pink and granular (*e.g.*, apocrine carcinoma). Stromal elements are also separable according to tinctorial characteristics, an example being the pale-blue mucinous matrix of a mixed tumor in contrast to the glassy, eosinophilic mantle that surrounds epithelial nests of a cylindroma.

Partially and Fully Cystic Tumors

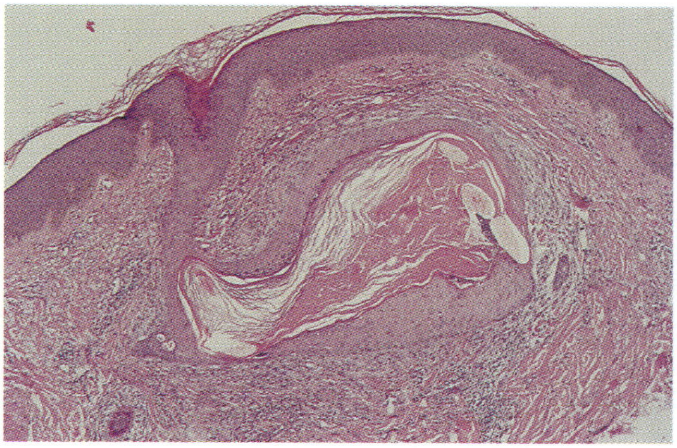

Figure 12–1. Epidermal inclusion cyst (*i.e.*, infundibular cyst). This cyst arises from the epithelium of the follicular infundibulum; therefore, its wall resembles surface epidermis.

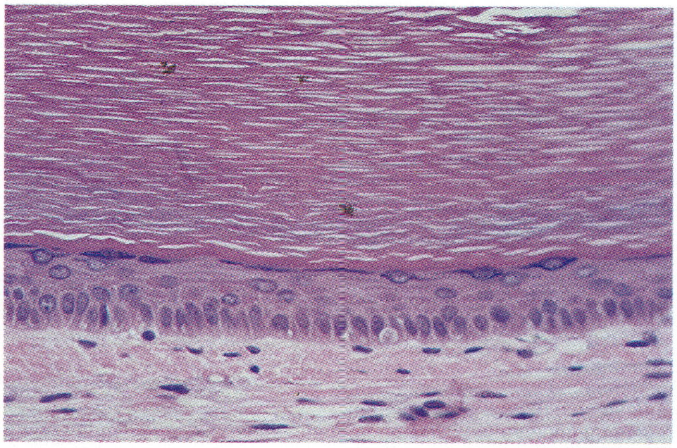

Figure 12–2. At higher magnification, the wall of an epidermal inclusion cyst has a thin but well-developed stratum granulosum, and the keratin produced is laminated orthokeratin.

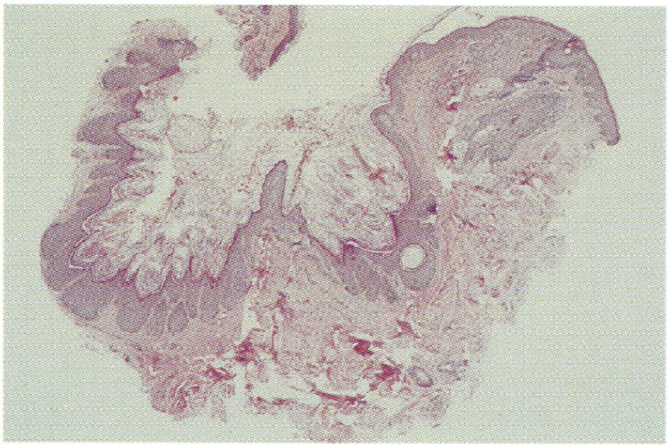

Figure 12–3. Pilar sheath acanthoma. The pilar sheath acanthoma is a dilated, relatively superficial invagination that produces laminated keratin similar to that within true infundibular cysts. The wall of the tumor typically has plate-like outgrowths of glycogenated infundibular epithelium.

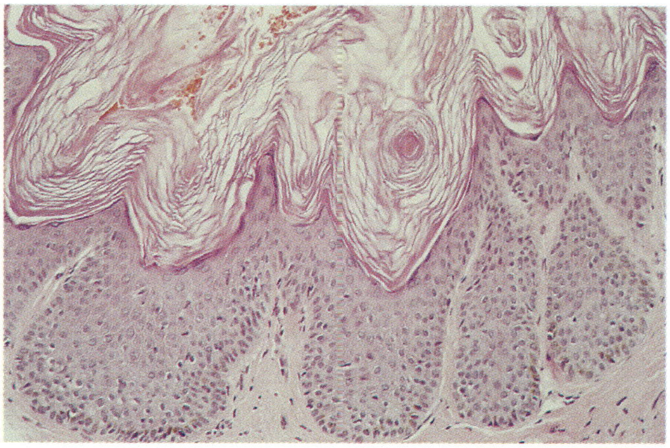

Figure 12–4. Higher magnification of the wall of the pilar sheath acanthoma in Figure 12–3.

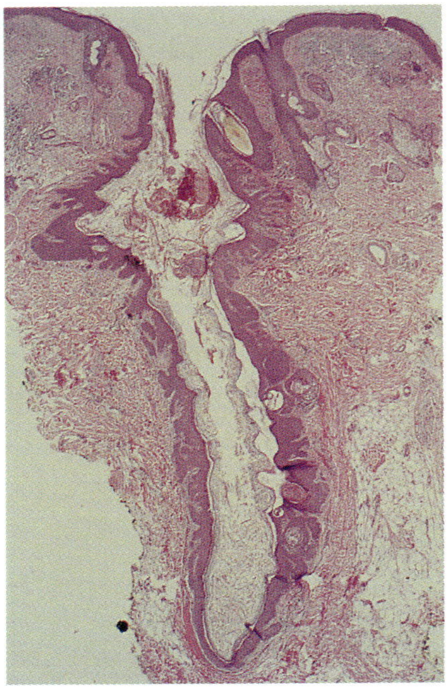

Figure 12–5. The dilated pore of Winer, on the other hand, is a deeper, conical invagination; plate-like outgrowths similar to those in pilar sheath acanthoma are also observed.

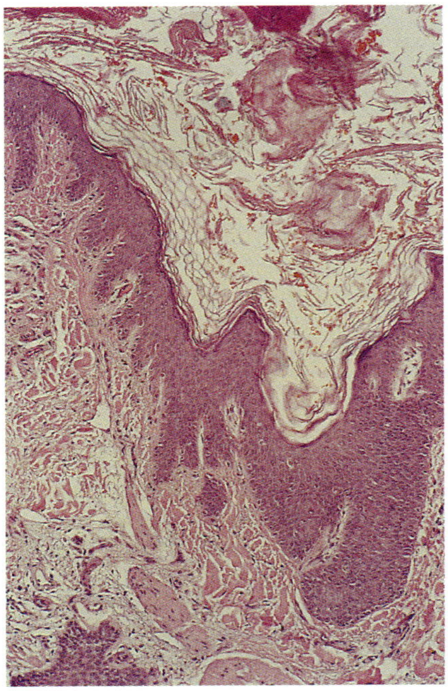

Figure 12–6. Higher magnification of the dilated pore shown in Figure 12–5.

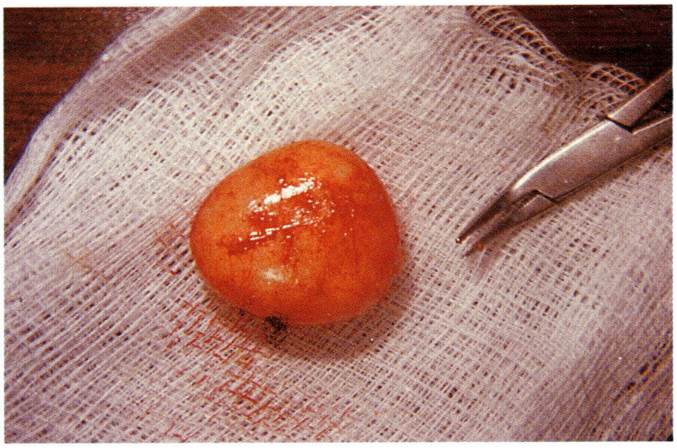

Figure 12–7. Trichilemmal (pilar) cyst. These tumors, also called wens and sebaceous cysts, are often shelled out as a cosmetic surgical maneuver or as a result of pain produced after partial rupture.

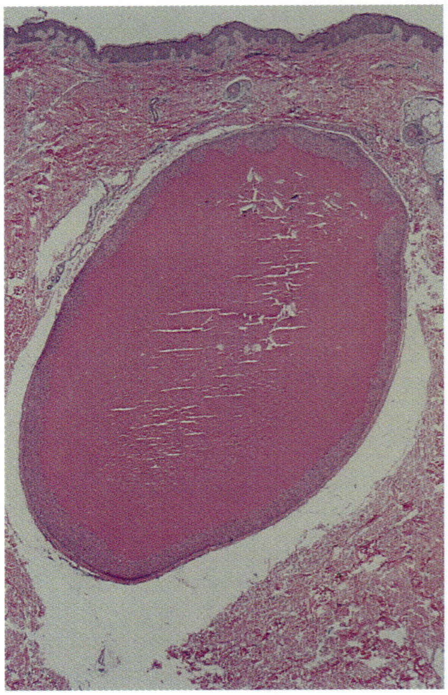

Figure 12–8. At scanning magnification, the trichilemmal cyst is filled with homogeneous keratin admixed with lipid.

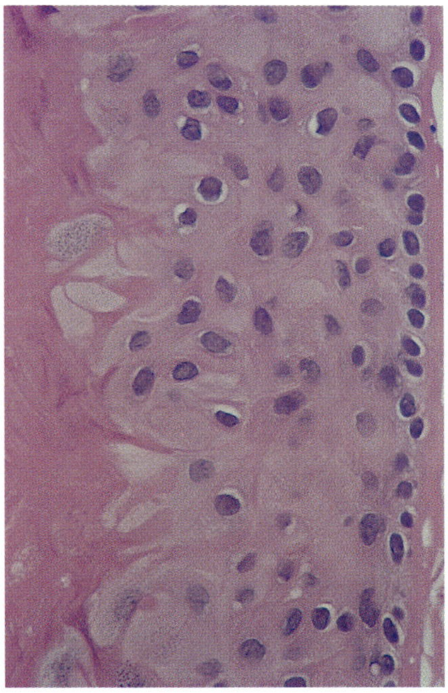

Figure 12–9. The wall of the trichilemmal cyst recapitulates the portion of the follicle deep to the infundibulum, where trichilemmal, not surface epidermal, keratinization normally occurs. Accordingly, keratin is formed abruptly, without an intervening granular cell layer *(left).* Note also the rounded contour of pale cyst epithelial cells as they interface with the cyst contents.

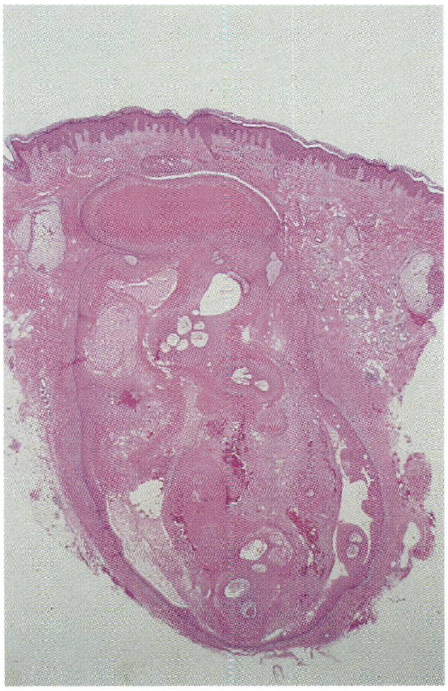

Figure 12–10. This proliferating trichilemmal cyst shows many of the features depicted in Figures 12–7 through 12–9, although the epithelial elements have begun to proliferate, forming solid ingrowths into the cyst lumen. Over time, continued proliferation will expand the cyst, which will become filled with reactive epithelial elements admixed with zones of pressure necrosis (*i.e.,* pilar tumor). Differentiation from squamous cell carcinoma depends on recognition of the smooth outer contour of such tumors.

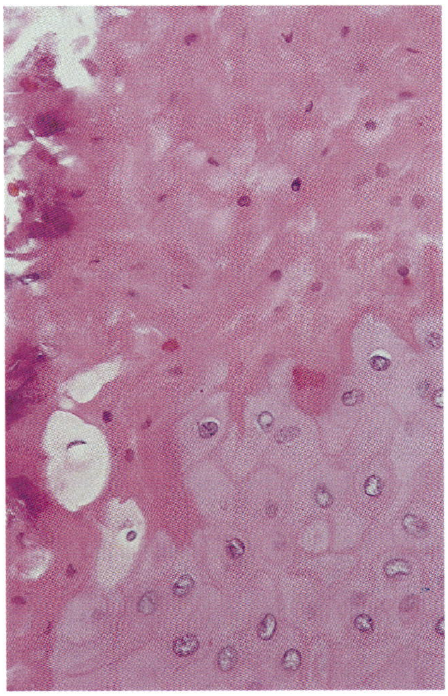

Figure 12–11. Differentiation from squamous cell carcinoma also depends on detection of zones in which trichilemmal keratinization is preserved.

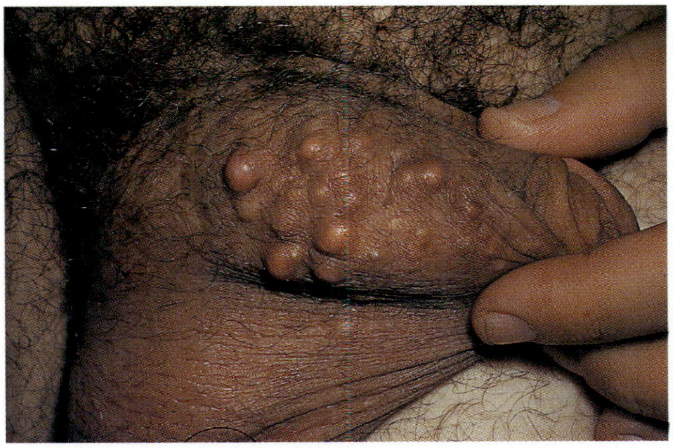

Figure 12–12. In the clinical form of steatocystoma, termed steatocystoma multiplex, multiple painless cystic nodules are observed, here on scrotal skin.

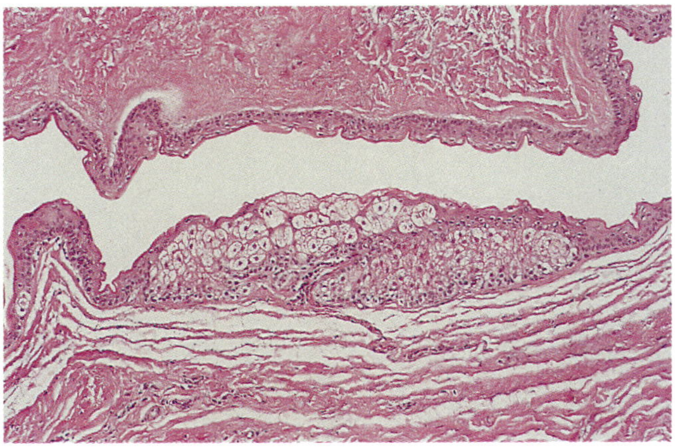

Figure 12–13. Histologic examination of steatocystoma reveals a cystic cavity filled with clear fluid and lined by flattened squamous cells.

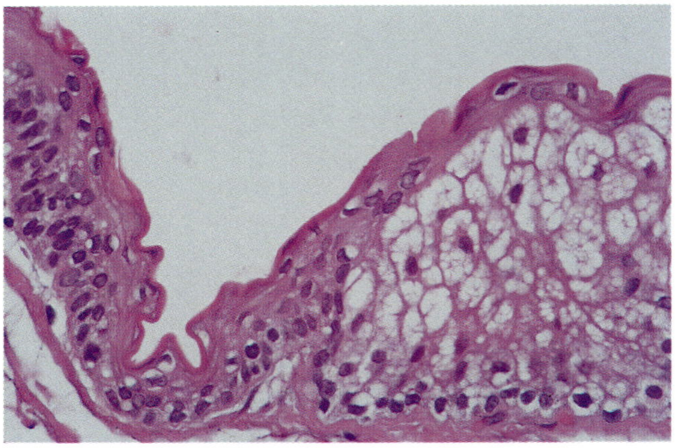

Figure 12–14. Distinguishing features of steatocystoma include compressed sebaceous lobules associated with the cyst wall (see also Fig. 12–13) and a hyalinized inner cuticle with a corrugated contour.

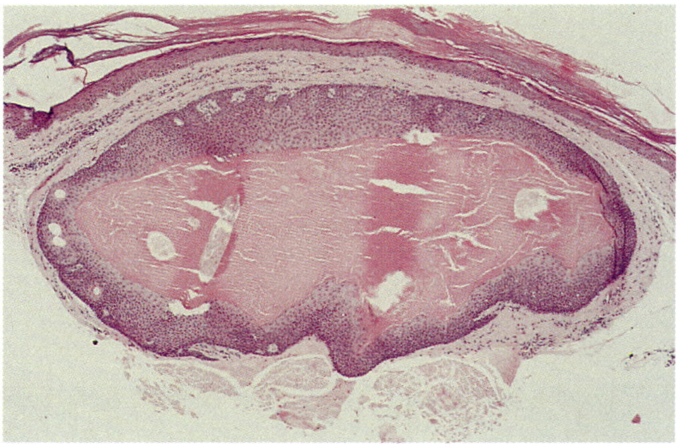

Figure 12–15. Hair matrix cysts are filled with amorphous, eosinophilic, keratinaceous material and lined by basaloid cells that recapitulate normal hair matrix and cortex.

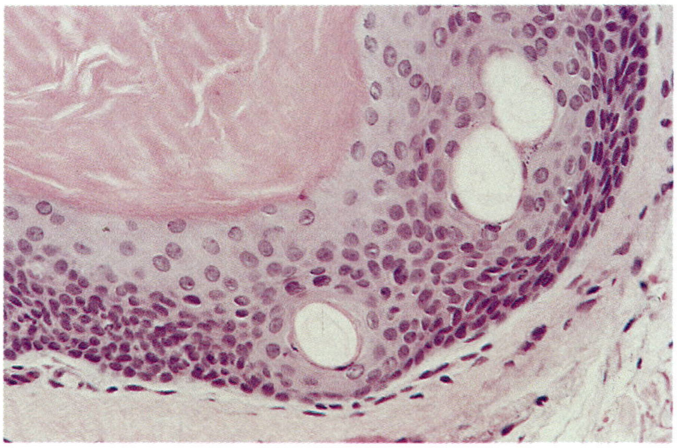

Figure 12–16. Occasionally, small cystic lumina may form within the wall of hair matrix cysts. Proliferative counterparts of these cysts may rupture and be responsible for the genesis of tumors called pilomatricomas.

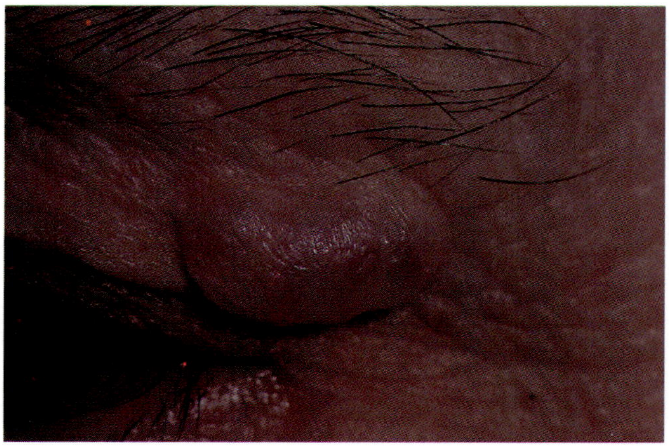

Figure 12–17. Apocrine cystadenoma. A semitranslucent, cystic nodule with a blue-gray hue arose on the eyelid.

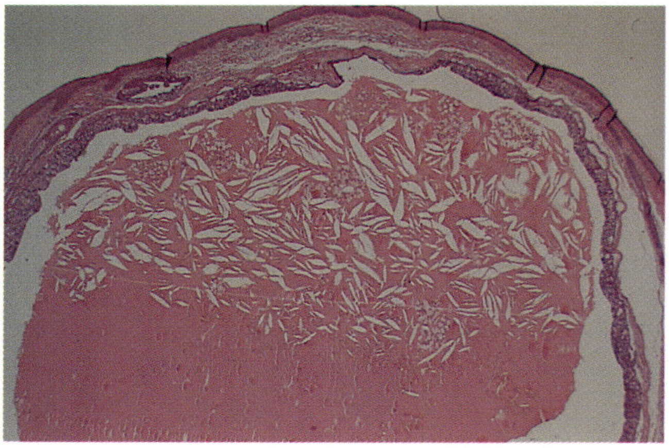

Figure 12–18. At low magnification, apocrine cystadenoma consists of a thin-walled cyst filled with eosinophilic fluid and cholesterol clefts.

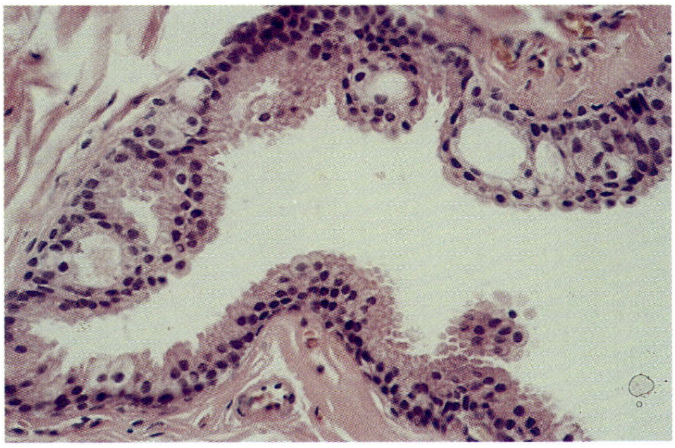

Figure 12–19. The lining of apocrine cystadenoma consists of several layers of apocrine-type epithelium, with formation of small papillations and epithelial bridges, and luminal zones of decapitation secretion.

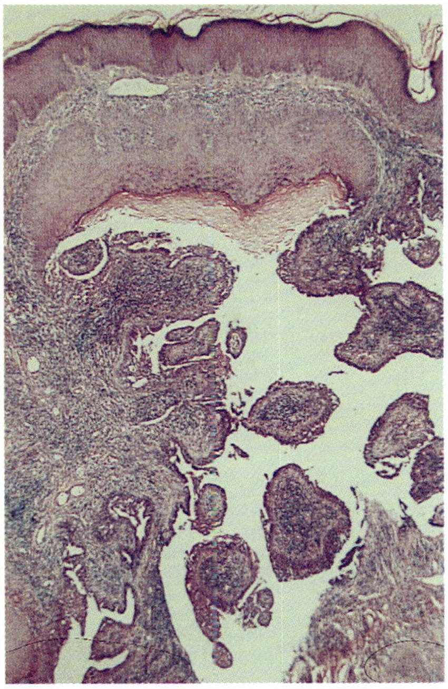

Figure 12–20. Syringocystadenoma papilliferum. This cystic and papillary adnexal tumor is characterized by an epithelial lining that may be squamous near the epidermal surface but becomes cuboidal to columnar over most of the cyst wall.

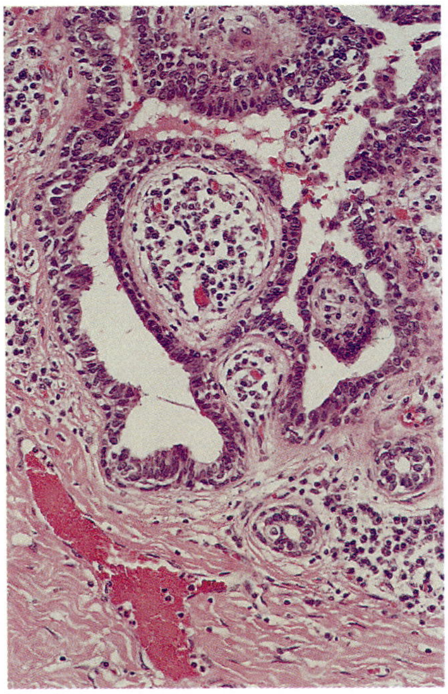

Figure 12–21. Generally in syringocystadenoma papilliferum there are two layers of epithelial lining cells with occasional foci of apocrine-type decapitation secretion. The stroma is typically rich in plasma cells and forms prominent internal papillations into the cyst lumen.

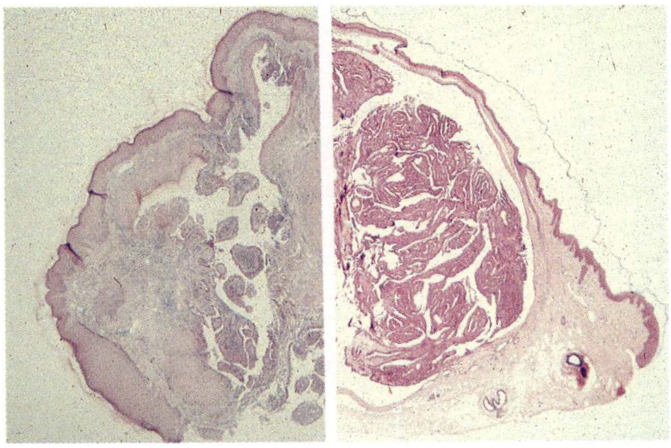

Figure 12–22. At scanning magnification, although hidradenoma papilliferum *(right)* has a cystic and papillary architecture that is similar to syringocystadenoma papilliferum *(left)*, it is devoid of a stroma filled with plasma cells.

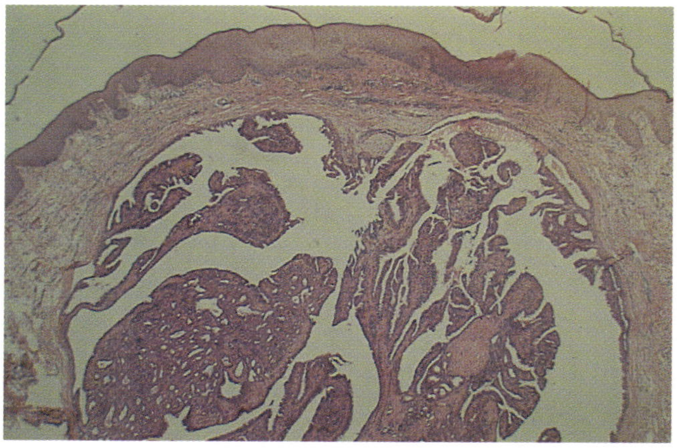

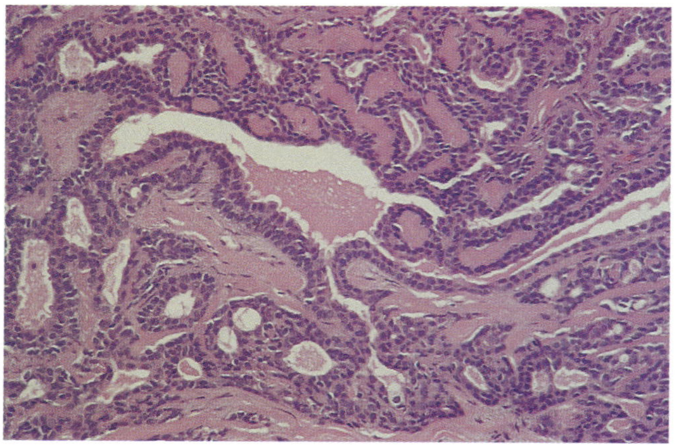

Figures 12–23 and 12–24. Hidradenoma papilliferum consists of a large cyst with internal papillations that nearly fill its lumen. The covering of the wall and its complex infoldings consist of two layers of cuboidal epithelial cells overlying a condensed, focally hyalinized fibrovascular stroma.

Tumors Forming Nests, Cords, and Ducts

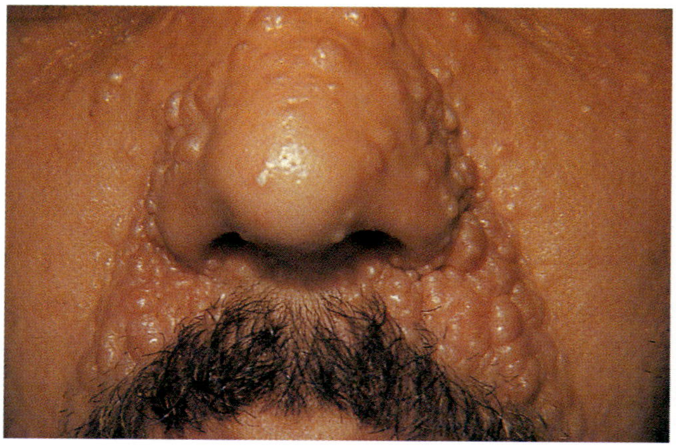

Figure 12–25. Multiple, dominantly inherited trichoepitheliomas bilaterally involve the nasolabial folds.

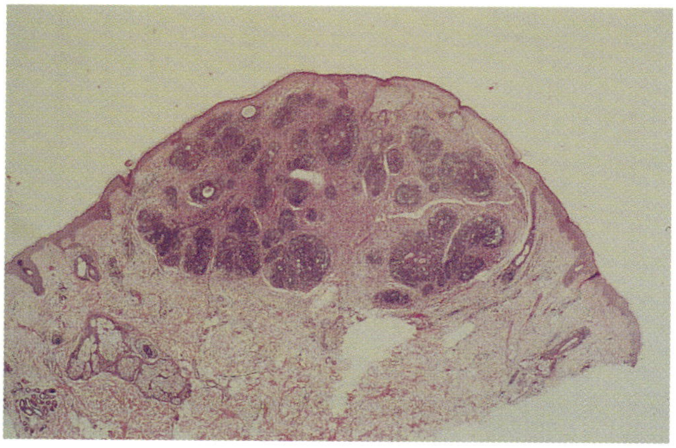

Figure 12–26. At scanning magnification, trichoepithelioma consists of nests and cords of basaloid cells forming small horn cysts.

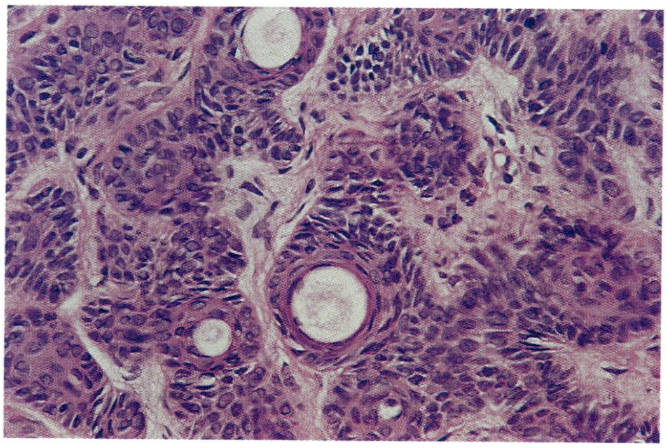

Figure 12–27. High magnification of lesion in Figure 12–26 reveals organoid nests of basaloid epithelial cells within a distinctive eosinophilic stroma. Unlike in basal cell carcinoma, individual cell necrosis, mitotic activity, and stromal-epithelial separation artifacts are not observed.

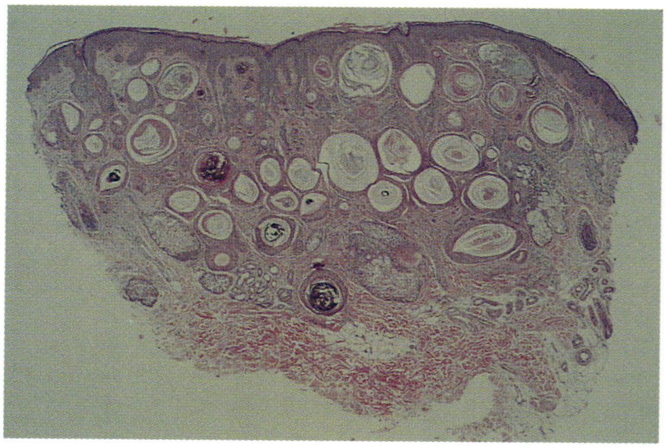

Figure 12–28. Tumors similar to trichoepitheliomas but termed trichoadenomas are characterized by a predominance of keratin-filled horn cysts.

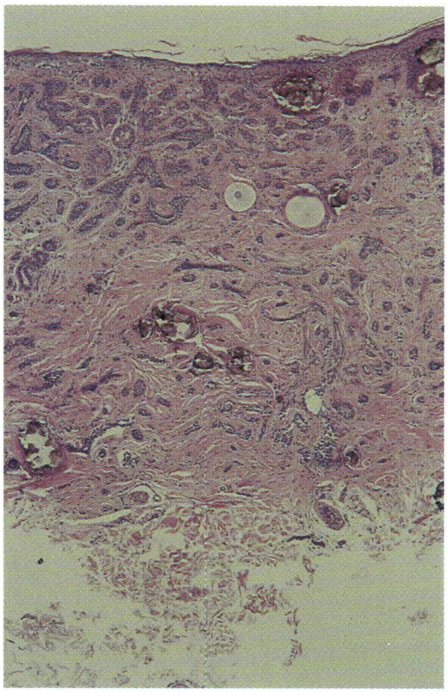

Figure 12–29. Desmoplastic trichoepithelioma. The features of symmetry, basaloid cords without necrosis of mitoses, and a distinctive fibrotic stroma devoid of separation artifact are maintained, although the stromal component predominates. This results in apparent compression of epithelial elements in a pattern that may resemble sclerosing basal cell carcinoma.

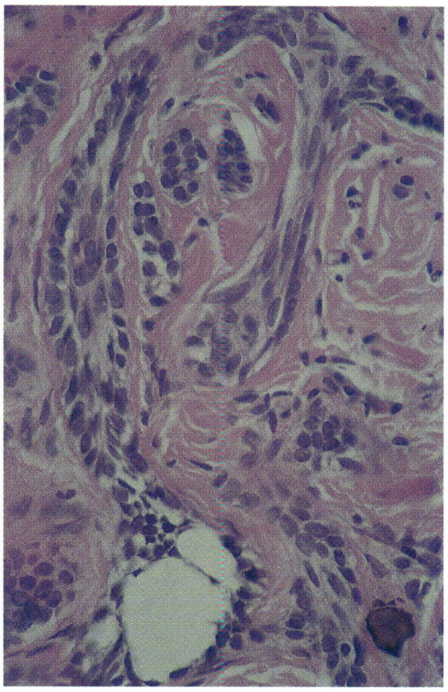

Figure 12–30. Higher magnification of the desmoplastic trichoepithelioma. Unlike in basal cell carcinoma, mitotic figures and individual cell necrosis are not observed. The separation that has occurred at the base is among the epithelial cells, not between stroma and epithelium.

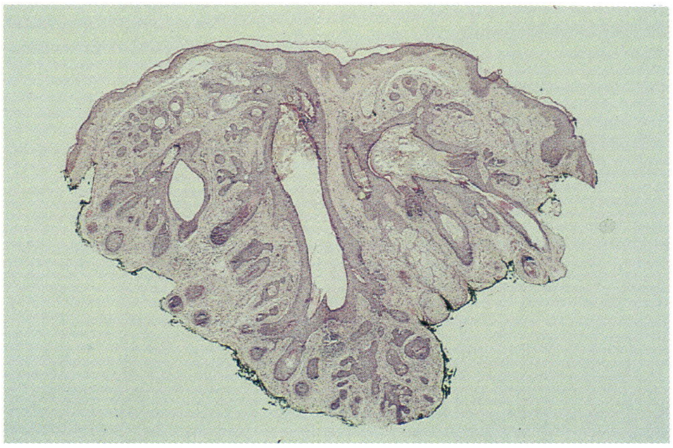

Figure 12–31. Trichofolliculoma. Low magnification reveals a central follicular infundibular plug from which radiating cords and branches of pilar epithelium sprout within a distinctive fibrotic stroma.

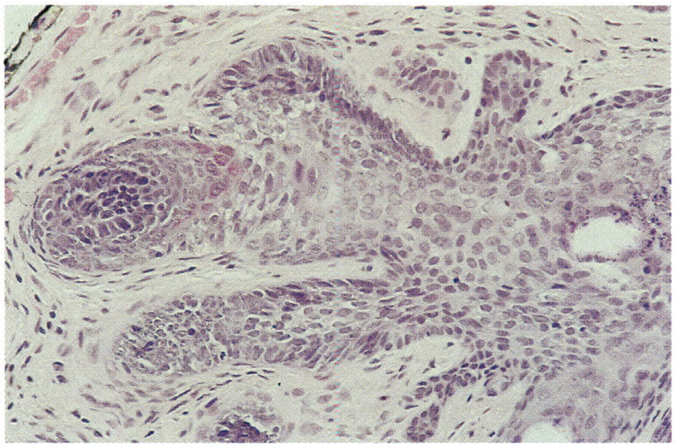

Figure 12–32. On closer inspection, hair matrix differentiation *(left),* hair cortex, and outer root sheath may be observed in trichofolliculoma . In addition, small hair shafts may be detected within central microcysts.

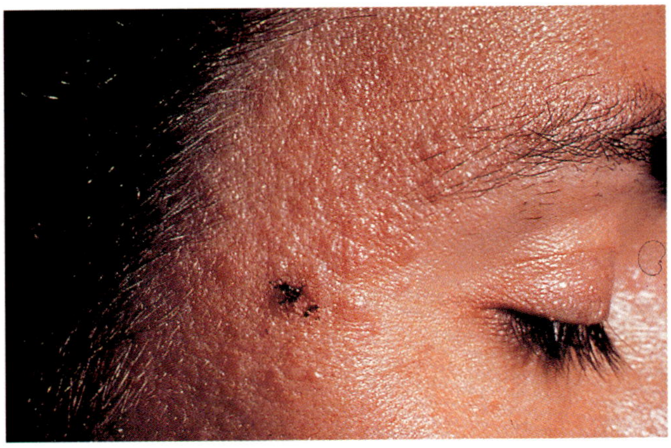

Figure 12–33. Syringoma. Multiple, small, flesh-colored papules are present on the temporal skin of this young woman.

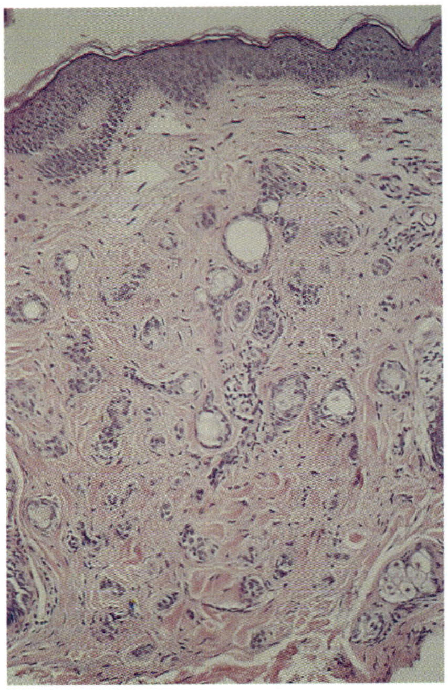

Figure 12–34. Histologically, syringoma is composed of small nests and cords of epithelium embedded within a dense, collagenous stroma.

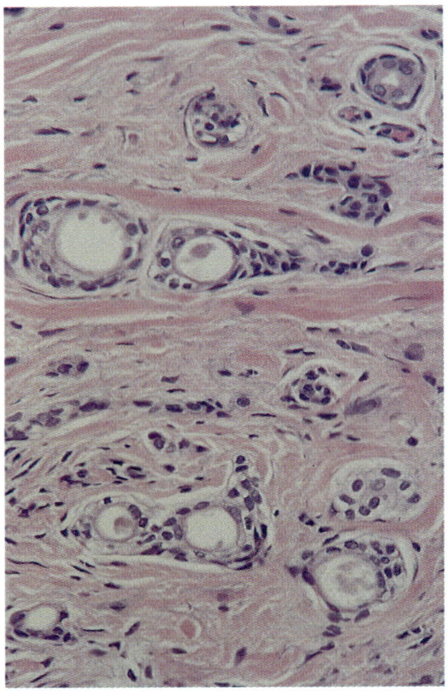

Figure 12–35. Individual cords of syringoma have central, eccrine-type lumina, and some cords have contours reminiscent of comma- or tadpole-like shapes.

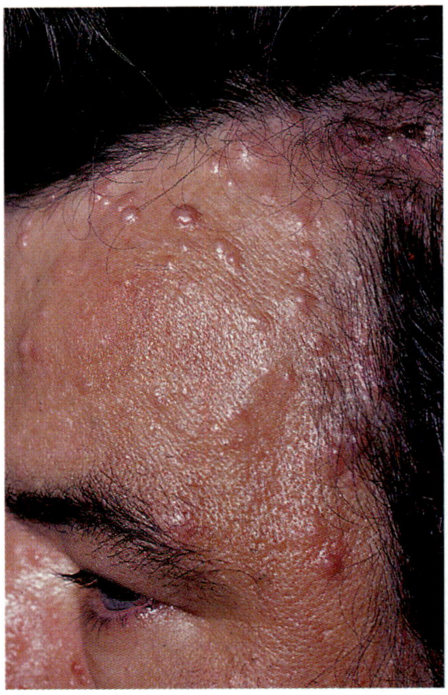

Figure 12–36. Early cylindroma lesions on the forehead and scalp. Over time, these may enlarge, become confluent, and produce a turban-like deformity.

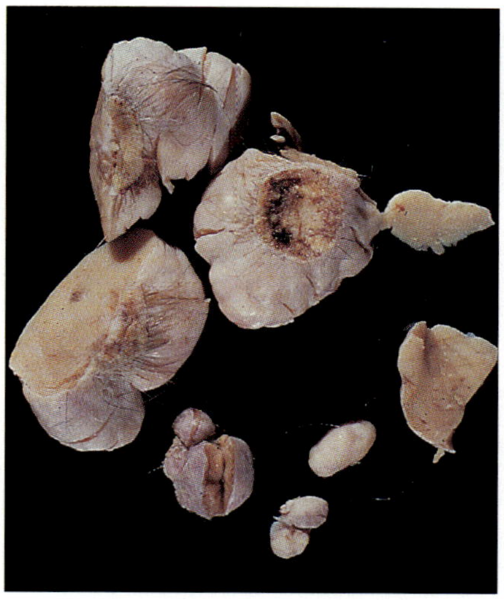

Figure 12–37. For the reason given in Figure 12–36, multiple cylindromas may be cosmetically removed and submitted for pathologic examination.

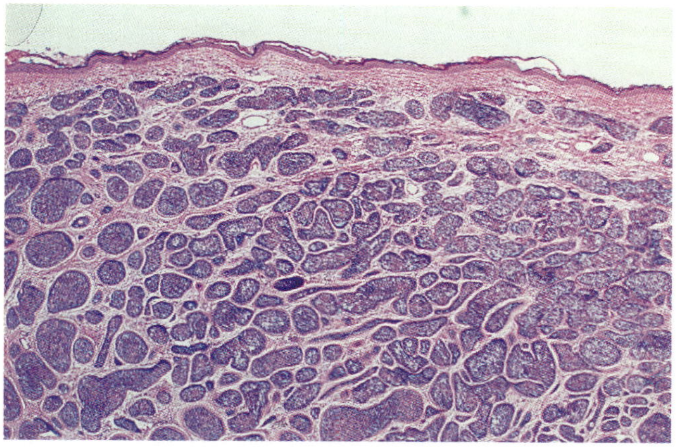

Figure 12–38. At scanning power, individual epithelial islands of cylindroma appear to interlock, as if they are pieces of a jigsaw puzzle. The islands are composed of small basaloid cells admixed with larger pale epithelial cells.

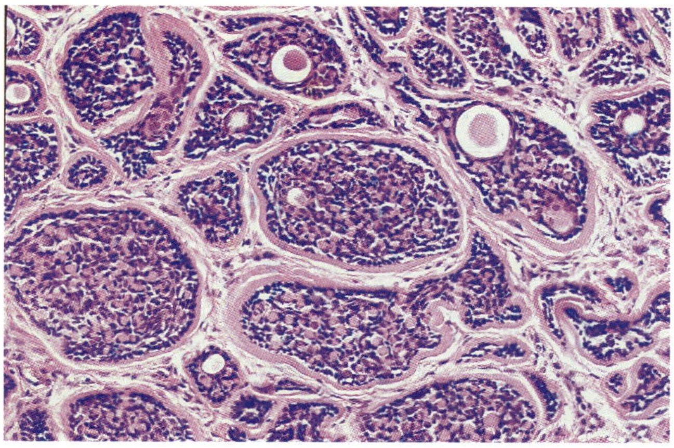

Figure 12–39. The epithelial islands of cylindroma contain small duct-like lumina and are surrounded by a cylinder or mantle of hyalinized basement membrane, which, over time, may become incorporated into islands as small, rounded, extracellular bodies.

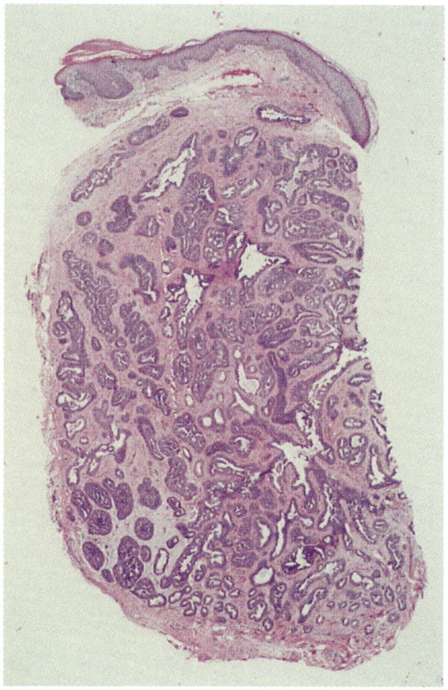

Figure 12–40. Papillary adenoma. The tumor is encased in a distinctive fibrotic stroma and consists of anastomosing epithelial nests with prominent glandular differentiation.

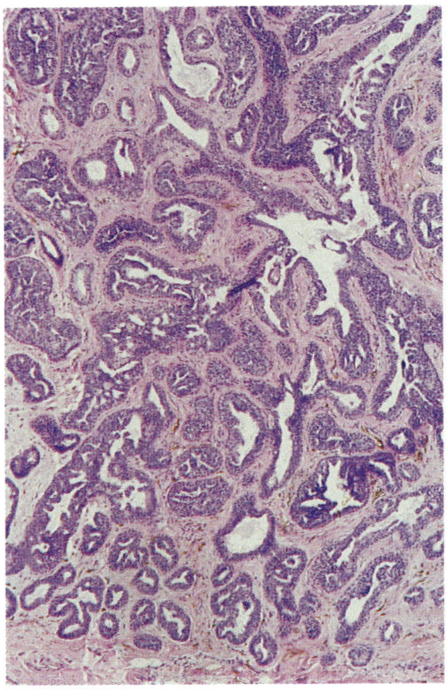

Figure 12–41. At higher magnification, papillary adenoma consists of small internal papillations with glands lined by one or two cuboidal epithelial layers. Foci of apocrine-type secretions also may be detected.

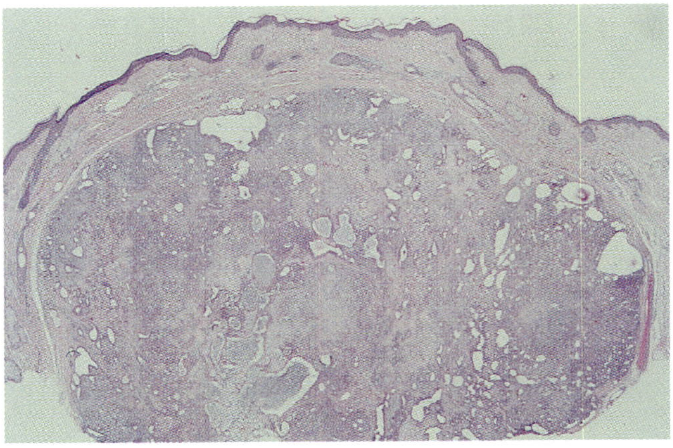

Figure 12–42. Mixed tumor. This symmetric nodule is largely composed of stroma in which small epithelial cords and ducts are dispersed.

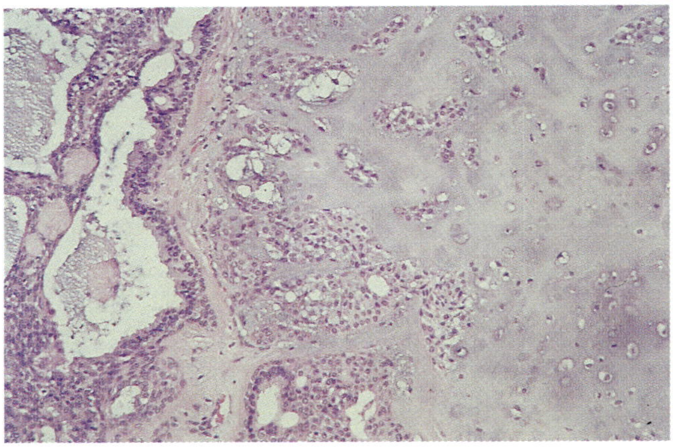

Figure 12–43. The stromal matrix of mixed tumor varies from myxoid to chondroid *(right)*. Epithelial elements show eccrine duct-like differentiation *(left)* and are lined by one or two cuboidal epithelial layers.

Tumors Forming Sheets and Nodules

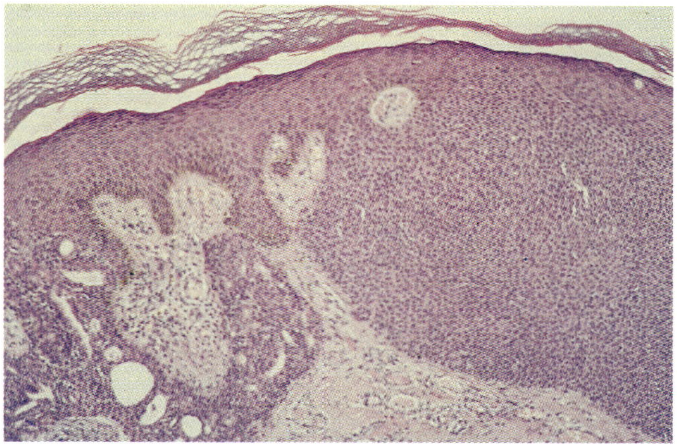

Figure 12–44. Poroma. Sheet-like downgrowths of epithelium are observed at scanning magnification.

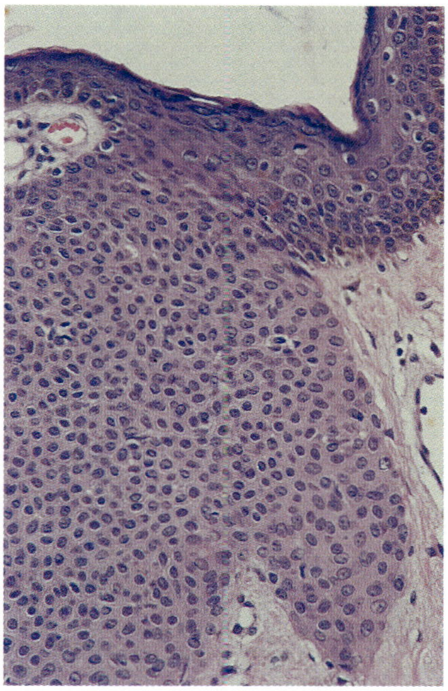

Figure 12–45. The cells forming these downgrowths in poroma are polyhedral but smaller than overlying normal or adjacent keratinocytes. Their cytoplasm is pale as a result of increased glycogen content.

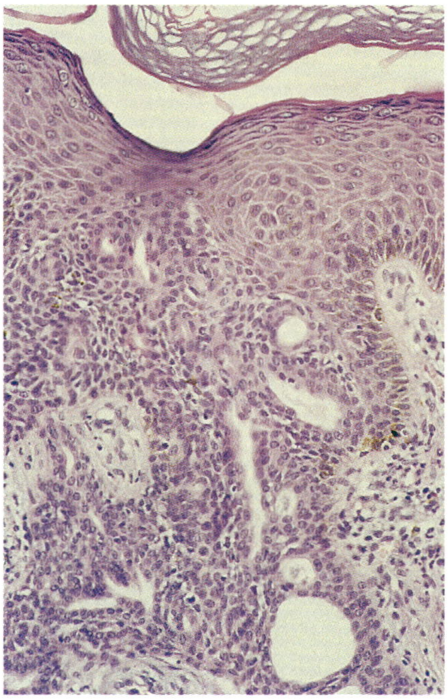

Figure 12–46. Foci of spiraling ductular differentiation *(center)* are also typically observed in poroma.

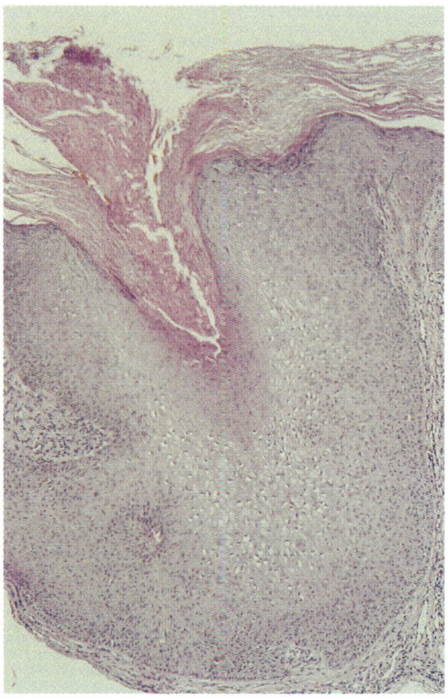

Figure 12–47. Trichilemmoma. There is plate-like downgrowth about a follicular infundibulum, which eventually may form an expansile nodule within the superficial and deep dermis.

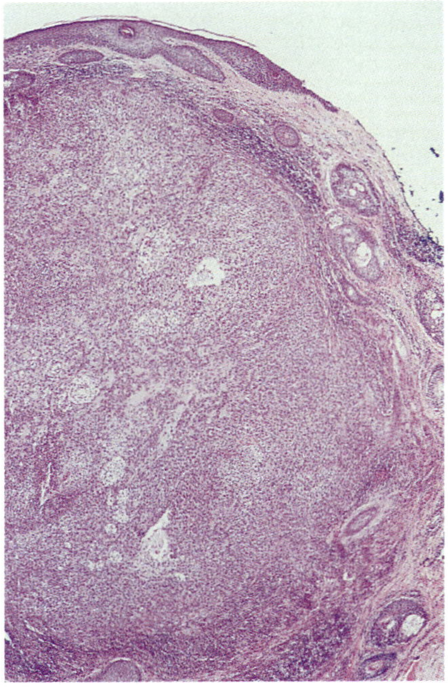

Figure 12–48. Nodular hidradenoma. There is a large cellular nodule within the dermis. The nodule may contain varying numbers of eccrine-type ducts, and invaginations of stroma frequently are markedly hyalinized.

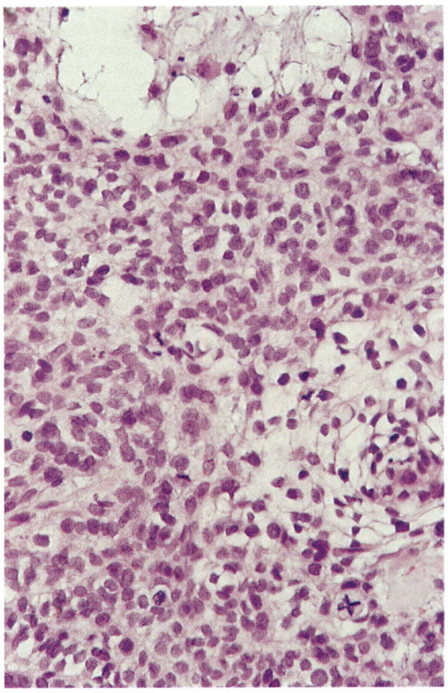

Figure 12–49. At higher magnification, nodular hidradenoma is characterized by foci of marked cytoplasmic glycogenation, which impart striking cytoplasmic clearing. Tumors in which this cytologic change predominates have been termed clear cell hidradenomas.

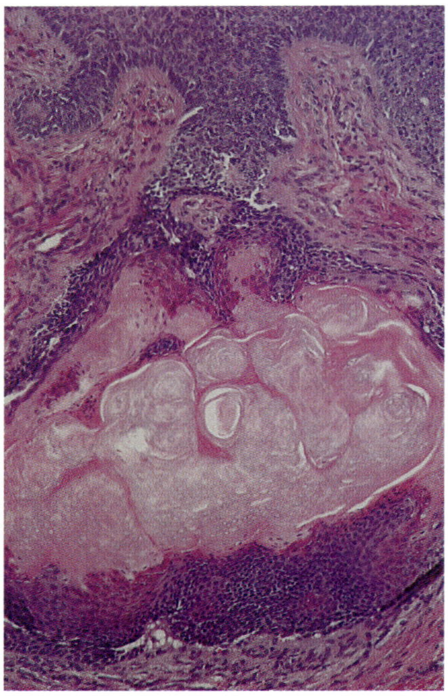

Figure 12–50. The pilomatricoma consists of a nodular aggregate of epithelial cells within a reactive desmoplastic stroma usually containing foreign body giant cells.

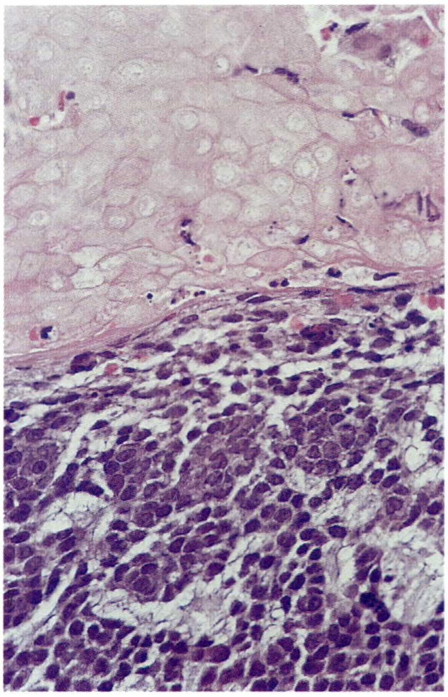

Figure 12–51. Diagnostic features of pilomatricoma include anucleate cells exhibiting hair cortex (*i.e.,* shadow cells; *top center*) and hair matrix *(bottom center)* differentiation. Foci of calcification and even ossification may be present.

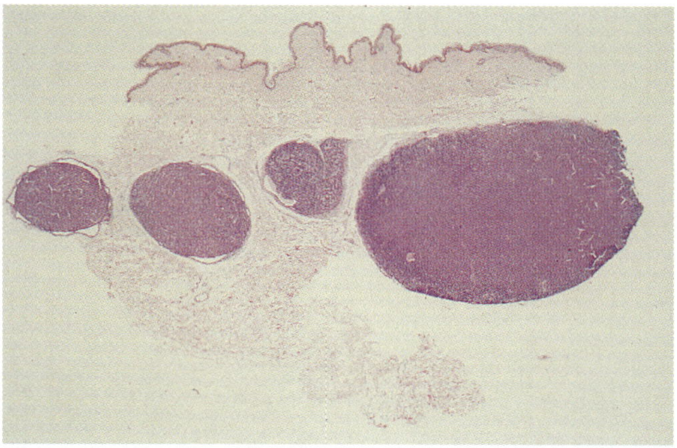

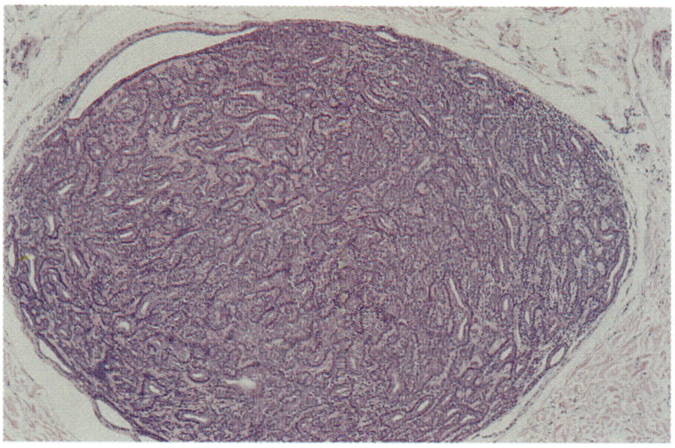

Figures 12–52 and 12–53. Solid variant of spiradenoma. Spiradenomas are nodular tumors composed of compacted cords of cuboidal epithelium.

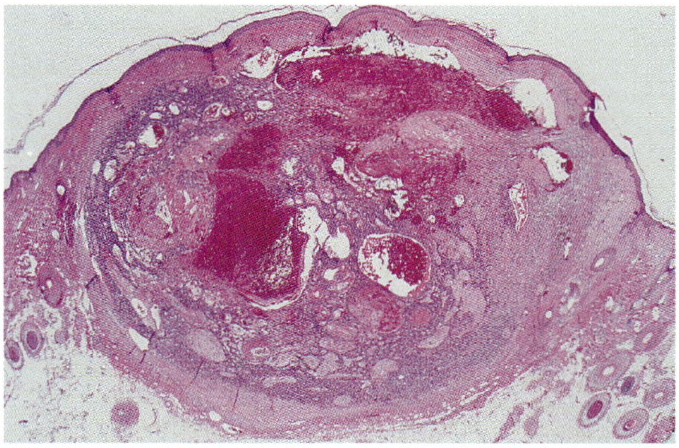

Figure 12–54. Vascular variant of spiradenoma; initial diagnostic impression at scanning magnification may include glomangioma.

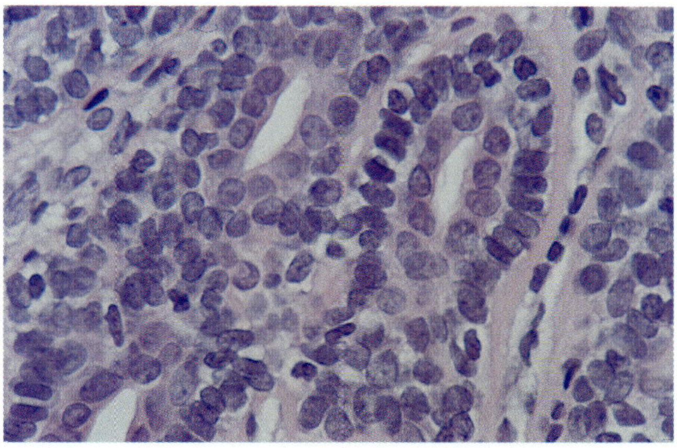

Figure 12–55. Small eccrine-type lumina and hyalinized matrix that often forms extracellular rounded bodies similar to those of cylindroma are routinely detected in spiradenoma. As in the case of cylindroma, the epithelial cells vary from small basaloid cells to larger, pale, epithelial elements.

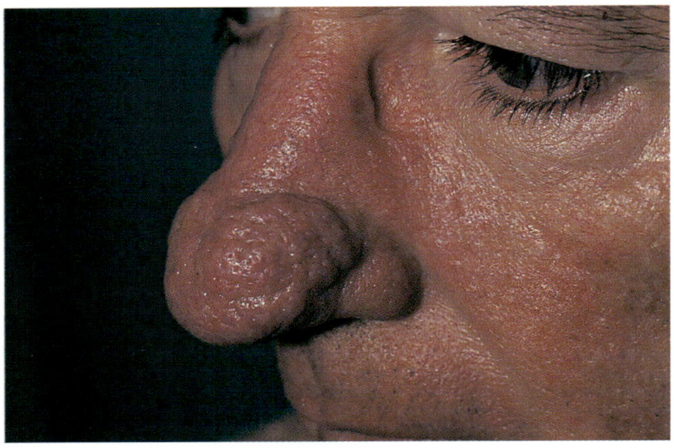

Figure 12–56. Sebaceous hyperplasia. Typical rhinophyma, or "W.C. Fields nose," is due to extensive sebaceous hyperplasia.

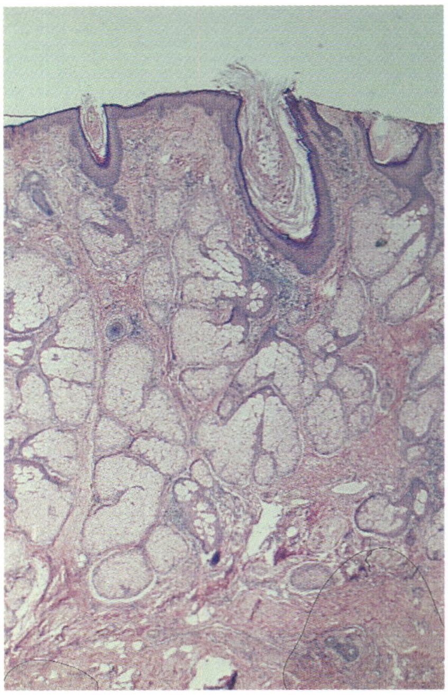

Figure 12–57. Histologically, the superficial and deep dermis is crowded with mature sebaceous lobules in sebaceous hyperplasia. Dilated and plugged follicular infundibula are also characteristically seen.

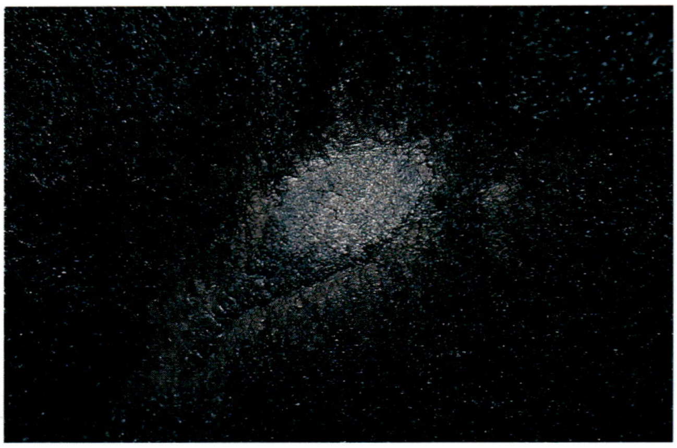

Figure 12–58. Nevus sebaceus. Alopecia is observed at the site of a verrucous plaque that has been present since birth.

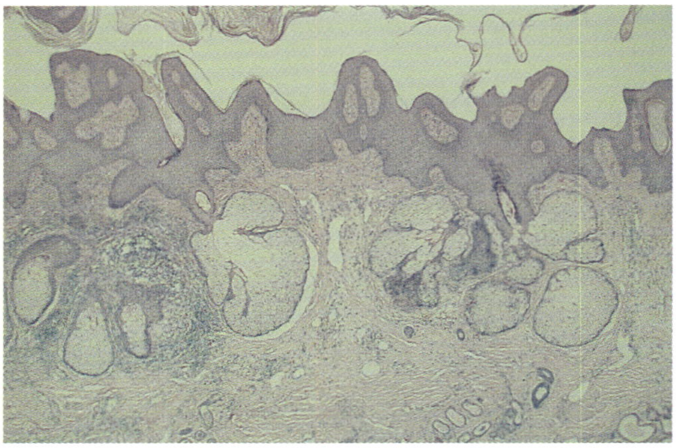

Figure 12–59. A biopsy specimen of nevus sebaceus reveals papillomatous epidermal thickening, focal sebaceous hyperplasia, and aberrant follicular buds.

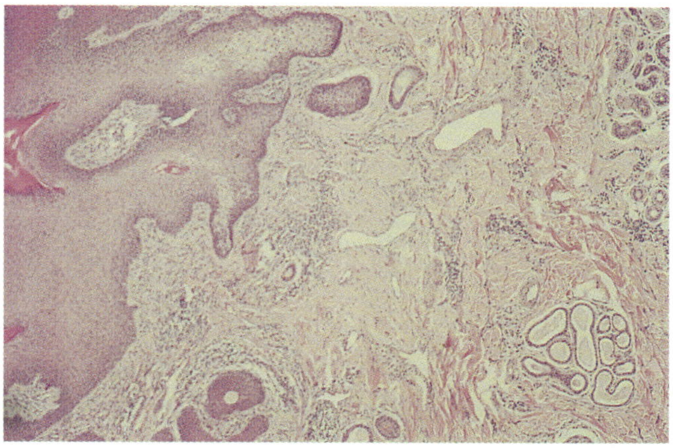

Figure 12–60. Often overlooked is the abnormal fibrovascular stroma, a form of dermal hamartoma that generally accompanies nevus sebaceus. Note anomalous apocrine differentiation for this anatomic site *(bottom left)*.

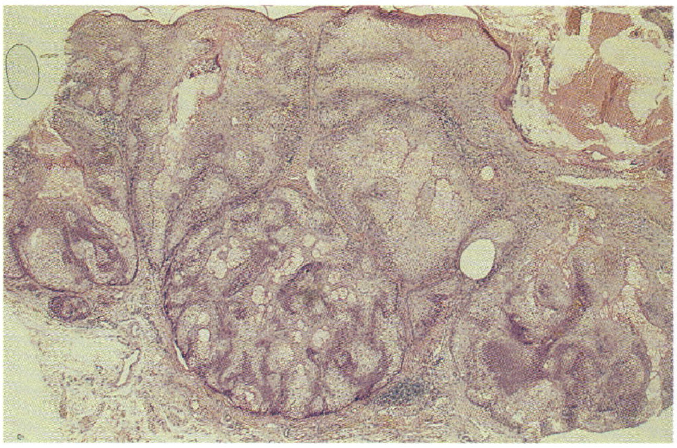

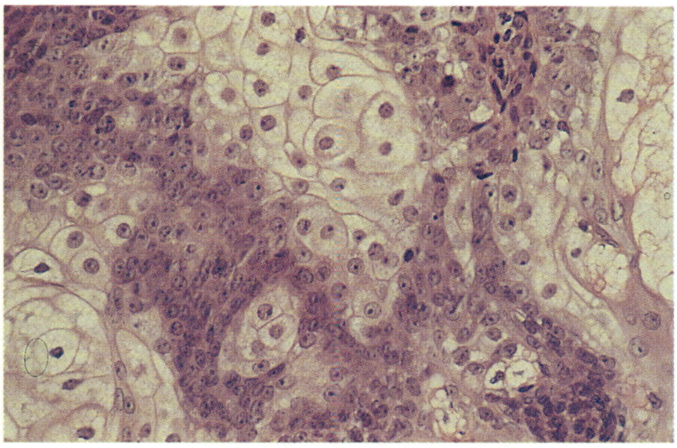

Figures 12–61 and 12–62. Sebaceous adenoma is an endophytic lobulated tumor with prominent central lipidization and only several layers of nonlipidized basaloid cells at the periphery.

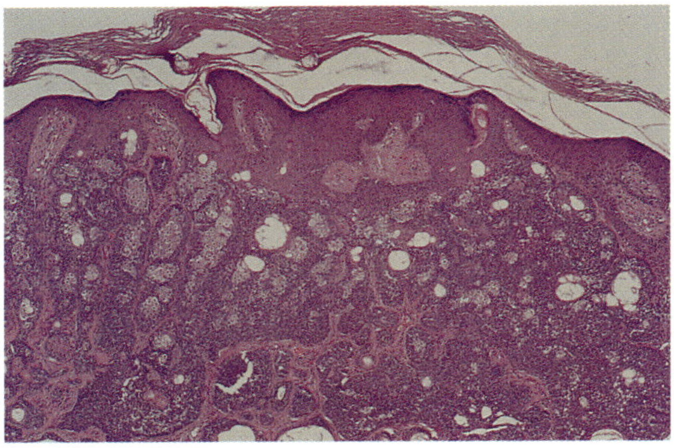

Figure 12–63. Sebaceous epithelioma has a similar architecture to adenoma, but increased basaloid elements (>50%).

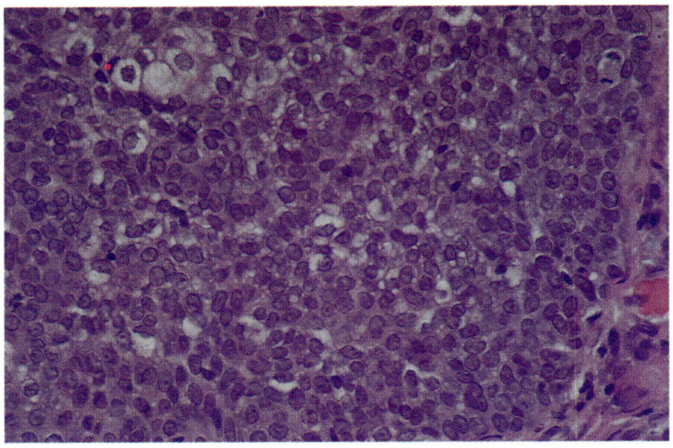

Figure 12–64. Basaloid cells predominate, and lipidization is only focally observed in sebaceous epithelioma.

Adnexal Carcinoma

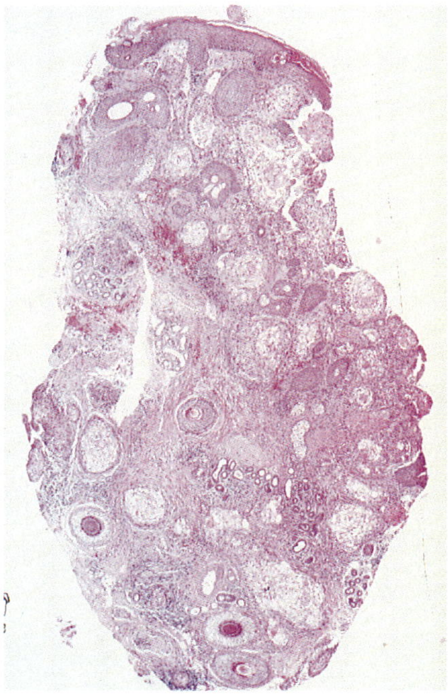

Figure 12–65. Sebaceous carcinoma. This is a poorly defined, deeply infiltrative neoplasm.

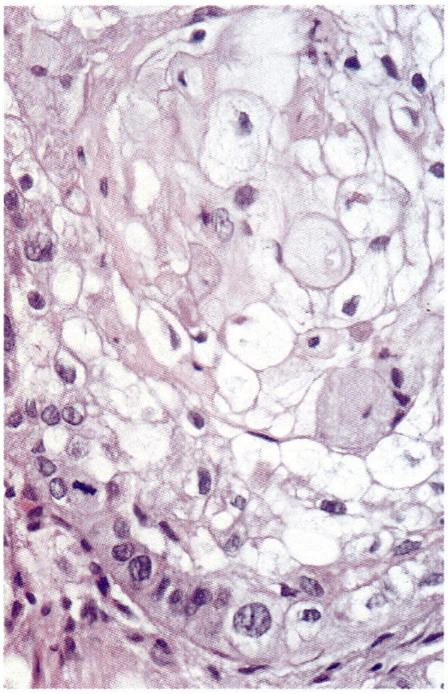

Figure 12–66. This sebaceous carcinoma shows regions of overt cytoplasmic lipidization. Other examples have a paucity of cytoplasmic lipid and more closely resemble poorly differentiated squamous cell carcinoma.

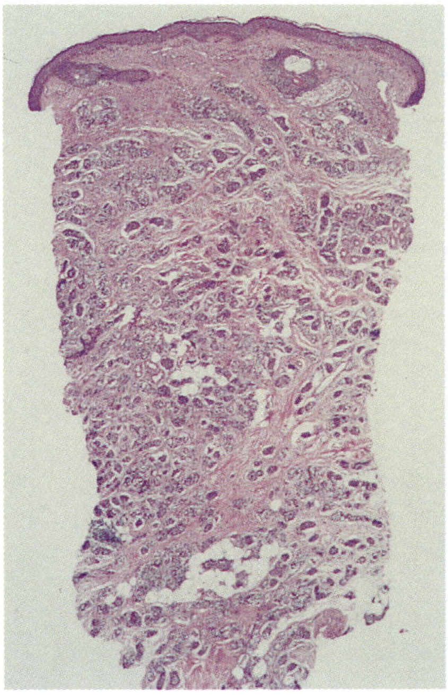

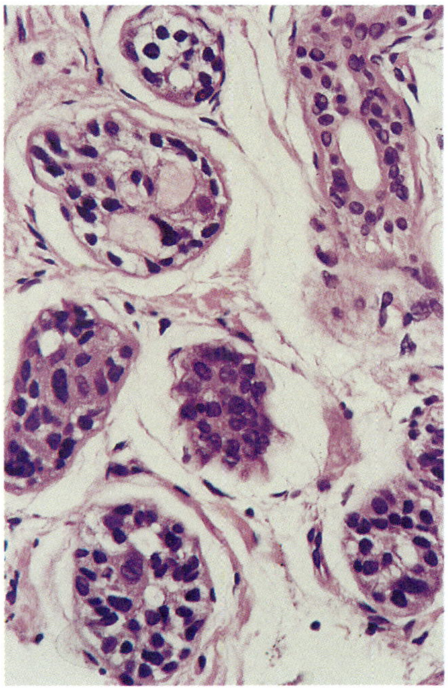

Figures 12–67 and 12–68. Eccrine carcinoma with foci of dermal ductular and secretory coil differentiation. Note the diffusely infiltrative pattern of growth (Fig. 12–67) and the striking nuclear hyperchromasia (Fig. 12–68).

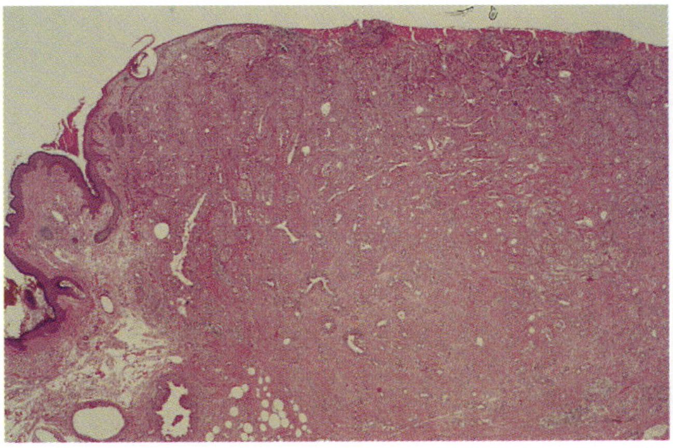

Figure 12–69. Apocrine carcinoma is a deeply invasive carcinoma composed of large epithelial cells with granular eosinophilic cytoplasm and focal lumen formation (see Fig. 12–70). Several regions demonstrated apocrine-type secretion. Although these findings are consistent with primary apocrine carcinoma, metastasis must be excluded, particularly from the breast, where primary adenocarcinomas may display apocrine features.

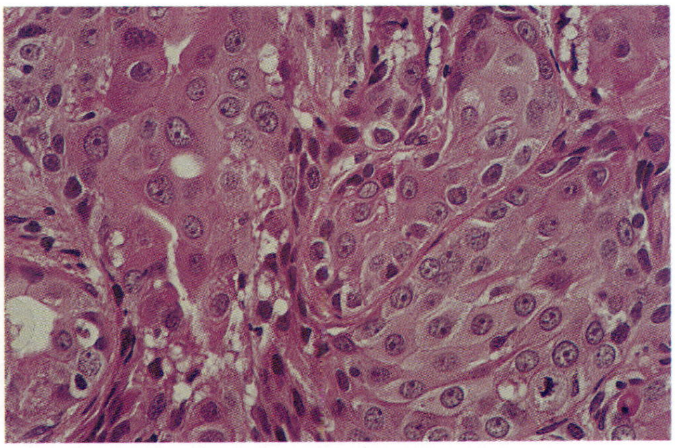

Figure 12–70. Large epithelial cells with granular eosinophilic cytoplasm and focal lumen formation characterize this apocrine carcinoma.

13

Melanocytic Tumors

Melanocytic hyperplasias and neoplasms are commonly removed for cosmetic and diagnostic reasons. Although most are benign, many may be confused clinically and histologically with malignant melanoma (heretofore referred to simply as melanoma), the most common potentially fatal neoplasm of the skin. On the other hand, numerous melanoma variants are mistaken daily for either benign nevi or other nonmelanocytic tumors. Despite these pitfalls, heightened clinical detection of early lesions has characterized recent advances in this area. Paradoxically, the incidence and mortality of patients with melanoma have sharply risen during recent years. Awareness of melanoma has resulted in more judicious clinical screening and biopsy of early precursor lesions, which may be typified by subtle or ambiguous histologic patterns. Accurate recognition of these patterns is critical to identification of lesions with significant premalignant or malignant potential and to their segregation from the numerous histologically similar hyperplasias and benign neoplasms of melanocytes.

Although most melanocytic nevi (*nevus* derives from Sanskrit root *-gna* and the Latin root *-gen,* both referring to *birth*) and melanomas are acquired during adolescence or adulthood, these lesions originate from a peculiar neoplastic transformation of pre-existing melanocytes. Melanocytes are dendritic, neural crest–derived cells that normally inhabit the basal cell layer of the epidermis. The purpose of these cells is the synthesis of photoprotective brown melanin pigment, and accordingly they are evenly dispersed in relatively low numbers (approximately 1 melanocyte per 10 contiguous basal keratinocytes in truncal skin not chronically actinically damaged), with their delicate melanin-laden dendrites extending toward the epidermal surface.

Hyperplasias of melanocytes are manifested clinically as diffuse hyperpigmentation (*e.g.,* tanning) or macular foci of cutaneous darkening (*e.g.,* lentigines). This is associated histologically with an increase in the ratio of melanocytes to basal keratinocytes (more than 1:10), often with increased melanization of the basal cell layer with thinning and elongation of the rete ridges. Linear hyperplasia of melanocytes within the basal cell layer is referred to as *lentiginous hyperplasia* (from the Latin *lenticula,* referring to a lentil-shaped spot). Lentiginous melanocytic hyperplasia characterizes simple lentigines and may be an integral component of certain acquired nevi, including dysplastic nevi. Nevus cell transformation refers to the poorly understood phenomenon whereby dendritic melanocytes become rounded cells that no longer tend to grow in lentiginous patterns but rather nest in aggregate, initially along the dermal-epidermal junction (junctional nevi). These cells eventually may "invade" the underlying dermis, first as nests and later as cords and single cells, to become compound nevi. Eventually, the junctional component is lost, producing pure dermal nevi.

The concept of *melanocytic atypia* deserves special attention. For this atlas, atypia connotes abnormal architectural or cytologic development but not necessarily premalignant alteration. Therefore, nevi recurring in scars, very old nevi with degenerative ("ancient") changes, and nevi with deep, penetrating patterns are, in a sense, atypical. On the other hand, atypical nevi that share some degree of architectural or cytologic similarity with melanoma are further categorized as exhibiting *dysplasia* and are regarded as potentially premalignant.

Melanoma may evolve from benign melanocytes or, more likely, from fields of progressive hyperplasia followed by dysplasia. This concept of tumor progression based on melanocytes has provided a conceptual basis for understanding the origins and natural evolution of a number of neoplastic systems. Early melanoma tends to grow within the epidermis along the lines or radii of a circle (radial growth) and does not form expansive nests or nodules, even at a microscopic level (nontumorigenic growth). With progression, tumor growth extends vertically into the underlying dermis (vertical growth), where melanoma cells form expansive and coalescent nests and nodules (tumorigenic growth). These simple concepts are of critical biological importance because they define stages in the evolution of melanoma with (vertical growth) and without (radial growth) capacity for metastatic spread.

The colors of melanocytic lesions are important at both clinical and histologic levels. Although most nevi are uniformly tan to brown, certain variants may be pink to red (spindle and epithelioid cell nevi) or even blue to black (blue nevi). Dysplastic nevi, on the other hand, are characteristically variegated tan, brown, and black, and in melanoma, this tendency may produce focal blue-gray and red hues. Histologically, colors are also important in identifying subtypes of nevus and melanoma cells. Generally, nevus cells have pale-pink cytoplasm, for example, whereas cells of spindle and epithelioid cell nevi have a typical blue-gray cytoplasm, and blue nevus cells are filled with particulate brown pigment. The nuclei of dysplastic and malignant melanocytes are usually darker blue than their benign counterparts, the result of progressive clumping and condensation of heterochromatin. Extremely basophilic aggregates of cells associated with the dermal components of nevi and melanomas often signify the presence of a brisk associated lymphocytic infiltrate, a feature that may be of prognostic importance in the latter and may be confirmed at higher magnification.

Evolution of Nevi

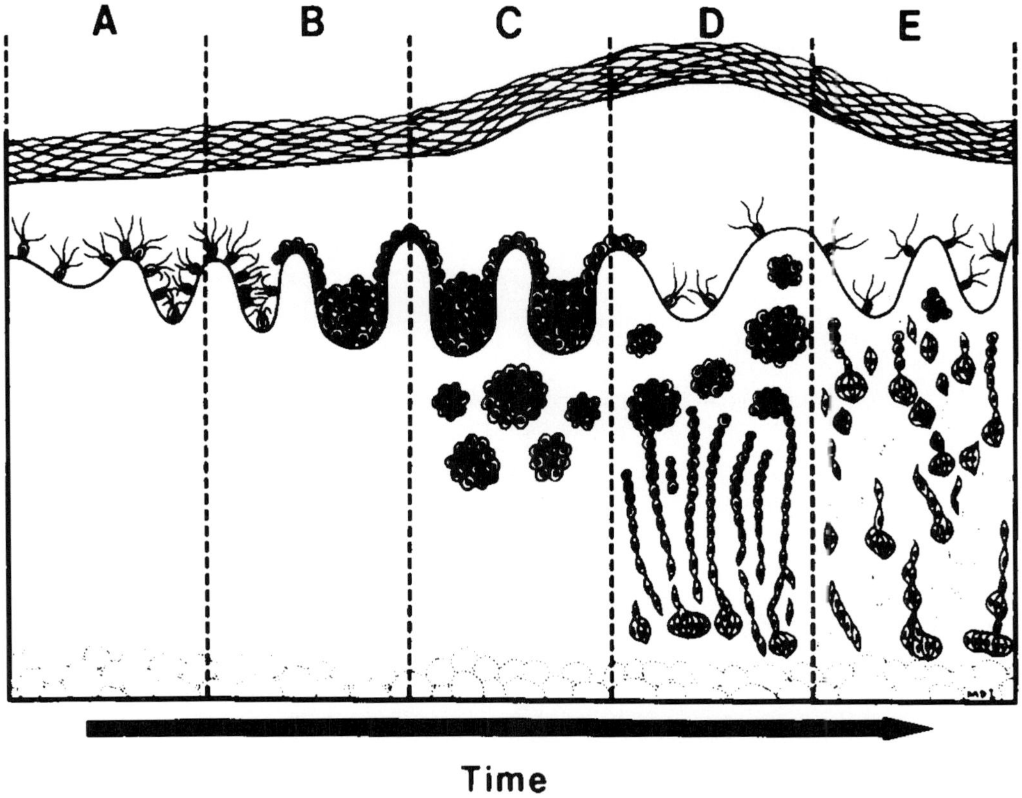

Figure 13–1. Natural evolution of a melanocytic nevus. Proliferation of normal melanocytes along the dermal-epidermal junction *(A)* leads to lentiginous hyperplasia and eventual nevic cell transformation to form a lentiginous junctional nevus *(B)*. Nested nevic cells at rete tips, over time, grow as nests within the underlying dermis to form a compound nevus *(C)*. The intraepidermal component then involutes *(D)*, and the purely dermal nevus that remains undergoes maturation, as evidenced by diminution in the size of cells at the base and eventual diffuse neural transformation of nevic cells within the dermal compartment *(E)*. A minority of nevi will show aberrant growth, developing dysplastic, potentially premalignant features (see Fig. 13–39).

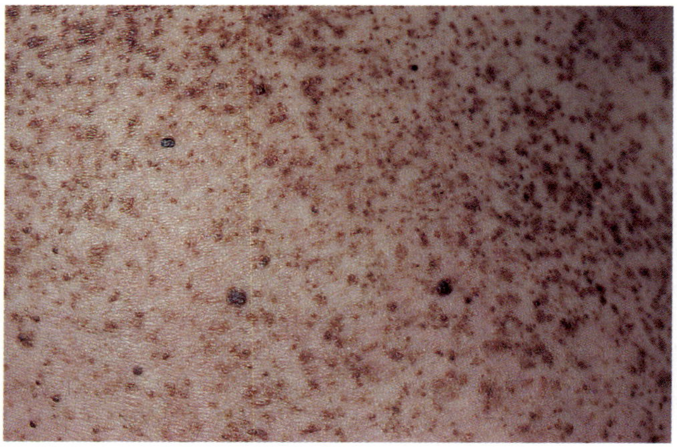

Figure 13–2. Melanocytic hyperplasia. Multiple lentigines are present in sun-exposed skin.

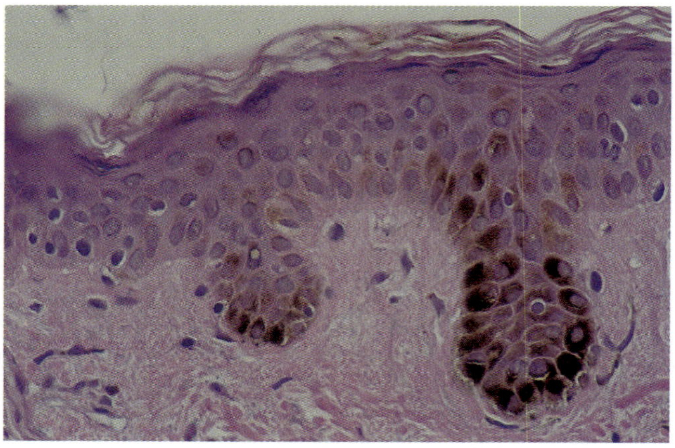

Figure 13–3. Melanocytic hyperactivity begins as increased pigment donation to basal keratinocytes, resulting in increased basal layer melanization and macular hyperpigmentation, referred to as a freckle or ephelis.

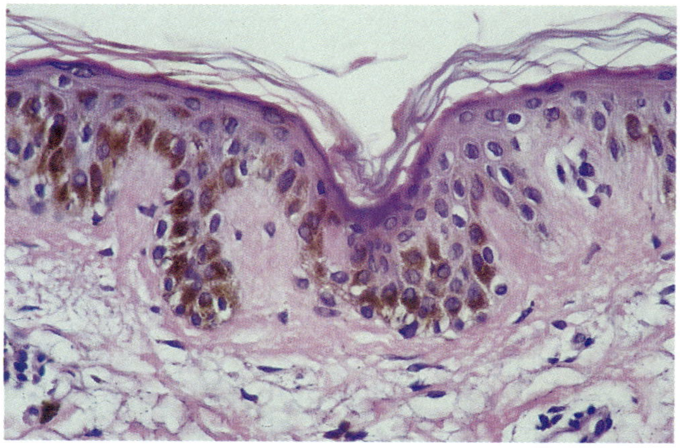

Figure 13–4. True melanocytic hyperplasia usually occurs in association with basal cell layer hyperpigmentation and is manifested by increased numbers of melanocytes at rete tips, producing a lentigo clinically. Unlike a freckle, a lentigo will appear slightly raised with side lighting.

Junctional Nevus

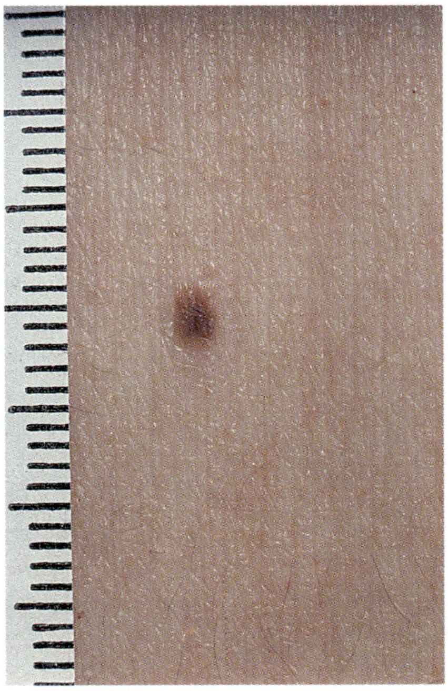

Figure 13–5. Clinically, junctional nevi are small, slightly elevated, uniformly colored, brown papules.

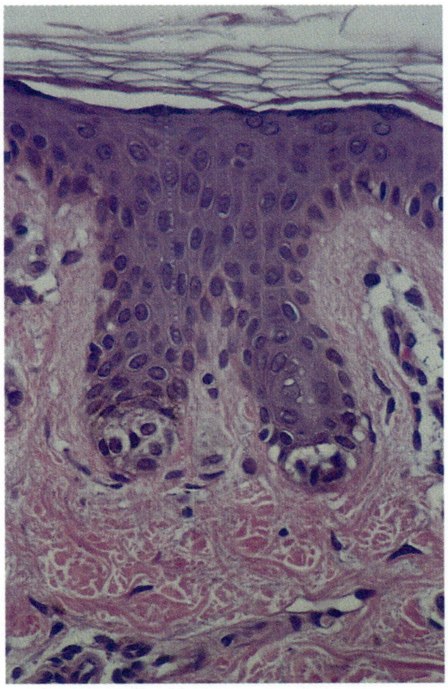

Figure 13–6. Histologically, there are small, rounded nests of nevus cells at the tips of the epidermal rete ridges. There is absence of dermal fibrosis or bridging of nests, evidence of aberrant growth.

Compound Nevus

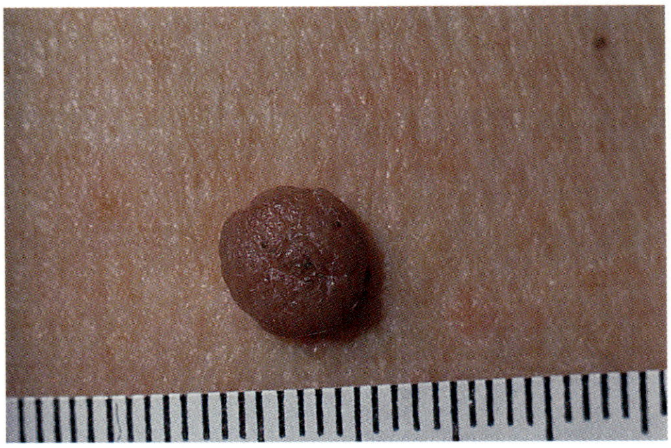

Figure 13–7. In contrast to lentigo and junctional nevus, the compound nevus is more raised and dome shaped. Note the uniform pigment distribution and symmetry, which are indicators of the benign nature of this process.

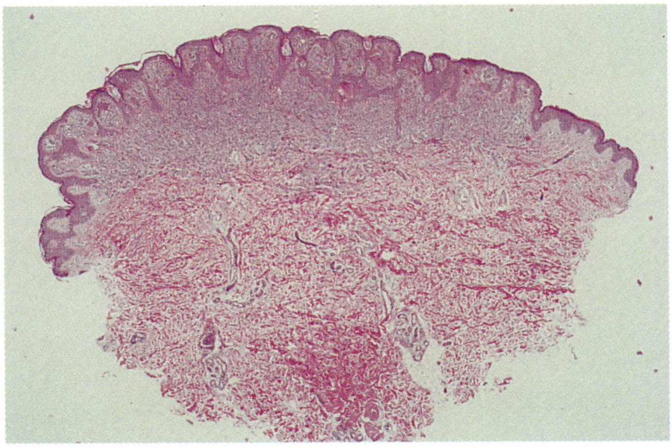

Figure 13–8. Histologic cross section of a compound nevus shows a symmetric proliferation of cells at the dermal-epidermal junction and within the superficial dermis. There often is associated epidermal hyperplasia.

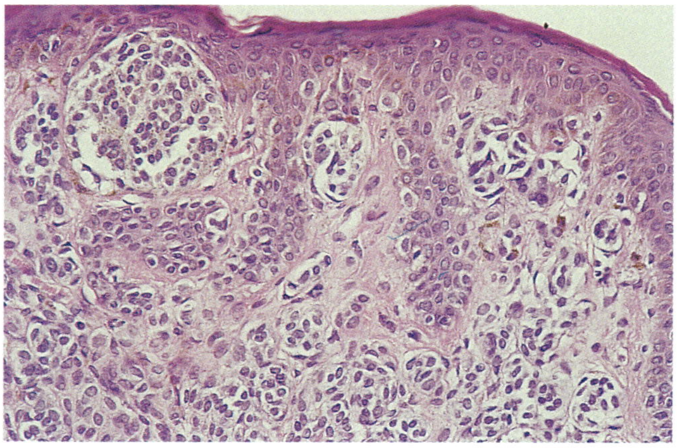

Figure 13–9. The nevus is composed of both junctional and dermal nevus cell nests. The dermal nevus nests are routinely smaller than those located at the dermal-epidermal junction.

Dermal Nevus

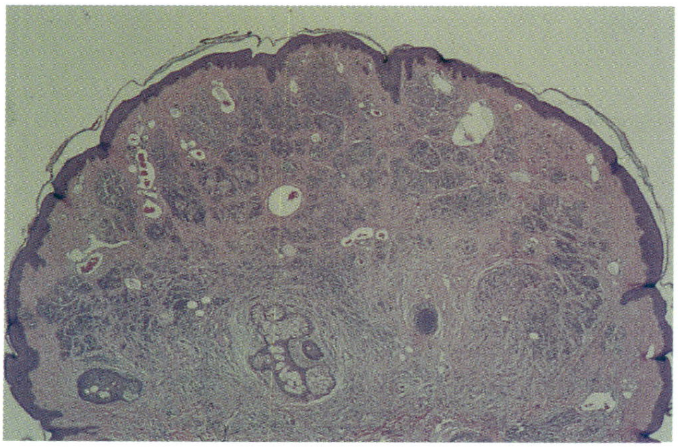

Figure 13–10. Scanning magnification of a dermal nevus reveals nests within the superficial and deep dermis.

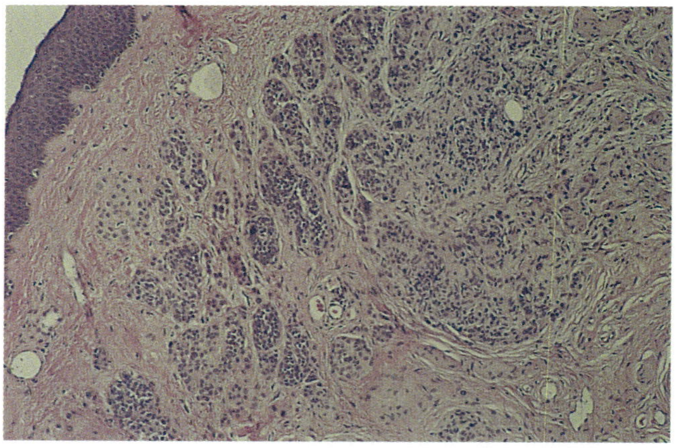

Figure 13–11. The nevus cells grow in superficial nests and mid-dermal cords and as deep dermal, relatively small spindle cells exhibiting neural differentiation *(extreme right).*

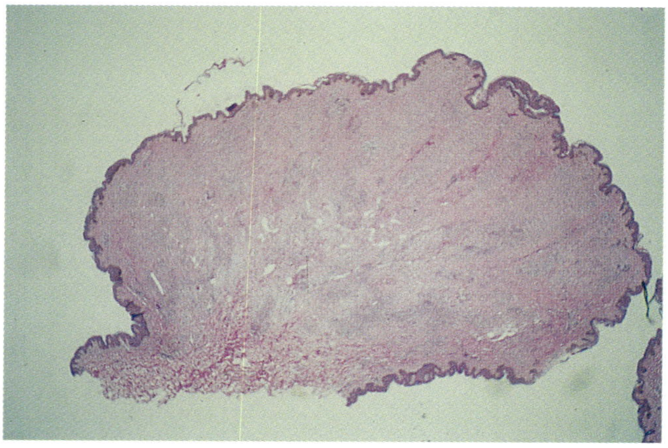

Figure 13–12. At low magnification, a dermal nevus with neurotization could be mistaken for a pedunculated neurofibroma.

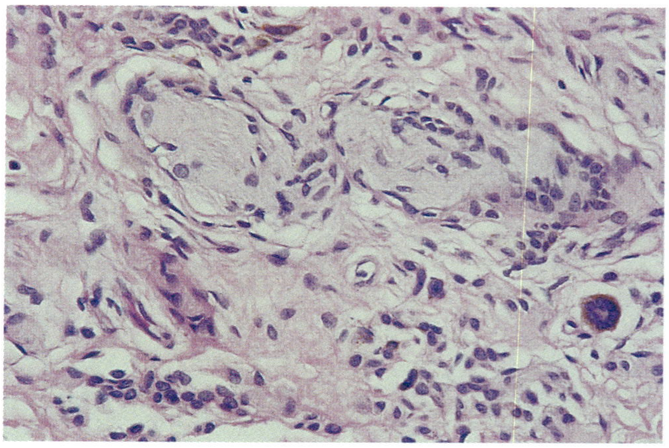

Figure 13–13. At higher magnification, nevus cells are fusiform and show prominent neural differentiation, including formation of Meissner corpuscle-like structures. Differentiation from tumors of true neural origin often depends on detection of residua of conventionally nested nevus cells just beneath the dermal-epidermal interface.

Congenital Nevus

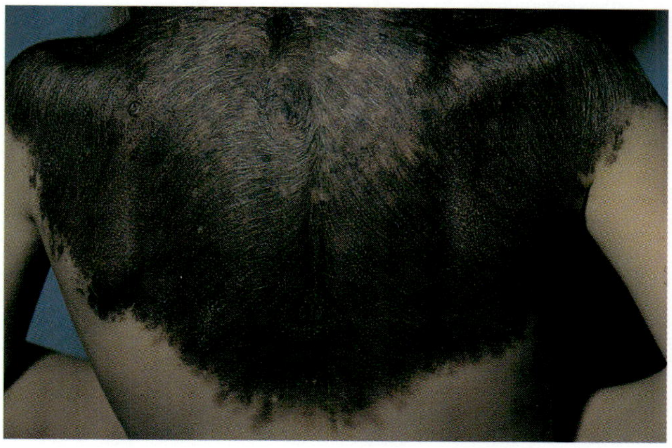

Figure 13–14. Large, garment-type congenital melanocytic nevi may cover large regions of the body surface and show extensive trichogenesis.

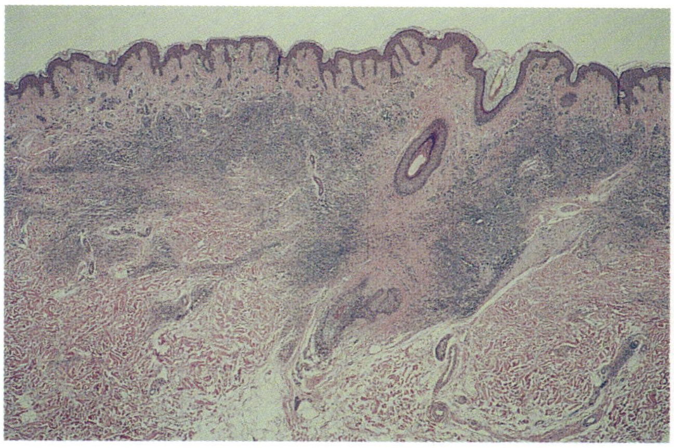

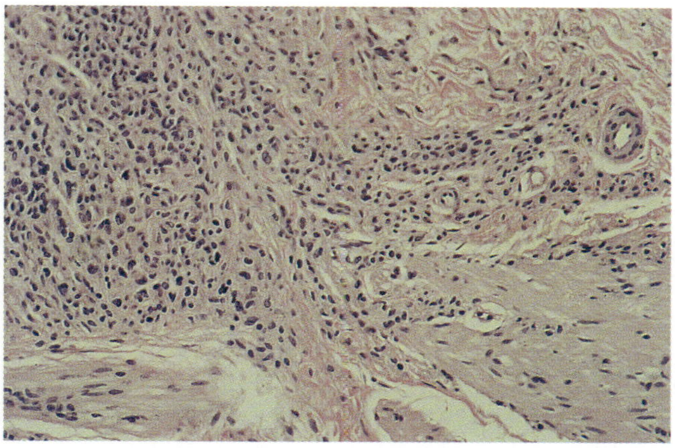

Figures 13–15 and 13–16. A clue to diagnostic recognition of congenital melanocytic nevi at scanning magnification is the diffusely permeative quality of the dermal component. Congenital melanocytic nevi also commonly show extension about eccrine ducts and neurovascular bundles, nest formation within adnexal epithelium, invagination into lymphatic lumina (see Fig. 13–17), and involvement of neural adventitia (see Fig. 13–18).

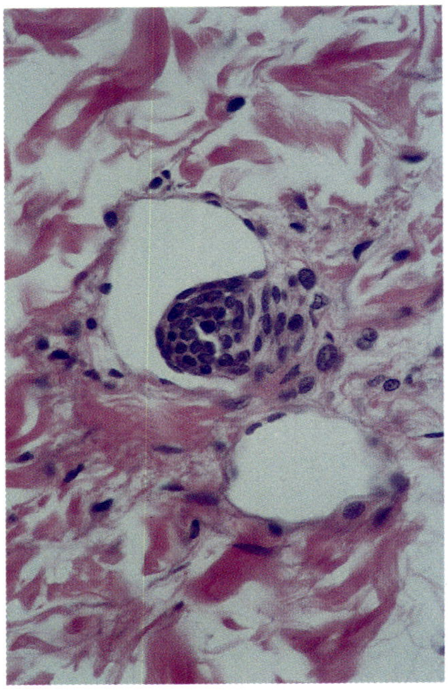

Figure 13–17. Invagination of melanocytic nevi into lymphatic lumina.

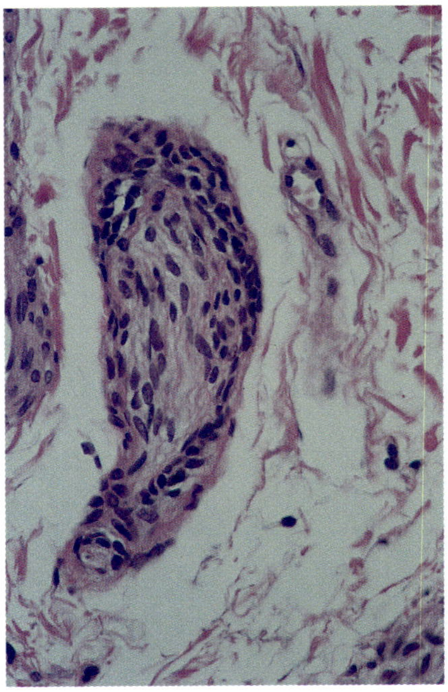

Figure 13–18. Involvement of neural adventitia.

Blue Nevus and Variants

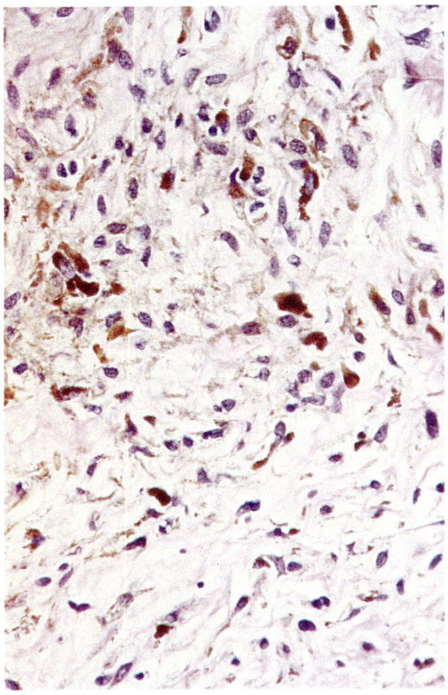

Figure 13–19. Ordinary blue nevi are characterized by proliferation of highly dendritic pigmented nevus cells within a fibrotic, superficial to mid-dermal stroma. These cells must be differentiated from pigment-laden histiocytes, which do not display prominent, melanin-containing dendrites.

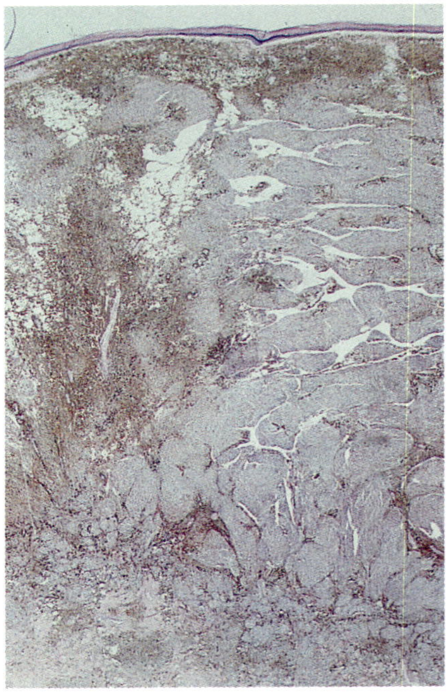

Figure 13–20. The cellular blue nevus contains pigmented regions that are typical of ordinary blue nevus (*left;* see also Fig. 13–19) and more cellular areas (*right;* see also Fig. 13–21) typical of this variant form. These lesions may show expansile, asymmetric growth into the deep dermis and subcutis, mimicking melanoma.

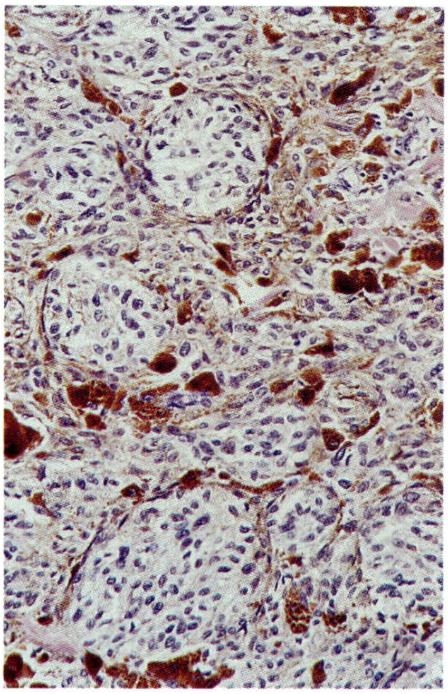

Figure 13–21. Cellular blue nevi are composed of large, nonpigmented epithelioid cells, often admixed with pigmented dendritic cells.

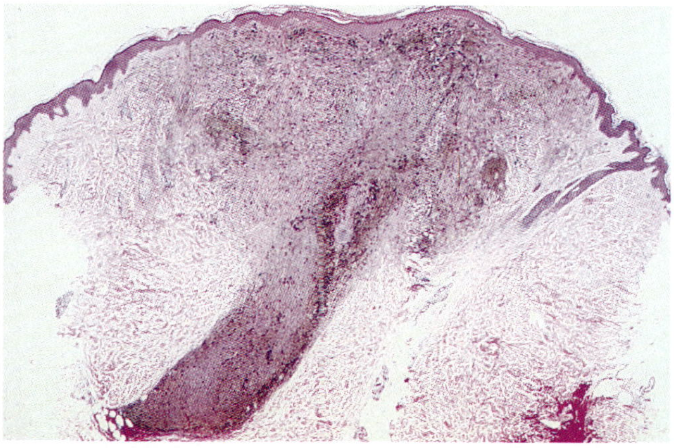

Figure 13–22. The contour of deep penetrating nevi, like that of cellular blue nevi, is asymmetric, with deep extension by tongues pushing into the subcutaneous fat.

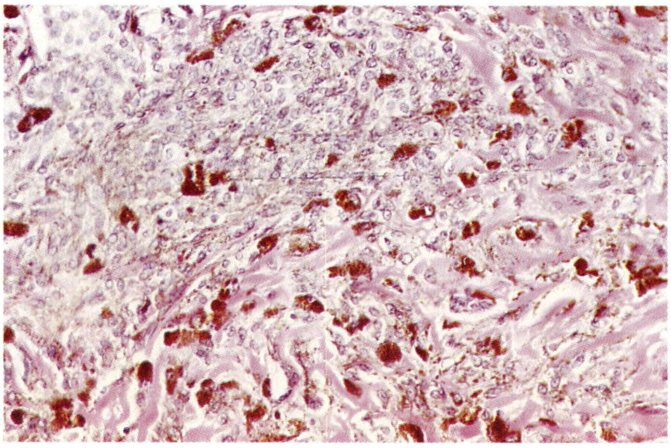

Figure 13–23. Like cellular blue nevi, lesions are composed of pigmented and relatively nonpigmented cells, although the former tend to be nondendritic in deep penetrating nevi.

Halo Nevus

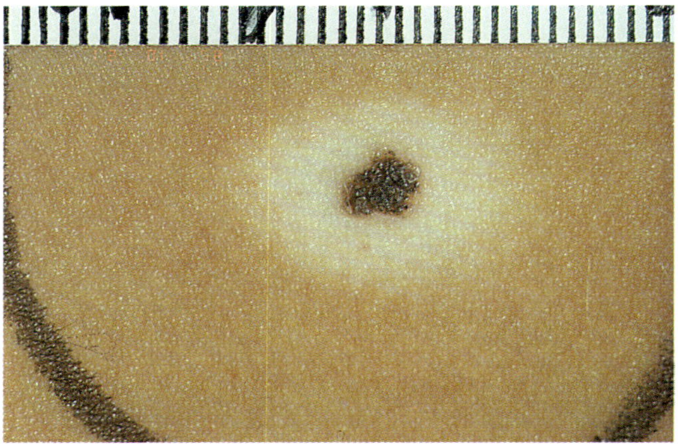

Figure 13–24. Halo nevus. A compound nevus is surrounded by a symmetric, vitiligo-like halo.

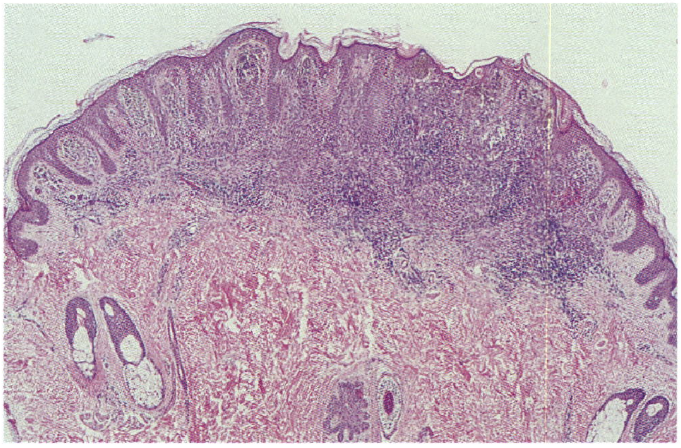

Figure 13–25. At low magnification, a relatively symmetric compound nevus appears abnormally basophilic because of the associated lymphocytic infiltrate.

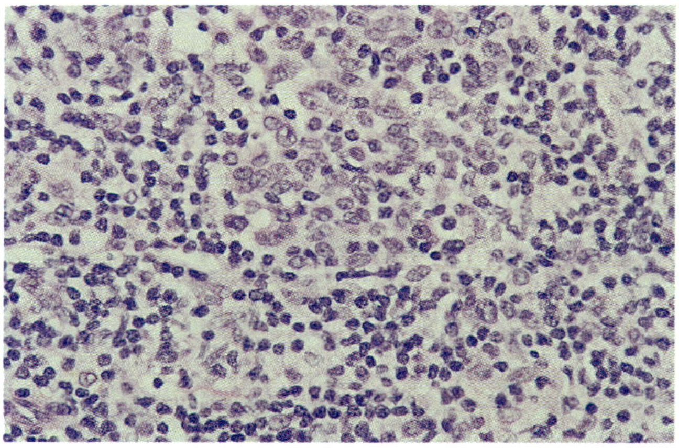

Figure 13–26. At higher power, individual nevus cells are surrounded by swarms of infiltrating lymphocytes. The normally nested contours of the nevus cell aggregates are jagged and irregular, presumably as a result of partial inflammatory regression induced by the cytotoxic immune response.

Spindle and Epithelioid Cell Nevus

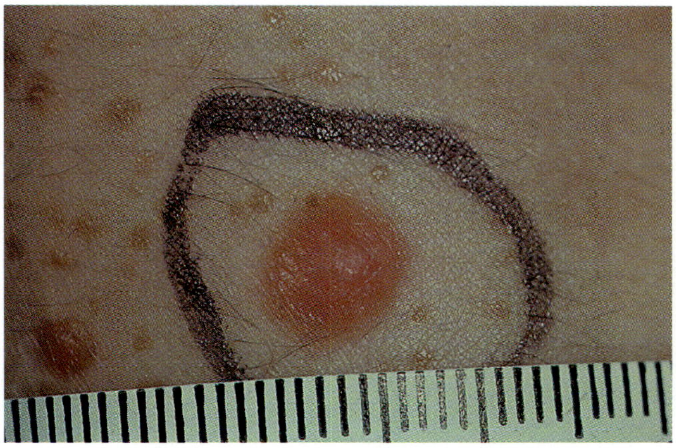

Figure 13–27. Spindle and epithelioid cell nevus. This rounded, dome-shaped nevus is pink to deep red clinically and here is surrounded by a shower of satellite nevi.

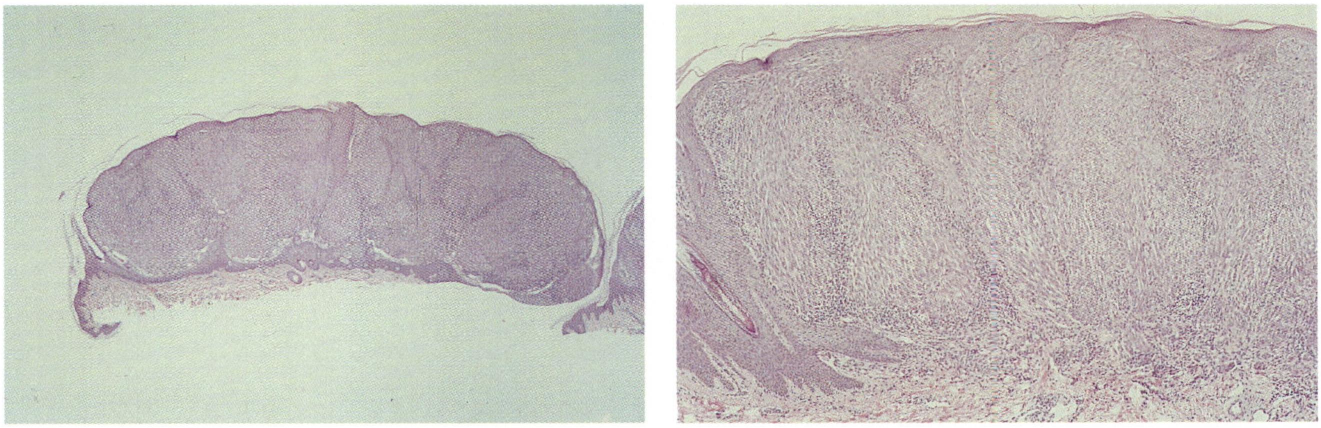

Figures 13–28 and 13–29. Although nevus nests along the dermal-epidermal junction appear large and coalescent, the lesion is bilaterally symmetric on scanning magnification, and significant pagetoid spread is not observed.

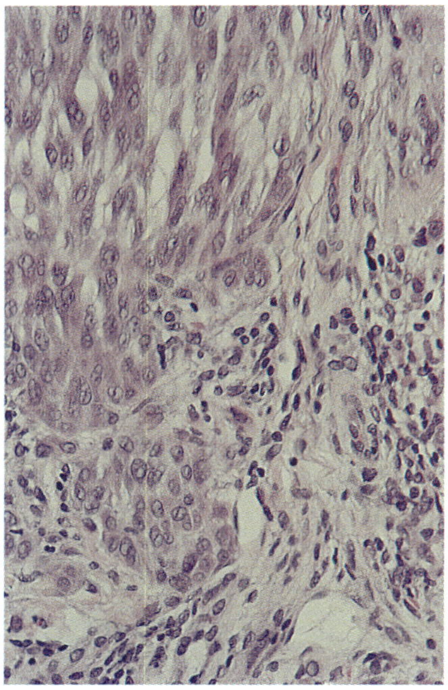

Figure 13–30. At higher magnification, epithelioid and fusiform cells are arranged in fascicles to produce a "raining-down" pattern. The stroma may be inflamed and often shows hyalinization and proliferation of dilated vessels.

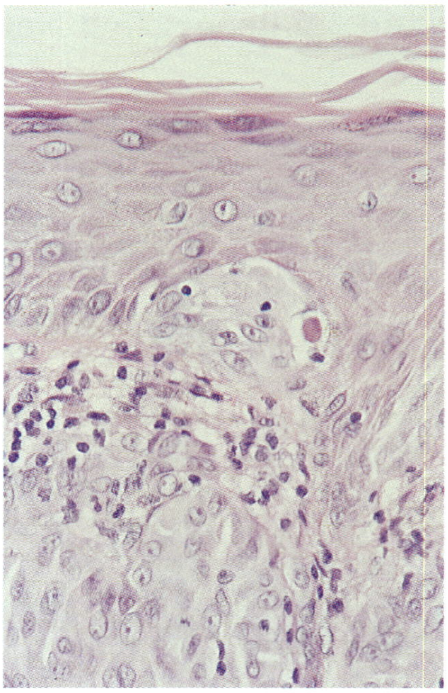

Figure 13–31. Along the dermal-epidermal junction, small eosinophilic bodies (*i.e.,* Kamino bodies) representing degenerated nevus cells are frequently observed.

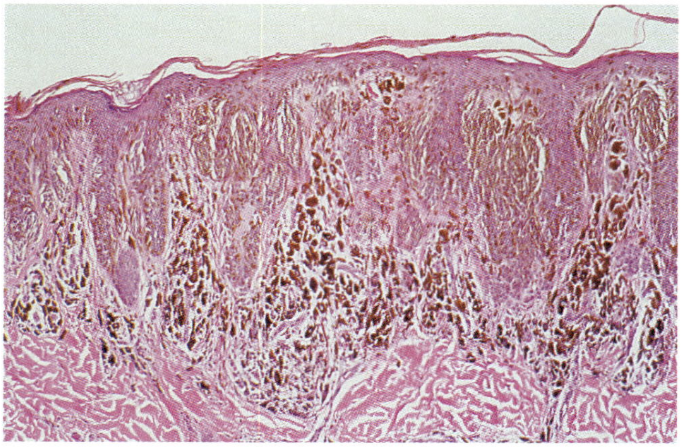

Figure 13–32. Pigmented spindle cell nevus. These relatively superficial lesions retain some of the architectural and cytologic features of ordinary spindle and epithelioid cell nevi and therefore may be mistaken for dysplastic nevi or malignant melanoma. Lesions are generally symmetric, composed predominantly of fascicles of spindle cells along the dermal-epidermal junction, and have marked melanin pigmentation, both within nevus cells and within aggregates of melanophages along the base of the dermal component.

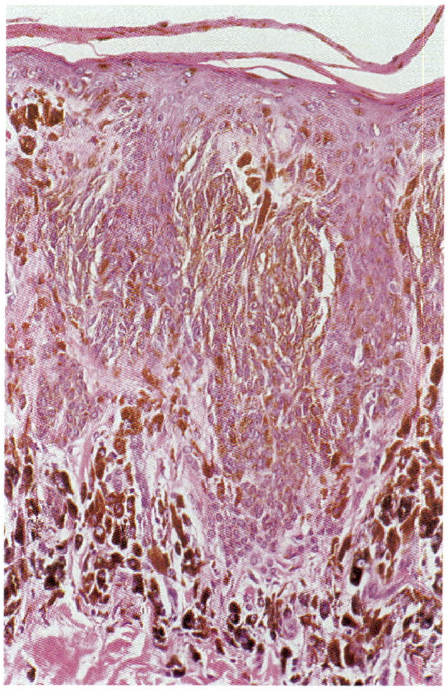

Figure 13–33. Pale Kamino body in pigmented spindle cell nevus is present along the dermal-epidermal junction. Note the architectural similarity to its relative, the spindle and epitheloid cell nevus, and the abundant dermal pigmentation due to the melanophages.

Recurrent Nevus

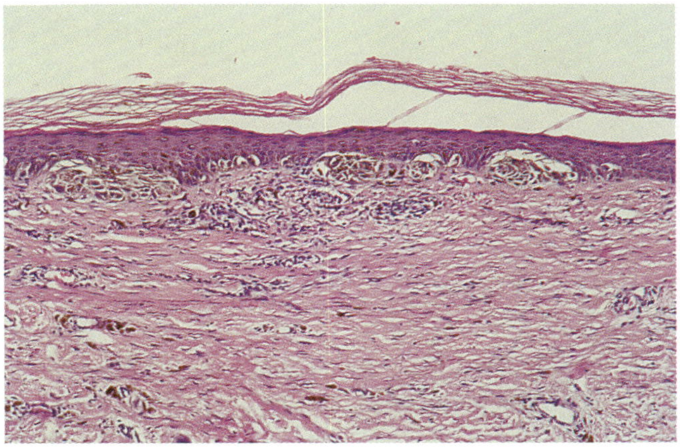

Figure 13–34. This recurrent nevus lesion is characterized by primarily intraepidermal nevic cell growth overlying a healing scar.

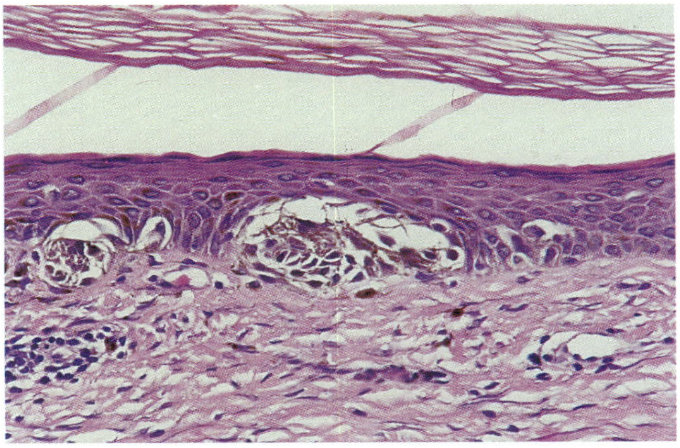

Figure 13–35. Nevus cells may be dyshesive and grow in irregular and coalescent nests composed of pigmented cells of variable shapes and sizes; true cytologic atypia or significant pagetoid spread, however, is not observed.

Processing Artifacts in Nevi

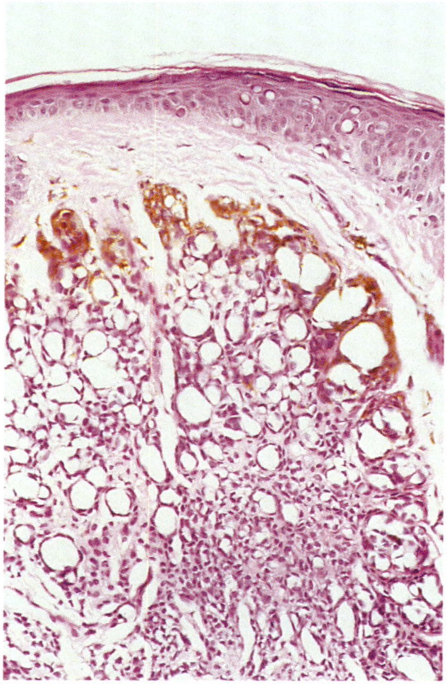

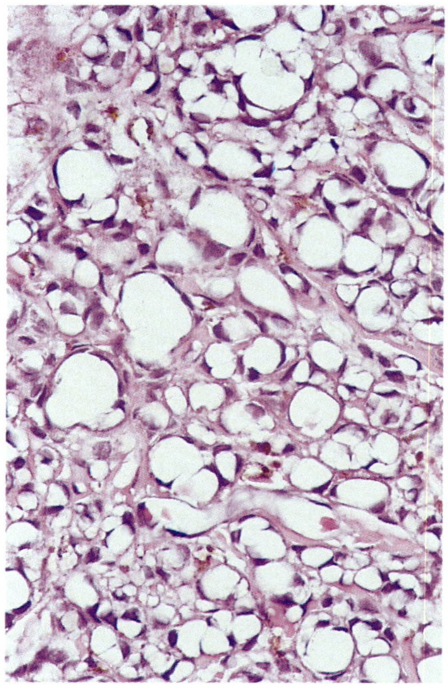

Figures 13–36 and 13–37. Common processing artifacts in nevi. Coarse vacuolization occurs as a result of freezing followed by thawing of tissue transported in formalin. This artifact is usually seen in winter months and should not be confused with balloon cell change in melanoma or with metastatic signet-ring cell carcinoma. Note that in Figure 13–36 even the more resilient keratinocytes show early vacuolization.

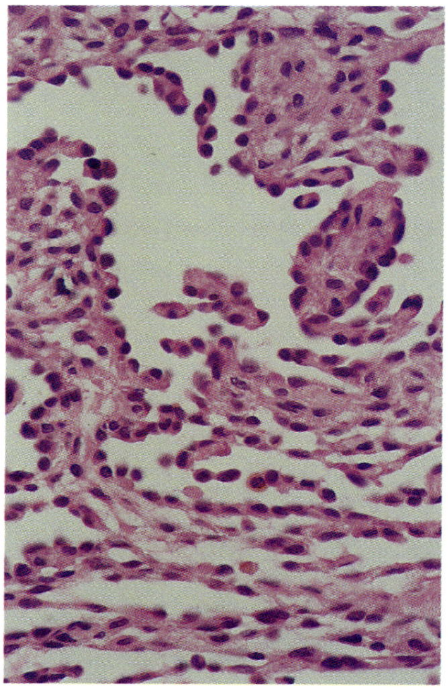

Figure 13–38. Lymphatic-like spaces are present in a dermal nevus as a result of dyshesion consequent to tissue preparation. The phenomenon may have a structural basis in impaired cell-cell adhesion between dermal nevus cells arranged in cords and is responsible for the "venetian-blind" pattern of clefts seen in the dermal components of some ordinary acquired melanocytic nevi.

Tumor Progression to Melanoma

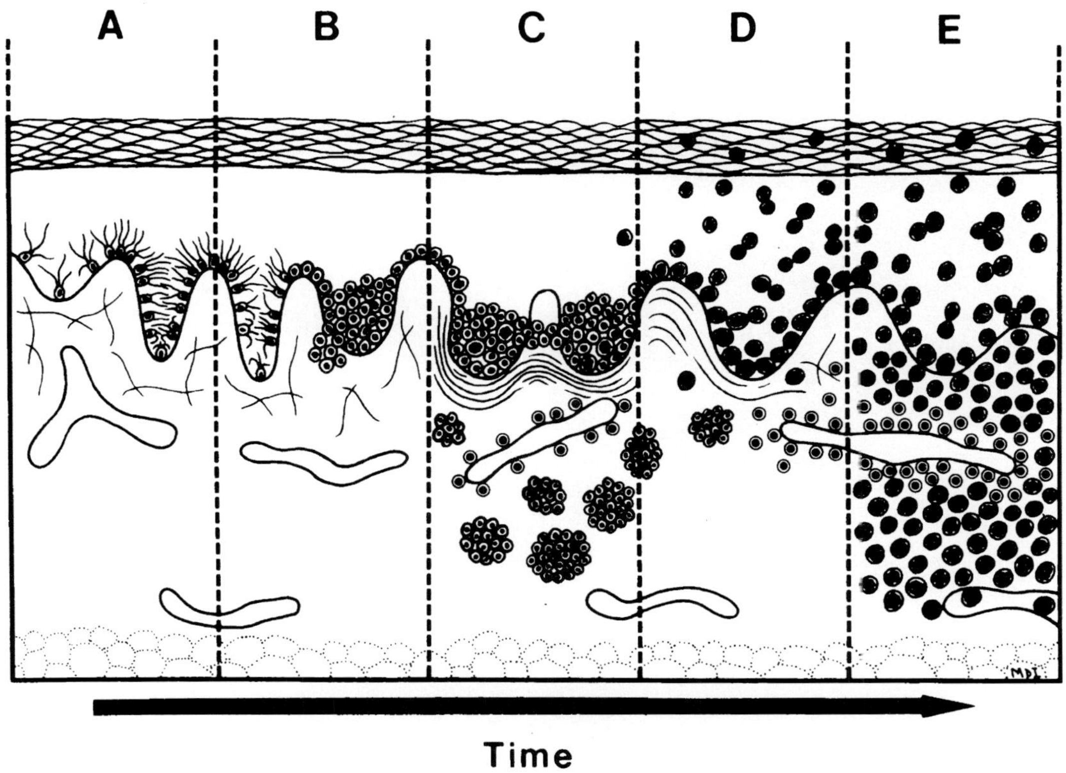

Figure 13–39. Tumor progression to malignant melanoma. Normal melanocytes along the basal cell proliferate in lentiginous fashion *(A)* and eventually undergo nevus cell transformation *(B)*. Aberrant nevus cell growth *(C)*, consisting of enlarged, coalescent nests; random cytologic dysplasia; and reactive stromal alterations, including lymphocytic infiltrate and lamellar fibroplasia, heralds the development of a lesion with the potential for further neoplastic progression, as opposed to involution to a neurotized dermal nevus, as is the case for most melanocytic nevi. Progression results in the emergence of a clone of malignant cells *(D)* with the ability to proliferate only within or in close proximity to the epidermal layer (*i.e.,* radial growth phase melanoma). *E,* Eventually, additional clones emerge with the ability to grow deeply into the dermis as tumorigenic nodules. Such cells also may acquire the ability to invade lymphatic spaces and spread to lymph nodes. Systemic dissemination depends on the ability to enter blood vessels and to metastasize to nonlymphoid viscera. Some melanomas appear to arise independent of a nevus cell intermediate and thus may progress from stage A directly to stage D.

Dysplastic Nevus

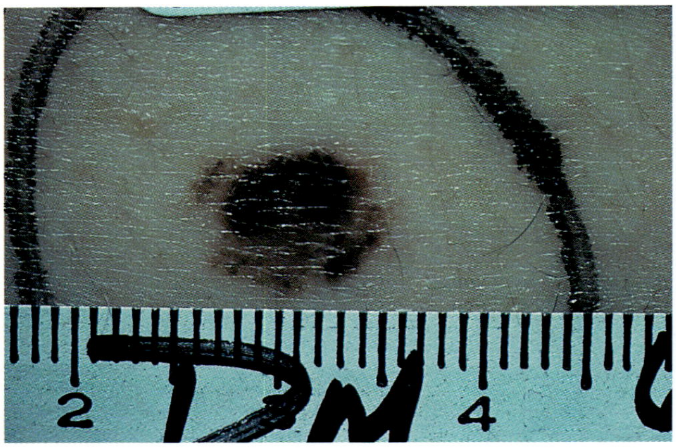

Figure 13–40. The clinical lesion in dysplastic nevus is a large (*i.e.*, more than 6 mm), asymmetric, variably pigmented plaque with an irregular, notched border.

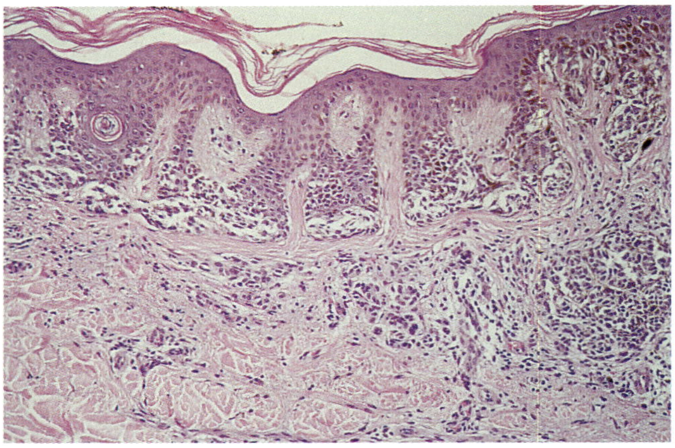

Figure 13–41. Histologically, there is a lentiginous compound nevus with prominent bridging of nevus nests across adjacent epidermal rete ridges. Some nests also arise aberrantly in inter-rete spaces.

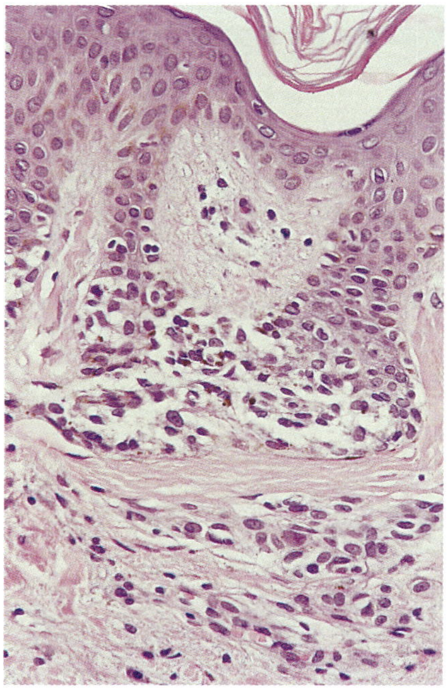

Figure 13–42. Bridging of nests is associated with lamellar fibrosis of the underlying papillary dermis as well as a variable lymphoid response with pigment incontinence. Cells within the nests show focally enlarged, angulated, hyperchromatic nuclei. This is clearly a very different clinical and histologic picture than that observed for the majority of acquired melanocytic nevi (see Figs. 13–5 through 13–13).

Superficial Spreading Melanoma

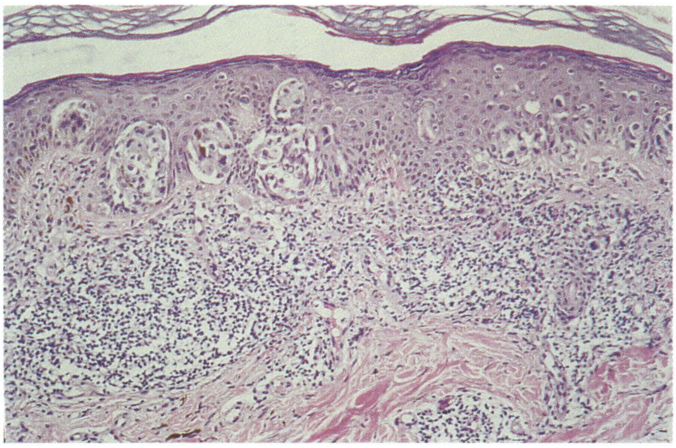

Figure 13–43. Malignant melanoma: Superficial spreading radial growth. At scanning magnification, there are irregular nests within the epidermis associated with an underlying lymphoid infiltrate.

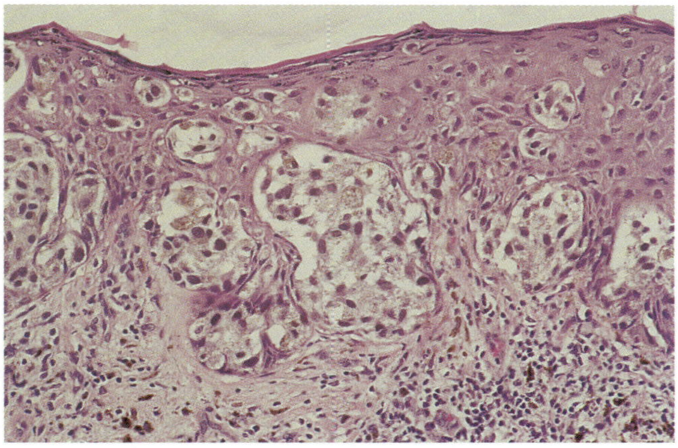

Figure 13–44. Malignant melanoma: Superficial spreading radial growth. At medium-power magnification, irregular and enlarged nests, as well as single cells, are present at all layers of the epidermis, whereas melanocytes in normal skin proliferate along the basal cell layer, and benign nevus cells form nests confined to rete tips.

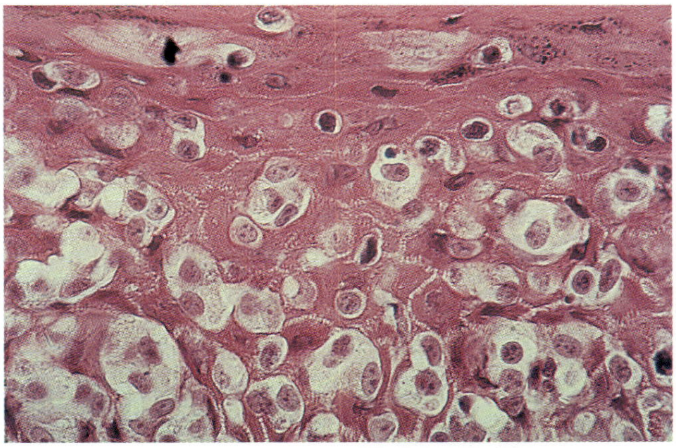

Figure 13–45. Marked pagetoid spread by cells showing fully evolved anaplasia consisting of nuclear enlargement, coarsely clumped and peripherally aggregated heterochromatin, and prominent nucleoli. Pagetoid spread extends upward to involve the stratum granulosum; this event is almost never observed for the rare pagetoid cells that may be seen in some nevi (*e.g.*, spindle and epithelioid cell nevi).

Lentigo Maligna Melanoma

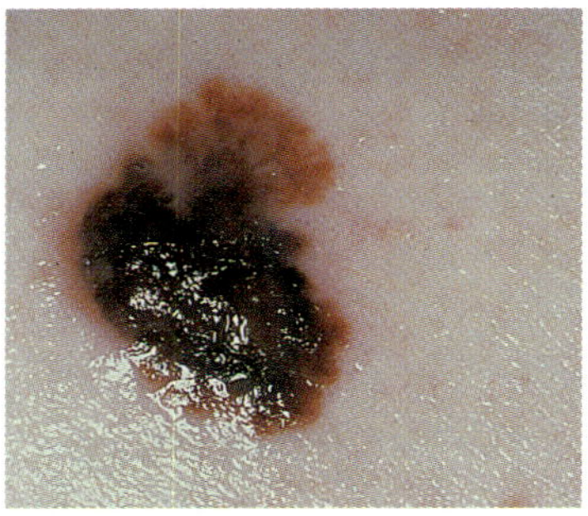

Figure 13–46. Melanoma: Lentigo maligna radial growth pattern. A different pattern of radial growth characterizes lentigo maligna, a dark, irregular ink spot–like, flat plaque that occurs on the sun-damaged facial skin of elderly individuals.

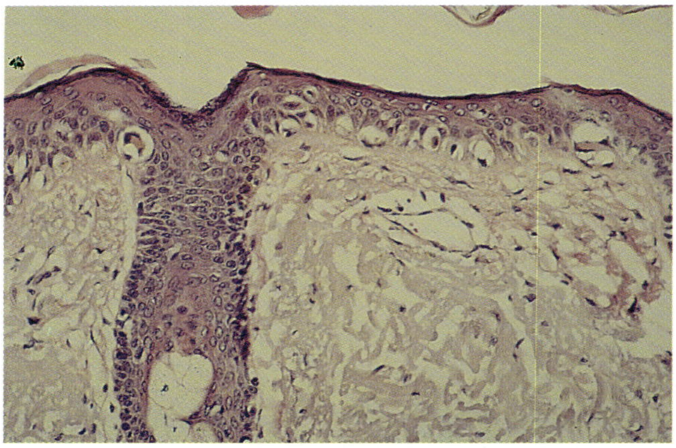

Figure 13–47. Histologically, there is contiguous lentiginous proliferation of dyshesive, variably shaped, malignant melanocytes located within an atrophic epidermal layer and involving the infundibular basal cell layer of hair follicles. The dermis typically shows solar elastosis. This form of radial growth is distinctive in its clinical appearance, its indolent and prolonged growth characteristics before the onset of vertical spread, and the histologic morphology of its radial and vertical growth phase, the latter of which frequently contains spindle cells.

Acral-Mucosal Lentiginous Melanoma

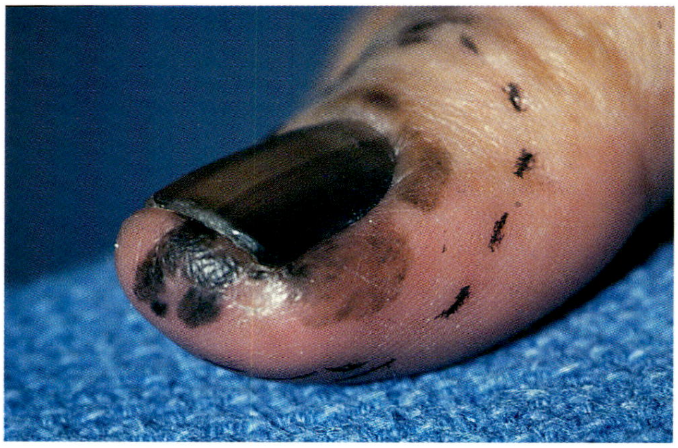

Figure 13–48. Melanoma: Acral-mucosal lentiginous radial growth. Melanomas involving the digits, particularly the nail bed and the mucosal and paramucosal epithelium, often show distinctive clinical and histologic features. Both radial and vertical growth may remain flat and heavily pigmented, obscuring clinical detection of the latter.

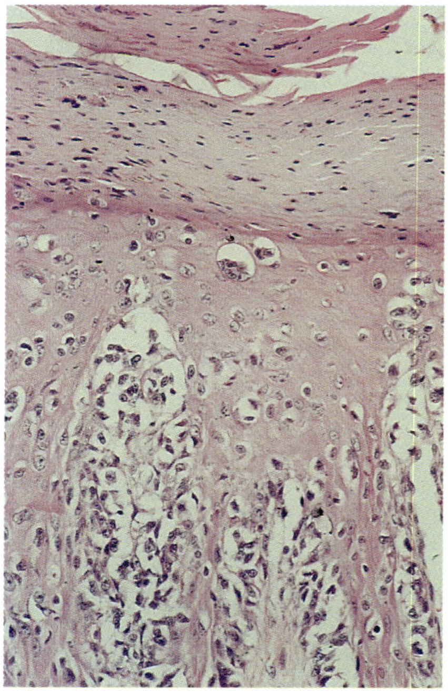

Figure 13–49. On microscopic examination, the radial growth phase of these lesions resembles that of lentigo maligna, although the malignant cells generally affect a hyperplastic rather than an atrophic epidermal layer. In addition, some acral melanomas also have heavily melanized, relatively thick dendrites that course upward through the thickened epidermis.

Vertical Growth Phase Melanoma

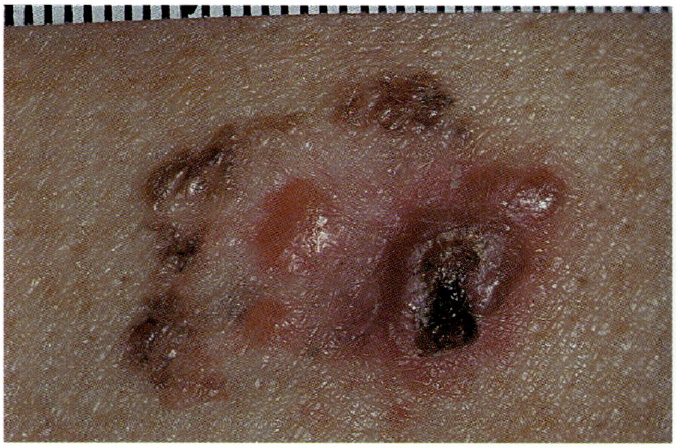

Figure 13–50. Melanoma: Vertical growth phase. Development of a nodule within an irregular pigmented plaque heralds the onset of vertical growth. In this case, there is a prominent zone of regression; the lighter nodule central to the regression was composed of a tumoral aggregate of lymphocytes, testimony to the extent of the inflammatory response.

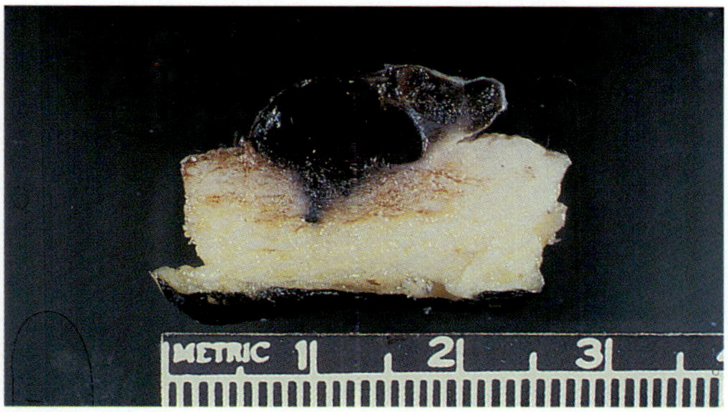

Figure 13–51. Cross section cf a heavily pigmented, vertical growth phase melanoma shows extensive involvement of the dermis and early involvement of the superficial subcutis.

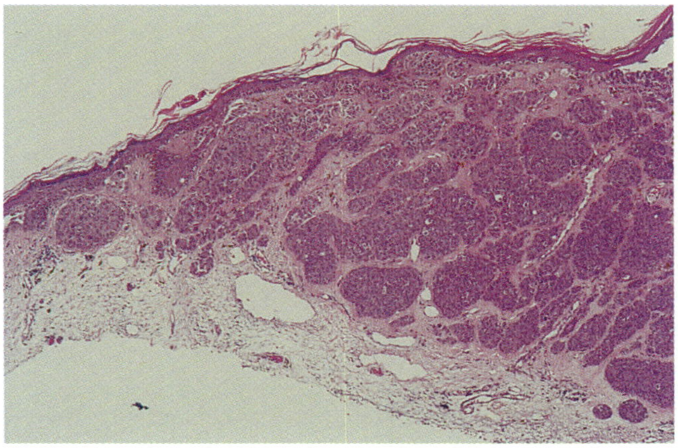

Figure 13–52. The microscopic appearance of vertical growth phase melanoma is characterized by downward tumorigenic growth of malignant cells, which expand the papillary dermis and extend into or through the reticular dermis. Note that the dermal nests are considerably larger than ordinary nevus cell or melanoma cell nests that occur at the dermal-epidermal junction, a finding that constitutes tumorigenic growth inherent to vertical growth phase disease.

Melanoma Variants

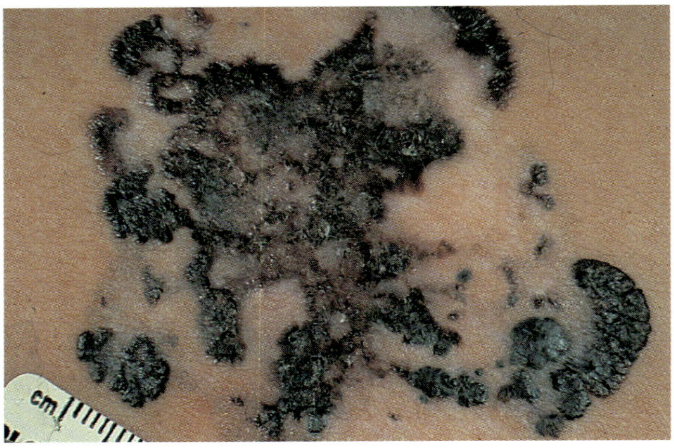

Figure 13–53. Regression in melanoma. Extensive regression has produced a "moth-eaten" clinical appearance in the superficial spreading melanoma.

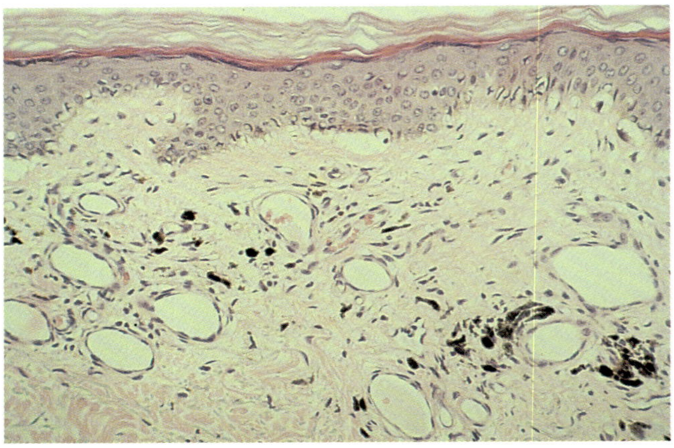

Figure 13–54. Examination of the nonpigmented regions internal to the tumor plaque in Figure 13–53 show increased numbers of widely dilated vessels within a fibrotic dermis containing numerous melanophages. Inflammation is minimal at this site, where regression is complete. This may be the only finding at sites where entire lesions have regressed.

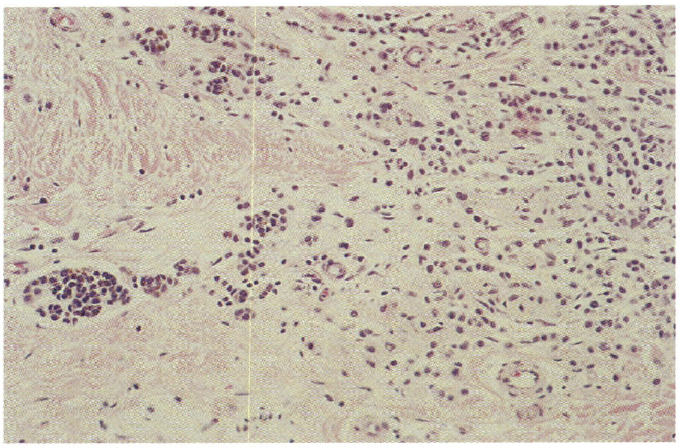

Figure 13–55. Melanoma with small cell differentiation. This vertical growth phase nodule has a permeative pattern of dermal infiltration suggestive of a congenital melanocytic nevus.

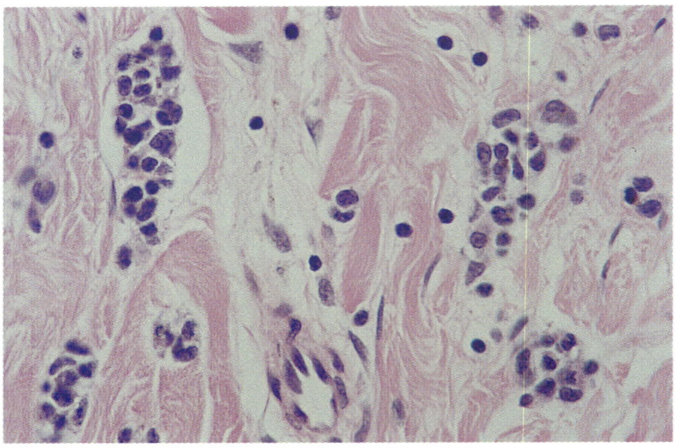

Figure 13–56. Individual cells in Figure 13–55, however, show nuclear contour angulation and diffuse hyperchromasia. Occasional mitoses are also present (not shown).

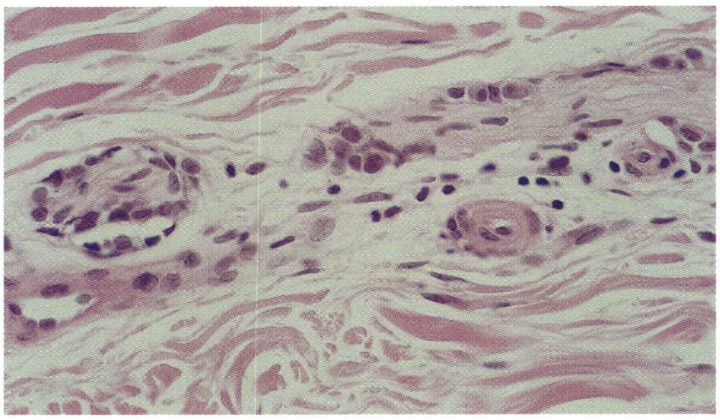

Figure 13–57. Perineural spread assists in establishing the diagnosis of small cell melanoma, although perineural patterns also may occur in congenital nevi.

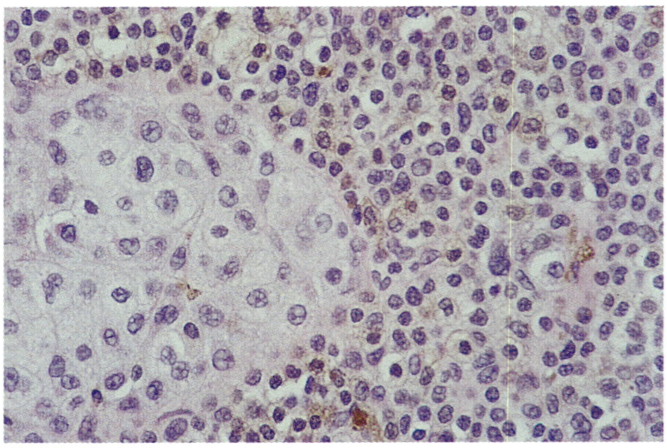

Figure 13–58. Zones where small melanoma cells *(right)* show apparent transitions with larger, more conventional melanoma cells *(left)* also assist in establishing the diagnosis in small cell melanoma variants.

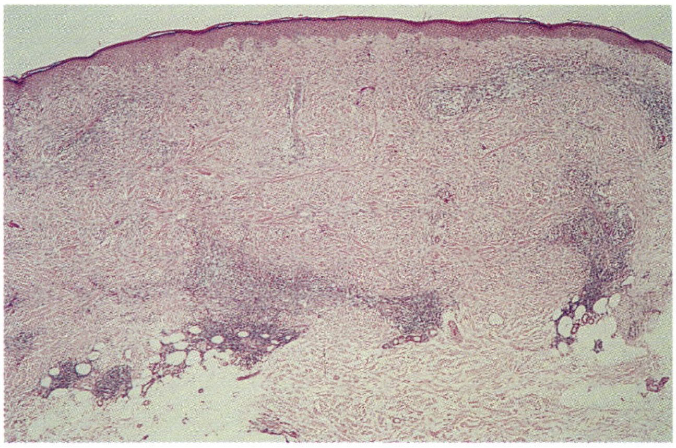

Figure 13–59. Melanoma with spindle cell differentiation. Spindle cell desmoplastic and neurotropic vertical growth phase melanomas often arise in association with lentigo maligna and acral-mucosal lentiginous radial growth. A helpful diagnostic feature at scanning magnification is the presence of lymphoid inflammatory infiltrates defining the perimeter of an otherwise vague vertical growth phase nodule.

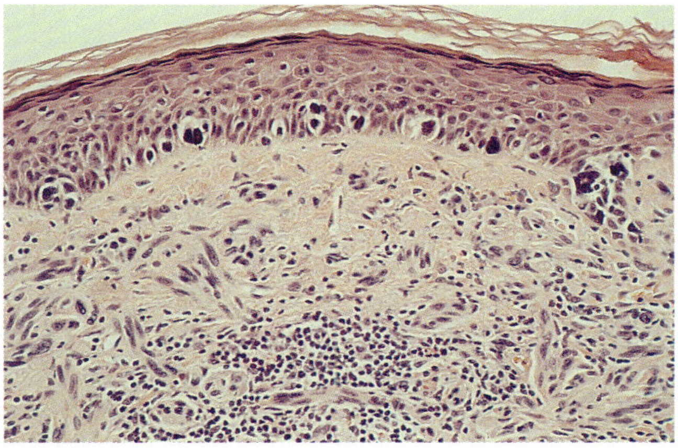

Figure 13–60. In amelanotic lesions of spindle cell melanoma, confirmation of melanocytic origin may depend on detection of residual radial growth along the dermal-epidermal interface.

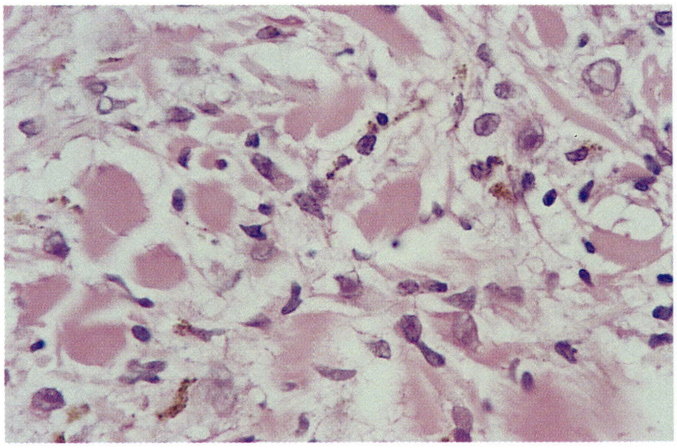

Figure 13–61. Individual cells of spindle cell melanoma may infiltrate collagen bundles diffusely and show bland nuclei with subtle hyperchromasia. Mitotic figures are generally detected after careful study.

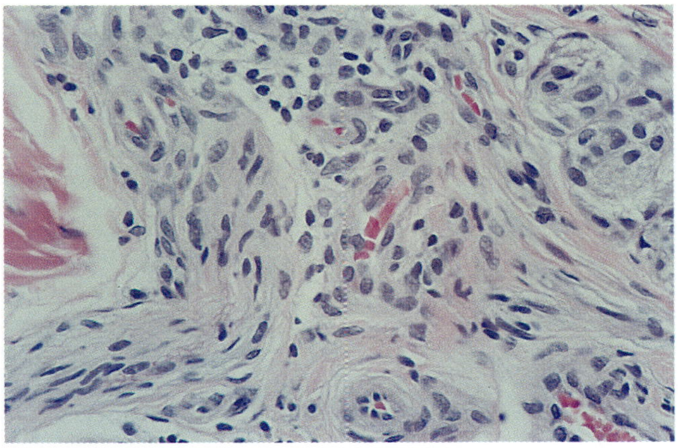

Figure 13–62. Zones of true neural invasion characterized by dermal nerve bundles rendered hypercellular by infiltration by malignant spindle cells are also a helpful diagnostic feature in spindle cell melanoma of the neurotropic type.

Metastatic Melanoma

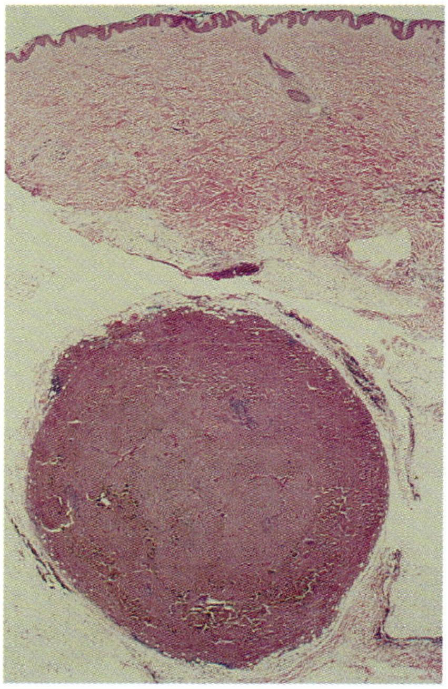

Figure 13–63. Metastatic melanoma. Histologically, there is a large, expansile tumor nodule within the subcutis.

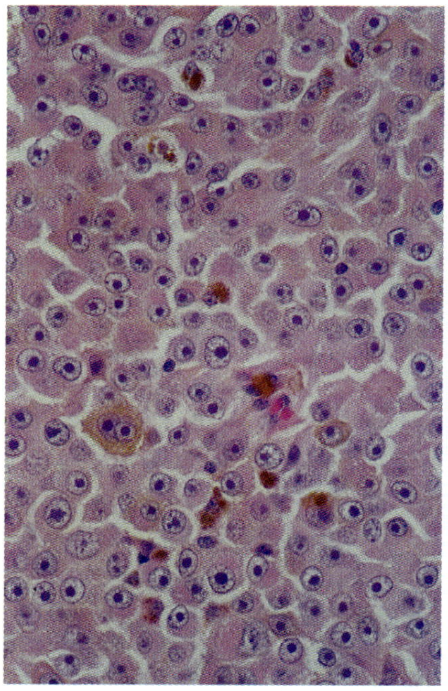

Figure 13–64. On higher magnification, this tumor nodule is composed of epithelioid malignant cells containing focal melanin pigmentation. Occasionally, metastases will home to the epidermal layer (*i.e.*, epidermotropic metastases), where they form nests and mimic nevi or primary melanoma. Careful inspection for cellular anaplasia and dermal mitotic activity and close correlation with clinical history are mandatory for such lesions.

Monsel Reaction Mimicking Melanoma

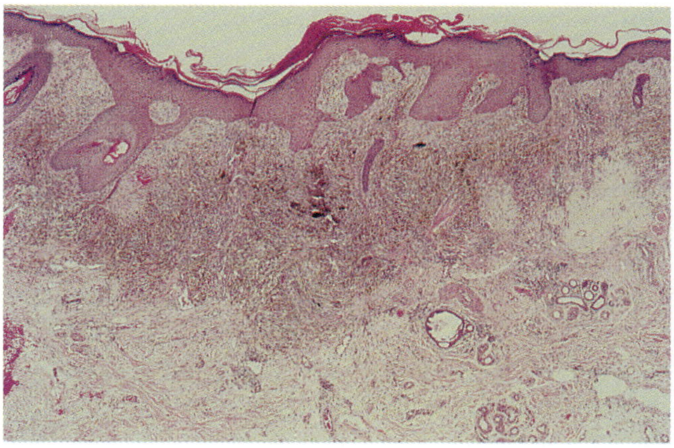

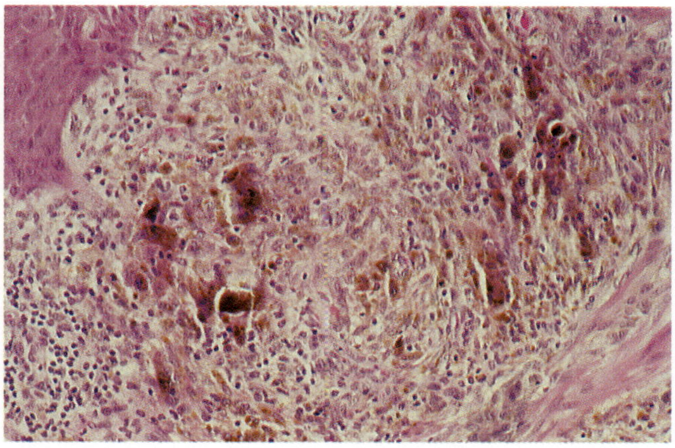

Figures 13–65 and 13–66. Monsel reaction at melanoma excision site. An excised biopsy site shows epidermal hyperplasia and a brisk dermal reaction consisting of plump fibroblasts and activated epithelioid histiocytes associated with clumped as well as particulate intracytoplasmic brown pigment. Although this histologic picture may resemble that of residual melanoma entrapped within dermal scar tissue, its origin as a cellular reaction to iron-containing Monsel solution is confirmed by Prussian blue stain.

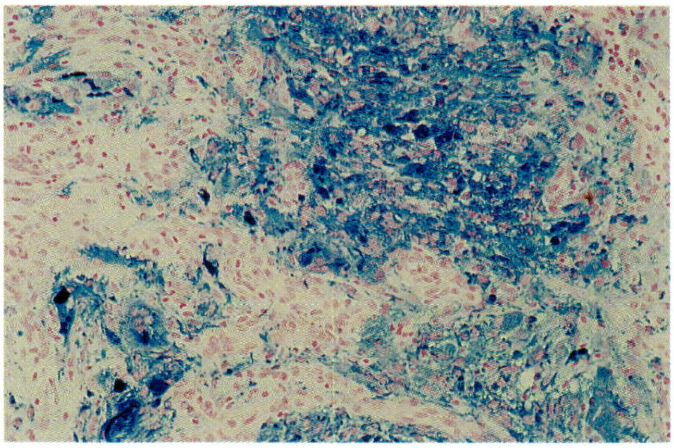

Figure 13–67. Prussian blue stain reveals that all of the intracellular and extracellular pigment is particulate iron.

14

Lymphoproliferative Tumors

Although the notion that skin is a lymphoid organ has emerged only during the past decade, it has gained wide acceptance as a basis for understanding cutaneous immunity and lymphoproliferative neoplasms. Working in concert with draining lymph nodes, the skin is the residence of specialized lymphocytes, histiocytes, and mast cells that comprise the skin-associated lymphoid tissue (SALT). Benign proliferations of normal lymphohistiocytic constituents of skin, dysplastic proliferations, and frank malignancy commonly occur and present significant diagnostic difficulties, particularly when there is no associated lymph node involvement.

Integral to understanding the histopathology and immunoarchitecture of hyperplastic conditions and neoplastic lymphoproliferative neoplasms of the skin is an appreciation of correlative processes in lymph nodes. Because infiltration of the epidermis by atypical and malignant lymphohistiocytic cells often results in cytologic and architectural distortion not seen in lymph nodes, distinctive diagnostic challenges are encountered when lymphoproliferative lesions present primarily in the skin. These challenges have been partially addressed by the recent emergence of sophisticated molecular biologic techniques for the analysis of clonal lymphoid proliferations. Thus, the accurate diagnosis of lymphohistiocytic tumors of the skin frequently requires a multifaceted approach that combines routine immunohistochemistry and molecular analytical techniques.

With the exception of cutaneous T-cell lymphoma (CTCL), the majority of non-Hodgkin lymphomas involving the skin cannot be accurately subclassified based on skin biopsy alone. Thus, although skin biopsy serves to alert the clinician of the probability of a lymphoproliferative disorder, careful systemic search for primary lymphoid involvement and, if found, subsequent nodal biopsy will often permit definitive classification.

Clinical recognition of hematopoietic malignancy of the skin may depend on detection of "plum-colored" nodules (*e.g.,* B-cell lymphoma) or green-yellow papules or nodules (*e.g.,* granulocytic leukemia or chloroma), and thus the wavelengths of light reflected by the infiltrated skin are diagnostically important. Because dermal lymphocytic infiltrates generally are observed as zones of deep blue at scanning magnification, the pattern of these zones has permitted generation of diagnostic algorithms based in part on tinctorial characteristics. For example, although most malignant T-cell infiltrates first appear as broad horizontal blue regions directly beneath the dermal-epidermal interface, malignant B-cell infiltrates tend to form coalescent nodular aggregates within the mid- to deep dermis. Reactive mixed lymphocytic infiltrates may show discrete foci or pale-pink pallor, the result of localized proliferation of maturing B cells (germinal centers) or histiocytic aggregation. Cutaneous plasmacytomas are characterized by cells with blue-purple cytoplasm, representing cells with abundant rough endoplasmic reticulum. True histiocytic infiltrates, including Langerhans cell histiocytosis, are typified by cells with abundant pale-pink cytoplasm.

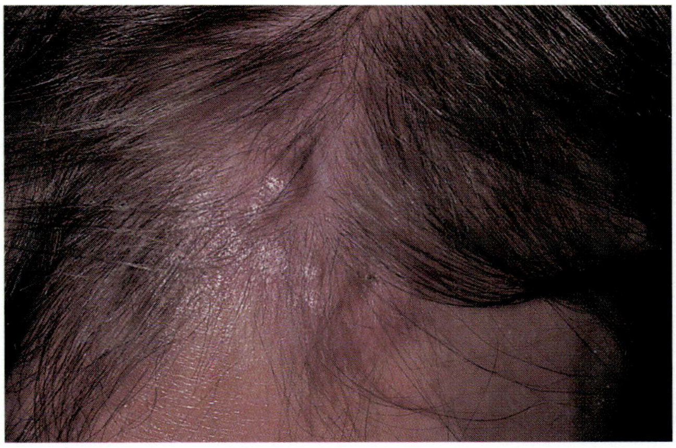

Figure 14–1. Cutaneous lymphoid hyperplasia. Firm, erythematous nodules on the posterior scalp raised the possibility of lymphoma in this middle-aged woman.

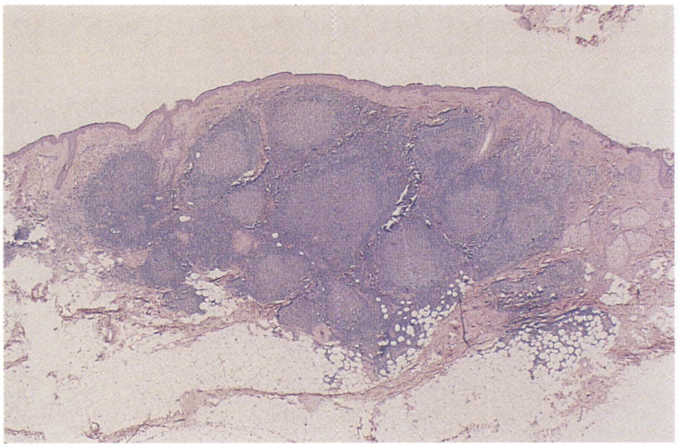

Figure 14–2. A biopsy specimen of a lesion similar to that shown in Figure 14–1 discloses aggregates of lymphoid follicles within the dermis.

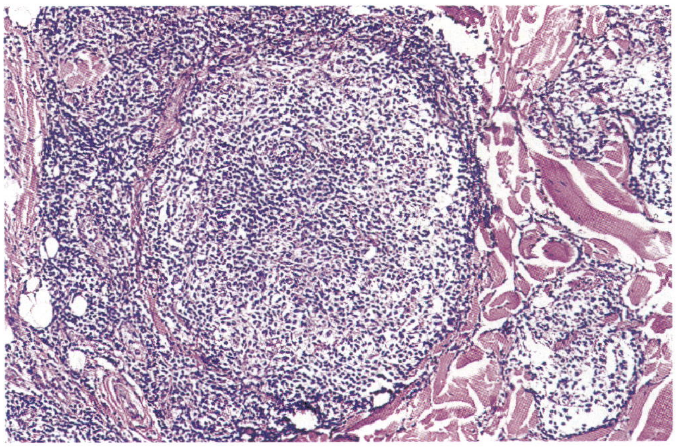

Figure 14–3. At higher magnification, larger cells (*i.e.,* B cells) comprise the central regions of the follicles, whereas smaller lymphoid cells (*i.e.,* T cells) are present about the perimeter.

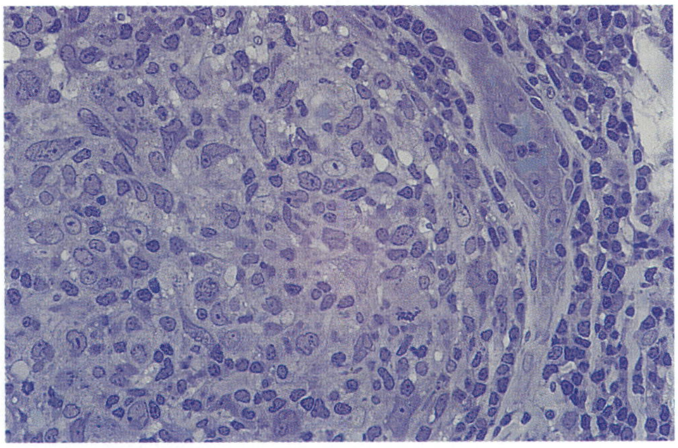

Figure 14–4. A spectrum of B-cell differentiation is observed within the more central component of a lymphoid follicle, consisting of smaller and larger lymphoid cells with both cleaved and noncleaved nuclei, occasional immunoblasts, and macrophages containing phagocytized basophilic material (*i.e.,* tingible body macrophages) in a 1 micrometer–thick section.

T-Lymphocyte Dyplasia ("Parapsoriasis")

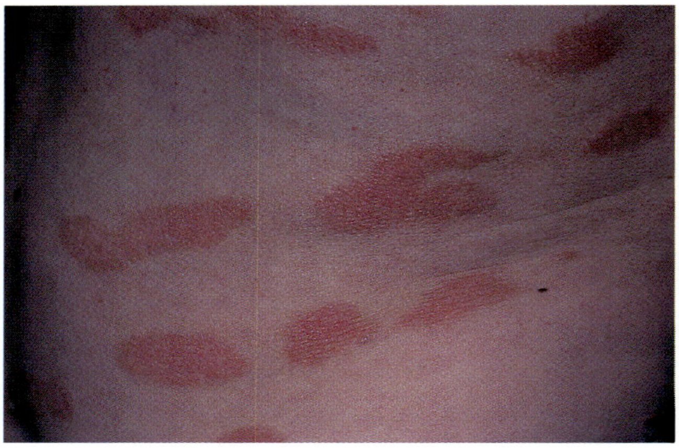

Figure 14–5. T-lymphocyte dysplasia. Often referred to as "parapsoriasis," these large patches and thin plaques are recalcitrant to treatment and may have a poikilodermatous appearance.

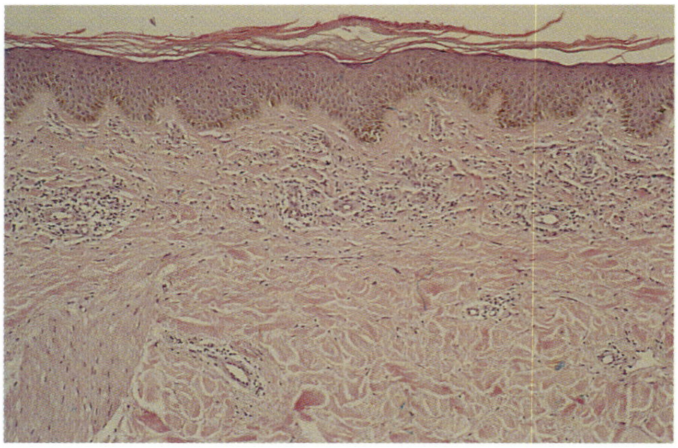

Figure 14–6. Histologically, there is a relatively sparse papillary dermal lymphocytic infiltrate beneath an epidermal layer showing diffuse mild hyperplasia and minimal spongiosis.

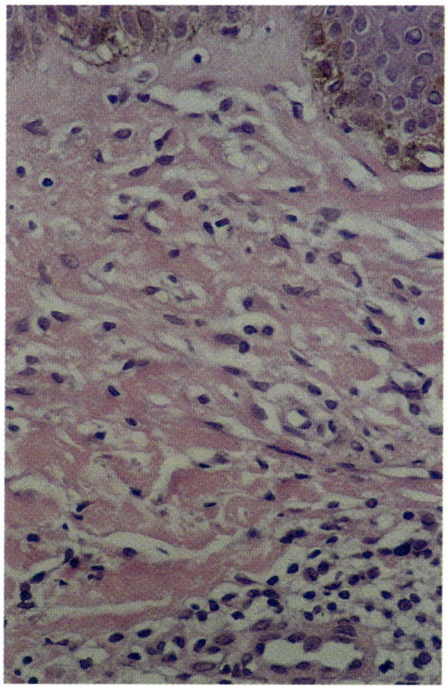

Figure 14–7. An important histologic clue is the interstitial pattern of lymphocyte infiltration within a diffusely fibrotic papillary dermis. At this juncture, lymphocytes are not predominated by atypical cells with irregular nuclear contours, nor is epidermotropism a prominent feature. Cell marker studies routinely fail to support malignancy in such lesions, although the lymphocyte trafficking pattern is not characteristic of a specific dermatosis (including guttate parapsoriasis, which represents a separate and distinctive entity) and shows signs of chronicity (papillary dermal fibrosis).

Cutaneous T-Cell Lymphoma, Epidermotropic Type

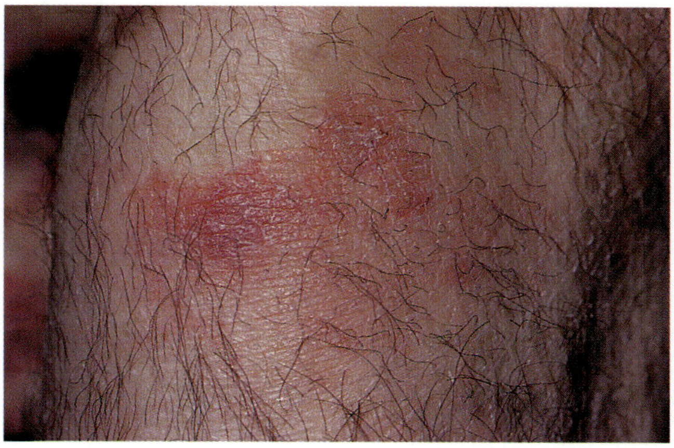

Figure 14–8. Cutaneous T-cell lymphoma, early epidermotropic type. The gross pathology is of a chronic, erythematous, scaling patch that is refractory to conventional anti-inflammatory treatment.

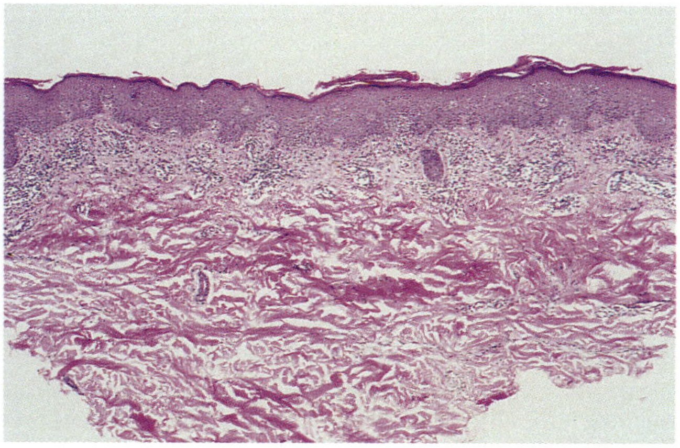

Figure 14–9. Histologically, there is a sparse band of lymphocytes within a fibrotic papillary dermis, a finding also observed in T-cell dysplasia.

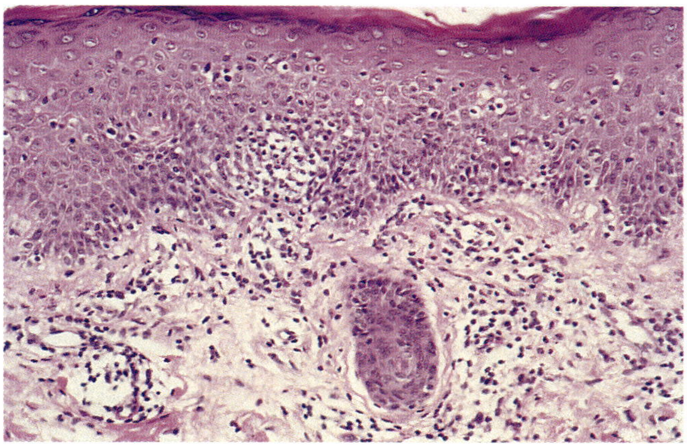

Figure 14–10. Single-cell and clustered epidermotropism is a prominent feature of cutaneous T-cell lymphoma.

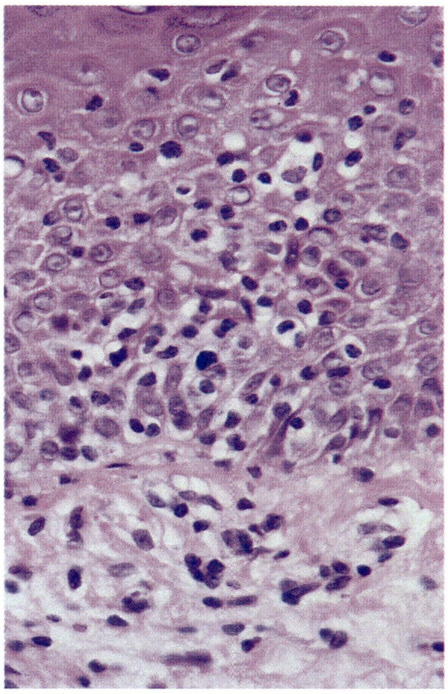

Figure 14–11. Epidermotropic cells contain hyperchromatic nuclei with irregular, infolded contours.

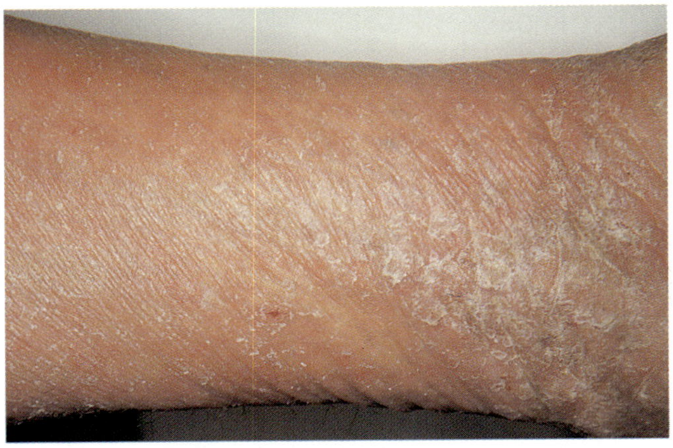

Figure 14–12. Cutaneous T-cell lymphoma, advanced epidermotropic type. The clinical appearance at this juncture is predominated by thickened erythematous plaques covered by adherent white scale.

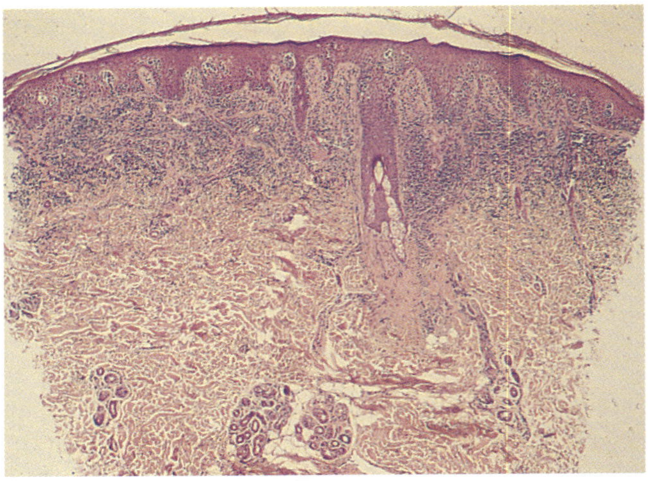

Figure 14–13. At scanning magnification, there is a dense band of lymphocytes within the superficial dermis associated with variable epidermal hyperplasia.

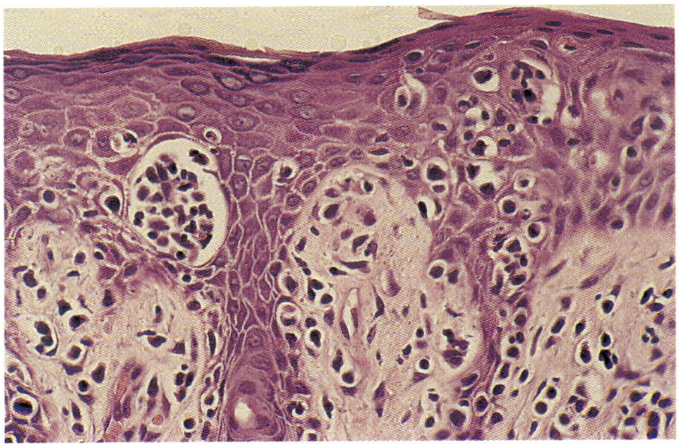

Figure 14–14. Closer inspection of the portion of the epidermis enclosed in Figure 14–13 shows well-developed microabscesses of enlarged lymphocytes containing hyperchromatic nuclei. Similar cells are easily detected in the underlying dermis.

Cutaneous T-Cell Lymphoma, Nonepidermotropic Type

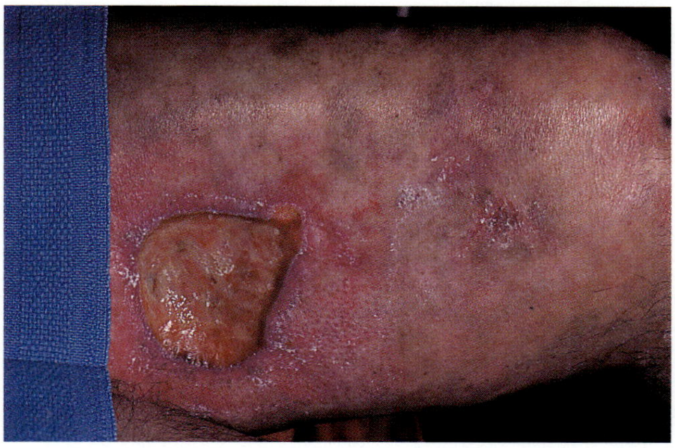

Figure 14–15. Cutaneous T-cell lymphoma (CTCL), nonepidermotropic type. An ulcerated nodule *(left)* has developed within a plaque *(center)* of epidermotropic CTCL.

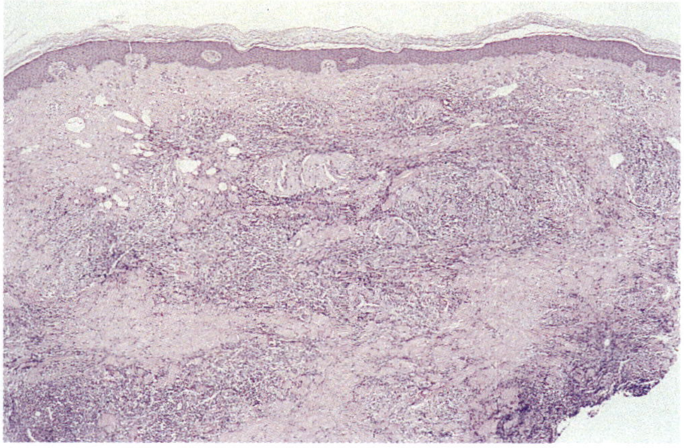

Figure 14–16. Typical lesions show diffuse infiltration of superficial and deep dermis by malignant lymphoid cells, sometimes accompanied by eosinophils and plasma cells. Note the sparing of the epidermal and papillary dermal layers.

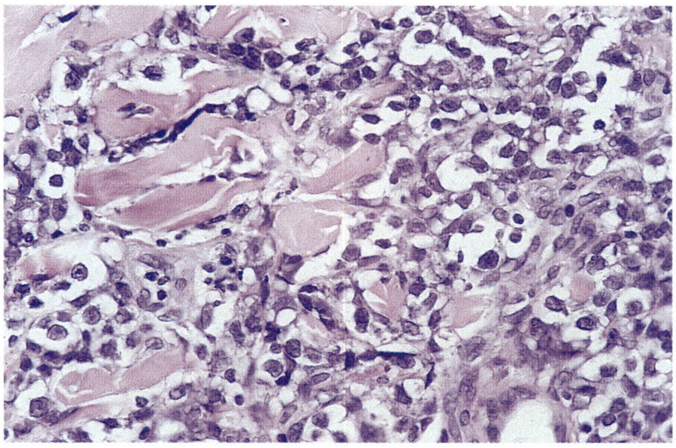

Figure 14–17. High magnification reveals malignant cells infiltrating between dermal collagen bundles. Although some lesions are characterized by Sézary cells within the dermis, many contain cells that have undergone transformation to large malignant lymphoid elements that cannot be reliably differentiated from malignant B cells without the assistance of cell marker analysis.

Cutaneous B-Cell Lymphoma

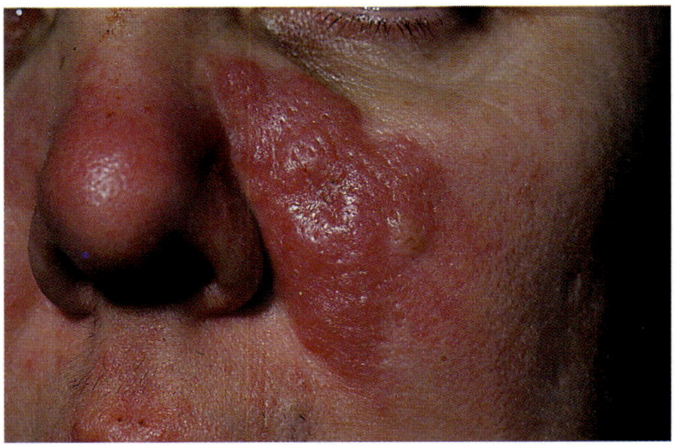

Figure 14–18. Cutaneous B-cell lymphoma, nodular large cell (follicular) type. A firm, plum-colored facial lesion is devoid of significant clinical evidence of epidermal involvement (*e.g.*, scale).

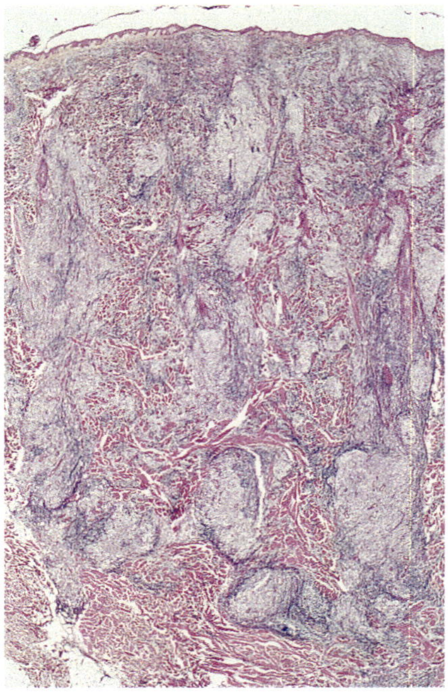

Figure 14–19. The infiltrate has a vaguely nodular quality and is deeply invasive at low magnification.

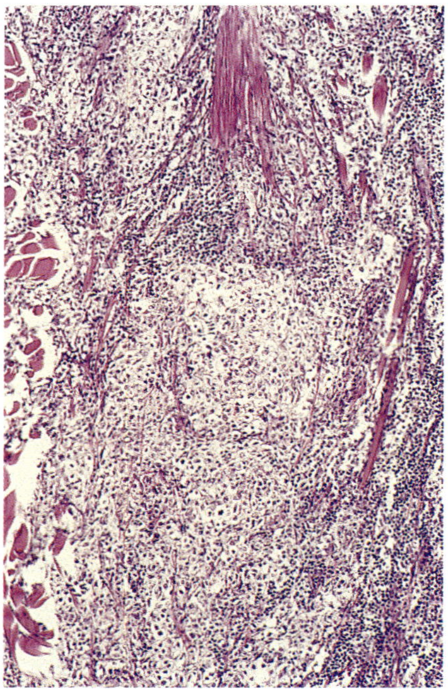

Figure 14–20. Higher-power magnification of one of the nodular areas in Figure 14–19 reveals reactive small lymphocytes at the periphery of discrete aggregates of large, malignant lymphoid cells.

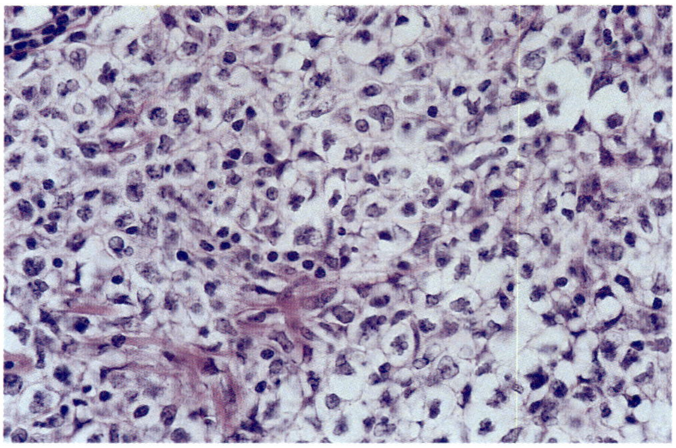

Figure 14–21. Further magnification of cells shown in Figures 14–19 and 14–20 demonstrates nuclear pleomorphism and chromatin aggregation consistent with anaplasia.

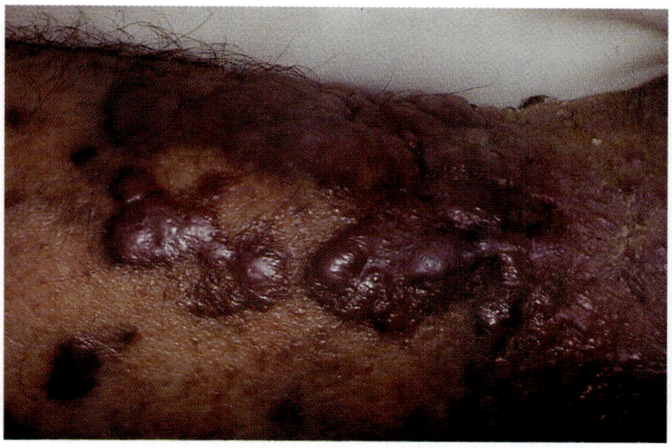

Figure 14–22. Cutaneous B-cell lymphoma, mixed small and large cell type. Clinically, lesions are coalescent red-purple nodules covered by an attenuated, shiny epidermal surface.

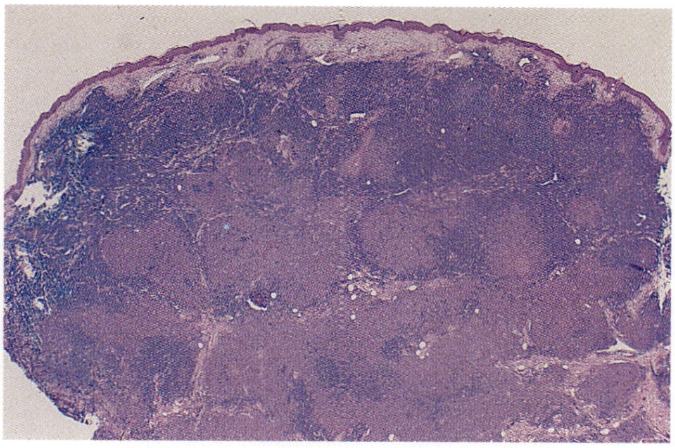

Figure 14–23. An overview of one of the smaller nodules reveals nodular aggregates of cells filling the dermis but sparing the papillary dermis *(top center)* and epidermis.

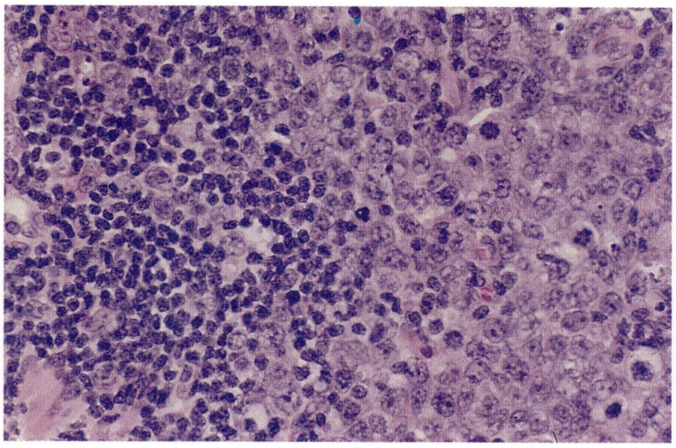

Figure 14–24. High magnification demonstrates two populations of malignant cells: one composed of monomorphous aggregates of smaller cells with diffuse nuclear hyperchromasia *(right)* and the other composed of larger malignant cells *(left)* similar to those demonstrated in Figures 14–20 and 14–21.

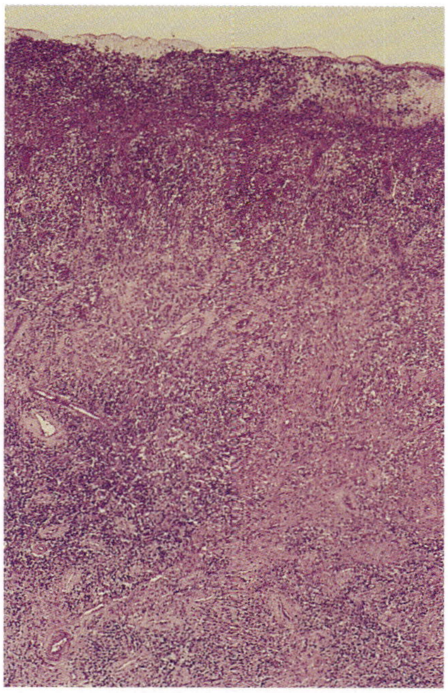

Figure 14–25. Cutaneous plasmacytoma. An ulcerated and destructive dermal infiltrate has a diffuse, permeative pattern of infiltration (ulcer surface at *top*).

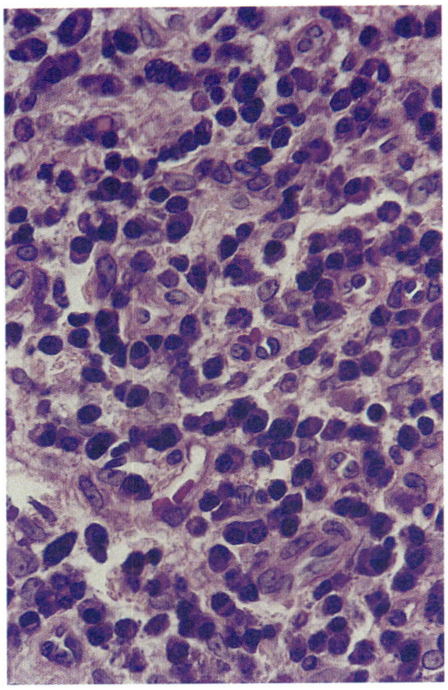

Figure 14–26. Higher magnification reveals that many of the infiltrating cells show eccentric, hyperchromatic nuclei consistent with plasmacytoid differentiation. Based on a skin biopsy specimen alone, the diagnosis was consistent with malignant lymphoma with plasmacytoid features.

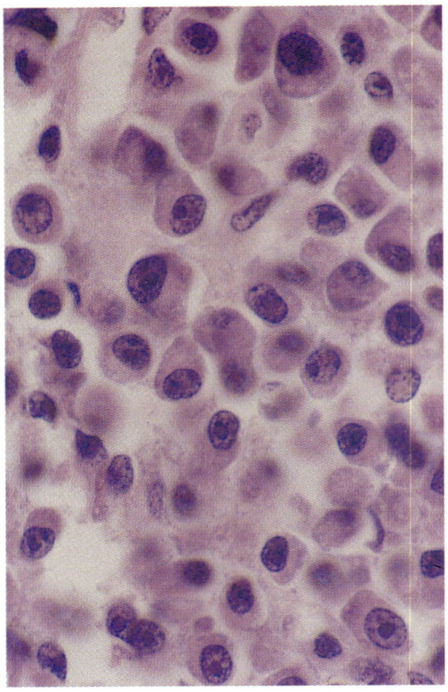

Figure 14–27. Cutaneous involvement by multiple myeloma shows more mature plasma cells with prominent, pleomorphic nuclei and focal nuclear hyperchromasia.

Leukemia Cutis

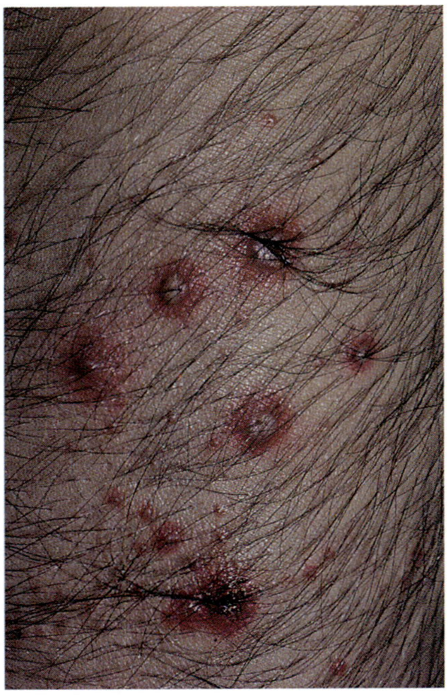

Figure 14–28. Leukemia cutis. Hemorrhagic nodules are present in a patient with acute myelogenous leukemia.

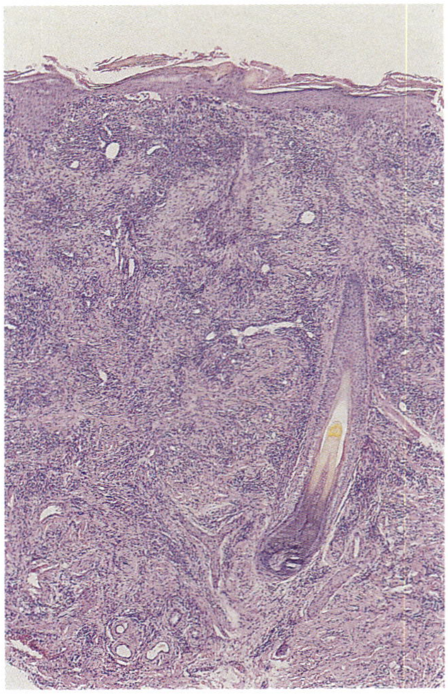

Figure 14–29. There is diffuse interstitial dermal involvement by leukemic cells; the complete absence of an angiocentric pattern of infiltration raises the possibility of hematopoietic malignancy.

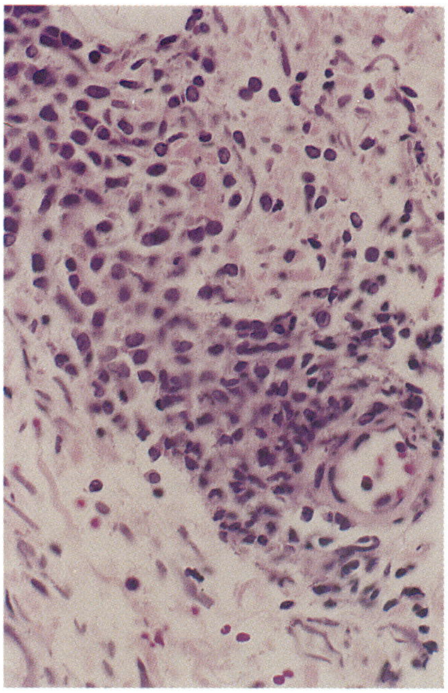

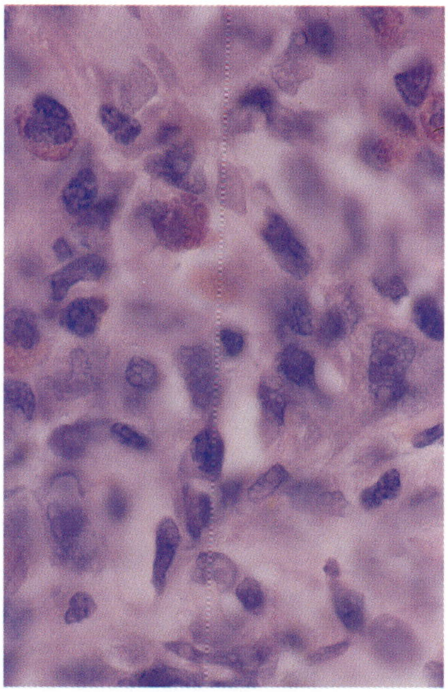

Figure 14–30. Hyperchromatic mononuclear cells within the dermal interstitium resemble lymphoma cutis; the finding of a malignant cell *(bottom right)* within a vessel lumen, however, warrants consideration of leukemia cutis, which occasionally presents as cutaneous lesions even before overt dissemination in the peripheral blood.

Figure 14–31. Confirmation of acute myelogenous leukemia is made by detection of myeloblasts with eosinophilic cytoplasmic granules (*i.e.*, eosinophilic myeloblasts; *bottom half*).

Langerhans Cell Histiocytosis

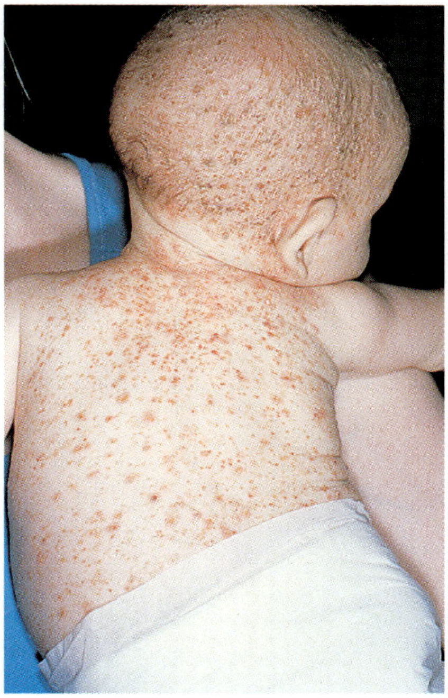

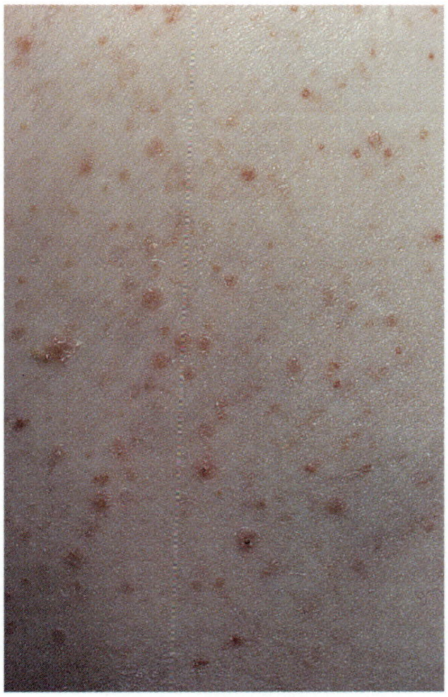

Figures 14–32 and 14–33. Langerhans cell histiocytosis (histiocytosis X). Eczematous papules mimic infantile seborrheic dermatitis.

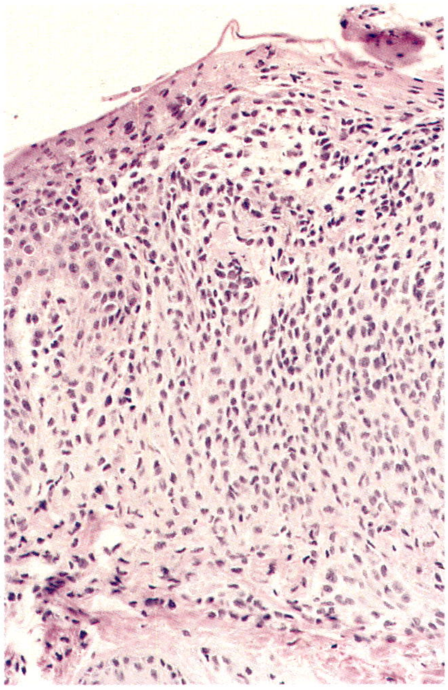

Figure 14–34. A superficial and mid-dermal mononuclear cell infiltrate with foci of epidermotropism is present.

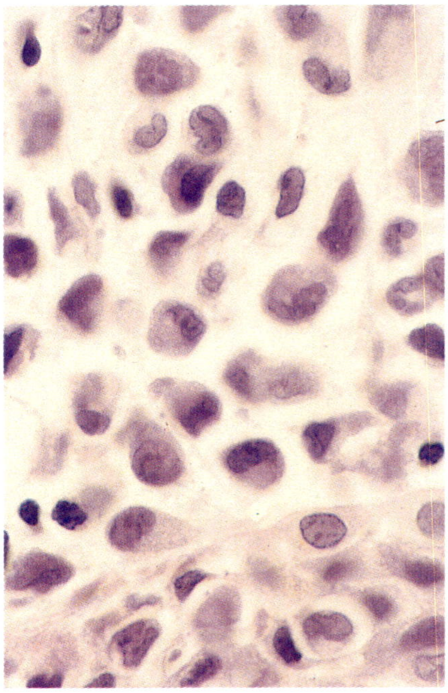

Figure 14–35. The infiltrating cells have pale, focally infolded nuclei and abundant cytoplasm relative to lymphocytes.

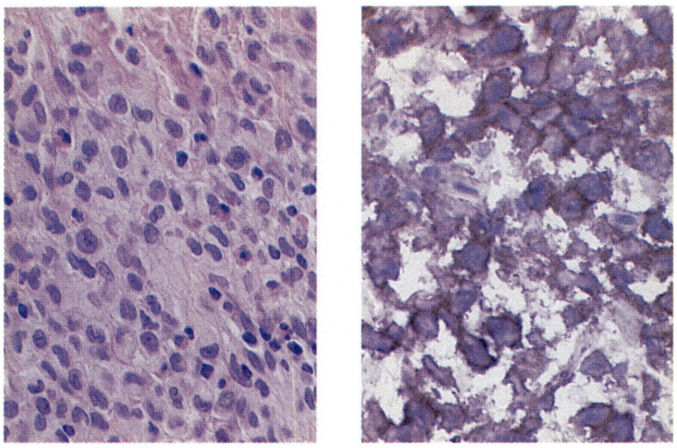

Figure 14–36. Langerhans cell histiocytosis (histiocytosis X): special studies. The histiocytoid dermal infiltrate in paraffin sections *(left)* may be stained for S100 protein or in frozen sections for the cell surface glycoprotein CD1a *(right)*.

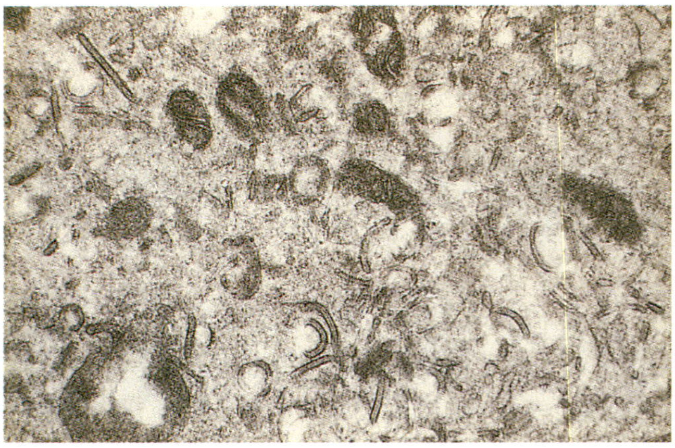

Figure 14–37. Diagnostic electron microscopy reveals characteristic rod-like and tennis racquet–shaped Birbeck granules within tumor cells.

Regressing Atypical Histiocytosis

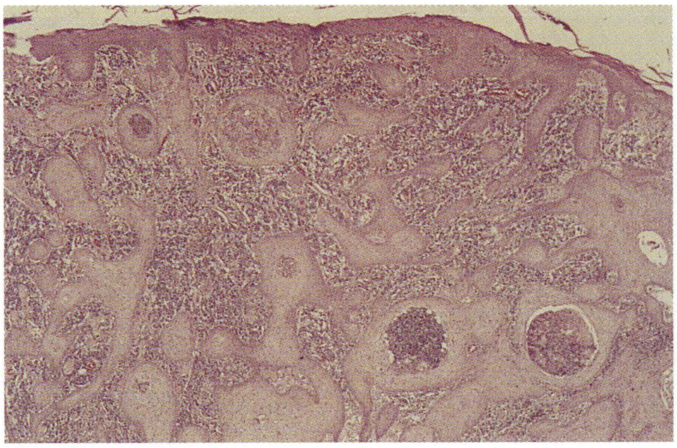

Figure 14–38. Regressing atypical histiocytosis. Active lesions show a brisk dermal infiltrate of atypical cells associated with marked overlying epidermal hyperplasia, a finding often associated with growth factors elaborated by an active immune or reparative response.

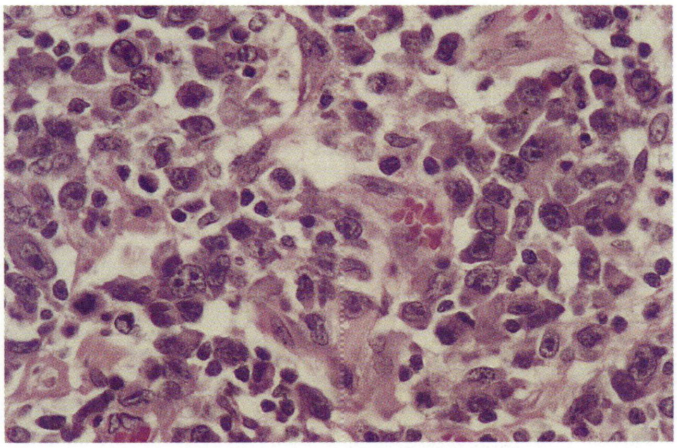

Figure 14–39. At progressively higher magnifications, the infiltrative component is composed of enlarged, anaplastic lymphoid cells with an associated infiltrate of reactive benign lymphocytes. Many of the atypical cells share characteristics with Reed-Sternberg variants and are Ki-1 positive by immunohistochemistry.

Mastocytoma

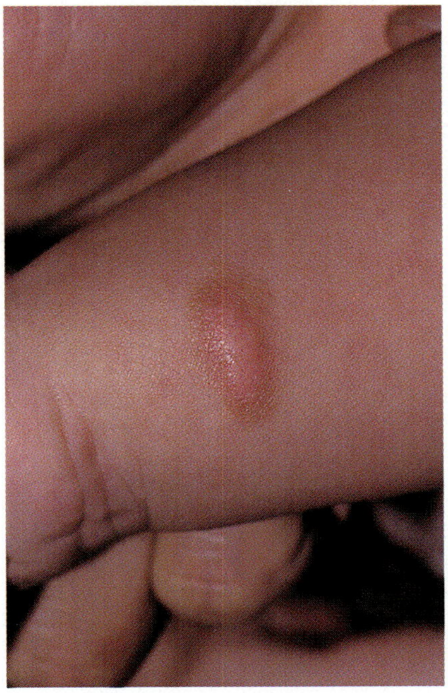

Figure 14–40. Solitary cutaneous mastocytoma. A dull-pink nodule from the upper extremity of a 1-year-old child.

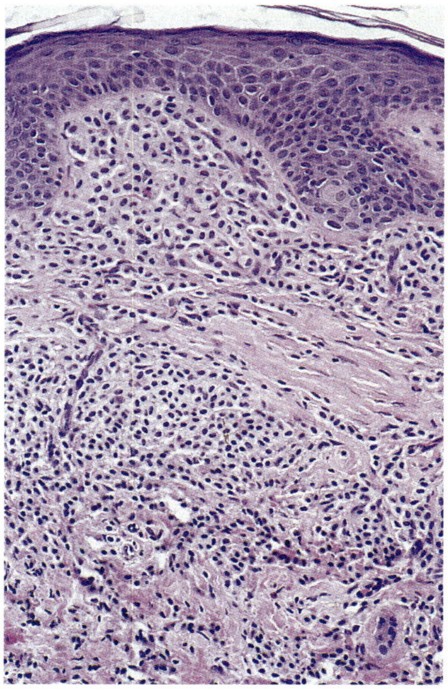

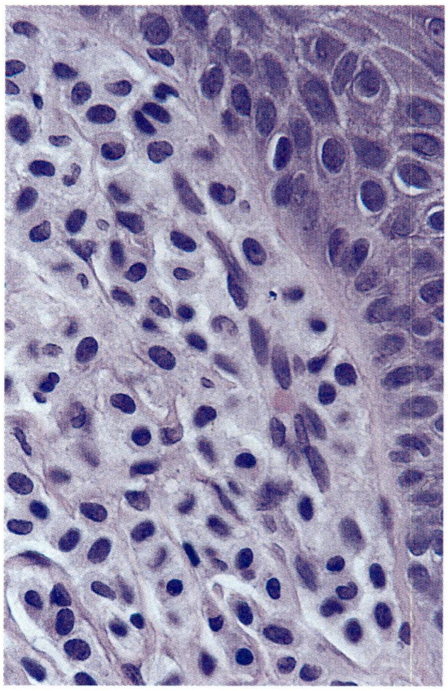

Figures 14–41 and 14–42. The monomorphous dermal infiltrate of solitary mastocytoma is devoid of epidermotropism and is characterized by cells containing evenly spaced nuclei due to a peripheral rim of apparently rigid cytoplasm (*i.e.,* "fried-egg" cells).

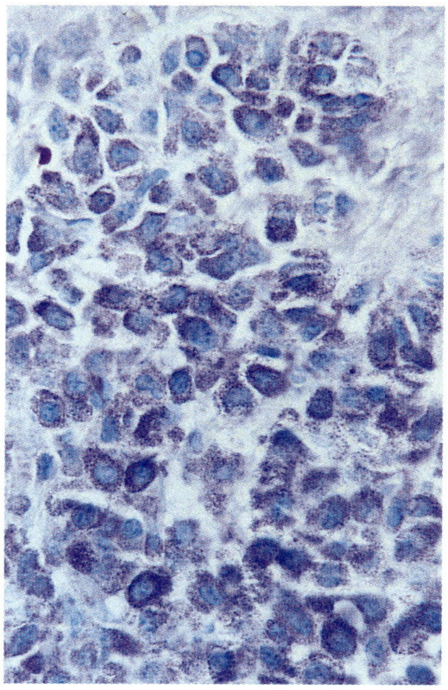

Figure 14–43. Staining with toluidine blue or with Giemsa reagent reveals metachromatic cytoplasmic granules typical of mast cells.

Xanthogranuloma

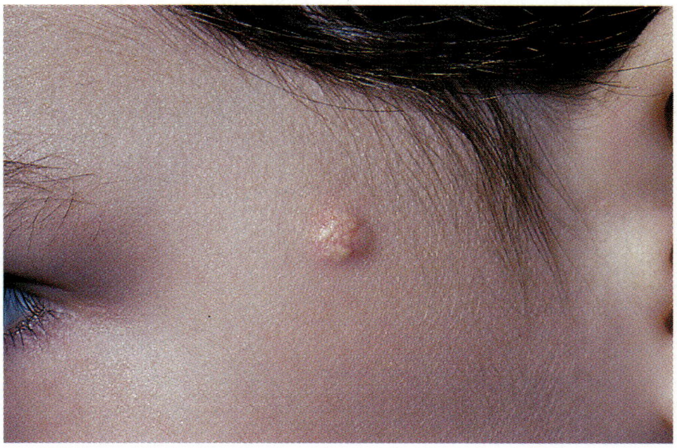

Figure 14–44. Xanthogranuloma. There is a yellow-white, firm nodule on the temporal skin of this 4-year-old girl.

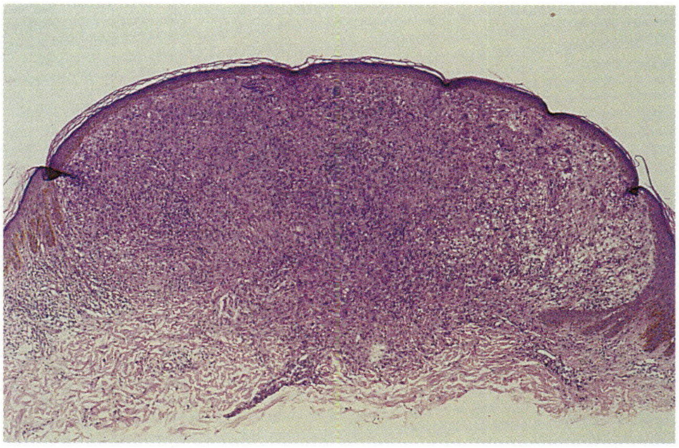

Figure 14–45. A biopsy specimen reveals a superficial and deep dermal infiltrate of mononuclear cells.

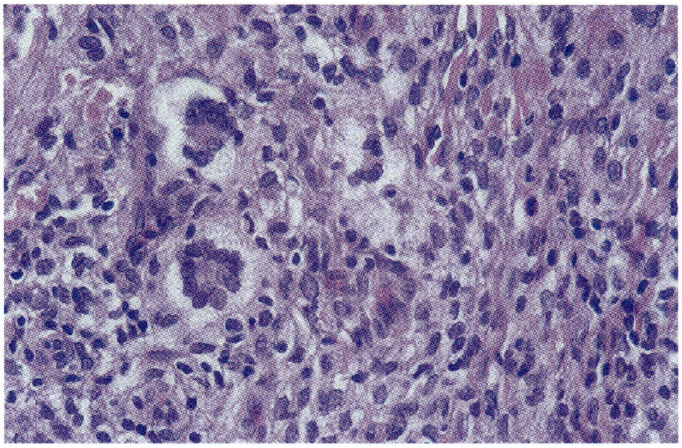

Figure 14–46. On higher magnification, the infiltrate demonstrates characteristic Touton giant cells *(left).* These cells are characterized by a wreath of nuclei surrounded by a rim of cytoplasmic vacuolization. Early lesions consisting primarily of focally lipidized histiocytes may be devoid of multinucleated cells and replete with eosinophils.

Reticulohistiocytoma

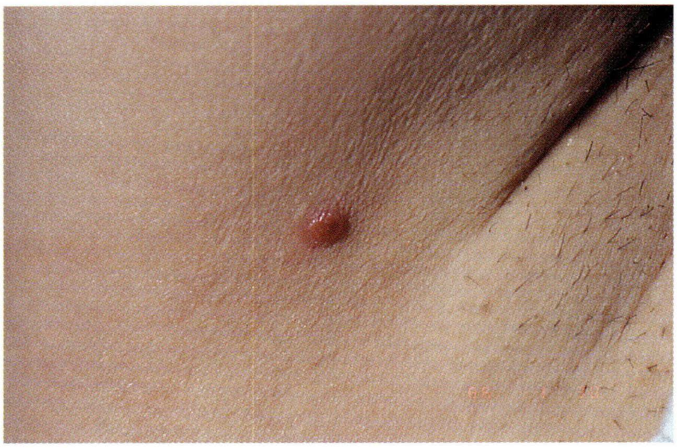

Figure 14–47. Reticulohistiocytoma. A small, firm, yellow-tan papule represents a solitary reticulohistiocytoma.

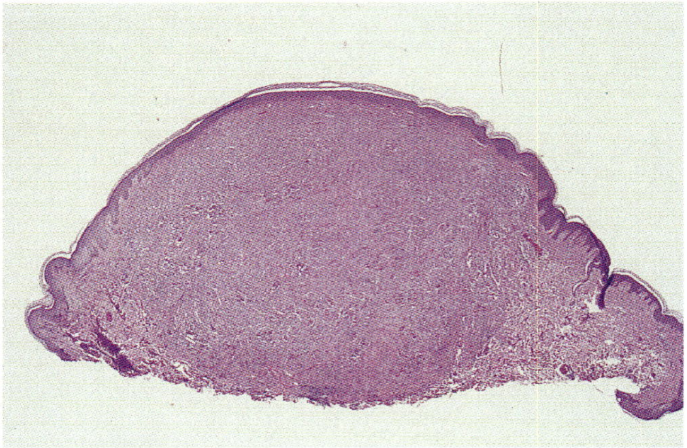

Figure 14–48. At low magnification, there is a proliferation of mononuclear and multinucleated intensely eosinophilic pink-purple cells within the superficial to mid-dermis.

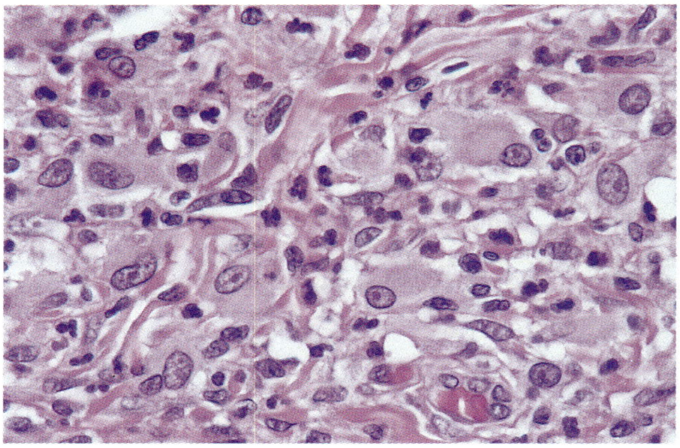

Figure 14–49. Cytologically, these cells contain one or more round, benign-appearing nuclei and ample quantities of bright-pink, periodic acid-Schiff–positive, granulated cytoplasm, which produces a ground-glass appearance.

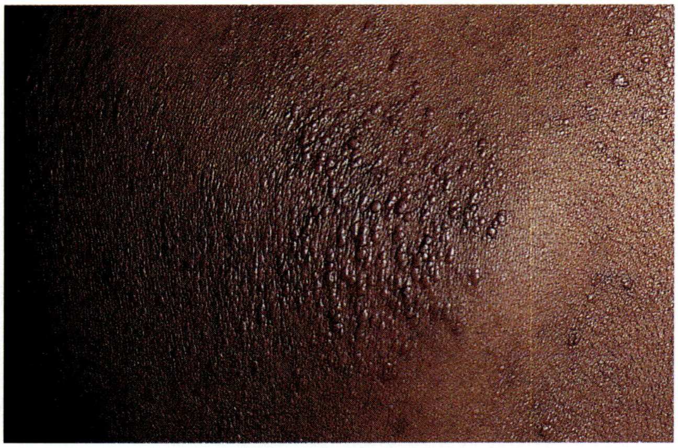

Figure 14–50. Multicentric reticulohistiocytosis. Multiple cutaneous papules representing reticulohistiocytomas are associated with destructive arthritis (see Fig. 14–51).

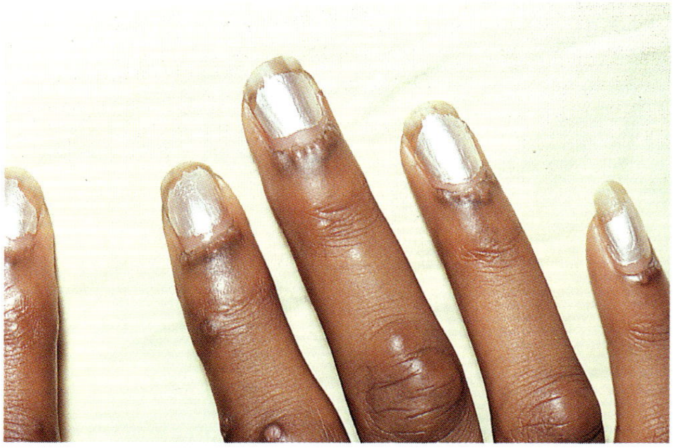

Figure 14–51. Destructive arthritis associated with reticulohistiocytomas.

15

Primary Mesenchymal Tumors

Mesenchymal tumors of the skin involve benign and malignant proliferations of endothelial cells, pericytes, and glomus cells; smooth muscle cells; cells of fibrohistiocytic origin; and neural and related supporting cells. The dermis is a fertile source for the development of such neoplasms, containing a plenitude of endothelium-lined vessels, vascular and erectile smooth muscle bundles, fibroblasts and fixed histiocytes, and neural elements. Many mesenchymal proliferations in the skin have counterparts in extracutaneous tissues (*e.g.,* leiomyomas, neuromas). However, in almost every case, mesenchymal neoplasms that arise in the dermis have distinctive clinical and/or histologic features that separate them from their extracutaneous counterparts.

In this section, the word *hamartoma* is used to refer to a malformation of mesenchymal elements normally expected to be present within the dermis. A hamartoma may therefore result from disordered or anomalous differentiation, structural organization, or quantity (too much or too little) of cellular elements. As is the case in all of dermatopathology, misnomers are easy to identify in the nomenclature of mesenchymal neoplasms of the skin. Perhaps the best example is Kaposi sarcoma, which is not a malignant mesenchymal tumor at all but rather a variably aggressive, multifocal angioproliferative process probably resulting from exposure of pre-existing vessels to anomalous growth factors. Such terms will not be abandoned because they have gained broad acceptance, and readers are aware of the potential deficits of the terminology.

Clinical detection of certain mesenchymal proliferations and neoplasms relies heavily on perception of color. For example, Kaposi sarcoma and angiosarcoma usually present as red to purple hemorrhagic patches, plaques, and nodules. Histologic recognition of primary mesenchymal tumors of the skin also may depend in part on characteristic tinctorial properties detected at both scanning and higher magnifications. A good example is the differential diagnosis of leiomyoma and other, non-smooth muscle spindle cell tumors of the skin. Smooth muscle cells typically have a deep-pink cytoplasm, which separates them from most fusifirm endothelial, fibroblastic, and neural cells. Trichrome staining reveals the cells to be bright red, whereas intervening collagen fibers are characteristically green-blue. More definitive confirmation of smooth muscle differentiation may be obtained through the use of immunoperoxidase techniques ("brown stains"), where smooth muscle cells are reactive with antibodies for smooth muscle actin. Similar examples can be cited for all other classes of neoplasms of cutaneous mesenchyme.

Vascular Tumors

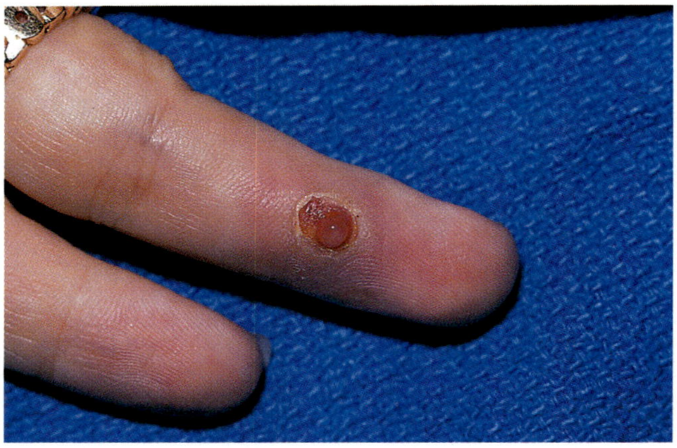

Figure 15–1. The clinical pyogenic granuloma lesion consists of an ulcerated, gelatinous mass of raised, proliferating tissue.

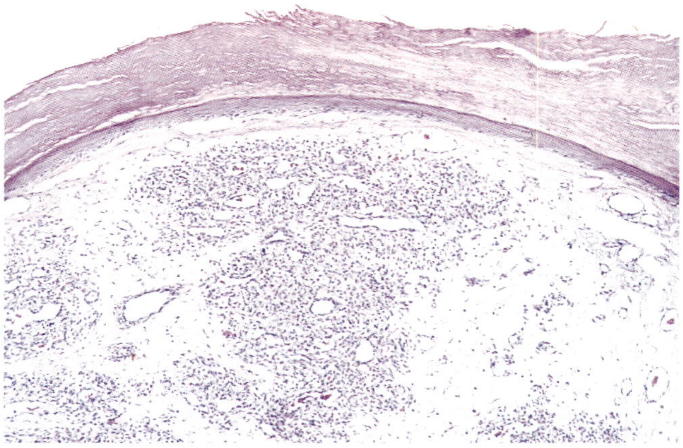

Figure 15–2. Earlier lesions of pyogenic granuloma are characterized by lobulated aggregates of capillaries within an edematous and frequently inflamed stroma.

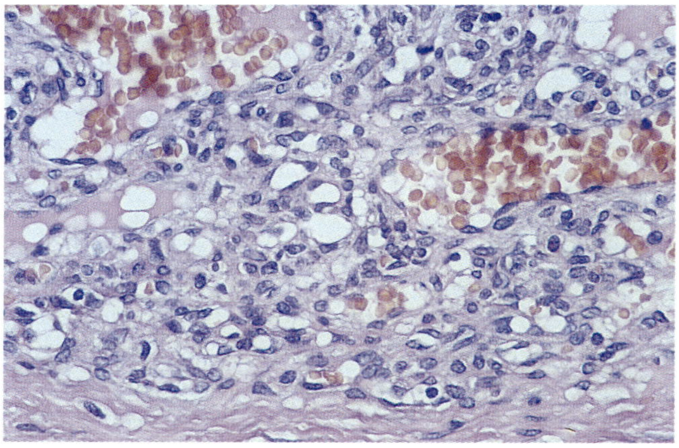

Figure 15–3. Older lesions of pyogenic granuloma may display dense aggregates of benign vessels that are indistinguishable from capillary hemangioma.

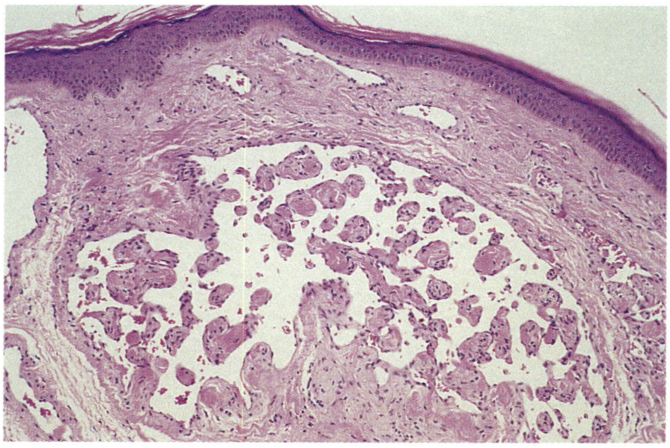

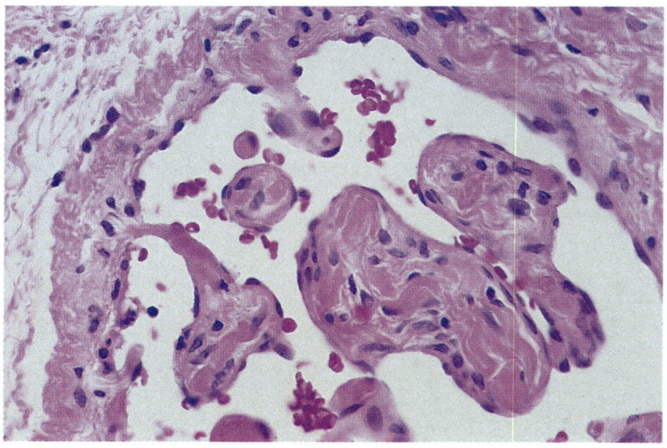

Figures 15–4 and 15–5. Intravascular papillary endothelial hyperplasia. Like pyogenic granuloma, this reactive endothelial hyperplasia is characterized by proliferation of benign endothelial cells at sites of inflammation or trauma. Intravascular papillary endothelial hyperplasia is characterized by papillary projections lined by flattened endothelium within the lumen of a dilated vessel showing perivascular fibrosis and hemosiderin deposition.

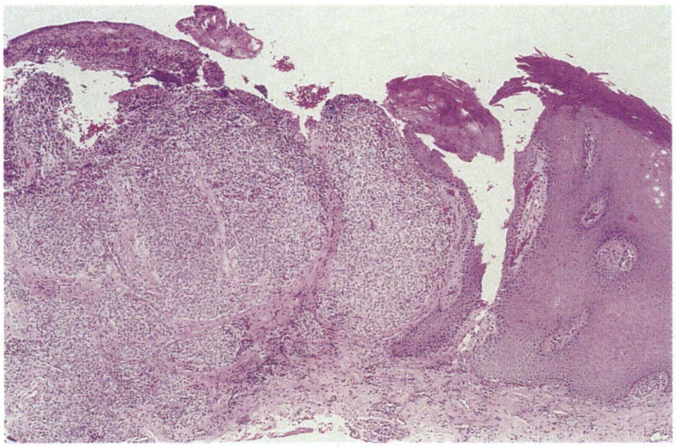

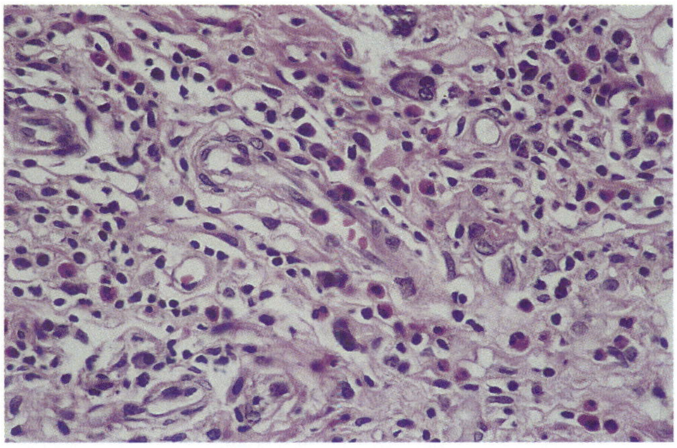

Figures 15–6 and 15–7. Epithelioid hemangioma is characterized in this lesion by a zone of ulceration with underlying granulation tissue containing numerous lymphocytes, eosinophils, and large epithelioid cells both within the stroma and lining the lumens of involved blood vessels.

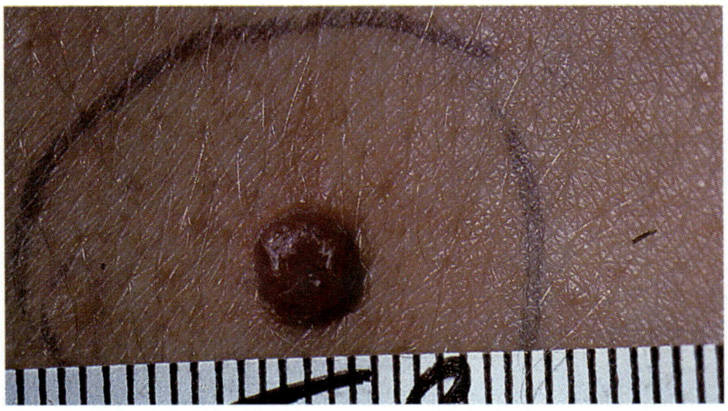

Figure 15–8. Hemangioma. A symmetric, cherry-red papule that, on examination of a biopsy specimen, disclosed numerous benign vessels within the superficial dermis.

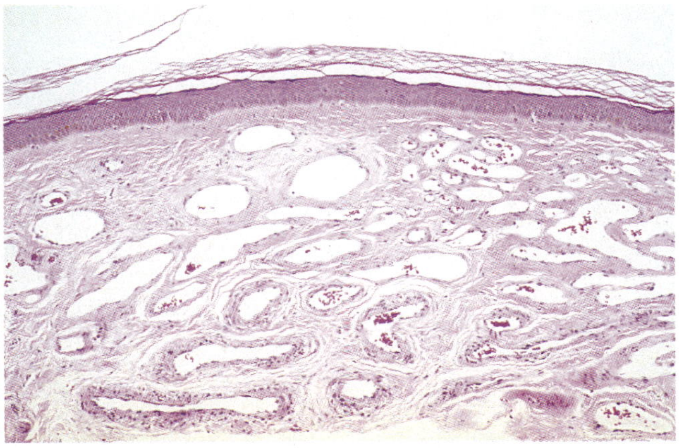

Figure 15–9. Hemangiomas with mixed capillary, arterial, and venous components are characterized by dilated, thick-walled superficial dermal vessels. These lesions result from either long-standing pressure gradients due to chronicity or arteriovenous shunts.

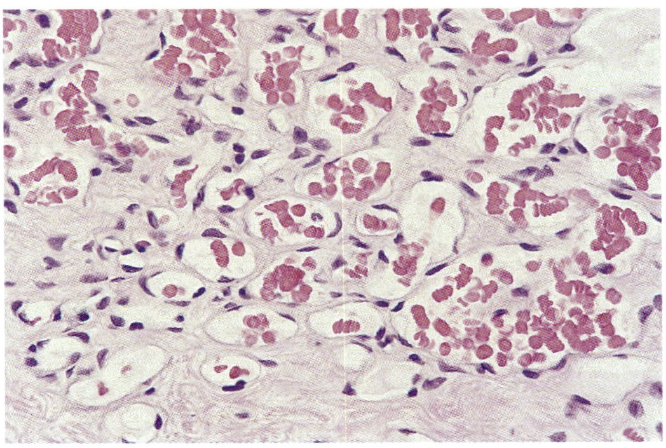

Figure 15–10. Capillary hemangioma, consisting of closely aggregated, thin-walled vessels lined with benign, flattened, endothelial cells.

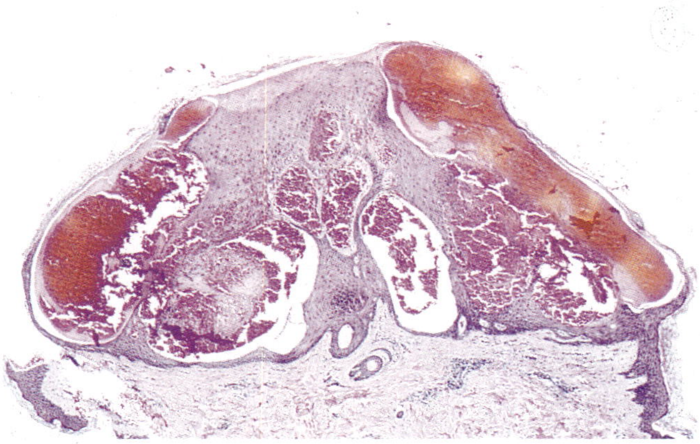

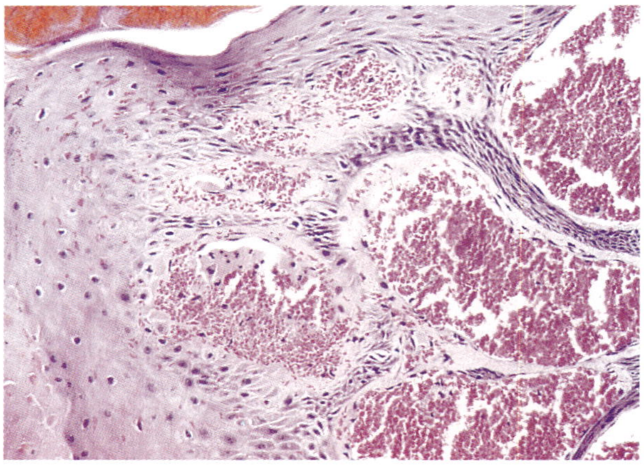

Figures 15–11 and 15–12. Angiokeratoma. Variably dilated, thin-walled vascular channels, many containing organizing thrombi, are present within the superficial dermis. Characteristic features include overlying verrucous epidermal hyperplasia, which embraces the underlying vascular tumor, and invagination of vessels into the epidermal layer such that some vessels appear to be floating within the epidermis, which is devoid of associated dermal stroma.

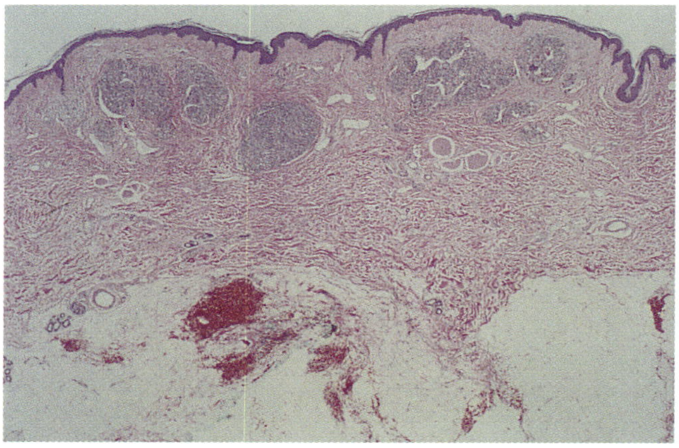

Figure 15–13. Acquired tufted hemangioma. At scanning magnification, discrete aggregates of cells are visible in the superficial dermis.

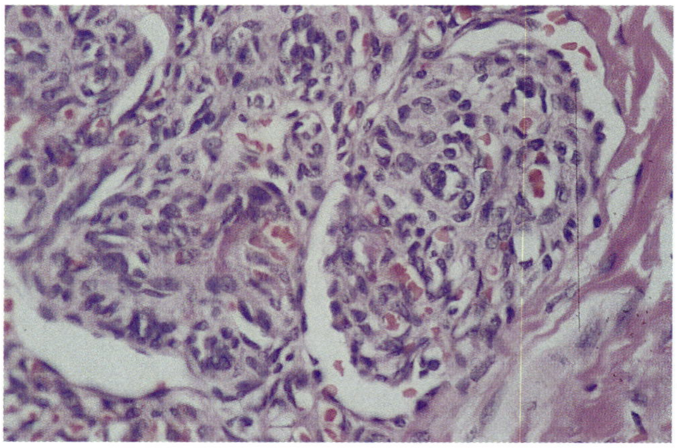

Figure 15–14. At increased magnification, the aggregates in Figure 15–13 are observed to contain plump pericyte-like cells that focally bulge into vascular spaces, creating characteristic semilunar contours.

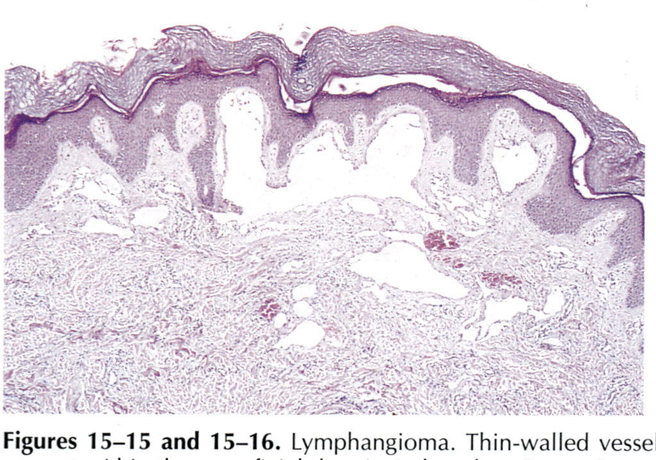

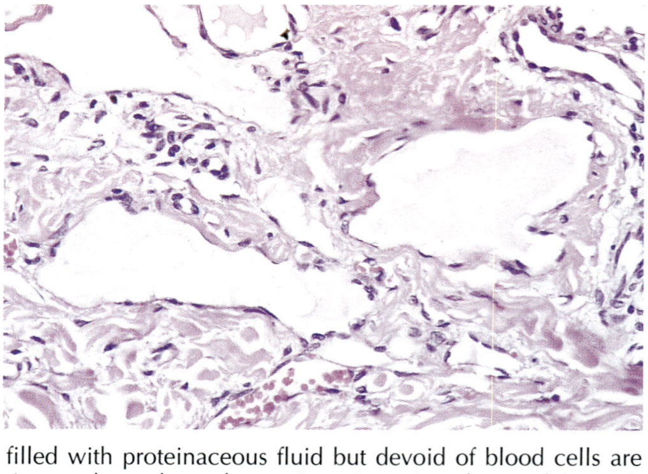

Figures 15–15 and 15–16. Lymphangioma. Thin-walled vessels filled with proteinaceous fluid but devoid of blood cells are present within the superficial dermis. In lymphangioma circumscriptum, these channels may invaginate into the overlying epidermal layer in a manner similar to that seen in angiokeratoma.

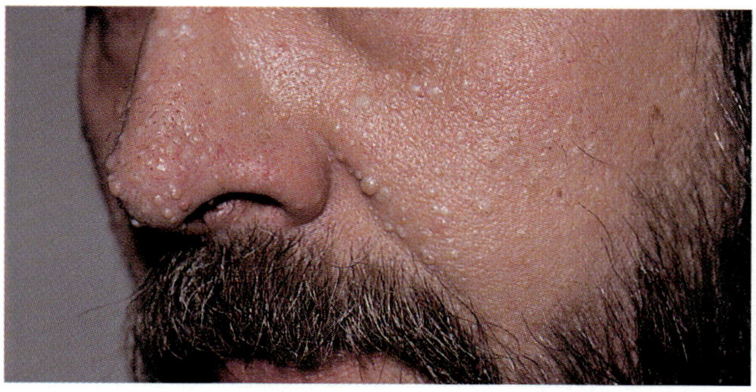

Figures 15–17. Angiofibroma. Multiple angiofibromas, also called fibrous papules and erroneously termed adenoma sebaceum, on the nasal and facial skin of a patient with tuberous sclerosis.

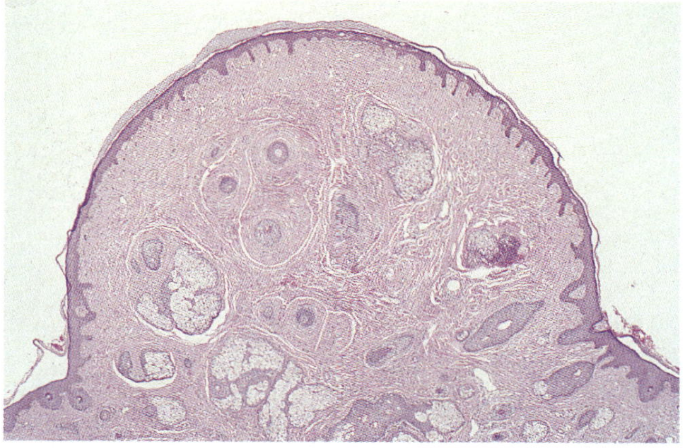

Figure 15–18. The dome-shaped papules of angiofibromas are formed as a result of dermal fibrovascular proliferations.

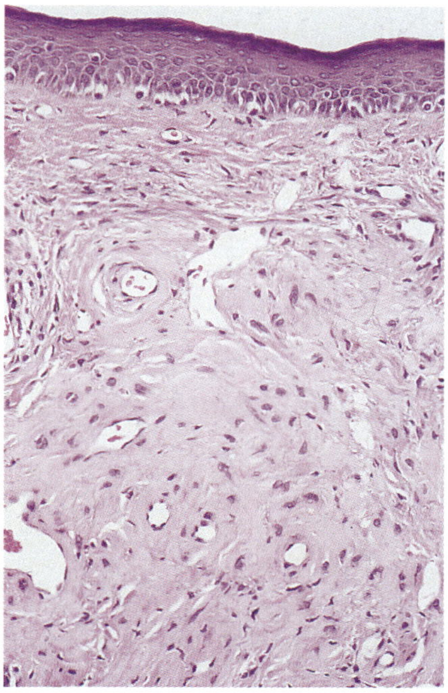

Figure 15–19. The dermal fibrovascular proliferations of angiofibromas contain small vessels and plump stellate cells within the superficial dermis (see Fig. 15–20).

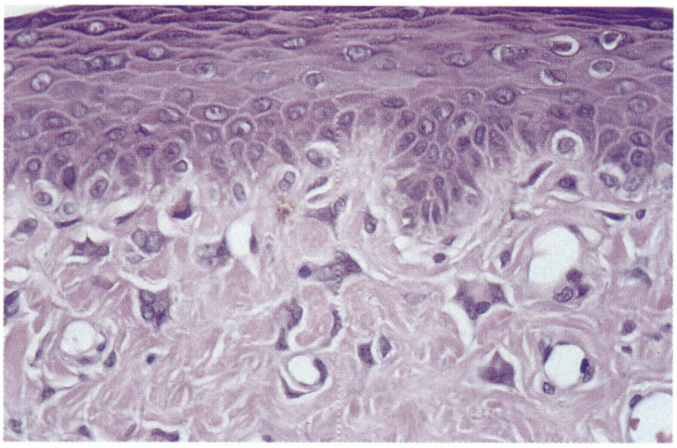

Figure 15–20. The plump stellate cells within the superficial dermis of angiofibromas stain for S100 protein and some are believed to be of melanocytic derivation.

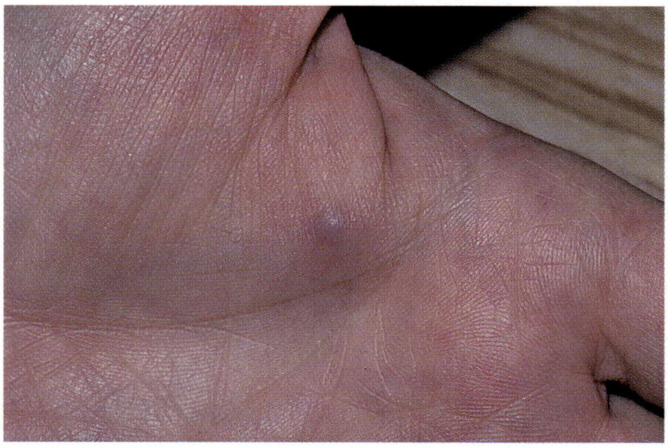

Figure 15–21. Glomangioma. A painful dermal nodule with a purple hue is present on the palm skin.

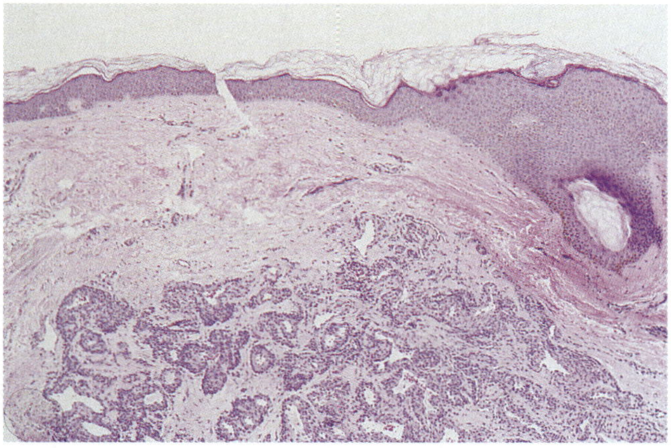

Figure 15–22. Biopsy of a glomangioma similar to the lesion in Figure 15–21 reveals a collection of mid-dermal vessels surrounded by a cuff of pericytes, imparting the impression of glandular differentiation at low magnification.

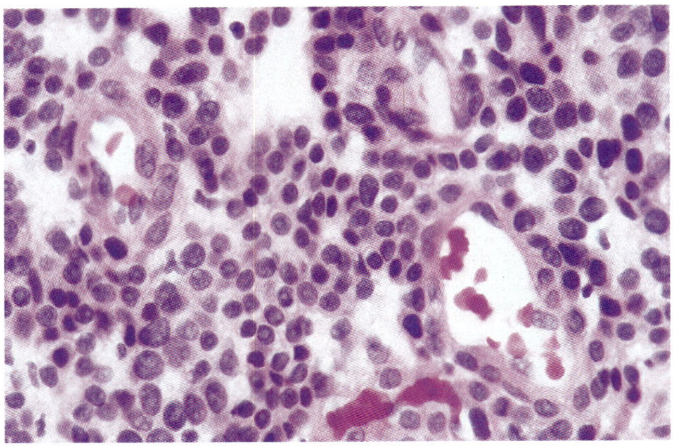

Figure 15–23. At higher magnification, glomangiomas are characterized by monomorphic aggregates of rounded-to-cuboidal pericytes containing nevus-like nuclei and intimately associated with an angiomatous dermal proliferation of small vessels.

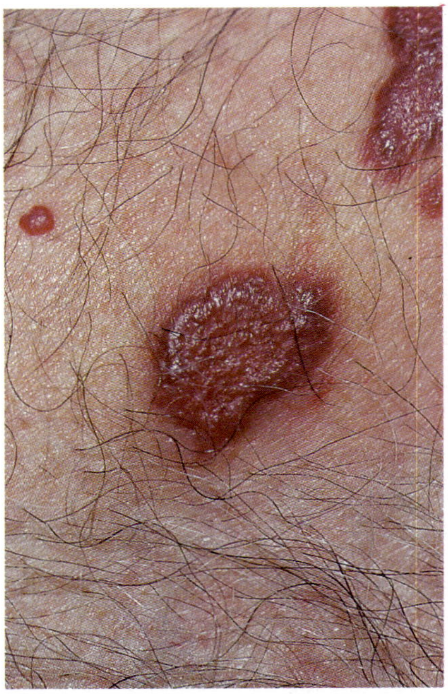

Figure 15–24. Kaposi sarcoma: Patch-plaque stage. An intensely erythematous, nonblanching plaque is present on the truncal skin of a human immunodeficiency virus–positive patient.

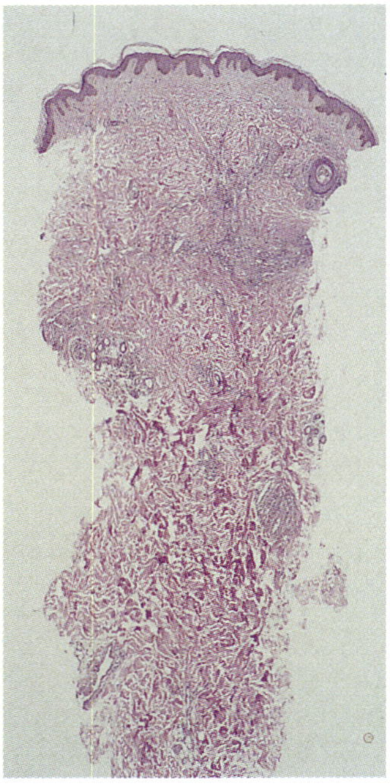

Figure 15–25. At scanning magnification, early Kaposi sarcoma shows the impression of increased cellularity in the superficial and mid-dermis.

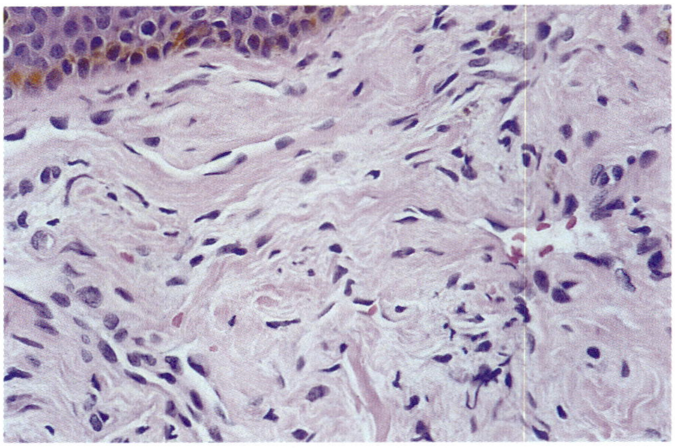

Figure 15–26. The dermal hypercellularity of early Kaposi sarcoma is the result of the proliferation of bland dendritic and spindle-shaped cells about superficial dermal vessels and vessels within periadnexal adventitia.

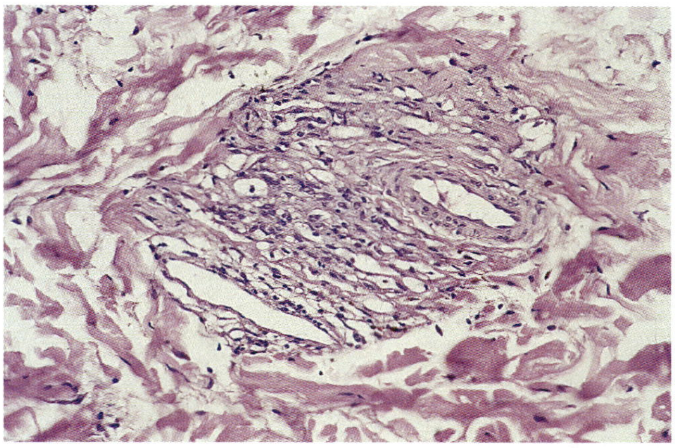

Figure 15–27. Occasional vessels demonstrate striking spindle cell proliferation within the perivascular space of Kaposi sarcoma lesions.

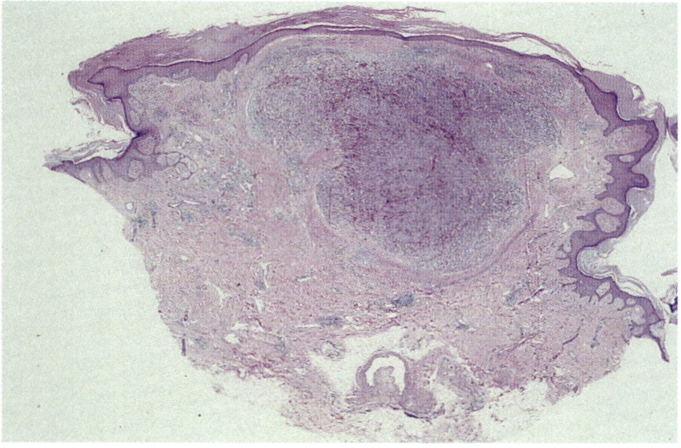

Figure 15–28. Kaposi sarcoma: Plaque-nodular stage. A forming mid-dermal nodule is composed of spindle cells.

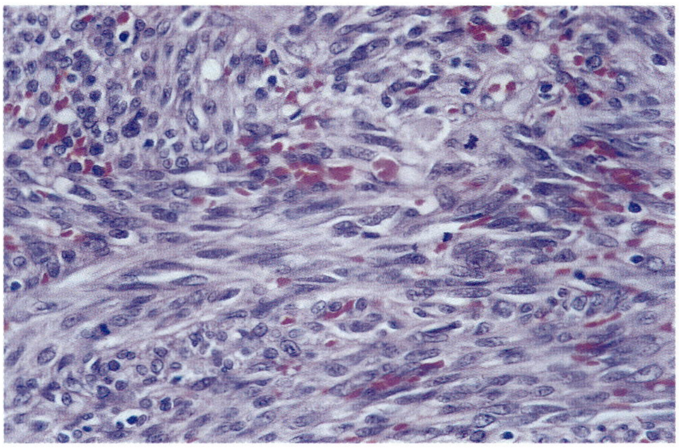

Figure 15–29. Higher magnification of nodular Kaposi sarcoma exhibits formation of slit-like spaces by cells with more nuclear pleomorphism and atypia than those of the earlier patch-plaque stage. A mitotic figure *(top right)* can be seen. Other features suggestive of this diagnosis (not illustrated) include "box car" alignment of erythrocytes within vascular spaces, intracytoplasmic hyaline droplets within tumor cells, and perivascular infiltrates of lymphocytes and plasma cells peripheral to the borders defined by neoplastic cells.

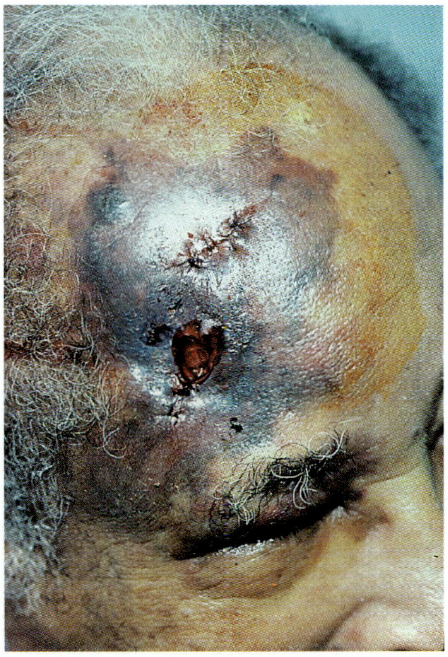

Figure 15–30. Angiosarcoma. This extensive purpuric, indurated plaque on the scalp is typical of a clinical lesion of angiosarcoma.

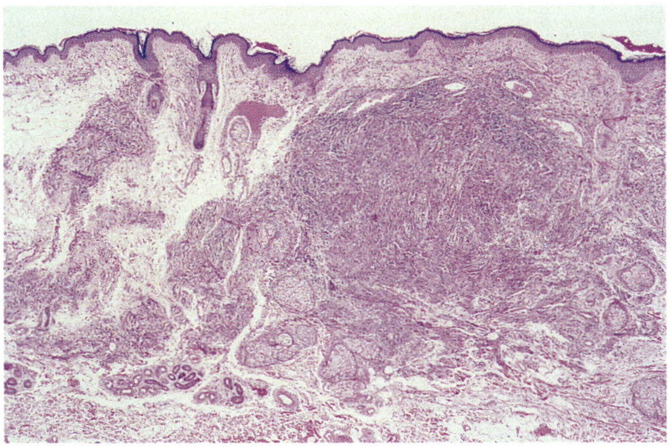

Figure 15–31. Scanning magnification of a biopsy specimen of angiosarcoma reveals coalescent aggregates of malignant spindle cells within the superficial and deep dermis.

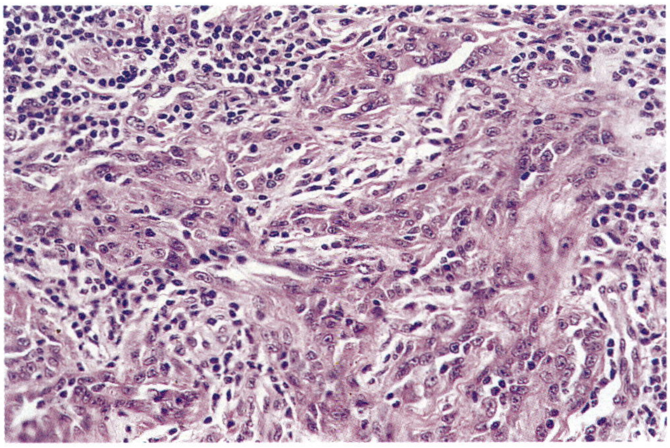

Figure 15–32. At higher magnification, atypical spindle cells of angiosarcoma are admixed with lymphocytes and form poorly demarcated vascular spaces.

Smooth Muscle Tumors

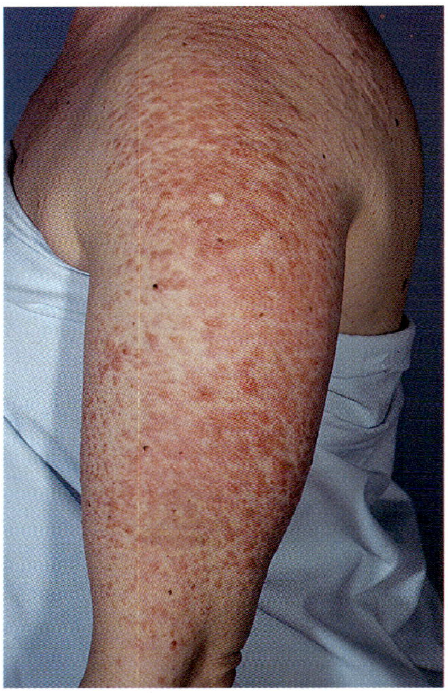

Figure 15–33. Leiomyoma: Multiple piloleiomyomas. This extremity is affected by multiple red-brown dermal nodules arranged in a linear plaque. These lesions are also referred to as arrector pili muscle hamartomas.

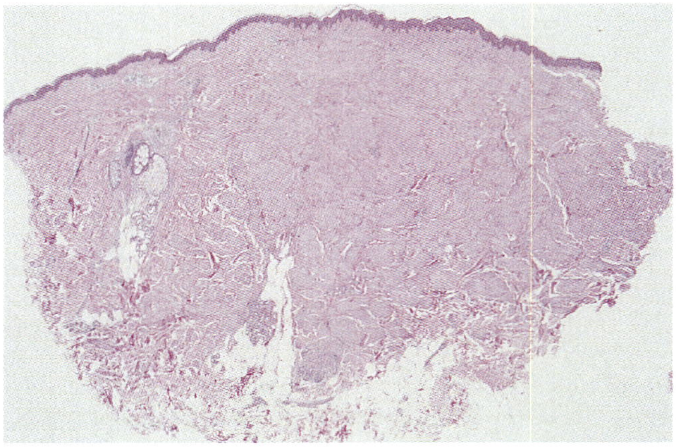

Figure 15–34. Histologically, piloleiomyomas demonstrate multiple smooth muscle bundles insidiously infiltrating dermal connective tissue.

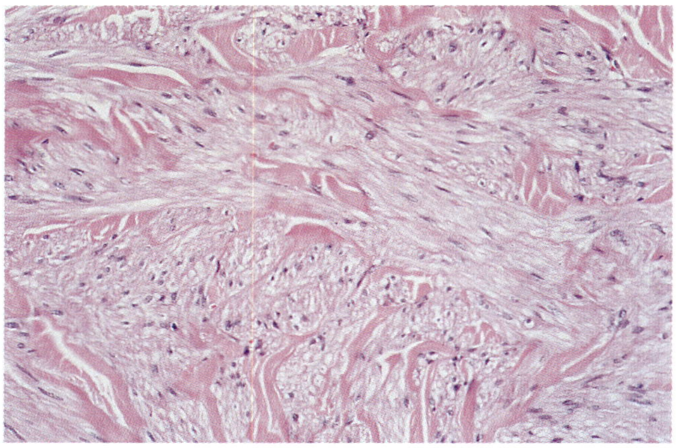

Figure 15–35. At high magnification, smooth muscle cells of piloleiomyoma have elongated, cigar-shaped nuclei with rounded ends in longitudinal section, and in cross section their cytoplasm appears deep pink and vacuolated. Cutaneous angioleiomyomas contain similar cells but form well-circumscribed, vascularized dermal or subcutaneous nodules.

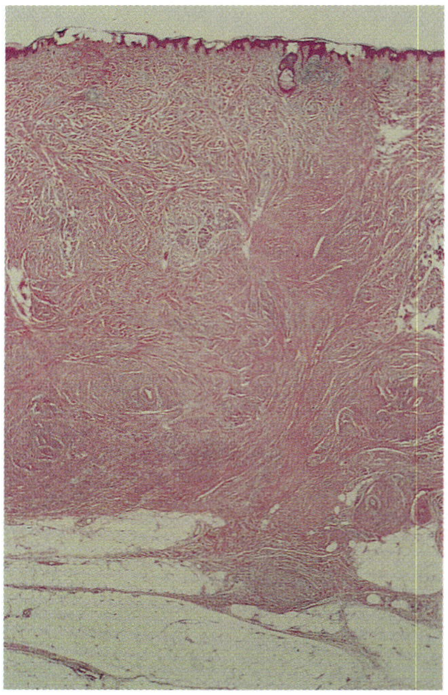

Figure 15–36. Leiomyosarcoma. The dermis is diffusely infiltrated by a spindle cell neoplasm that focally extends into subcutaneous fat.

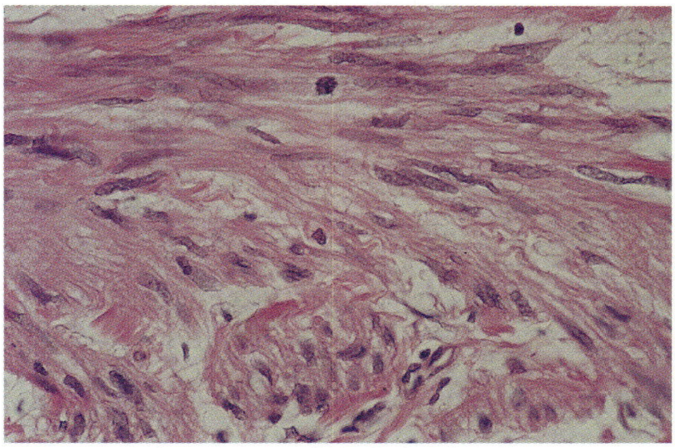

Figure 15–37. At high magnification, the fusiform cells composing leiomyosarcoma are characterized by elongated, cigar-shaped, hyperchromatic nuclei demonstrating numerous mitotic figures.

Fibrohistiocytic Tumors

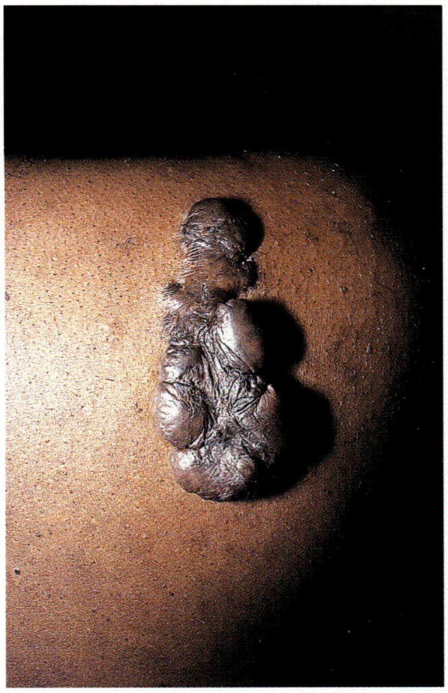

Figure 15–38. Keloid. This unique form of proliferative scar results in exophytic plaques and nodules at the sites of clinical and subclinical trauma in genetically predisposed individuals.

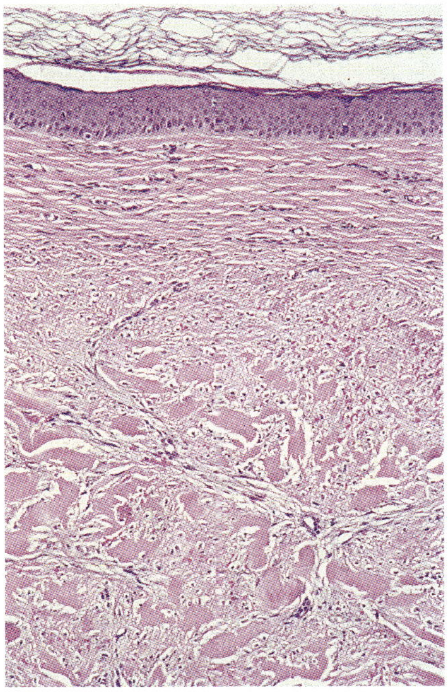

Figure 15–39. At scanning magnification, a keloid is characterized by mid-dermal and deep dermal sclerosis.

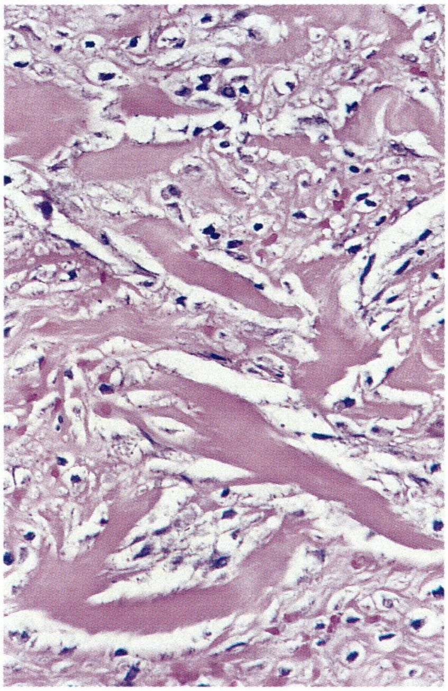

Figure 15–40. At high-power magnification, keloids demonstrate proliferating fibroblasts intermixed with hyalinized and thickened bundles of collagen, producing a zebra-stripe pattern.

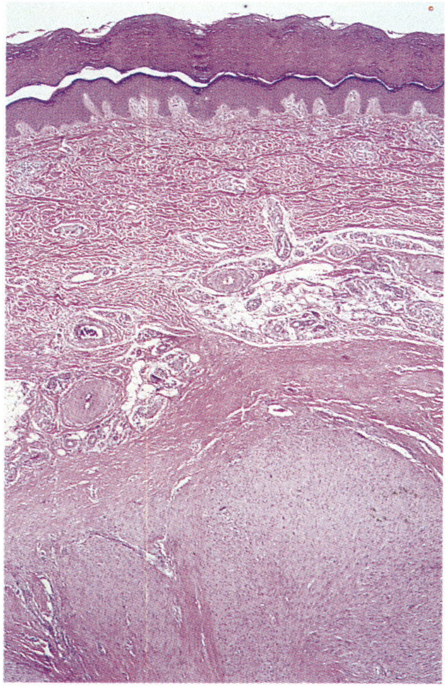

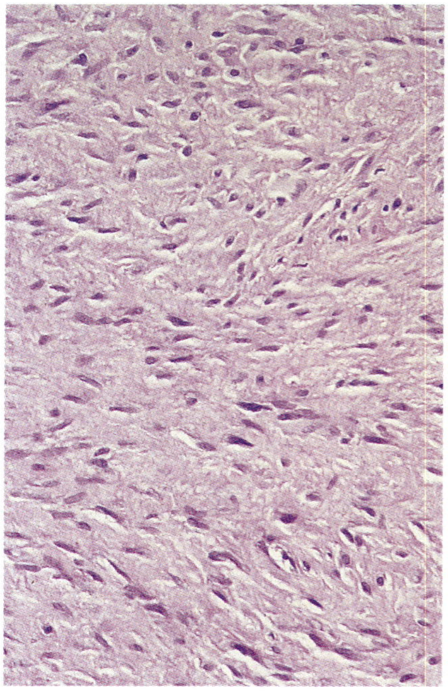

Figures 15–41 and 15–42. Hypertrophic scar. As opposed to a keloid, hypertrophic scars consist only of interlacing fascicles of fibroblasts and delicate collagen bundles within the mid-dermis and deep dermis. Thickened, hyalinized bands are not present.

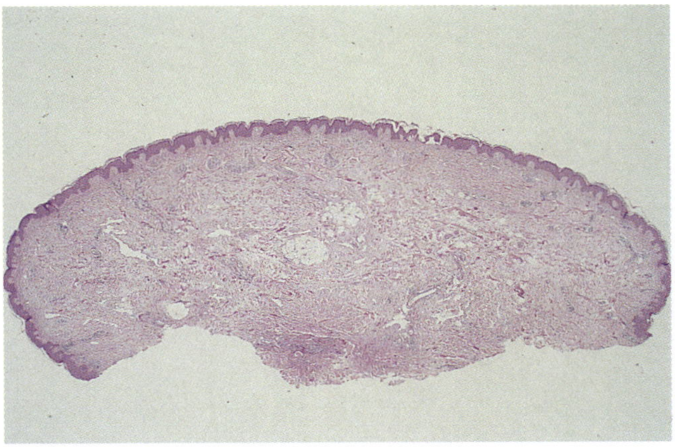

Figure 15–43. Connective tissue nevus (hamartoma). Low magnification reveals a subtle yet anomalous proliferation of vessels, collagen, and associated extracellular matrix elements, as well as lymphatics beneath a diffusely hyperplastic epidermis.

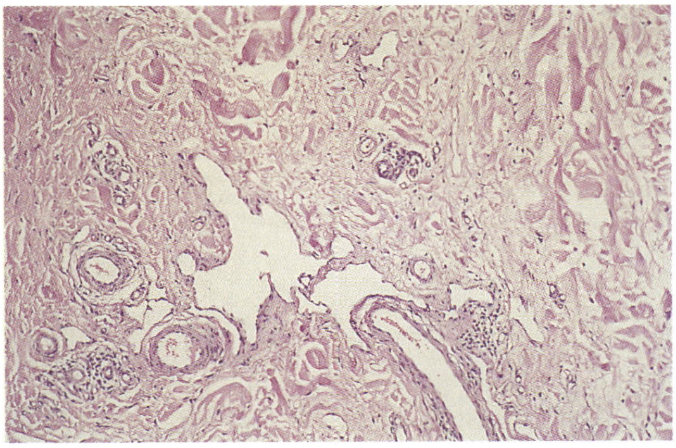

Figure 15–44. High magnification of the connective tissue nevus in Figure 15–43. Note anomalous blood vascular and lymphatic spaces, as well as abnormal collagen bundles of varying caliber.

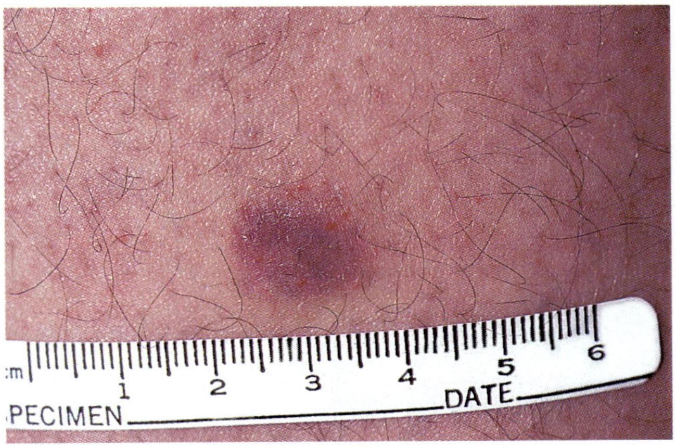

Figure 15–45. Benign fibrous histiocytoma (dermatofibroma). Clinically, these lesions appear as firm, brown papules found predominantly on the lower extremities. Inward compression produces dimpling, in contrast to vertical growth phase melanoma, which generally protrudes outward with this maneuver (*i.e.,* Fitzpatrick sign).

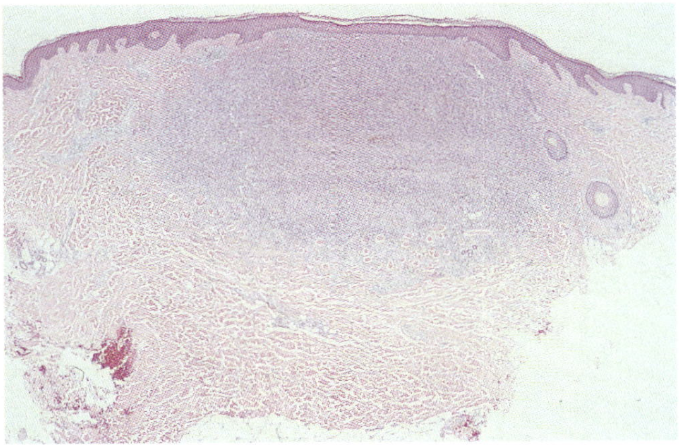

Figure 15–46. At scanning magnification, benign fibrous histiocytoma is characterized by a subtle spindle cell proliferation within the mid-dermis and deep dermis. The overlying epidermis is generally hyperplastic, although the portion of the epidermis most central to the tumor depicted is attenuated, owing to pressure atrophy.

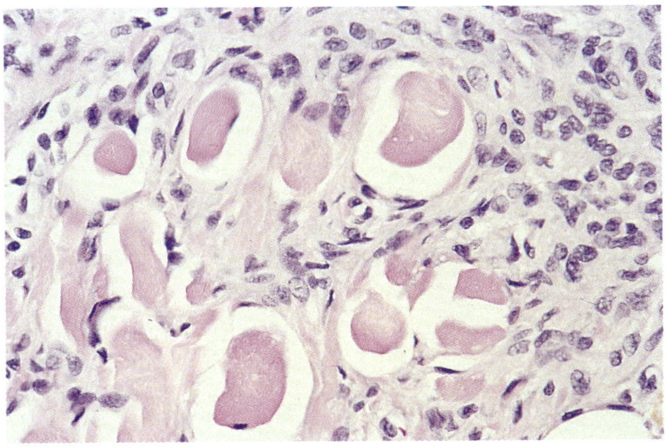

Figure 15–47. A peripheral region of a benign fibrous histiocytoma shows fusiform benign fibroblasts entrapping collagen bundles. Other dermal lesions that result in collagen bundle entrapment include early Kaposi sarcoma, early granuloma annulare, and metastatic carcinoma.

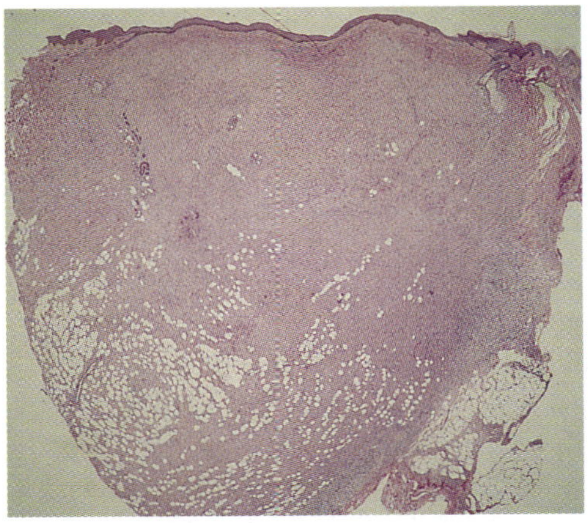

Figure 15–48. Dermatofibrosarcoma protuberans. There is diffuse dermal infiltration beneath an attenuated epidermis by a cellular spindle cell neoplasm that characteristically replaces subcutaneous fat to produce a honeycomb pattern.

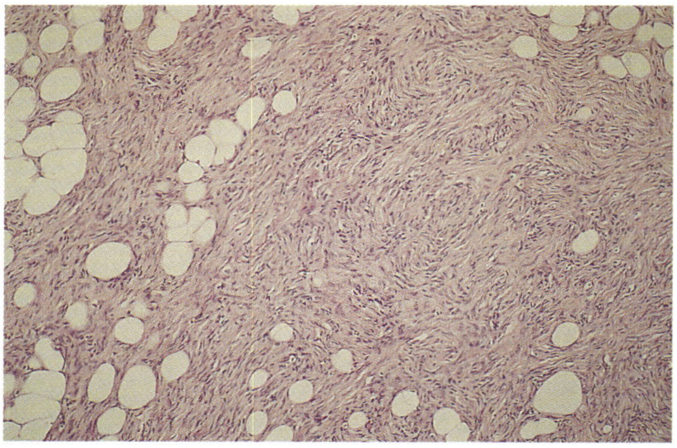

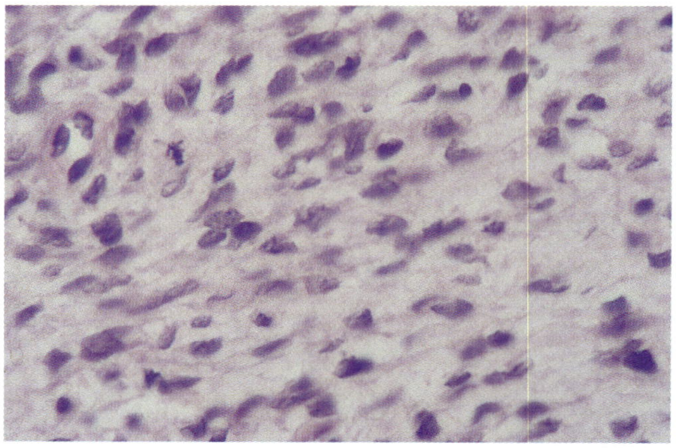

Figures 15–49 and 15–50. In dermatofibrosarcoma protuberans there is a storiform pattern, which also may be potentially present in benign fibrous histiocytoma, hypercellularity, and focal dermal mitoses (Fig. 15–50; *top left*).

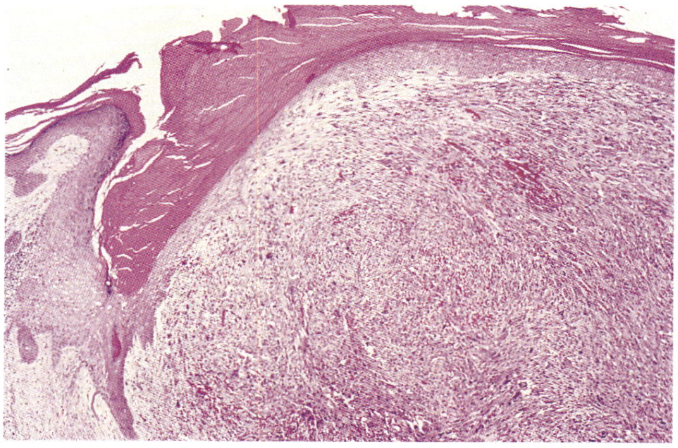

Figure 15–51. Atypical fibroxanthoma. A cellular neoplasm of highly pleomorphic cells is present within actinically damaged dermis and beneath an attenuated epidermal layer.

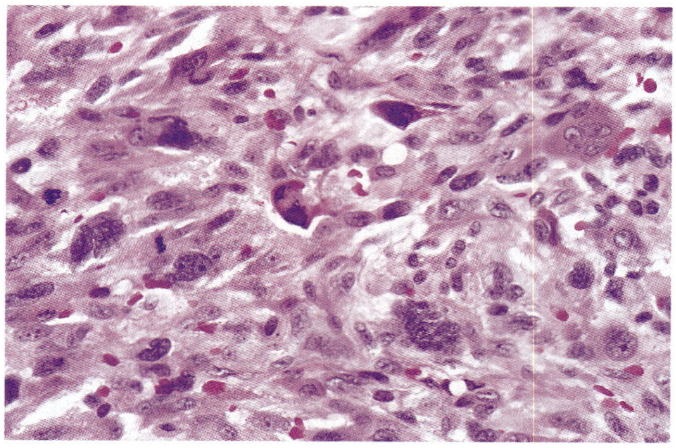

Figure 15–52. The cells comprising atypical fibroxanthoma consist of variably pleomorphic fibroblasts and histiocytes, some of which exhibit multinucleation, prominent hyperchromasia, and elaborate, frequent mitotic figures.

Neural Tumors

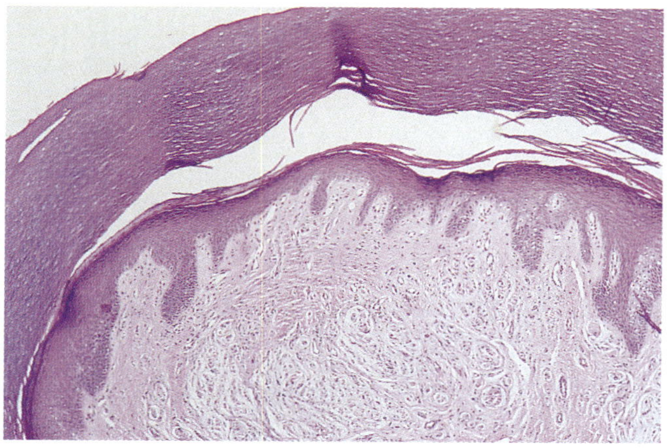

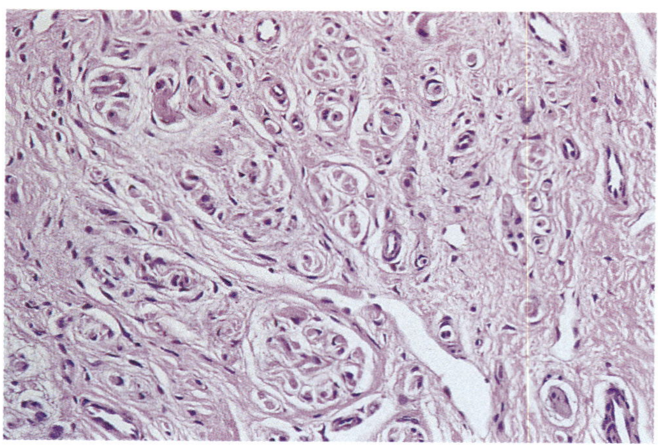

Figures 15–53 and 15–54. Traumatic neuroma. Numerous nerve fibers are embedded within a sclerotic dermis at a site of repeated trauma or inflammation.

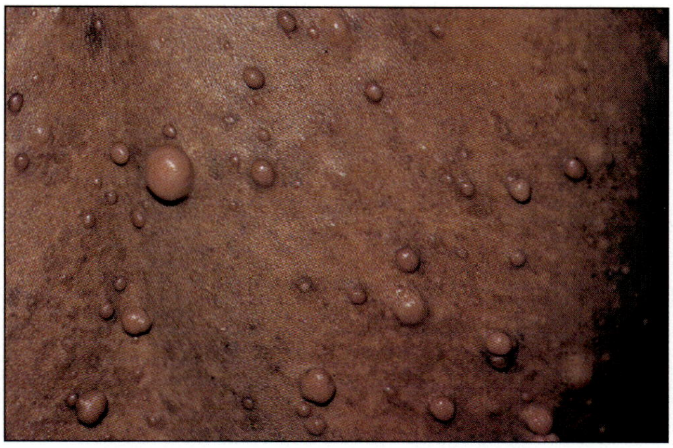

Figure 15–55. Multiple neurofibromas in the setting of neurofibromatosis. Individual lesions are sessile-to-pedunculated, soft, fleshy tumors.

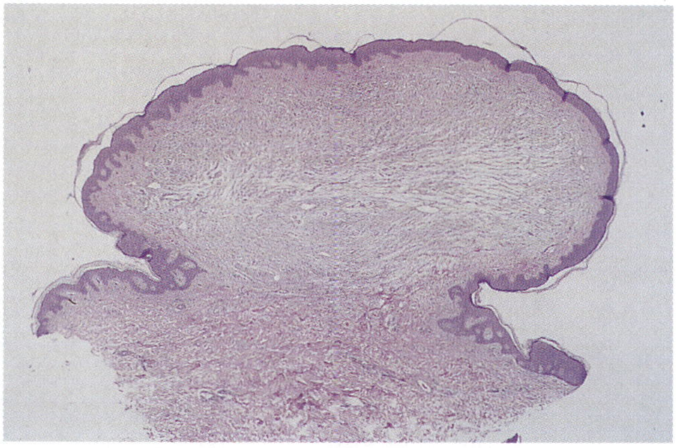

Figure 15–56. At low magnification, a pedunculated neurofibroma shows a loosely arranged stroma partially surrounded by a diffusely hyperplastic epidermal layer.

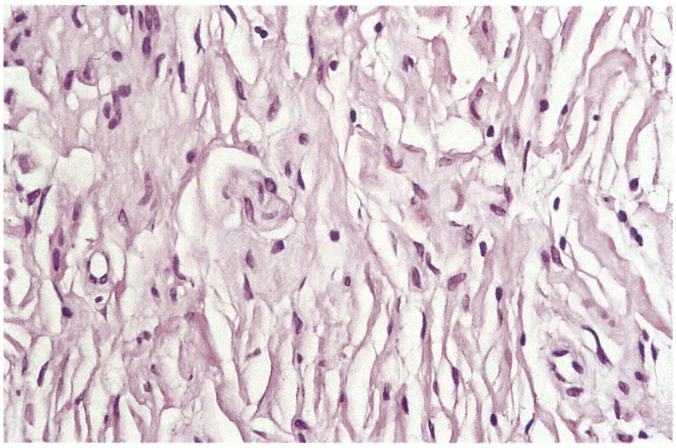

Figure 15–57. At higher magnification, small, bland spindle cells proliferate among wavy collagen bundles, mast cells, and occasional nerve fibers *(left, center).*

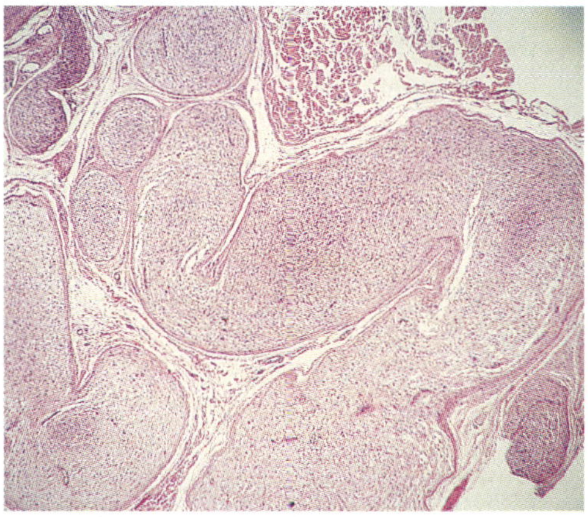

Figure 15–58. In a plexiform neurofibroma, a more specific marker for neurofibromatosis based on a solitary lesion, there are discrete, enlarged nerve bundles in serpiginous array within a loose connective tissue stroma.

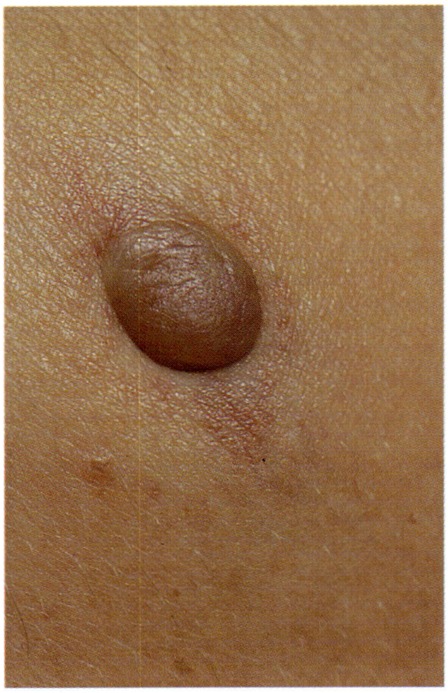

Figure 15–59. Neurolemmoma. This soft, fleshy nodule was formed by a well-demarcated tumor within the deep dermis and subcutis.

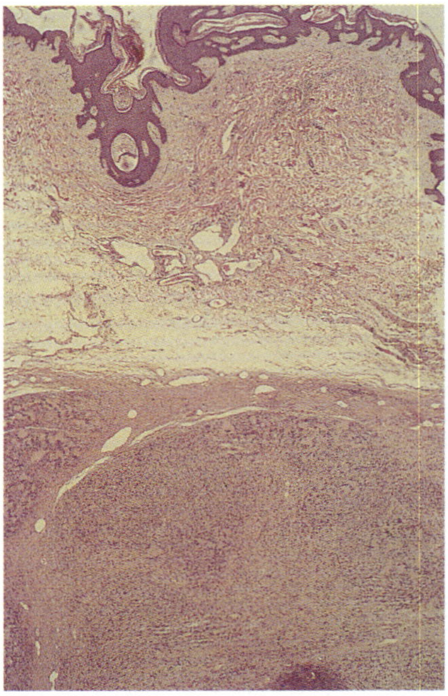

Figure 15–60. The tumor nodule of neurilemmoma is well circumscribed and composed of variably cellular regions surrounded by a fibrous mantle.

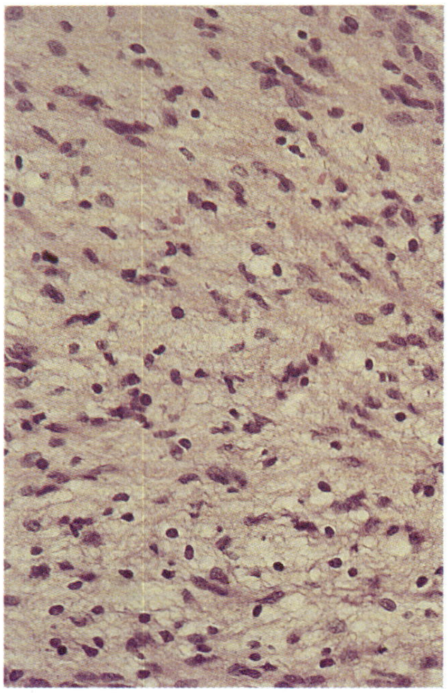

Figure 15–61. At higher magnification, the stroma of neurilemmoma is composed of neuroid spindle cells within a finely fibrillar matrix.

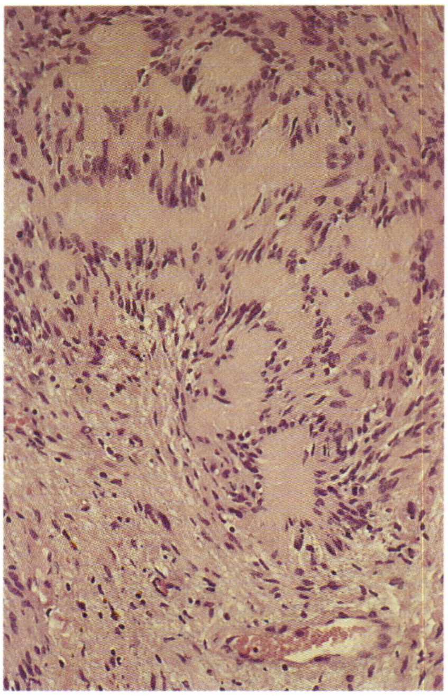

Figure 15–62. Neurilemmomas are also characterized by zones where spindle cells prominently palisade (*i.e.,* Verocay bodies).

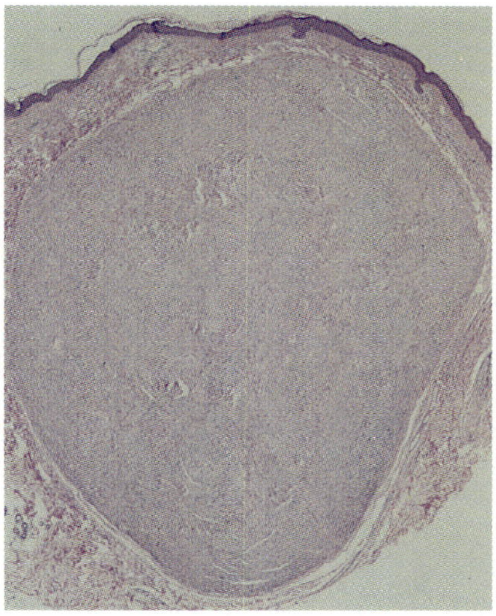

Figure 15–63. Palisaded encapsulated neuroma. This uniformly cellular dermal nodule is well demarcated.

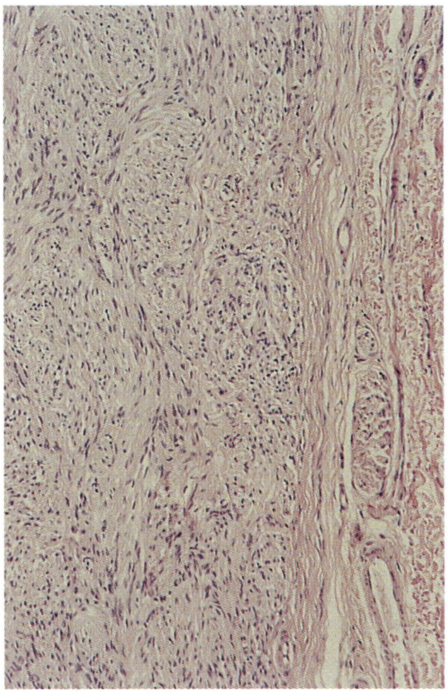

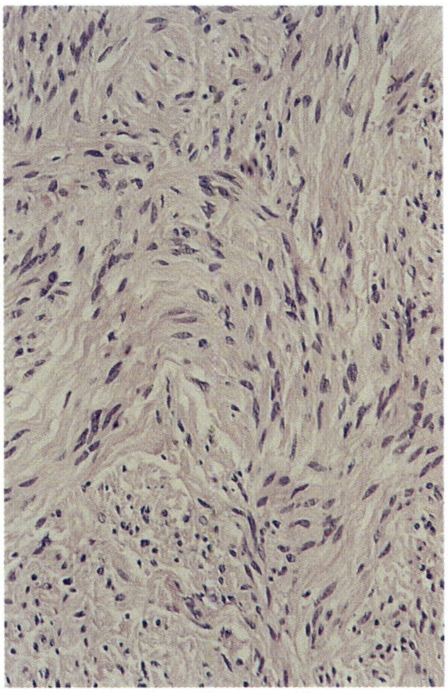

Figures 15–64 and 15–65. The dermal nodule of palisaded encapsulated neuroma is composed of spindle cells and axons in approximately a 50:50 ratio. Note the nerve fiber at the perimeter of the tumor (Fig. 15–64, *right center*).

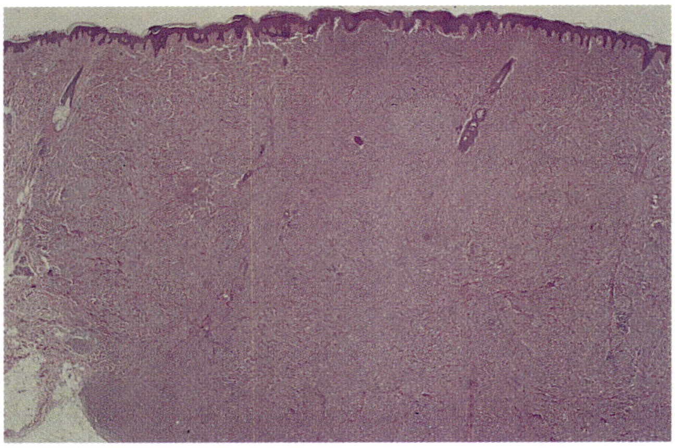

Figure 15–66. Granular cell tumor. At scanning magnification, the dermis is diffusely permeated by pale blue-pink cells beneath an epidermal layer showing marked hyperplasia.

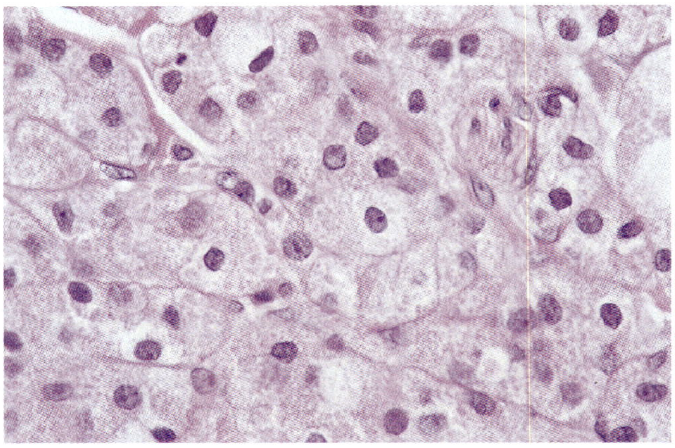

Figure 15–67. At high magnification, the cells of granular cell tumor have distinct cell membranes; finely granular, not vacuolated, cytoplasm; and centrally located, uniform, round nuclei.

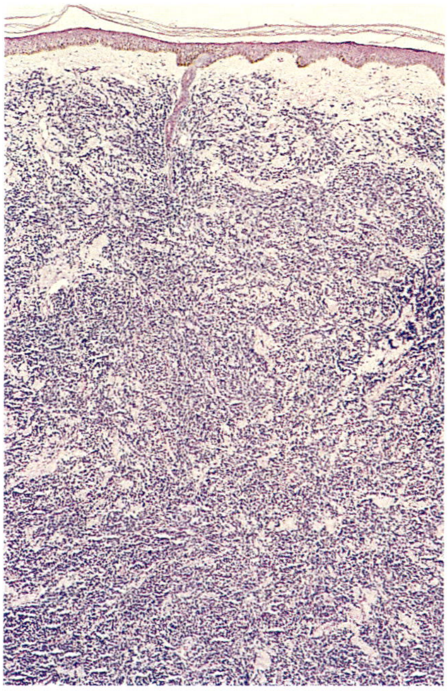

Figure 15–68. Neuroendocrine carcinoma. There are confluent nests and inconspicuous trabeculae of small, lymphocyte-like cells within the superficial and deep dermis.

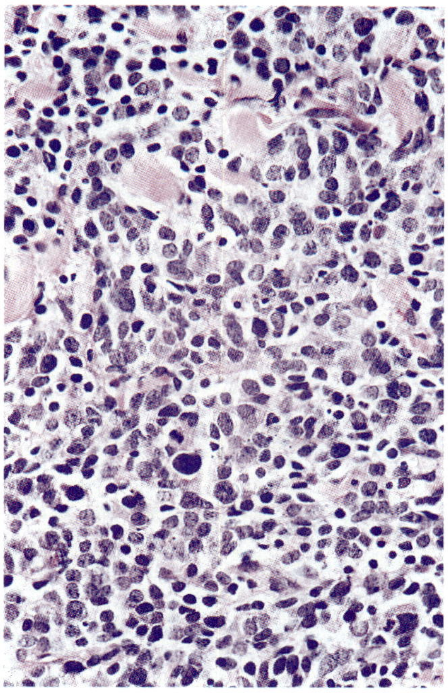

Figure 15–69. At higher magnification, neuroendocrine carcinoma is characterized by cells with scant cytoplasm, and nuclei are pleomorphic and exhibit numerous mitotic figures as well as prominent individual cell necrosis.

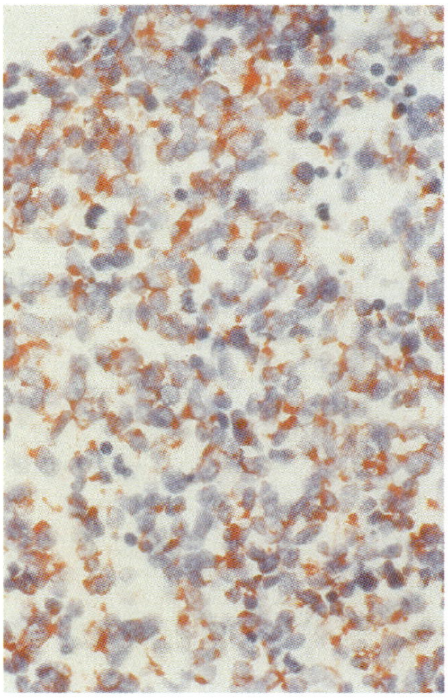

Figure 15–70. Immunohistochemical stain for cytokeratin reveals a characteristic perinuclear zone of positive staining in most cells of neuroendocrine carcinoma.

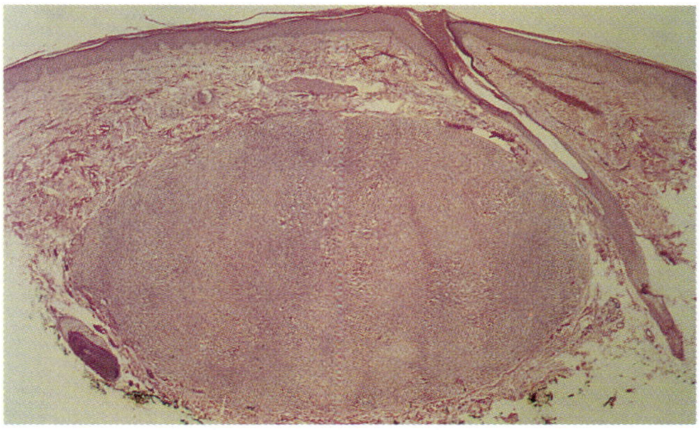

Figure 15–71. Neurothekeoma. The tumor is well circumscribed within the mid-dermis.

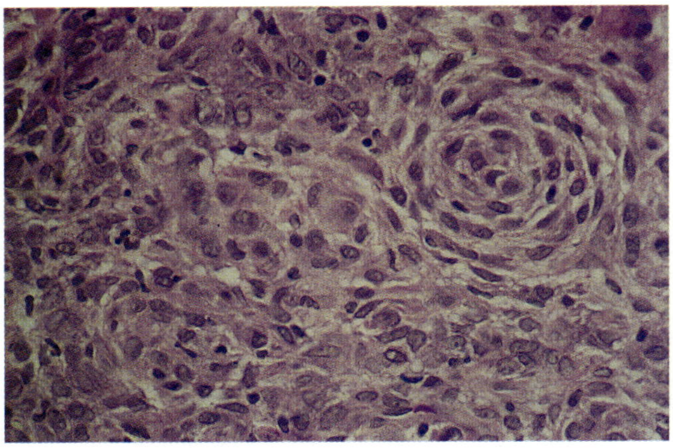

Figure 15–72. This epithelioid variant of neurothekeoma is composed of clustered nests of round-to-ovoid cells with variable nuclear pleomorphism and occasional mitotic figures. Other foci show cells embedded in a fibrillar matrix. Myxoid variants are composed predominantly of stellate and fusiform cells within a mucinous, myxoid stroma, as well as isolated foci of epithelioid cells.

Tumors of Adipose Tissue: Cutaneous Lipoma

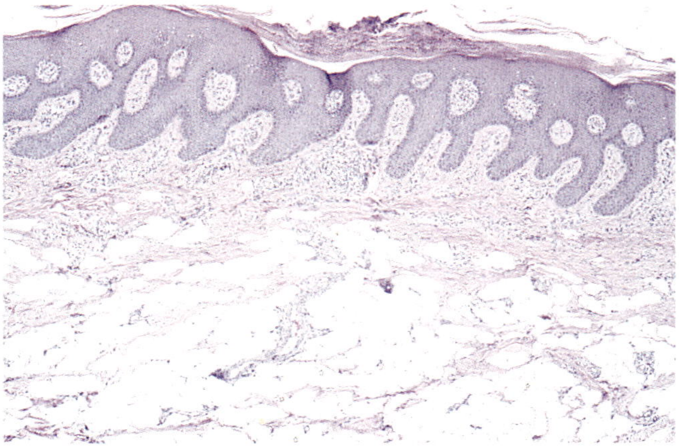

Figure 15–73. Lipoma and variants. Nevus lipomatosus superficialis with the lower two thirds of the dermis replaced by mature adipose tissue.

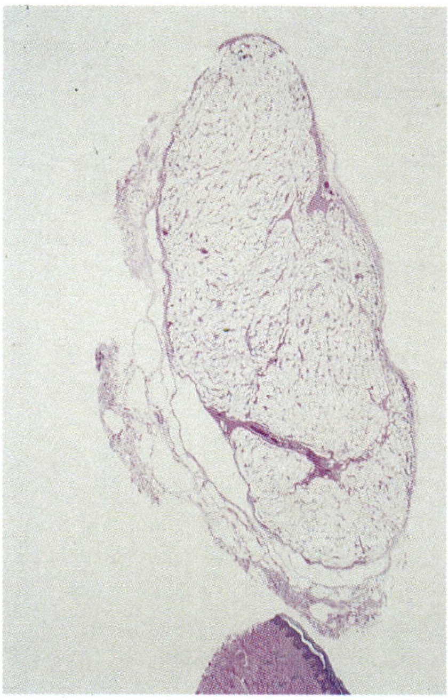

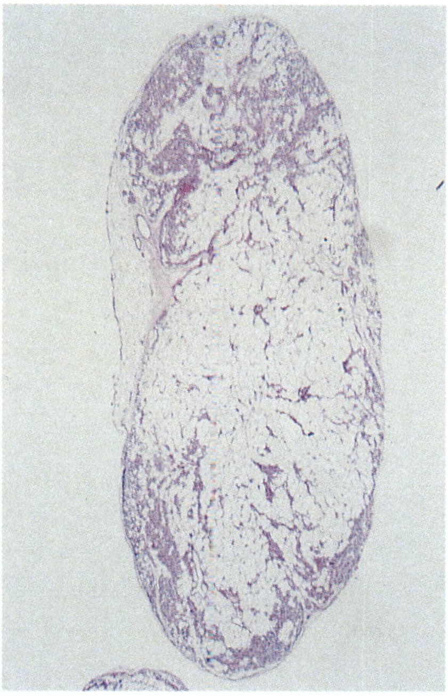

Figures 15–74 and 15–75. Although both lipoma (Fig. 15–74) and angiolipoma (Fig. 15–75) are well-defined encapsulated tumors of mature adipose tissue, only the latter has a significant component of small vessels, often containing thrombi (opaque anastomosing structures concentrated at the upper and lower poles of this ovoid tumor).

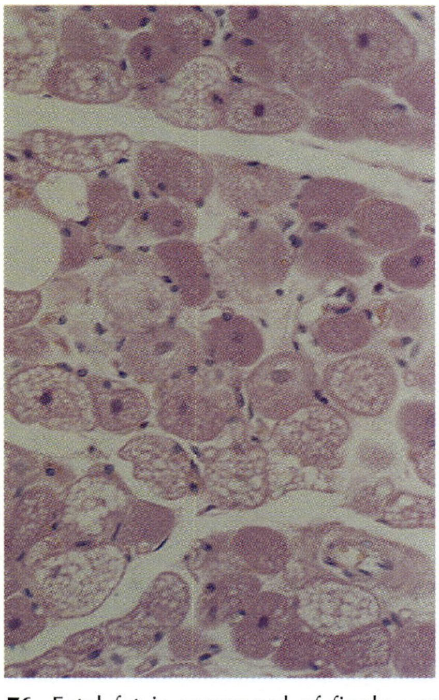

Figure 15–76. Fetal fat is composed of finely vacuolated to granulated adipocytes with a brown clinical appearance and an eosinophilic hue by routine histology. It is found in adults primarily as the main cellular constituent of the lipoma termed hibernoma.

16

Metastatic Tumors to Skin

Metastatic tumors to skin represent a diagnostically problematic and diverse group of neoplasms that may mimic primary carcinoma, melanoma, adnexal carcinoma, and sarcoma. Metastatic carcinoma to the skin is relatively uncommon, although the issue arises frequently enough in routine differential diagnosis that its brief consideration is warranted in this atlas. In women, breast carcinoma is the most frequent lesion to spread to skin, accounting for approximately two thirds of all metastases. Other primary sites that commonly involve the skin in women include colon cancer and carcinoma of the lung, ovaries, and melanoma. In men, lung cancer is the most common primary tumor to spread to the skin (approximately one fourth of all cases of cutaneous metastasis), followed by colon cancer; malignant melanoma; and oropharyngeal, renal, and gastric carcinoma.

Metastatic carcinoma may take a number of differing clinical forms, including diffuse dermal lymphatic spread and nodular aggregates of tumor within the dermis, or the pattern clinically may be dominated by a desmoplastic response. When diffuse lymphatic dissemination occurs, edema and inflammation (erythema or tan-brown discoloration) frequently are observed, producing brawny induration and a *peau d'orange* appearance to the epidermal surface. This latter feature results when superficial dermal edema occurs about follicular ostia, rendering them prominent and patulous. Emboli of tumor cells within blood vessels may lead to associated telangiectasia or overt zones of red-black tissue necrosis. Carcinomas that produce desmoplasia result in firm induration and, in some instances, depression of the involved site *(e.g., carcinoma en cuirasse).* Metastases may vary in size and shape, be flesh colored to hemorrhagic, and show ulceration. In summary, metastases may clinically mimic inflammation and edema, fibrosis, vasculitis, or a wide variety of primary cutaneous tumors.

Histologically, tinctorial characteristics are often of assistance in differential diagnosis of metastatic carcinoma. The stroma surrounding glandular epithelium of endometriosis, a condition that may mimic metastatic carcinoma to the dermis, for example, is densely packed by basophilic spindle cells, whereas the reactive desmoplastic stroma of certain forms of breast and colon cancer tends to be eosinophilic. Mucin-producing tumors may contain pale gray-blue pockets of cytoplasmic mucin or secrete similar materials into central lumens. As occurs with primary malignant tumors of skin, the degree of nuclear basophilia often correlates with clumping of heterochromatin within nuclei of metastatic malignant cells and therefore is of assistance in differentiating benign from malignant processes (*e.g.,* primary adnexal adenoma from metastatic carcinoma).

"Benign Metastases": Endometriosis

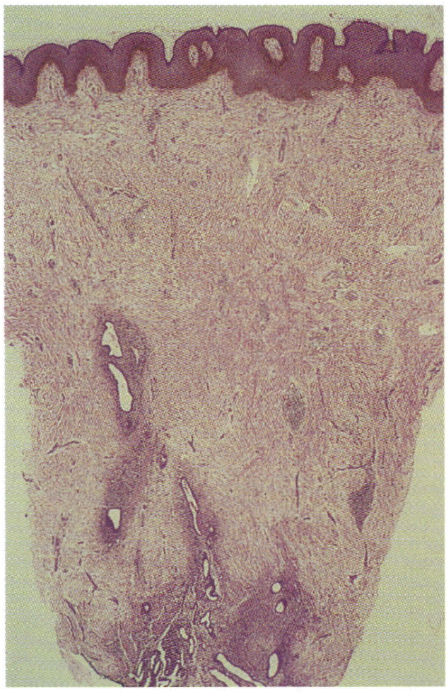

Figure 16–1. Cutaneous endometriosis. Within the mid-dermis to deep dermis, there are glands surrounded by a cellular cuff.

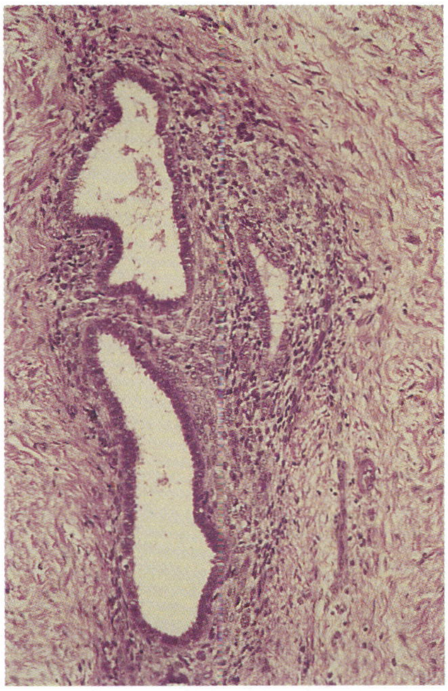

Figure 16–2. These glands, some of which show early cystic dilation, are composed of nonciliated columnar epithelium. The cuff does not represent inflammation or a desmoplastic response to metastasis but rather is normal endometrial stroma with foci of hemorrhage and hemosiderin deposition.

Metastatic Melanoma

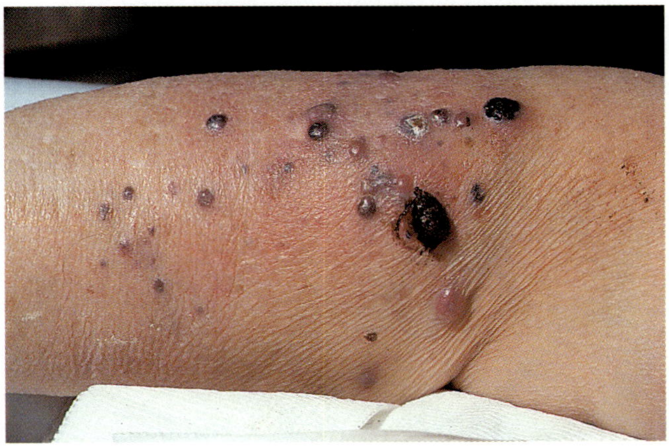

Figure 16–3. Epidermotropic metastases: melanoma. Multiple pigmented papules and nodules are covered by a shiny, focally ulcerated epidermal surface.

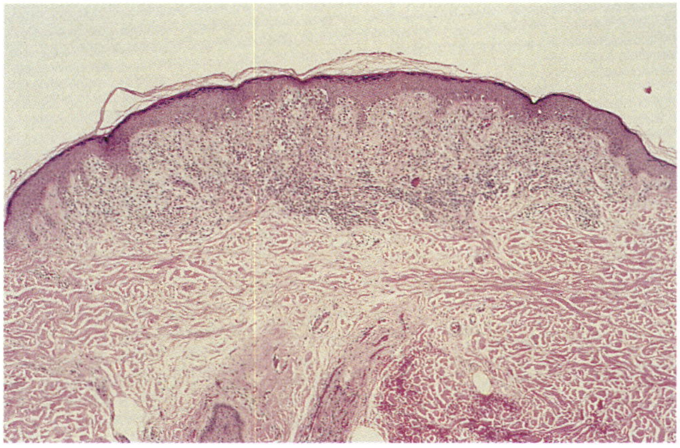

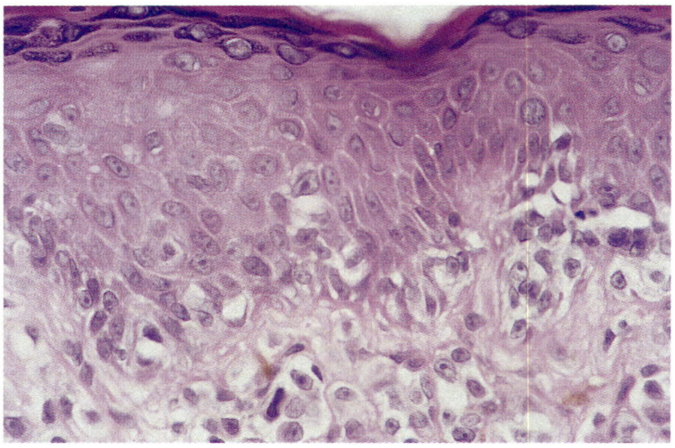

Figures 16–4 and 16–5. At scanning (Fig. 16–4) and midrange (Fig. 16–5) magnification, nested and solitary malignant melanocytes are observed along the dermal-epidermal interface with focal extension into the epidermal layer.

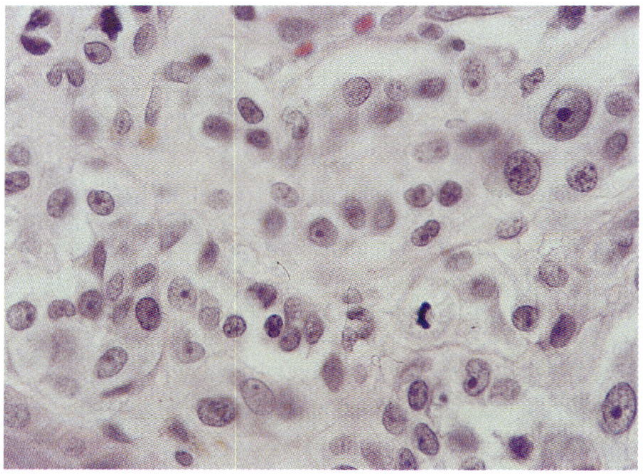

Figure 16–6. Although the silhouette portrayed in Figure 16–4 is deceptively symmetric, the cytology of the nodule shows variable cellular atypia of the nested melanoma cells and occasional mitotic figures *(center, right).*

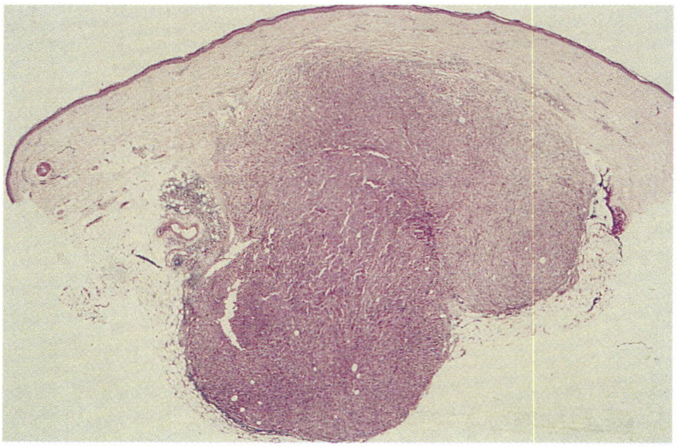

Figure 16–7. Amelanotic metastatic melanoma. An asymmetric tumor nodule within the deep dermis and subcutis is separated from the epidermal layer by a broad band of superficial and mid-dermal collagen.

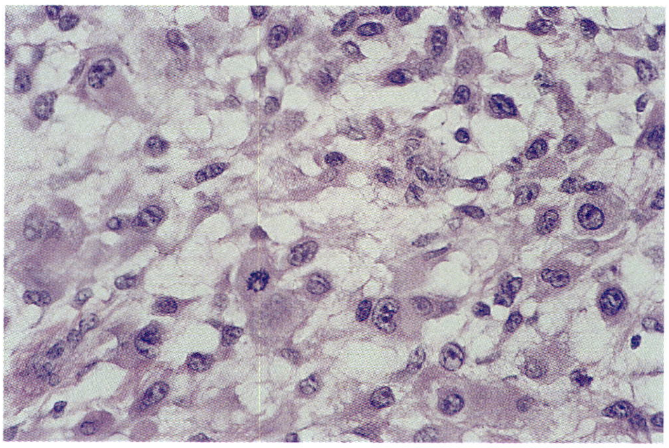

Figure 16–8. The tumor cells in the lesion depicted in Figure 16–7 are malignant in appearance but lack signs of differentiation such as intracellular pigment, intercellular junctions, or glandular differentiation.

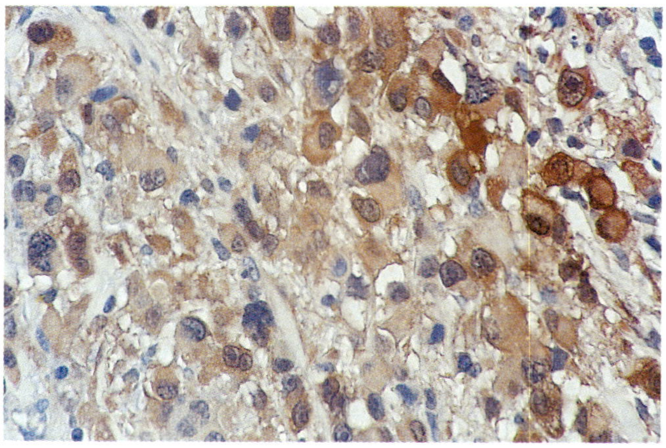

Figure 16–9. A panel of immunohistochemical stains reveals that many of the tumor cells strongly express S100 protein, as well as HMB-45 antigen (not shown), confirming the diagnosis of metastatic melanoma, nonepidermotropic type.

Metastatic Gastrointestinal Carcinoma

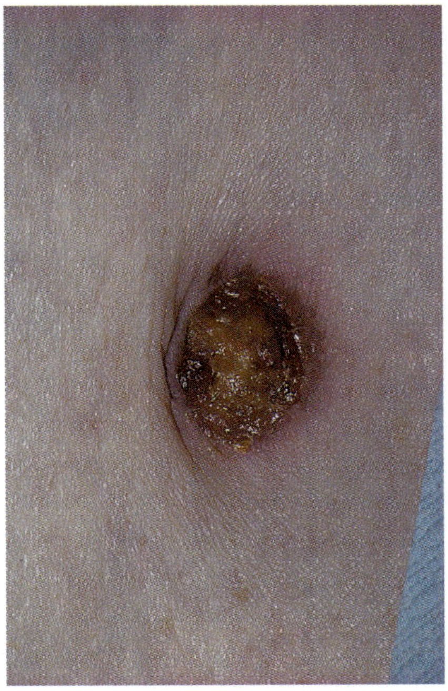

Figure 16–10. Metastatic gastrointestinal carcinoma. This ulcerated umbilical nodule was the first sign of internal gastrointestinal malignancy (*i.e.*, "Sister Mary Joseph" nodule).

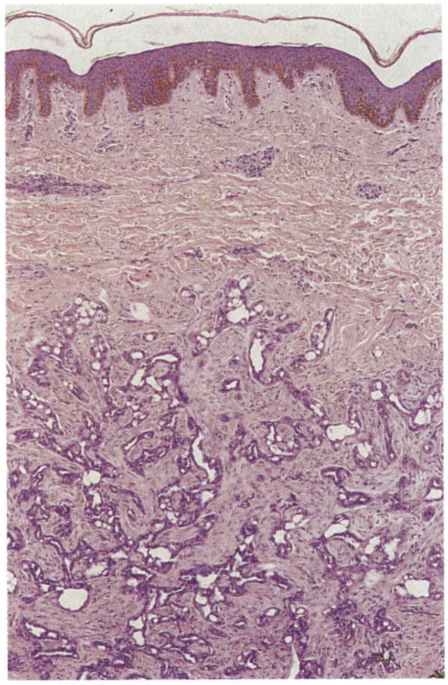

Figure 16–11. Irregular islands of gland-forming epithelium are proliferating within a distinctive fibrous stroma within the mid-dermis to deep dermis.

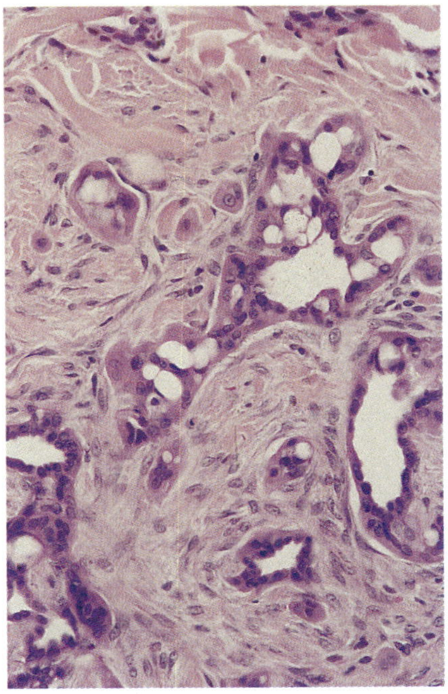

Figure 16–12. The nuclei are hyperchromatic and pleomorphic, and the glandular spaces are irregularly and abortively formed. The patient had pancreatic adenocarcinoma.

Metastatic Breast Carcinoma

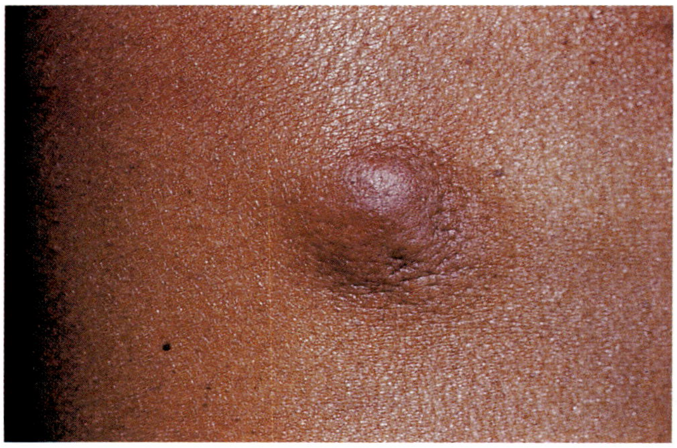

Figure 16–13. Metastatic intralymphatic carcinoma from the breast. This metastatic nodule is surrounded by a halo of edematous skin with patulous follicular orifices resembling the skin of an orange (*i.e., peau d'orange* appearance).

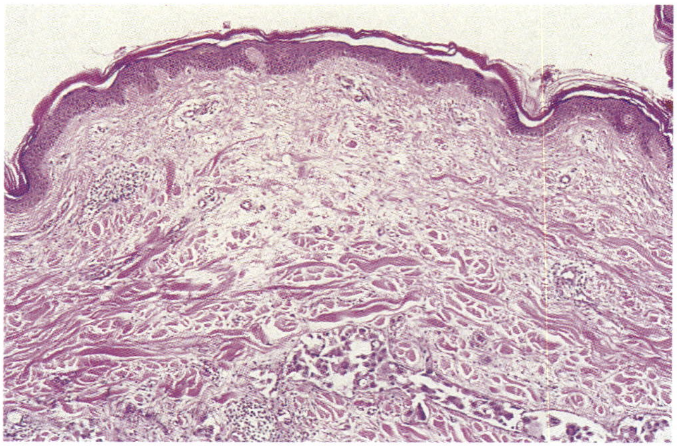

Figure 16–14. At low magnification, there is diffuse dermal edema; it may be easy to overlook the plug of tumor cells responsible for these changes *(bottom, center).*

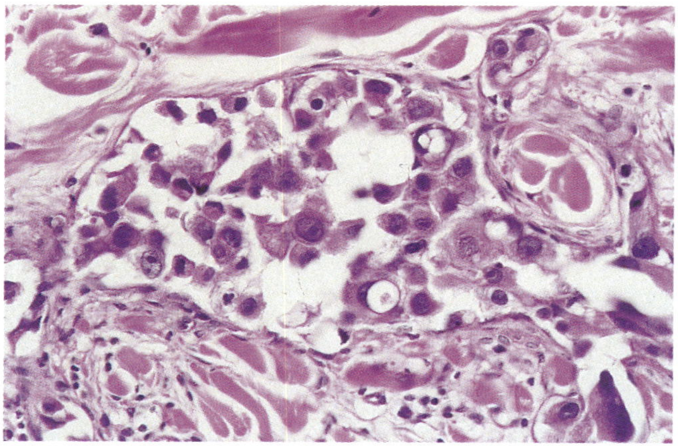

Figure 16–15. Within the widened lymphatic space, there are malignant cells, some of which show cytoplasmic vacuolization due to mucin. This pattern of local or distant spread has sometimes been called "inflammatory carcinoma."

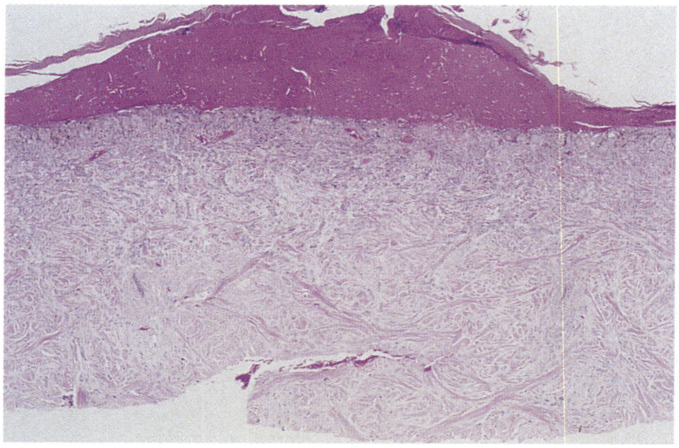

Figure 16–16. Metastatic small cell adenocarcinoma from the breast. This crusted lesion shows only subtle hypercellularity within the superficial dermis. As with most lesions, higher magnification than scanning is needed to ensure a correct diagnosis.

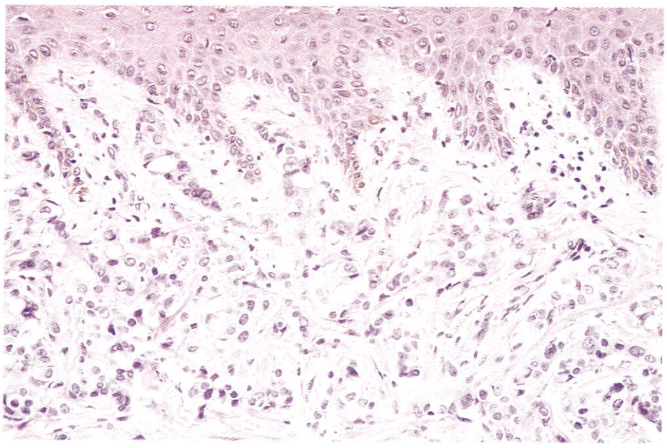

Figure 16–17. At midrange magnification, small cords of innocuous appearing cells are observed; some are reminiscent of dermal nevus cells.

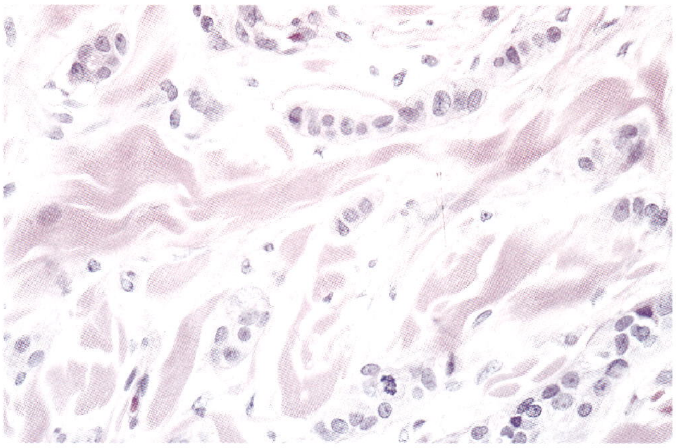

Figure 16–18. At high power, the cells are arranged in "Indian-file" configurations and contain oval nuclei with distinctive nucleoli. Occasional mitoses are present *(bottom, center).* Collectively, these findings are those of metastatic breast carcinoma of the small cell type (infiltrating lobular carcinoma).

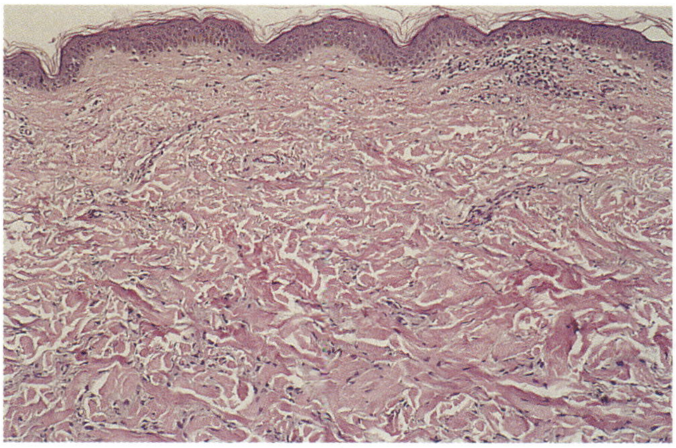

Figure 16–19. Metastatic adenocarcinoma from the breast: sclerosing or interstitial pattern. At scanning magnification, there is a vague impression of increased dermal cellularity, particularly in the deep dermis.

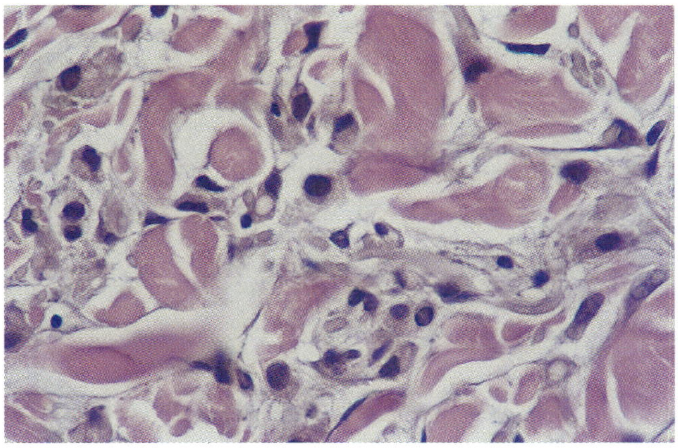

Figure 16–20. At high magnification, malignant cells with densely hyperchromatic nuclei and occasional intracytoplasmic vacuoles *(left, center)* insidiously infiltrate between collagen bundles. The pattern resembles the relation between cells and matrix seen in early granuloma annulare, dermatofibroma, or Kaposi sarcoma.

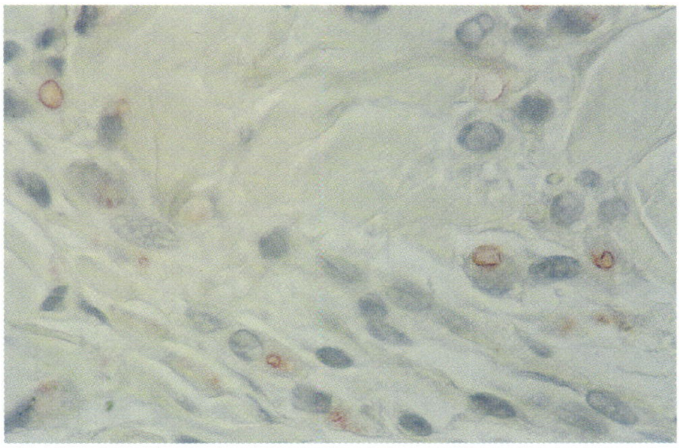

Figure 16–21. Immunohistochemistry for epithelial membrane antigen reveals that the vacuoles seen in Figure 16–20 represent intracytoplasmic lumina *(right, center),* confirming the impression of metastatic adenocarcinoma.

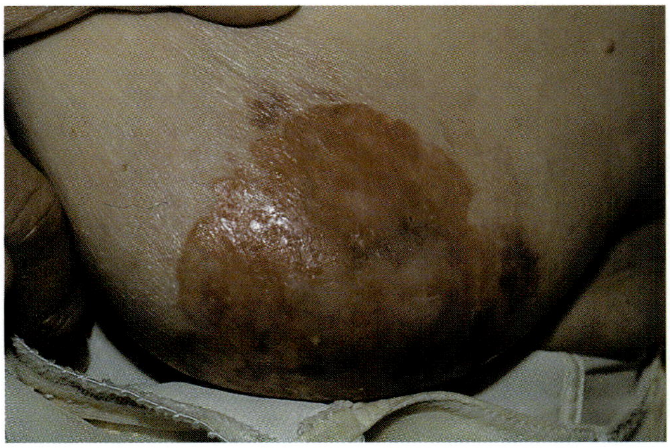

Figure 16–22. Paget disease. An eroded, oozing, erythematous plaque affects breast skin.

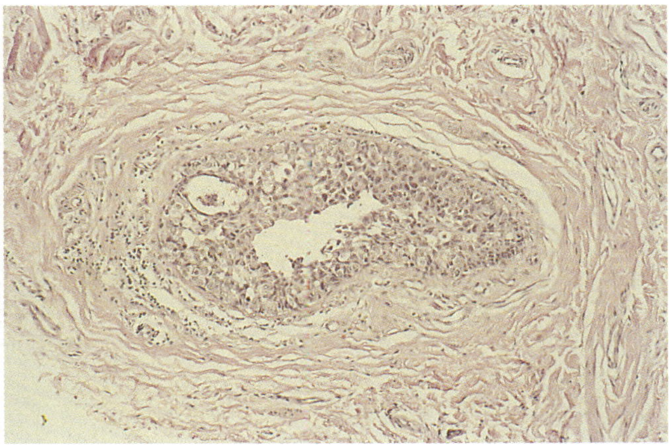

Figure 16–23. A focus of carcinoma in situ within an underlying breast duct is observed in a case of Paget disease.

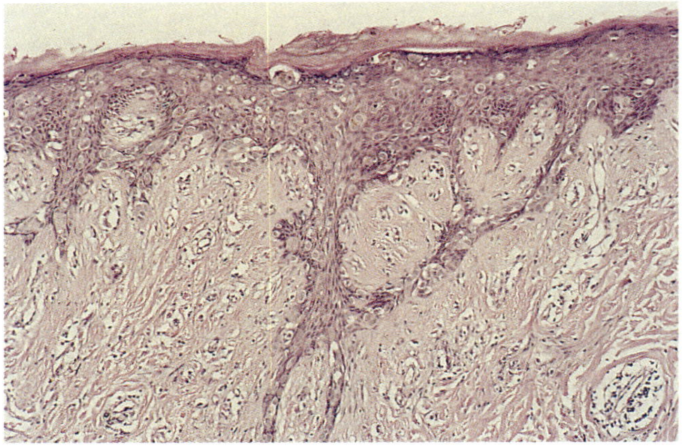

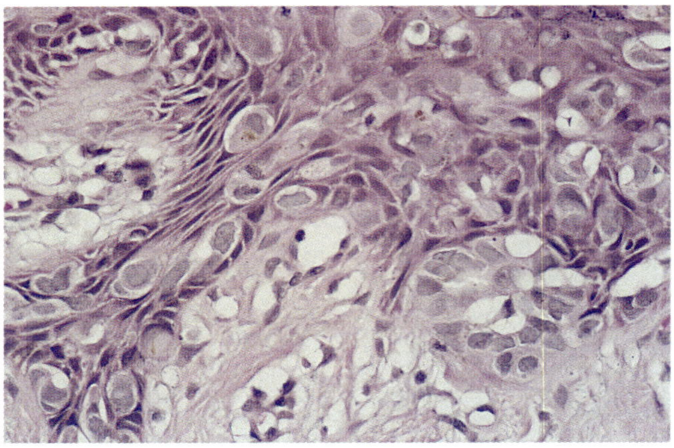

Figures 16–24 and 16–25. Similar adenocarcinoma cells are present throughout the overlying epidermal layer, a finding diagnostic of Paget disease and one that must be distinguished from intraepidermal growth in melanoma and squamous cell carcinoma. Paget cells are generally CEA+, S100−, and keratin−.

Metastatic Lung Carcinoma

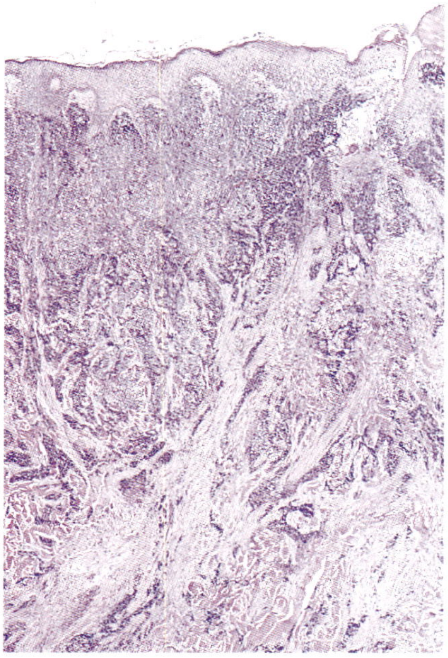

Figure 16–26. Metastatic lung carcinoma: Small cell type. Sheets, clusters, and strands of small, lymphocyte-like cells fill the papillary dermis and diffusely infiltrate the reticular dermis.

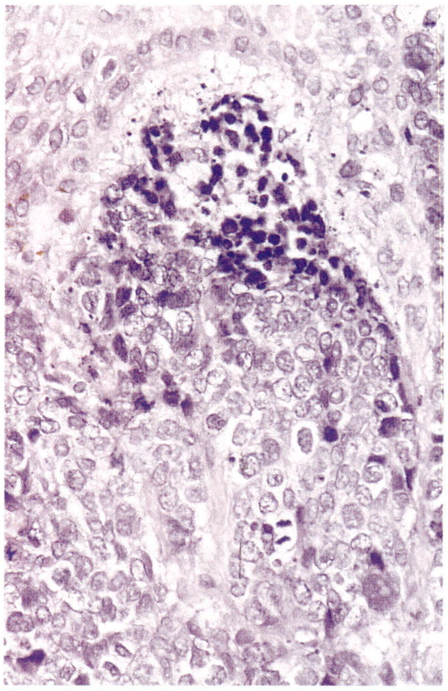

Figure 16–27. Polygonal dark and ovoid pale, small to intermediate-size tumor cells fill the papillary dermis but spare the epidermis *(top)*. There is tumor cell necrosis in the upper half of the field beneath the epidermis and a suggestion of molding between several adjacent cells. Mitotic figures *(bottom)* are also observed.

Metastatic Ovarian Carcinoma

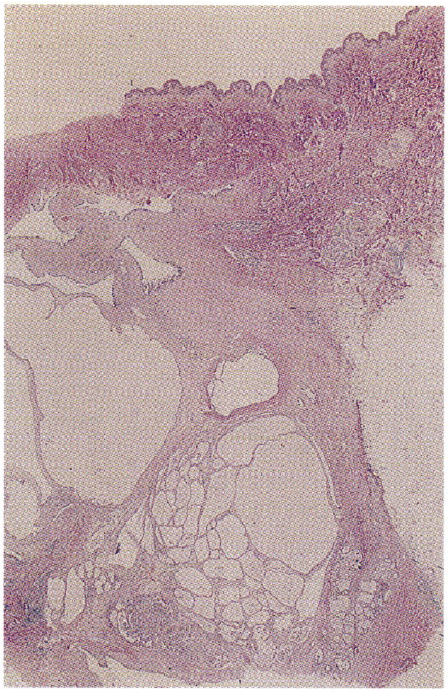

Figure 16–28. Metastatic ovarian papillary serous cystadenocarcinoma. At scanning magnification, within the deep dermis there are multiple, variably sized, epithelial-lined cysts filled with pale fluid or with complex papillary infoldings *(bottom)*.

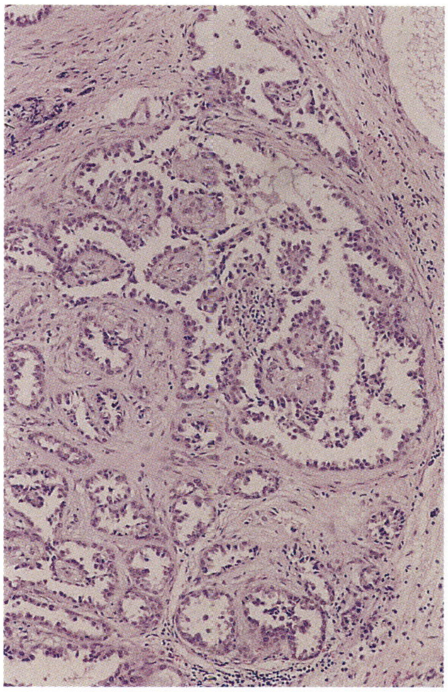

Figure 16–29. An epithelium-lined cystic structure filled with papillary processes, similar to the region in Figure 16–28, is composed of partially stratified epithelium overlying a fibrovascular core. Epithelial buds also are found within smaller cystic structures infiltrating the dermal stroma.

Metastatic Prostatic Carcinoma

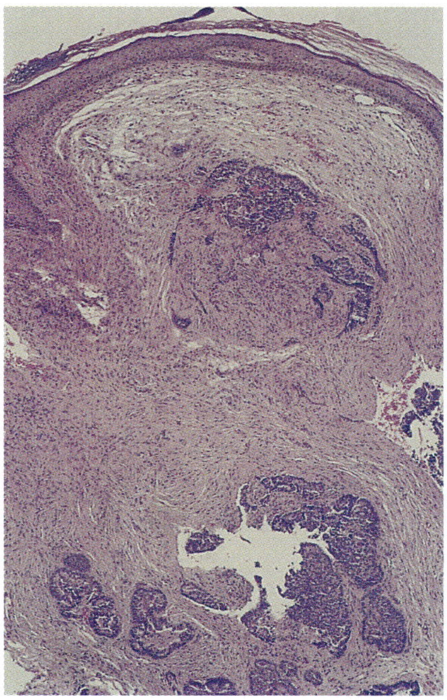

Figure 16–30. Metastatic prostatic adenocarcinoma. Irregular basaloid islands are present within a desmoplastic dermal stroma.

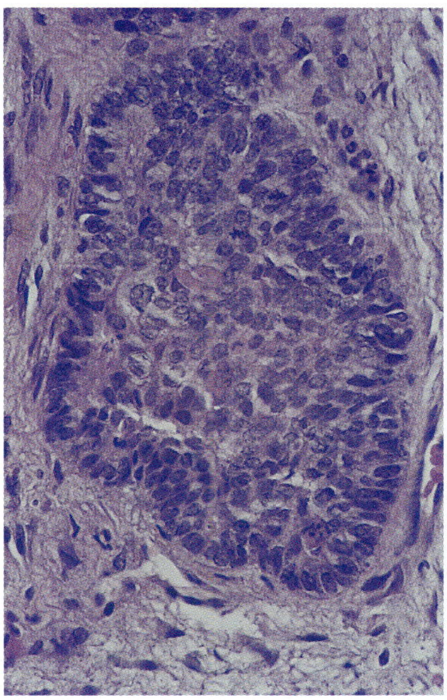

Figure 16–31. Although some regions demonstrate cribriform growth, this solid nest mimics basal cell carcinoma. Tumor cells are positive for prostatic acid phosphatase by immunohistochemistry.

Metastatic Renal Cell Carcinoma

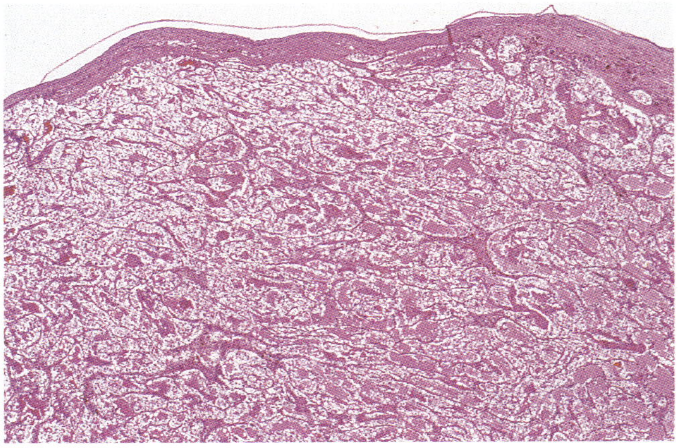

Figure 16–32. Metastatic renal cell carcinoma. Clear cells with a vascular stroma are present within the dermis and compress the overlying epidermis.

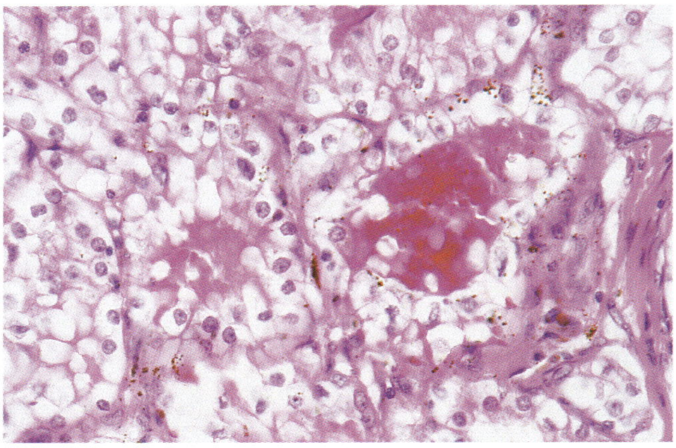

Figure 16–33. Tumor cells form glands and alveolar spaces, contain relatively uniform round-to-ovoid nuclei with distinct nucleoli, and exhibit a clear, highly glycogenated cytoplasm. Collapsed vessels form thin trabeculae that separate aggregates of tumor cells. Hemosiderin deposition confirms previous hemorrhage within this highly vascularized metastasis.

IV

Pigmentary, Systemic/Metabolic, and Degenerative Disorders

17

Cutaneous Pigmentary Disorders

Disorders characterized primarily by alterations in normal cutaneous pigmentation pose one of the most difficult challenges in diagnostic dermatopathology because related histologic changes are often exceedingly subtle or require special stains or analytic methods to fully appreciate the nature and extent of the underlying pathology. Frustration may arise due to apparent inconsistencies between the clinical appearance of lesions, which may be quite striking, and the corresponding histology, where remarkably little pigment represented in a 6μm-thick section accounts for the gross pathology.

Pigmentary disorders may arise from abnormalities at all levels of the integument (stratum corneum synthesis, epidermal cells, and dermal pigment deposits). Melanin, the principal endogenous pigment, is synthesized and deposited on melanosomes within melanocytes, which normally account for approximately 1 of every 10 basal cells along the dermal-epidermal interface. Clinical pigmentation, however, is not predominately the result of melanin within melanocytes. Rather, melanin that has been transferred to adjacent keratinocytes results in diffuse distribution of melanin throughout the lower epidermal layers and contributes most significantly to clinically overt skin color. Thus, alterations in melanin synthesis, melanocyte number, and the degree and even dispersion of melanin from melanocytes to keratinocytes may affect this normal pigmentation. Another physiologic determinant of cutaneous pigmentation is related to scavenger activity of superficial dermal macrophages normally concentrated about small vessels within the superficial vascular plexus. These cells normally take up epidermal melanin pigment and debris from degenerating keratinocytes, thus contributing to the programmed cell death, or apoptosis, that regulates epidermal turnover and equilibrium. Activity of these macrophages (melanophages) results in quantities of melanin within their cytoplasm that exceed their ability for degradation and, therefore, dermal pigment deposition. These macrophages also are able to take up exogenously introduced pigment, as in a tattoo, or blood-borne pigment, as in argyria.

Vitiligo

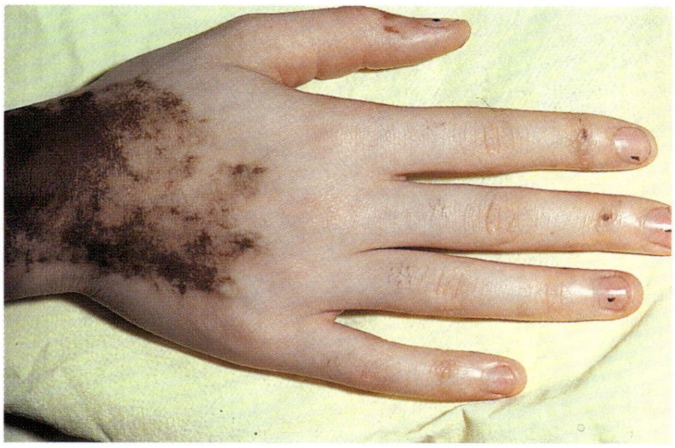

Figure 17–1. Vitiligo. Pigment loss on this hand is extensive, with only residual normal brown-black color on the wrist.

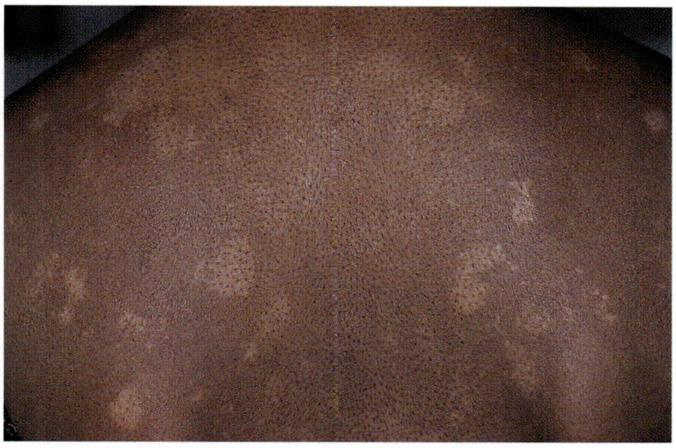

Figure 17–2. Repigmentation in a patient with vitiligo; note that the return of normal pigment within white macules is heralded by punctate pigmentation about follicular orifices.

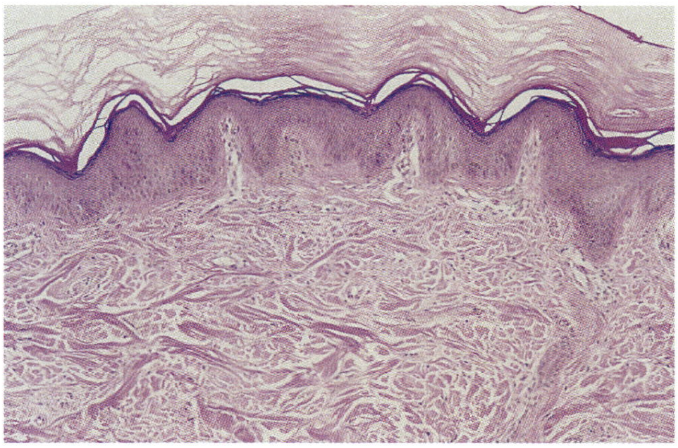

Figure 17–3. Routine histology of lesional vitiligo skin fails to disclose specific diagnostic abnormalities.

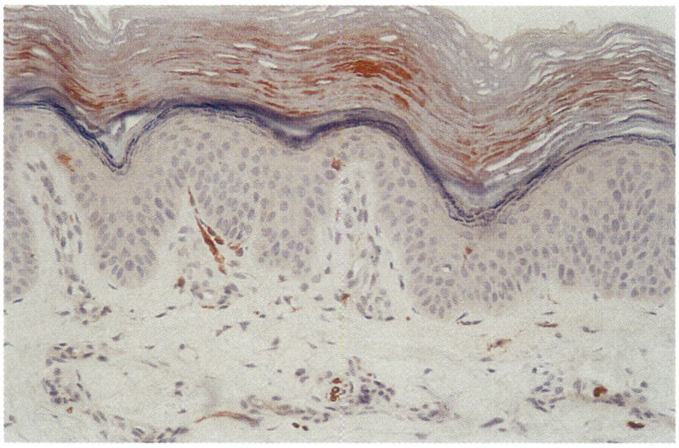

Figure 17–4. In vitiligo, S100 stain demonstrates marked reduction in S100-positive basal melanocytes, which populate the stratum basalis in approximately a melanocyte-to-keratinocyte ratio of 1:10. The papillary dermal nerve twig *(left, center)* serves as an internal positive control.

Albinism

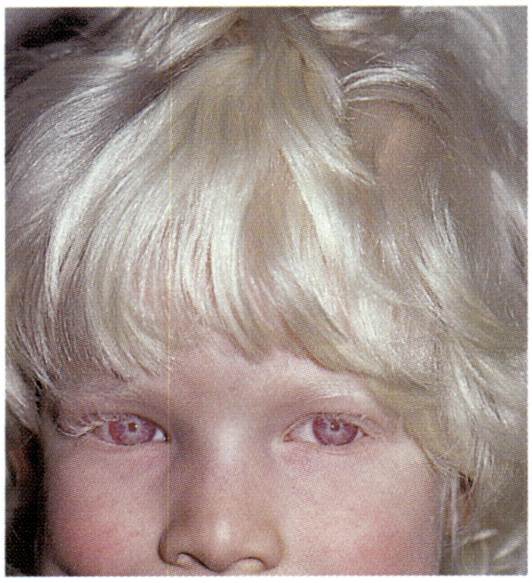

Figure 17–5. Albinism. Note the absence of pigment in skin and hair. The irises also are devoid of pigment.

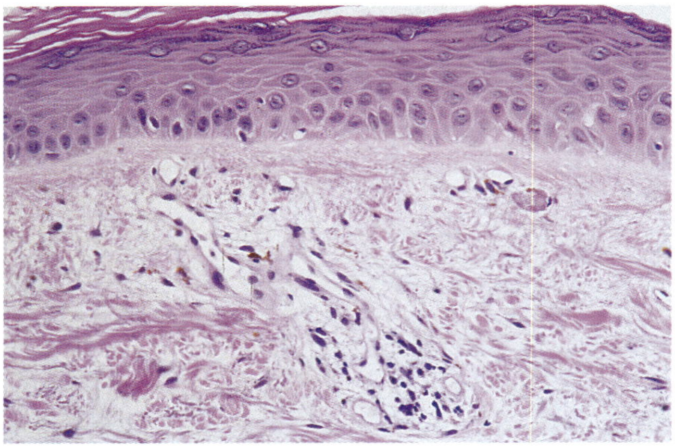

Figure 17–6. In contrast to vitiligo, in which melanocytes are absent, individual melanocytes along the dermal-epidermal junction in albinism are observed as cells with dense, small nuclei and a peripheral clear zone. Special stains for melanocyte antigens confirm this impression.

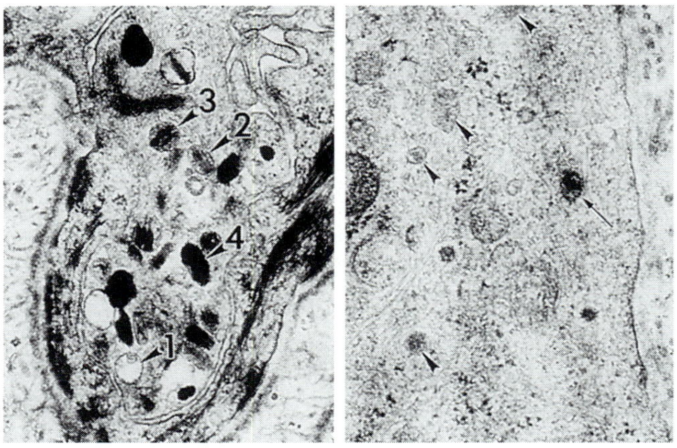

Figure 17–7. Electron microscopy of melanocytes in albinism. Normal melanocytes contain complete evolutionary stages of melanosomes, consisting of stage 1 through stage 4 organelles *(panel to left).* Stage 1 melanosomes are nonmelanized vesicular structures *(1),* whereas stage 2 melanosomes have a lattice-like internal structure with minimal melanization *(2).* Stage 3 melanosomes demonstrate moderate electron density in the lattice, indicating partial melanization *(3),* whereas stage 4 melanosomes are completely obscured by electron-dense melanin *(4).* Note the presence of nonmelanized *(arrowheads)* and melanized *(arrow)* melanosomes in melanocytes of albino skin *(panel to right).*

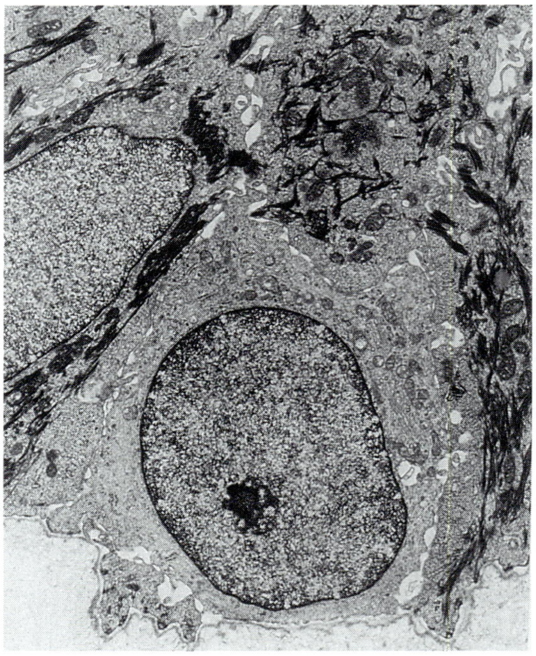

Figure 17–8. Electron micrograph of tyrosinase-negative albinism. A melanocyte within the basal cell layer is entirely devoid of even partially melanized melanosomes.

Pityriasis Alba

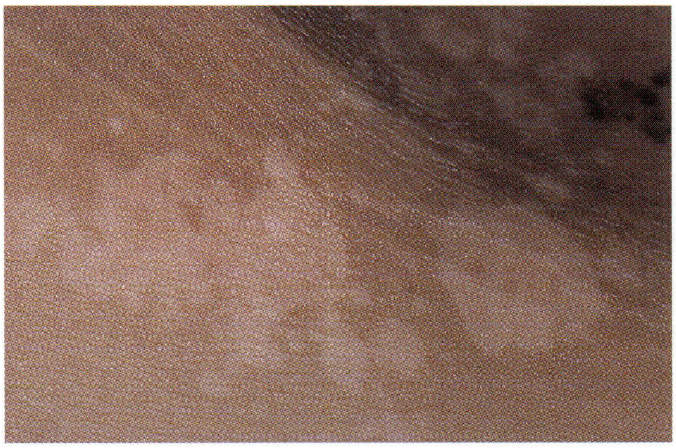

Figure 17–9. Pityriasis alba. Numerous coalescent macules show hypopigmentation.

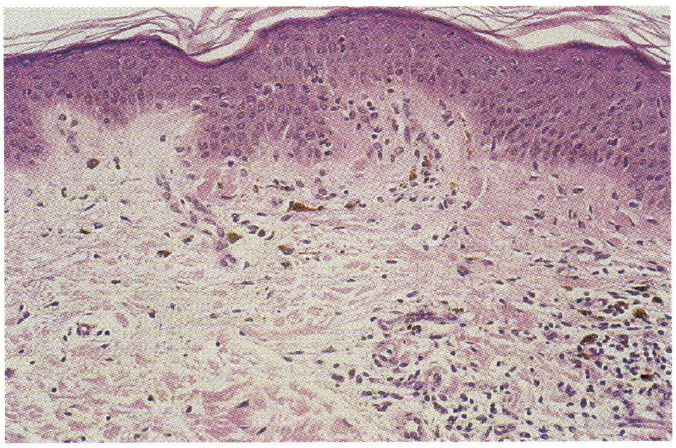

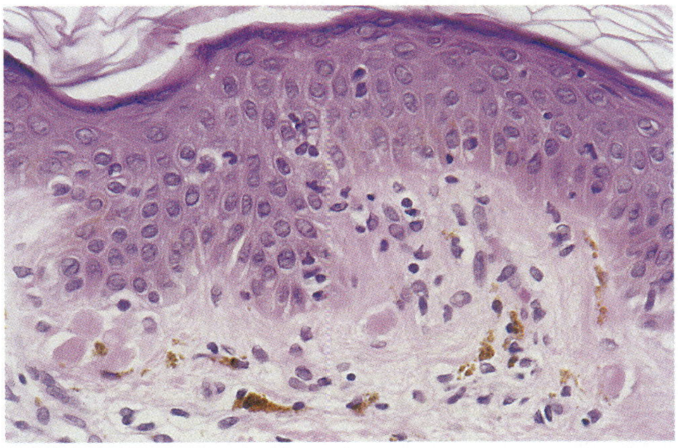

Figures 17–10 and 17–11. In pityriasis alba, evidence of an associated inflammatory dermatitis consists of a sparse, nonspecific, superficial, perivascular, lymphocytic infiltrate and zones of colloid body formation indicative of previous interface change (Fig. 17–11). In some lesions, spongiotic alterations predominate.

Tinea Versicolor

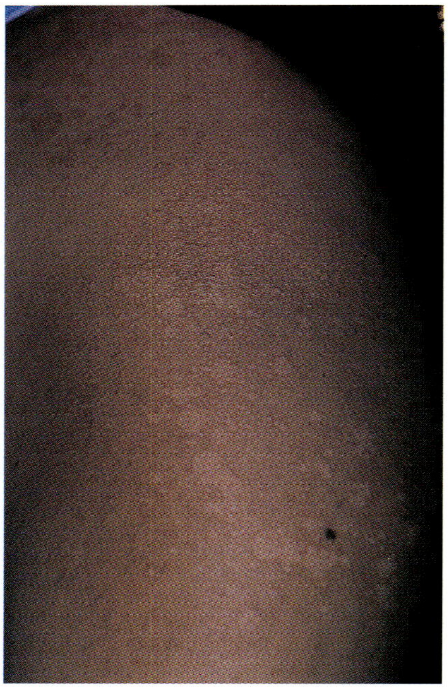

Figure 17–12. Tinea versicolor. Multiple hypopigmented macules are present on truncal skin; there is a velvety, adherent scale covering some of these macules.

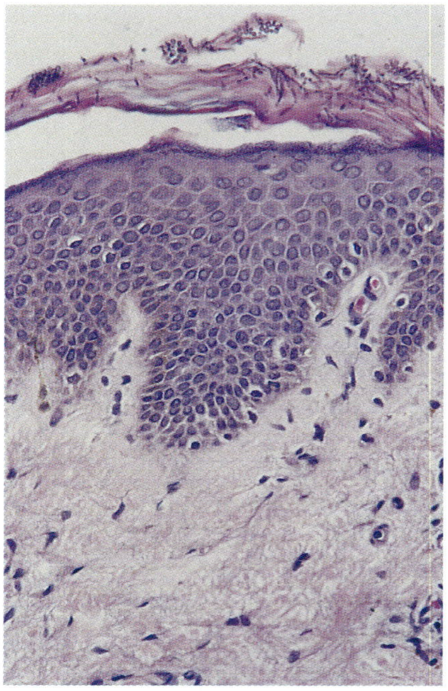

Figure 17–13. A biopsy specimen of tinea versicolor demonstrates small, basophilic, hyphal organisms within hyperkeratotic scale, even in routine hematoxylin and eosin stains.

Postinflammatory Hyperpigmentation

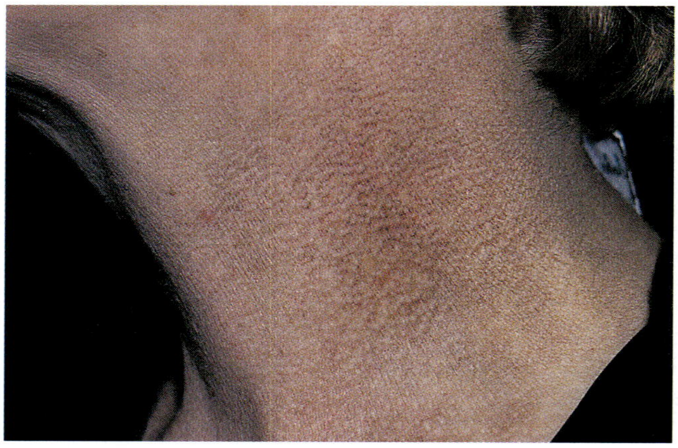

Figure 17–14. Postinflammatory hyperpigmentation. Chronic rubbing and a low-grade primary irritant effect to neck skin produced mottled hyperpigmentation.

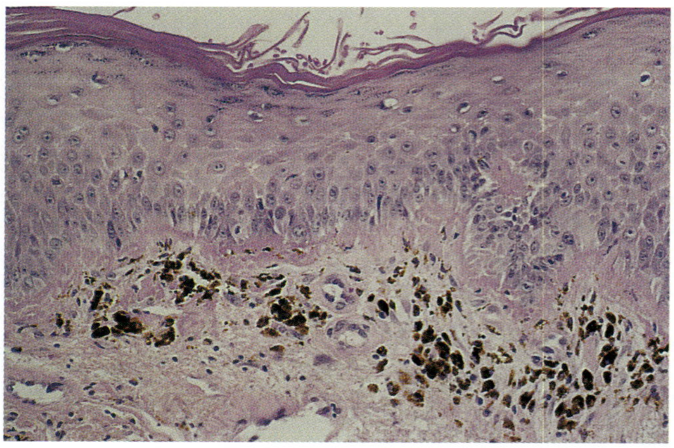

Figure 17–15. A biopsy specimen of postinflammatory hyperpigmentation reveals numerous brown, melanin-laden macrophages within the superficial dermis.

Café-au-lait Macule

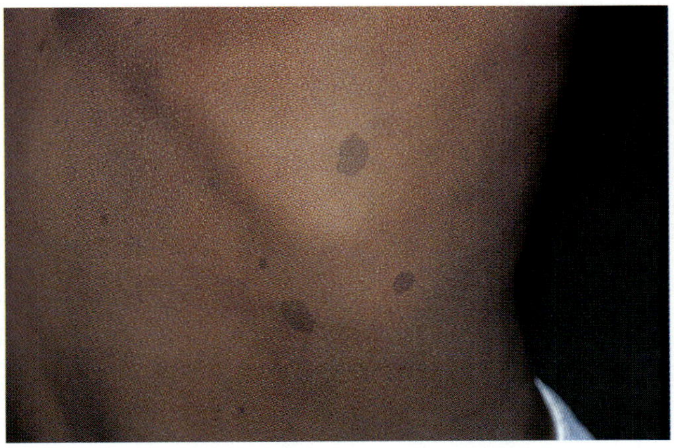

Figure 17–16. Clinical pathology of café-au-lait macules. Multiple coffee stain–like macules are present on the trunk of a patient with neurofibromatosis.

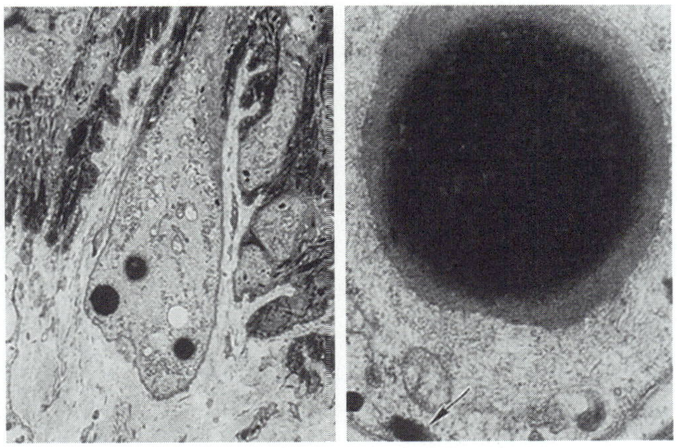

Figure 17–17. Macromelanosomes of café-au-lait macules. The primary microscopic defect in café-au-lait macules is the formation of macromelanosomes. Even by scanning or low-power magnification ultrastructure *(left),* these electron-dense, globoid bodies predominate in the cytoplasm of basal melanocytes. *Right,* Too large to be transferred to adjacent keratinocytes, these bodies are uniformly electron dense and many times greater in volume than normal melanosomes *(arrow, lower left corner).* Macromelanosomes probably form by condensation of normal melanosomes that are partially degraded by phagolysosomes.

Pigmented Localized Stasis

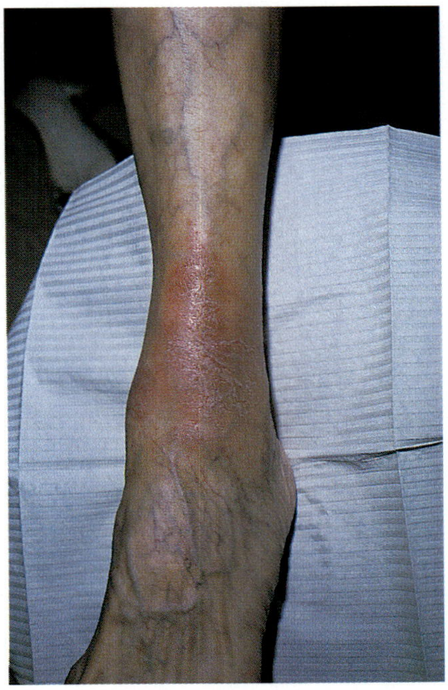

Figure 17–18. Hyperpigmentation due to localized stasis. The gross pathology of a lower extremity subjected to chronic stasis change is erythema admixed with zones of brawny, copper-colored hyperpigmentation.

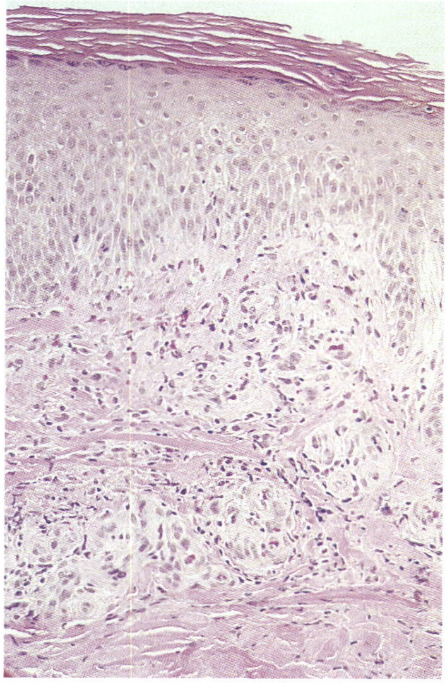

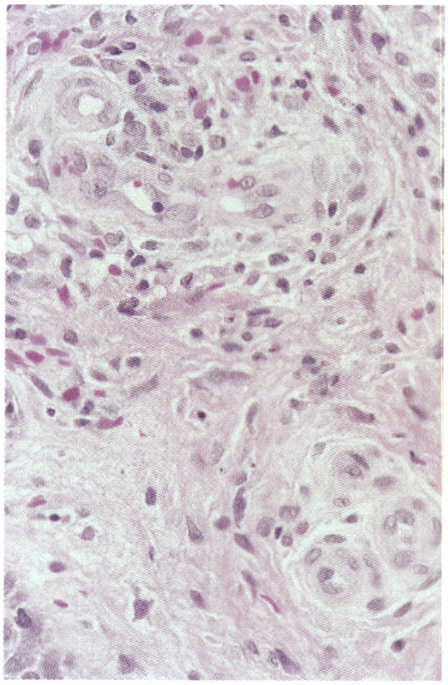

Figures 17–19 and 17–20. Histologically, stasis dermatitis is characterized by prominent vascular proliferation and fibrosis within chronically inflamed dermal papillae and papillary dermis.

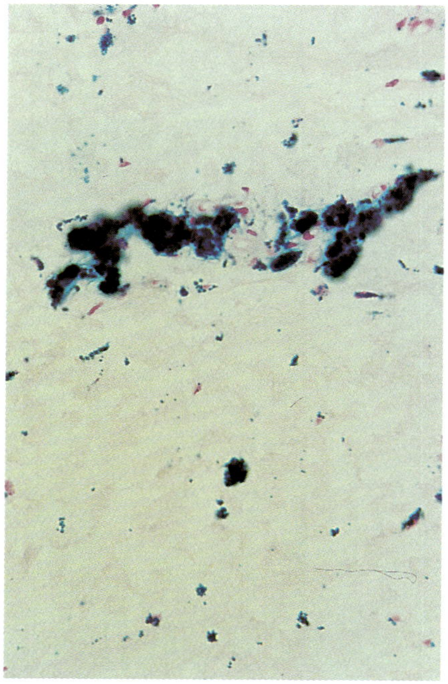

Figure 17–21. Stains for iron in stasis dermatitis reveal foci of particulate hemosiderin deposition, the result of chronic erythrocyte extravasation from the leaky vessels which proliferate as a consequence of this condition.

Drug-induced Hyperpigmentation

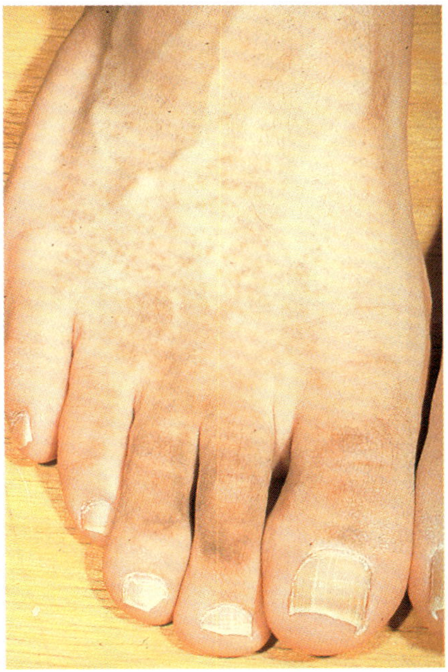

Figure 17–22. Drug-induced hyperpigmentation: Minocycline. The distal extremity of this young man shows mottled, confluent, brown macular hyperpigmentation. He had been treated with minocycline for facial acne.

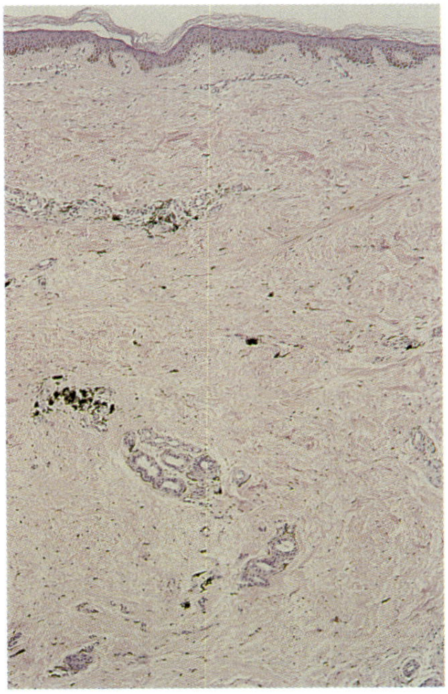

Figure 17–23. Histologically, minocycline-induced hyperpigmentation shows pigment-laden macrophages about superficial and deep dermal vessels *(left center)*. This pigment stains for iron, and the macrophages have been shown to contain elemental iron by energy-dispersive x-ray probe microanalysis.

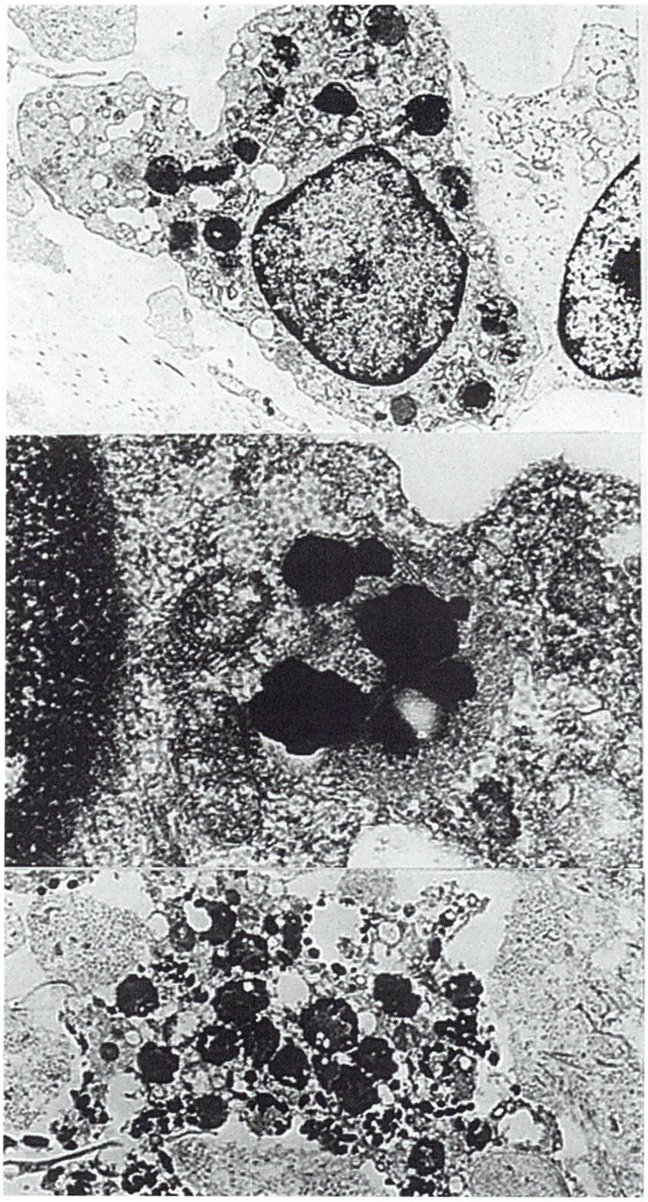

Figure 17–24. Ultrastructure of pigment within dermal macrophages in pigment incontinence. *Top,* Siderosomes (*i.e.,* phagolysosomes containing particulate iron) occurred as a result of minocycline ingestion. *Middle,* Argyria occurred as a result of silver ingestion. *Bottom,* Melanin phagolysomes are a result of postinflammatory hyperpigmentation. Although the electron-dense material within phagosomes is subtly different among these three groups, elemental analysis by x-ray probe methods is sometimes necessary for definitive identification.

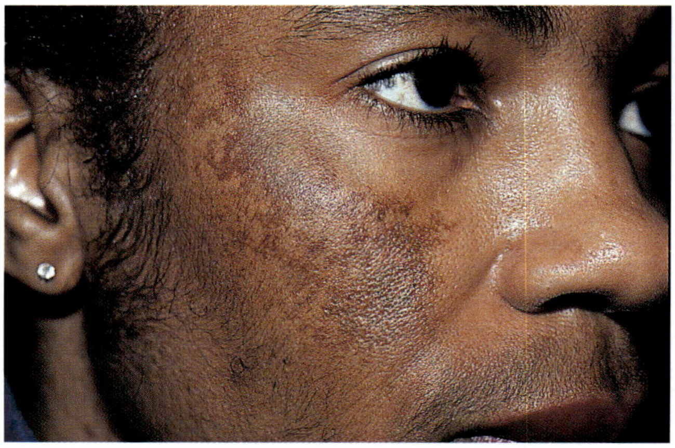

Figure 17–25. Melasma: Hyperpigmentation due to enhanced melanogenesis. The primary defect in this common condition appears to be the result of an altered threshold for melanogenesis. This results in increases in both epidermal and dermal melanin pigment deposition. Either epidermal melanin or dermal melanin may predominate in the clinical and histologic picture. The histology shows superficial dermal melanophages (see Fig. 17–15).

18

Maturational and Degenerative Disorders

The group of largely unrelated disorders illustrated in this section are reflective of the more common cutaneous conditions in which altered maturation or degeneration of dermal or epidermal elements is represented by histologic findings that are pivotal to accurate diagnosis. Several of the disorders, such as ichthyosis and porokeratosis, present clinically primarily as a result of abnormal formation of the most superficial skin layers. Others, such as anetoderma and keloids, result in gross pathology indicative of the absence or increased deposition of normal dermal constituents. These conditions, although linked together pathogenetically by anomalous development or lack of homeostatic maintenance, are unrelated, and their histologies share little common ground, impeding an algorithmic approach to their diagnosis. However, most occur commonly enough to produce confusion with a number of other dermatoses and even neoplasms illustrated in this atlas, and therefore it is prudent to be aware of their salient clinicopathologic characteristics.

Although conditions such as solar elastosis and keloids may be observed daily in a busy dermatopathology practice, others in the same category, such as anetoderma and ichthyosis, are only rarely observed. These latter conditions are biologically important, however, and because they do occur from time to time, awareness of their often subtle histologic characteristics is useful in differential diagnosis. The tinctorial properties of cutaneous maturational and degenerative disorders are equally subtle. For example, although lichenoid amyloidosis is evident as pale-pink material often deposited within tips of dermal papillae, lichen sclerosus produces similar, homogeneous pink pallor that replaces the papillary dermis. Special staining coupled with polarization microscopy, in the case of amyloidosis, alters its subtle appearance to bright "apple green" birefringence. Special stains may be required to "color" elements of dermal matrix to render visible subtle pathologic alterations. In anetoderma, for example, elastic tissue stains may be required to identify (render dark gray) elastic fibers that are eroded or diminished as part of this rare but fascinating pathologic process.

Ichthyosis and Congenital Keratoderma

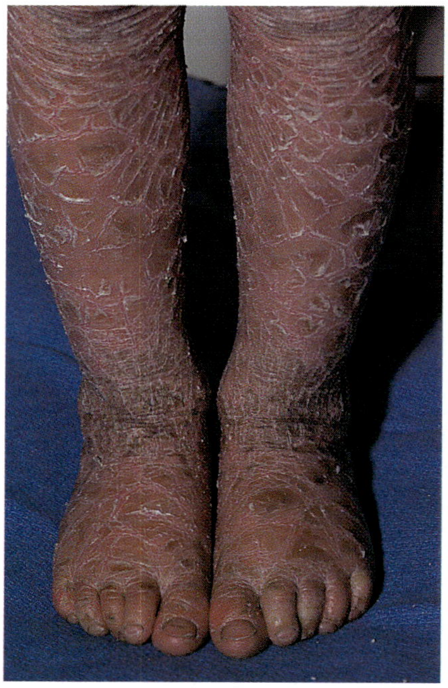

Figure 18–1. Lamellar ichthyosis is characterized by fish-like scales, each of which is composed of thousands of anomalous stratum corneocytes.

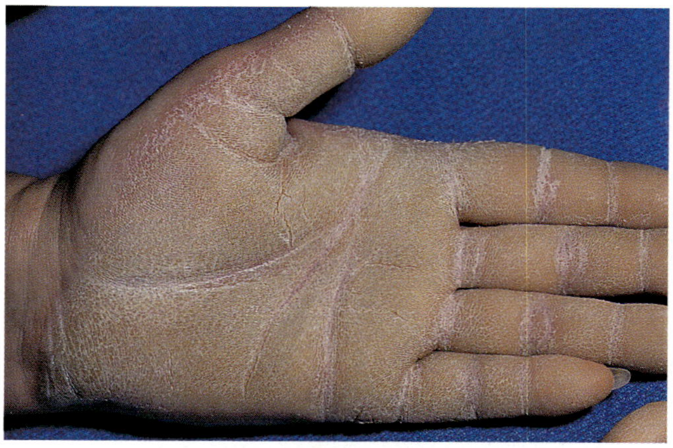

Figure 18–2. Palmar keratoderma is an autosomal dominant condition characterized by diffuse hyperkeratosis. Both ichthyosis and keratoderma result from thickening of the stratum corneum.

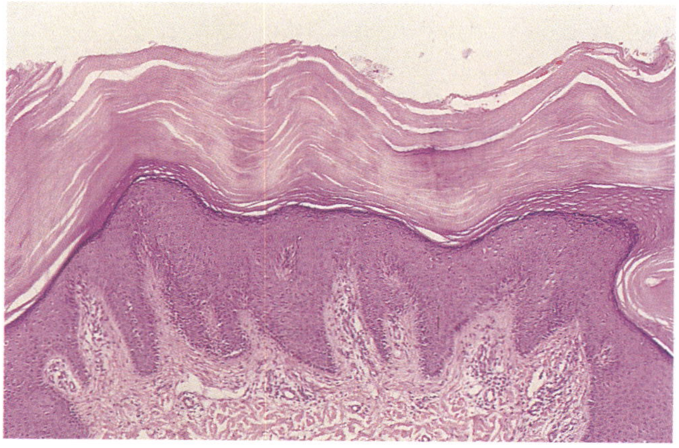

Figure 18–3. Lamellar ichthyosis demonstrates compacted hyperorthokeratotic stratum corneum, which accounts for the plate-like scales observed clinically in Figure 18–1.

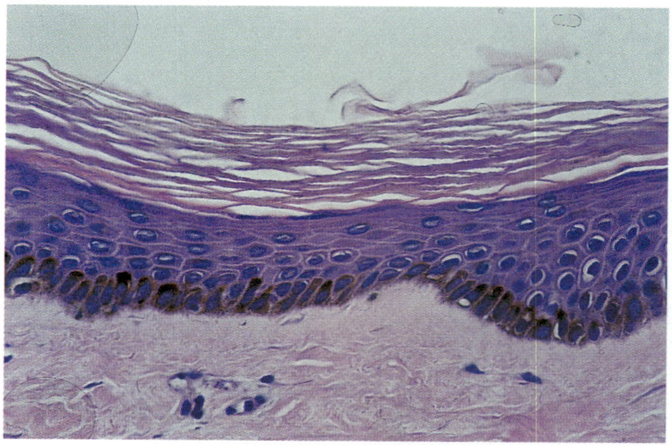

Figure 18–4. Ichthyosis vulgaris is associated with subtle compacted hyperkeratosis (note the complete absence of the normal basket-weave pattern) as well as marked thinning of the stratum granulosum.

Porokeratosis

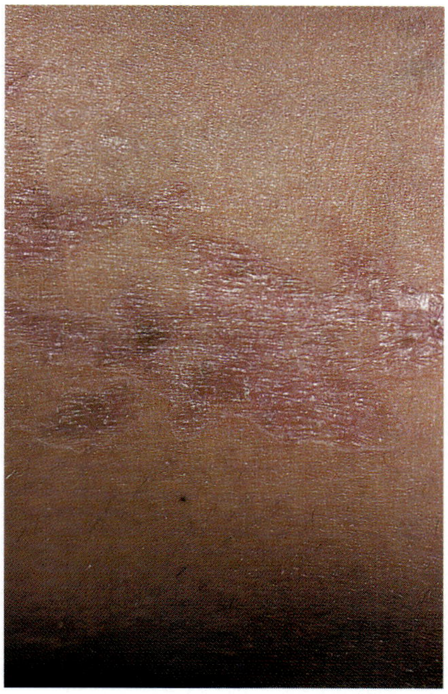

Figure 18–5. Porokeratosis, plaque type. Clinically, there is a well-defined plaque surrounded by a hyperkeratotic ridge at its perimeter.

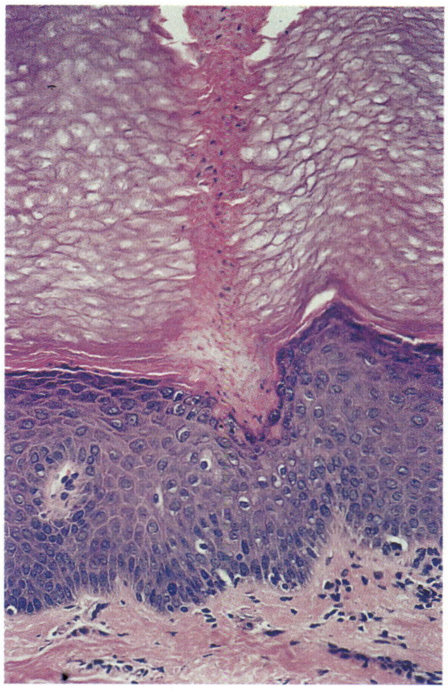

Figure 18–6. A biopsy specimen from the edge of a lesion shows a well-developed cornoid lamella typical of this condition. The lamella consists of a discrete tower of parakeratotic scale overlying a small invagination showing focal hypogranulosis.

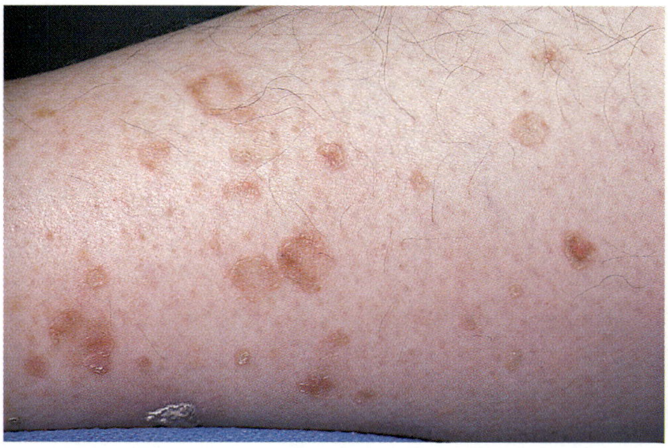

Figure 18–7. Porokeratosis, disseminated superficial actinic type. Multiple erythematous hyperkeratotic plaques are present on sun-exposed skin.

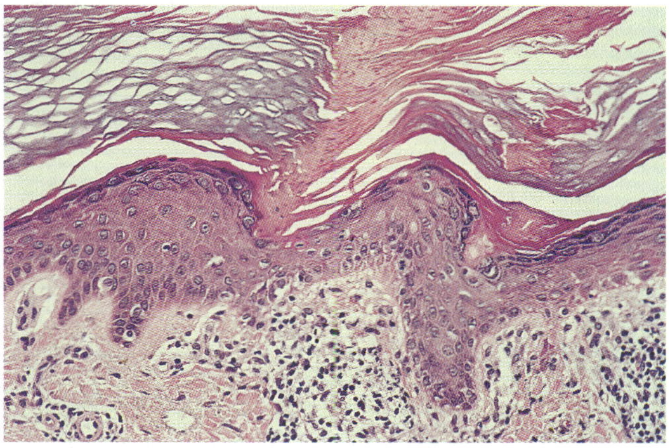

Figure 18–8. A biopsy specimen from the edge of one of the lesions reveals a cornoid lamella leaning inward toward a zone of epidermal atypia, variable atrophy, and a patchy, superficial dermal, inflammatory infiltrate.

Darier Disease

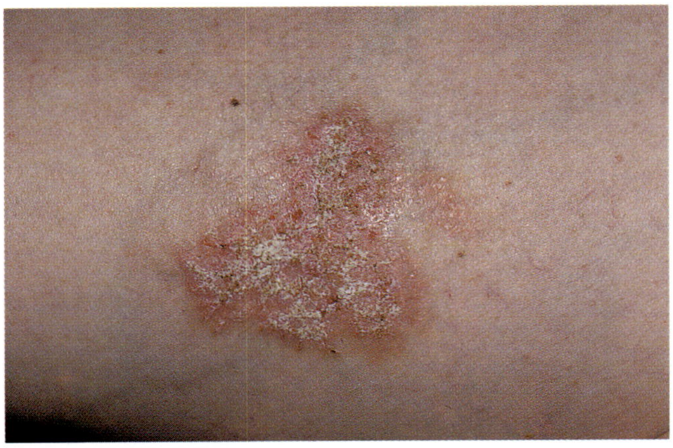

Figure 18–9. Darier disease (keratosis follicularis). This crusted erythematous plaque formed as a consequence of coalescence of multiple hyperkeratotic follicular papules.

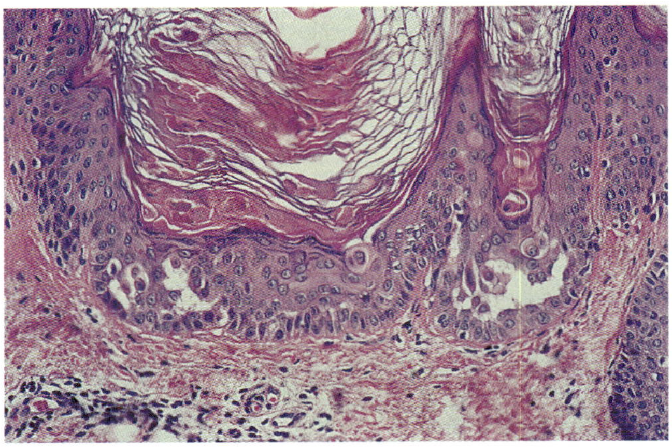

Figure 18–10. Histology of an early lesion demonstrates small foci of suprabasal acantholysis, verrucous epidermal hyperplasia, and hyperkeratosis.

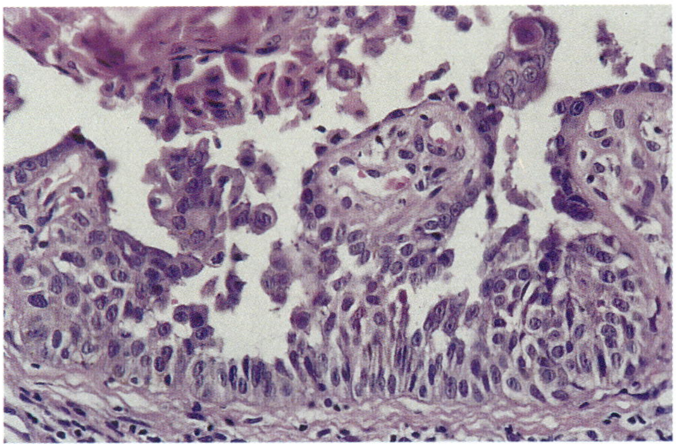

Figure 18–11. A more advanced lesion shows a suprabasal cleft containing rounded acantholytic cells near the base (*i.e.,* corps ronds) and condensed, smaller acantholytic cells near the surface (*i.e.,* corps grains).

Grover Disease

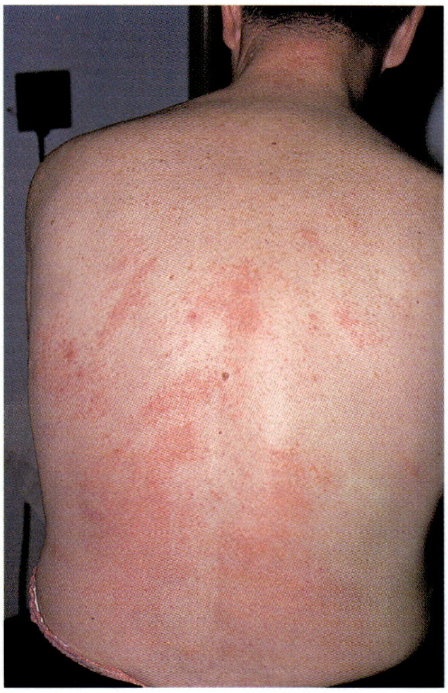

Figure 18–12. Grover disease (transient acantholytic dermatosis). The back of this patient is covered with numerous, slightly erythematous, hyperkeratotic papules.

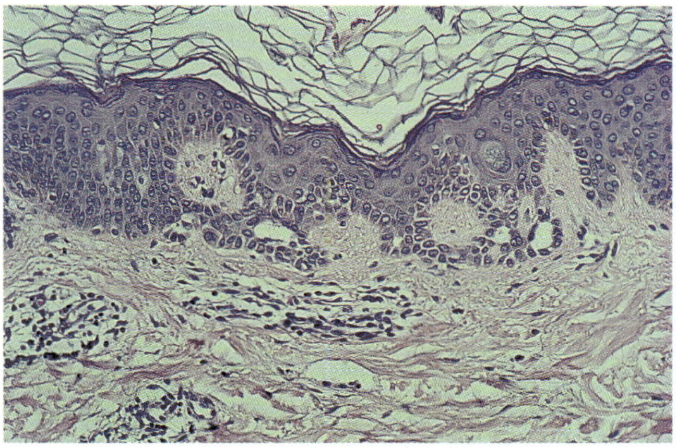

Figure 18–13. Early lesions show multiple microscopic foci of suprabasal acantholysis with minimal hyperkeratosis.

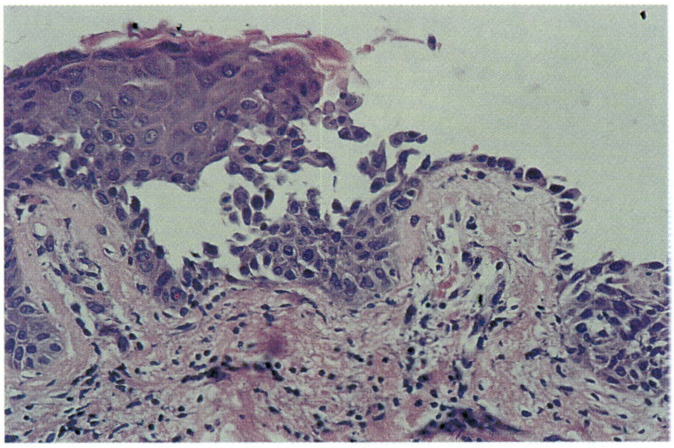

Figure 18–14. Advanced lesions may have well-developed suprabasal acantholytic clefts, but these are seldom as extensive as those seen in Darier disease and are not accompanied by significant verrucous epidermal hyperplasia.

Epidermolytic Hyperkeratosis

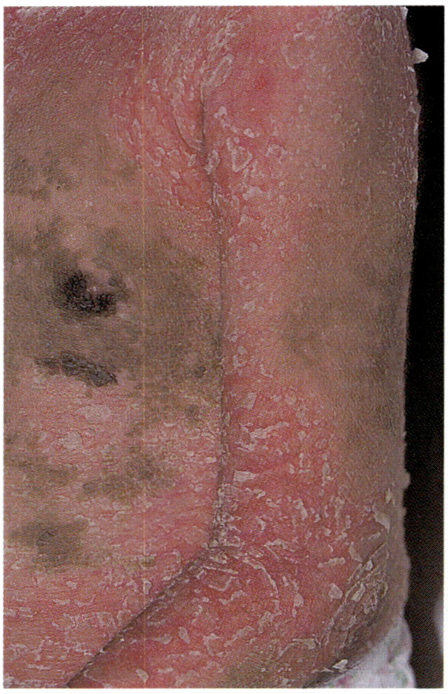

Figure 18–15. Epidermolytic hyperkeratosis. The gross pathology consists of marked hyperkeratosis and scaling, particularly in regions of flexural creases. Soon after birth, bullae and vesicles may also be observed.

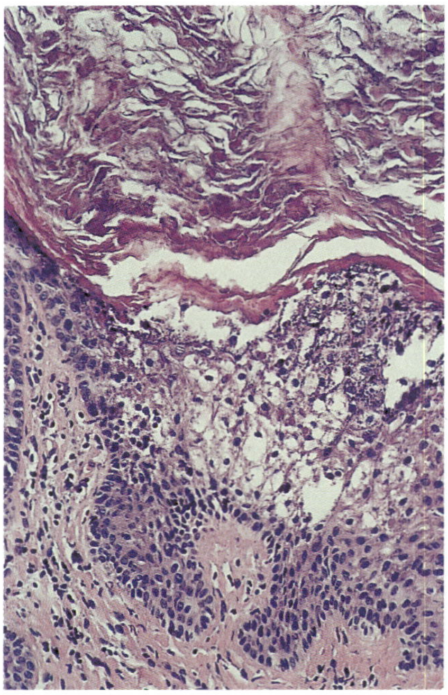

Figure 18–16. Histologically, there is cytoplasmic lysis of cells forming the midepidermis to upper epidermis, coarse keratohyalin granules associated with the formation of eosinophilic trichohyalin granules within the stratum granulosum, and marked overlying hyperkeratosis.

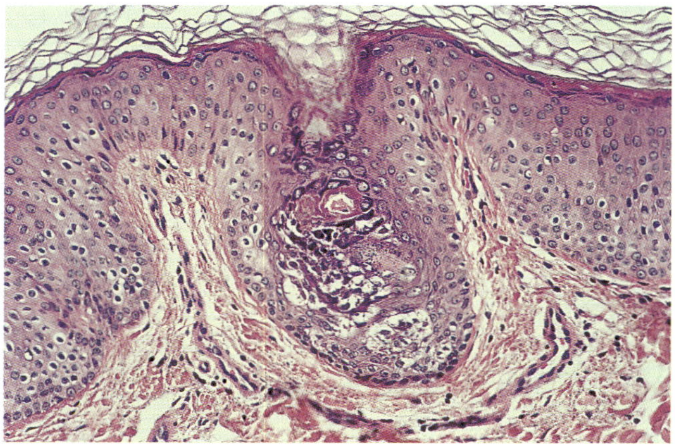

Figure 18–17. Focal involvement of a follicular infundibulum by epidermolytic hyperkeratosis.

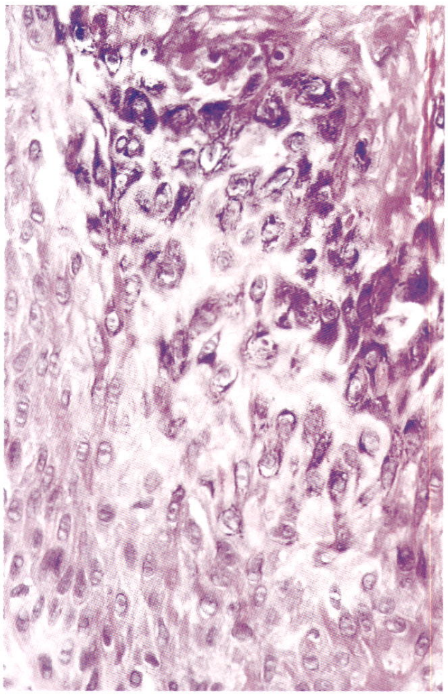

Figure 18–18. High magnification of prominent keratohyalin granules within the uppermost epidermal layers.

Lichenoid Amyloidosis

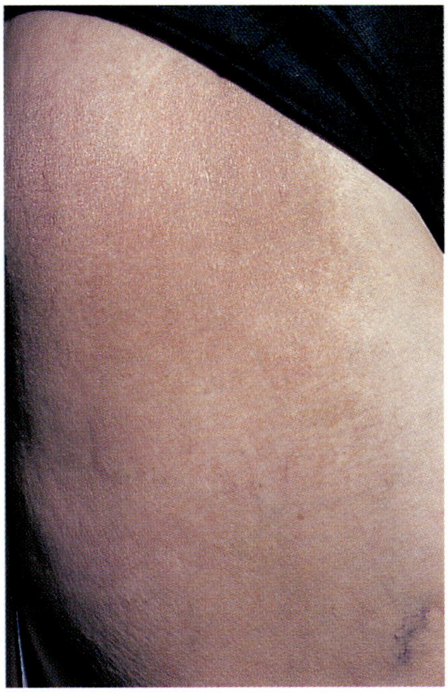

Figure 18–19. Lichenoid amyloidosis. Coalescence of small, red-brown papules on the lower extremity has produced an ill-defined, pigmented plaque. There is a central zone of relative sparing where residual papules are still observed.

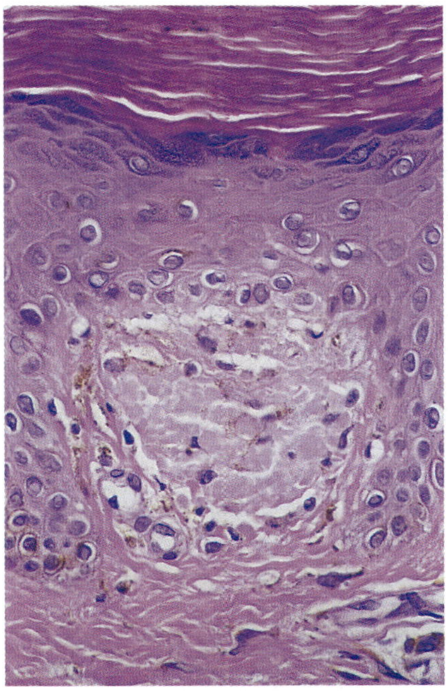

Figure 18–20. Small, rounded amyloid deposits are characteristically observed in dermal papillae and within the superficial layers of the papillary dermis.

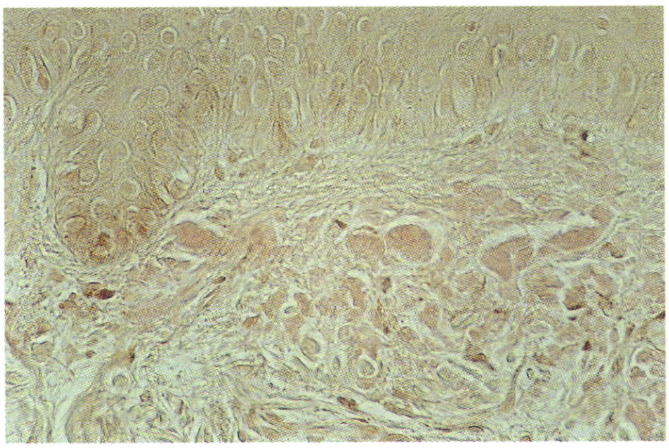

Figure 18–21. Congo red stain reveals dull red staining of amyloid deposits in the superficial dermis.

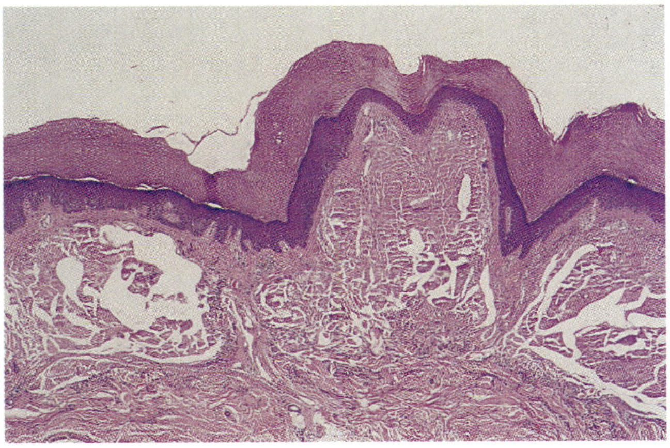

Figure 18–22. Amyloid within the superficial dermis must be distinguished from colloid milium, depicted here; note deposits of amyloid-like material associated with characteristic large clefts within the superficial dermis.

Lichen Sclerosus

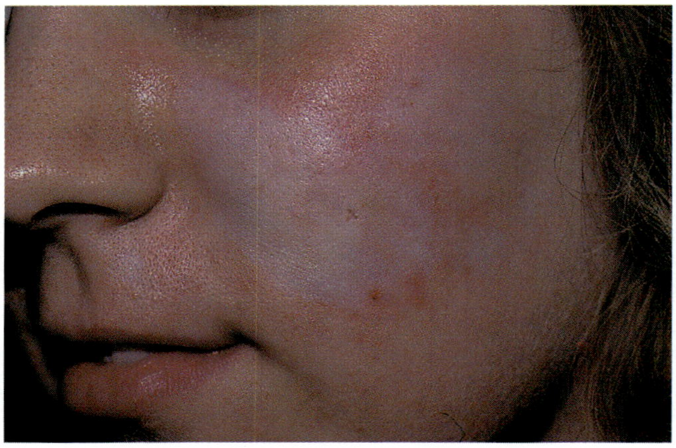

Figure 18–23. Lichen sclerosus. An indurated, white plaque involves facial skin. Dilated follicles containing keratotic material are focally visible within this plaque.

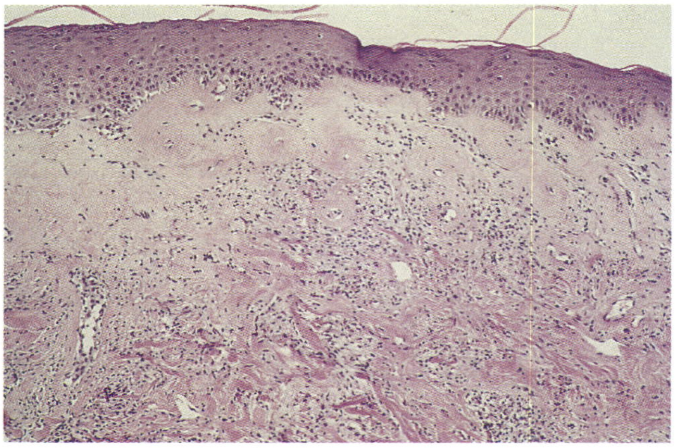

Figure 18–24. A biopsy specimen from a relatively early lesion reveals pale, hyalinized, superficial dermal collagen associated with a diffuse underlying lymphocytic infiltrate containing occasional plasma cells.

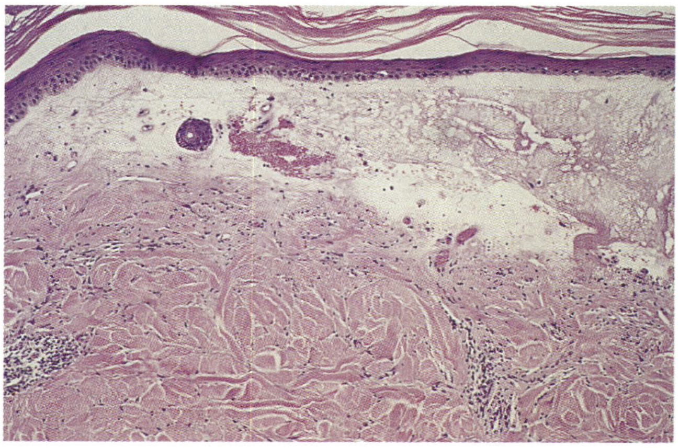

Figure 18–25. A biopsy specimen from an advanced lesion reveals marked pallor and hyalinization of the superficial dermis, associated with epidermal atrophy and hyperkeratosis.

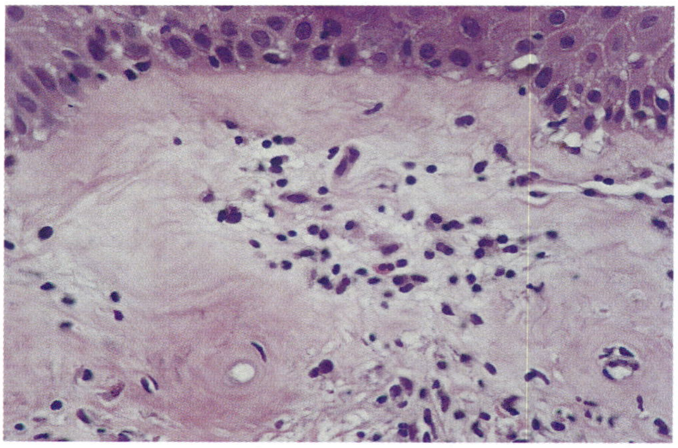

Figure 18–26. At higher magnification, collections of lymphocytes associated with melanophages are associated with the altered extracellular matrix. Foci suggestive of basal cell vacuolization are present within the overlying basal cell layer.

Chronic Radiation Dermatitis

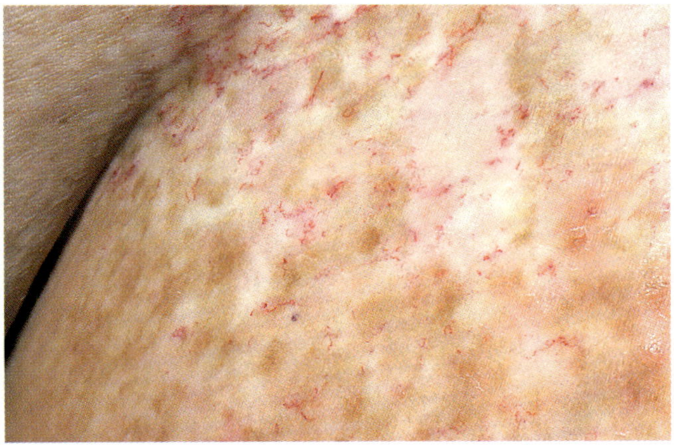

Figure 18–27. Chronic radiation dermatitis. Clinically, the skin appears poikilodermatous, or atrophic, with mottled areas of hypopigmentation and hyperpigmentation and associated telangiectasias.

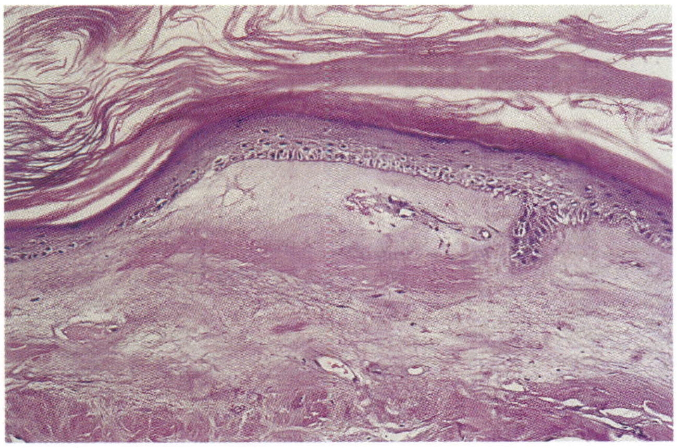

Figure 18–28. At low magnification, the superficial dermis and mid-dermis show variably dense sclerosis and hyalinization associated with epidermal atrophy and hyperkeratosis.

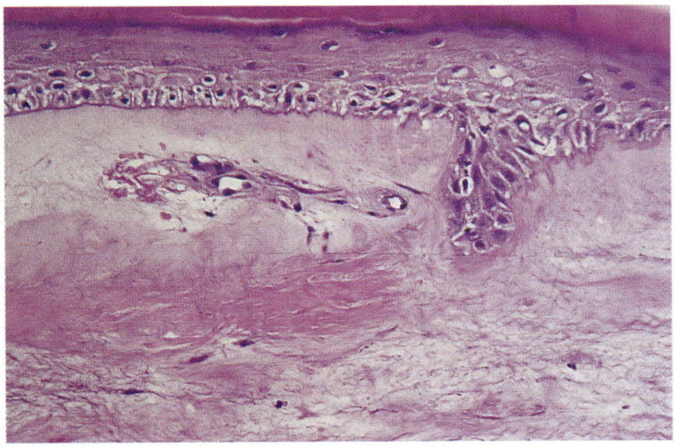

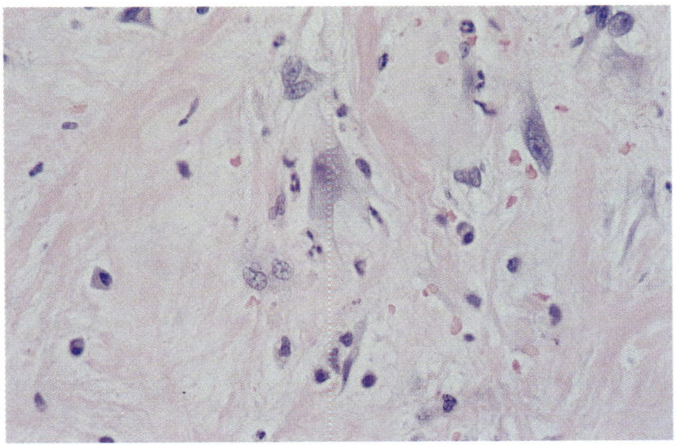

Figures 18–29 and 18–30. Within the altered collagen are endothelial cells and plump, stellate fibroblasts containing enlarged, hyperchromatic nuclei indicative of radiation effect.

Solar Elastosis

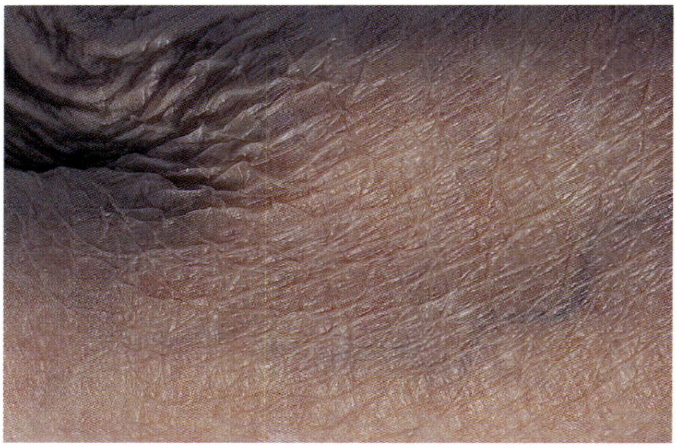

Figure 18–31. Solar elastosis. Chronically sun-damaged, elastotic skin may show premature loss of normal recoil and cohesive properties, resulting in wrinkles.

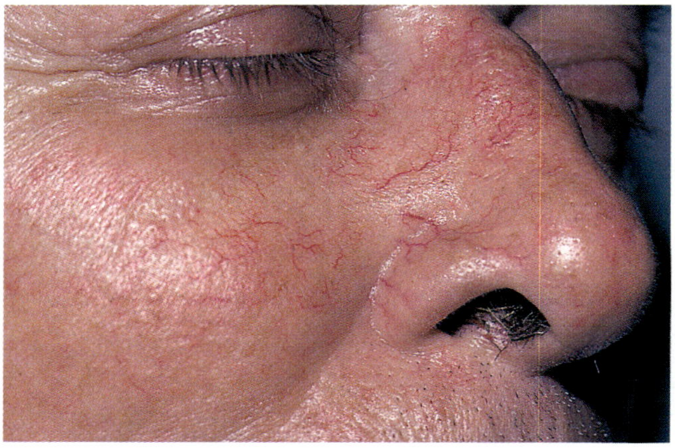

Figure 18–32. The result of solar elastosis also could be widely dilated blood vessels (*i.e.,* telangiectasias).

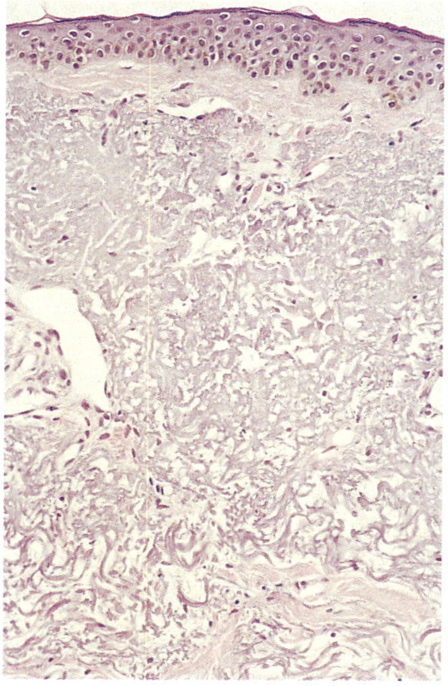

Figure 18–33. Histologically, elastosis is characterized by coarse aggregates of pale basophilic material within the superficial dermis and mid-dermis. Note the associated dilated vessels *(left center).*

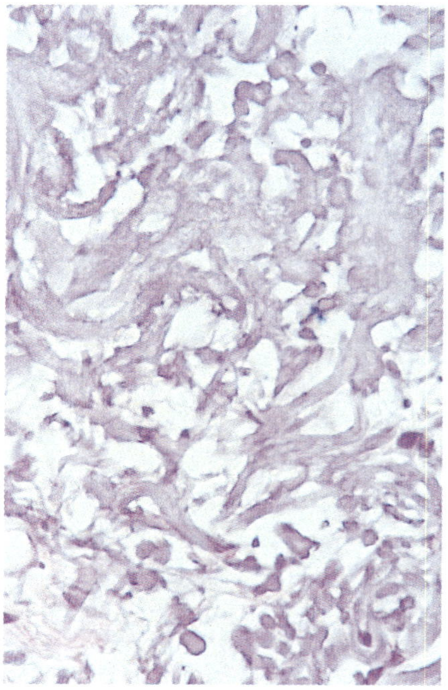

Figure 18–34. Also note the comparison between elastotic fibers *(top center)* and relatively normal, smaller fibers *(bottom).*

Pseudoxanthoma Elasticum

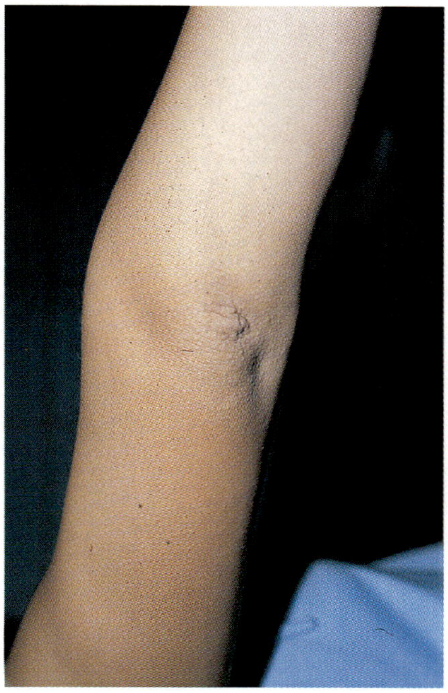

Figure 18–35. Pseudoxanthoma elasticum. Coalescent, yellow-tan papules involve the elbow skin.

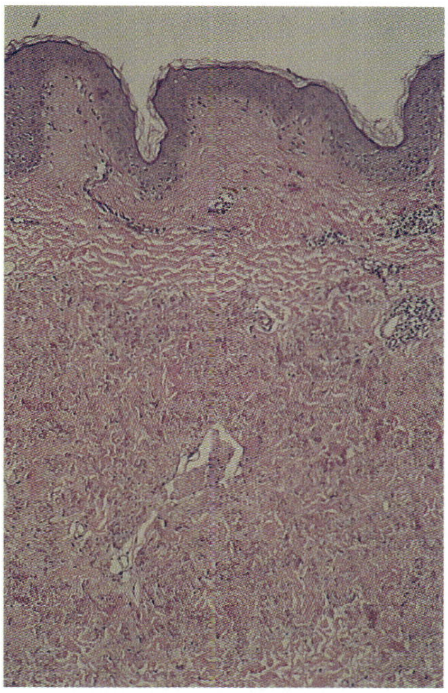

Figure 18–36. At low magnification, the mid-dermis and deep dermis are diffusely infiltrated by clumped, fragmented, markedly abnormal elastic fibers.

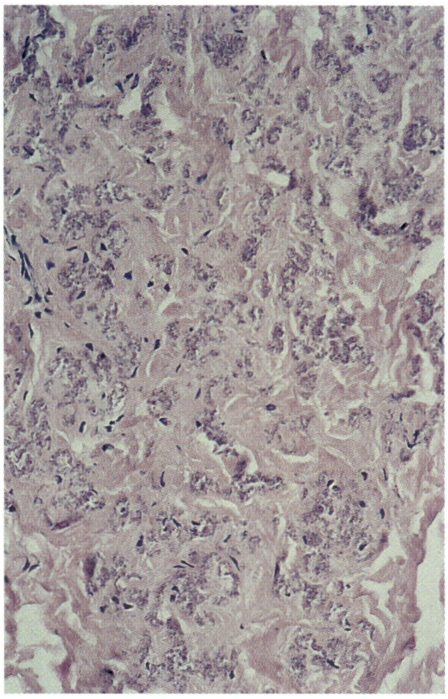

Figure 18–37. At higher magnification, many of the fibers have a pale-purple hue and a granular quality, which are indicative of early calcification.

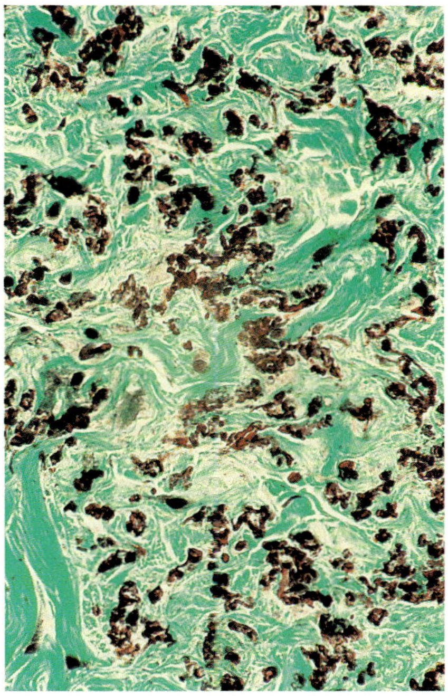

Figure 18–38. Elastic tissue stain of the abnormal fibers demonstrates the marked clumping and aggregation of the abnormal fibers.

Elastosis Perforans Serpiginosa

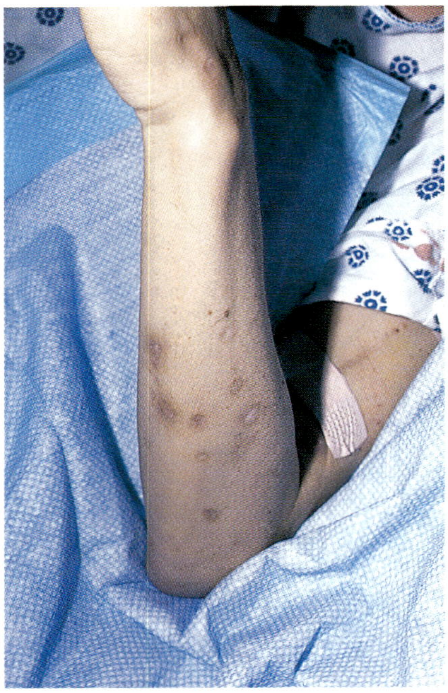

Figure 18–39. Elastosis perforans serpiginosa. In this patient, annular lesions formed by grouped hyperkeratotic papules are associated with marked postinflammatory hyperpigmentation.

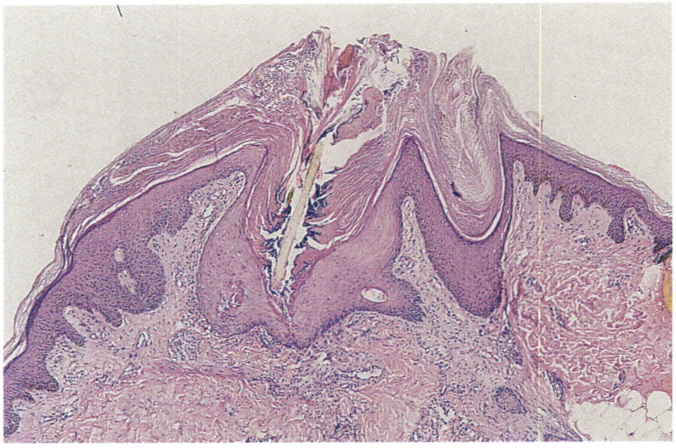

Figure 18–40. There is a broad, follicle-like invagination associated with hyperkeratosis and foci of perforation at the base of the lesion.

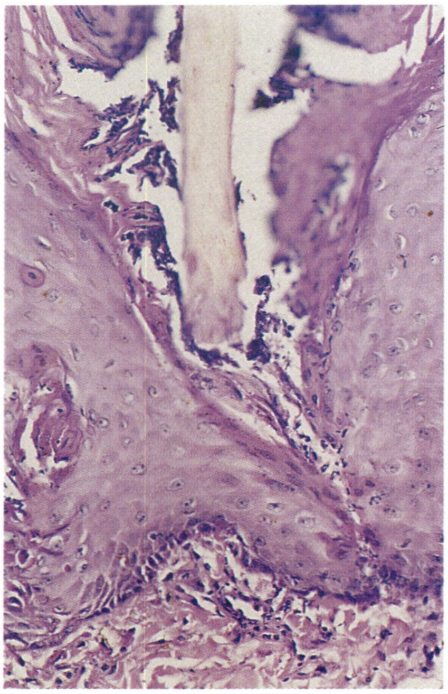

Figure 18–41. Transepithelial perforation is associated with extrusion of altered elastic fibers within the underlying dermis. Although a small hair shaft is secondarily entrapped, most lesions were discontinuous with follicular epithelium.

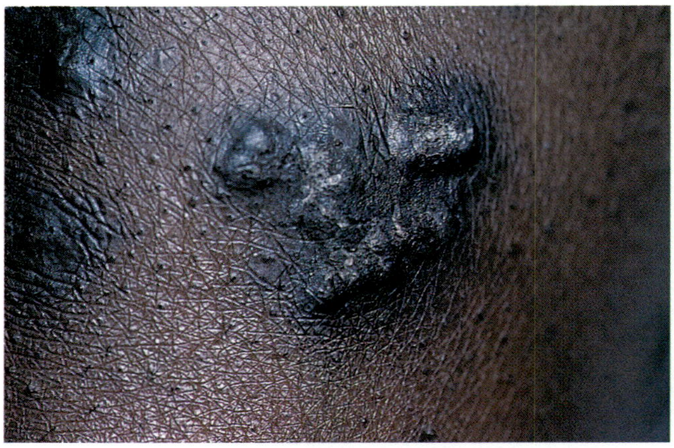

Figure 18–42. Elastosis perforans serpiginosa. Annular hyperkeratotic papules may be misdiagnosed as reactive epidermal and dermal alterations unless perforating disorders are considered and appropriate stains are obtained.

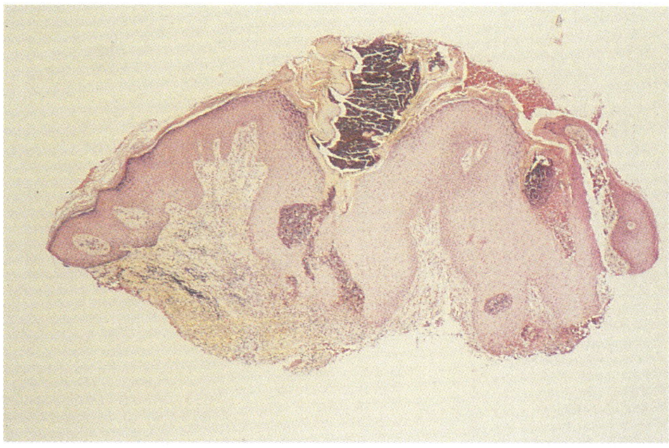

Figure 18–43. Low magnification of a lesional biopsy specimen shows altered elastic fibers within the hyperplastic epithelium and within the cornified plug being extruded.

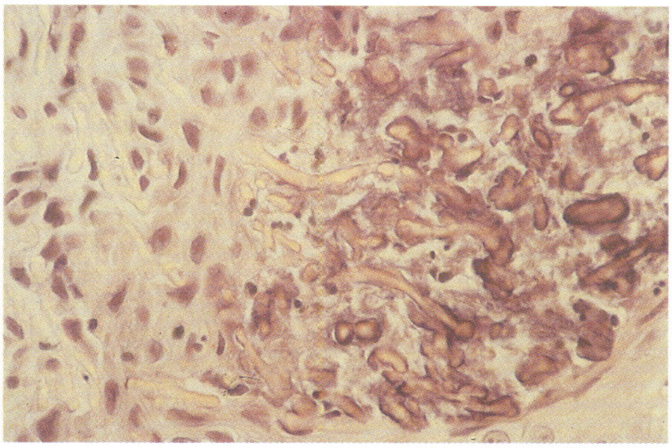

Figure 18–44. Higher magnification of the lesional biopsy in Figure 18–43. Altered elastic tissue fibers are observed adjacent to the site of perforation.

Reactive Perforating Collagenosis

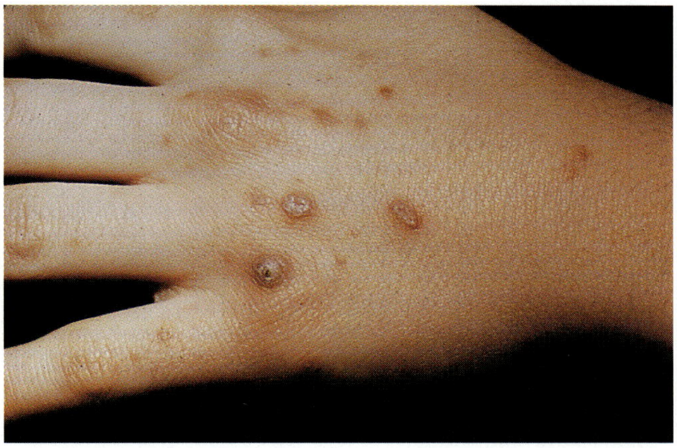

Figure 18–45. Reactive perforating collagenosis. Multiple hyperkeratotic papules, some with central umbilications, are present at sites of trauma on the dorsum of the hand.

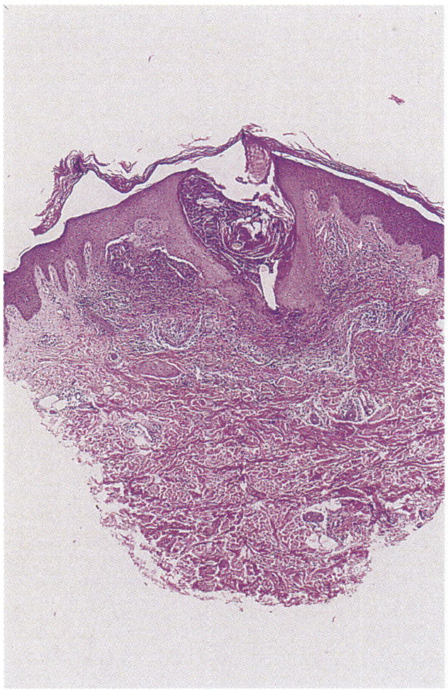

Figure 18–46. At scanning magnification, there is a cup-shaped depression filled with parakeratotic and hyperorthokeratotic scale and inflammatory debris.

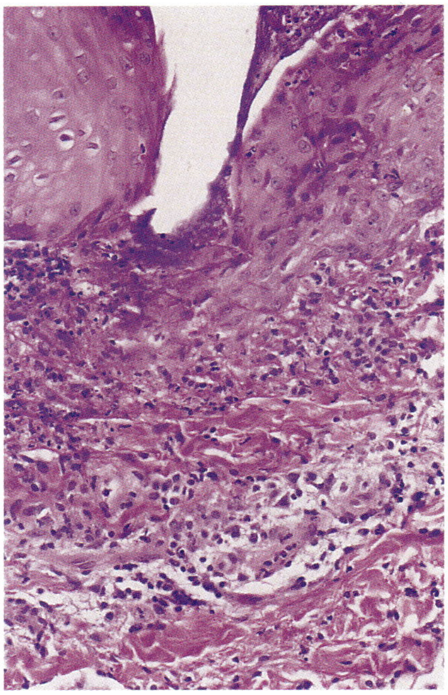

Figure 18–47. At the base of the depression, there is a site of transepithelial perforation of degenerating basophilic collagen bundles associated with mixed inflammatory cells.

Anetoderma

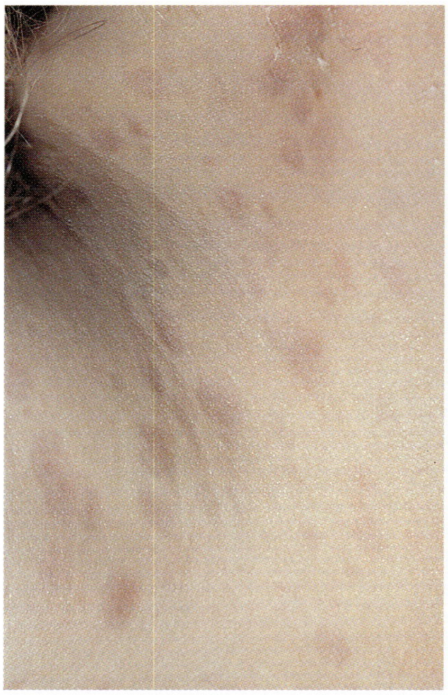

Figure 18–48. Anetoderma. Multiple atrophic plaques involve the upper trunk. Palpation yields a hernia-like defect because of diminished elastic recoil.

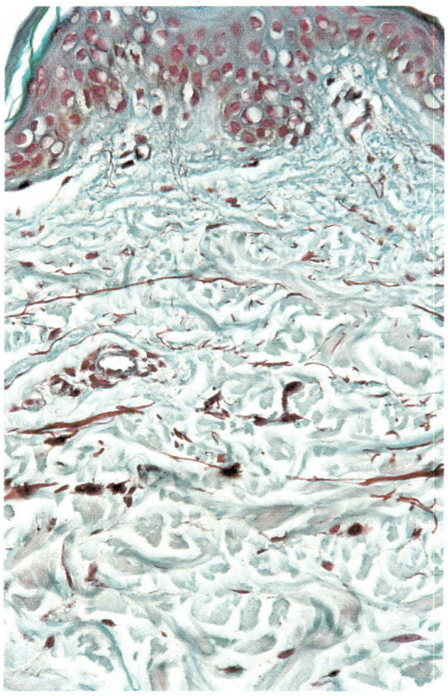

Figure 18–49. Elastic tissue stain reveals markedly attenuated elastic fibers within the superficial dermis and mid-dermis.

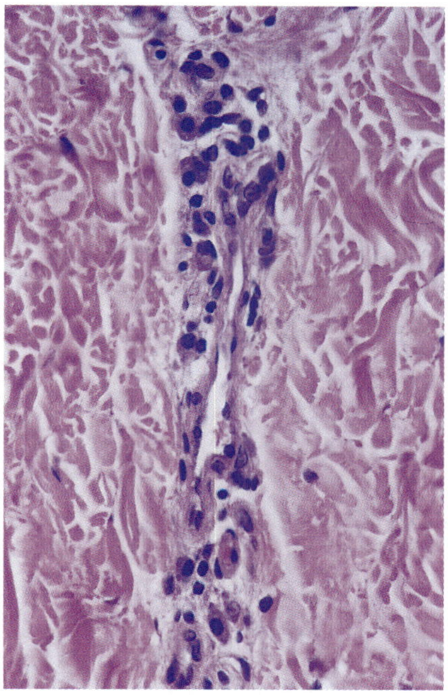

Figure 18–50. A variable perivascular lymphocytic infiltrate may be present, particularly in early lesions, in which loss of elastic fibers is generally less prominent.

Cutis Laxa

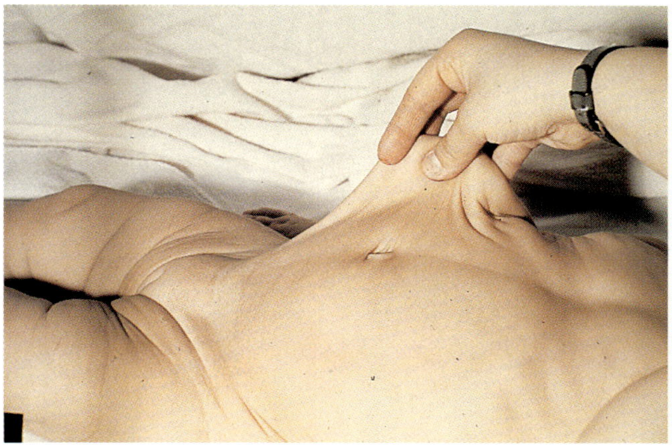

Figure 18–51. Cutis laxa. The skin of this patient is loose, pendulous, and without elastic recoil.

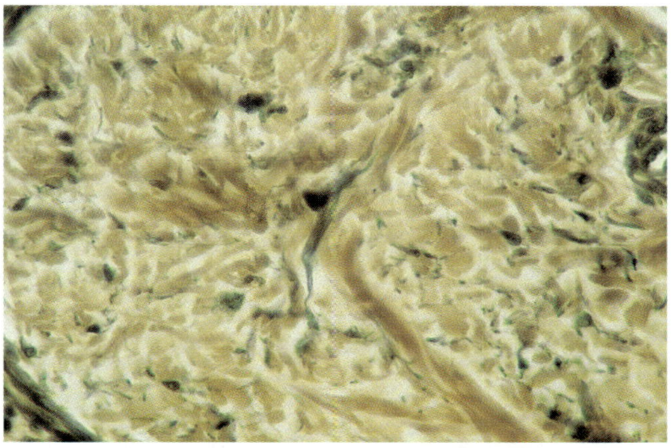

Figure 18–52. Elastic tissue stain of a biopsy specimen reveals diminished numbers of elastic fibers; those that remain often are focally thickened but characteristically tapered at the ends. Small, thin beaded fibers may also be detected.

Keloid

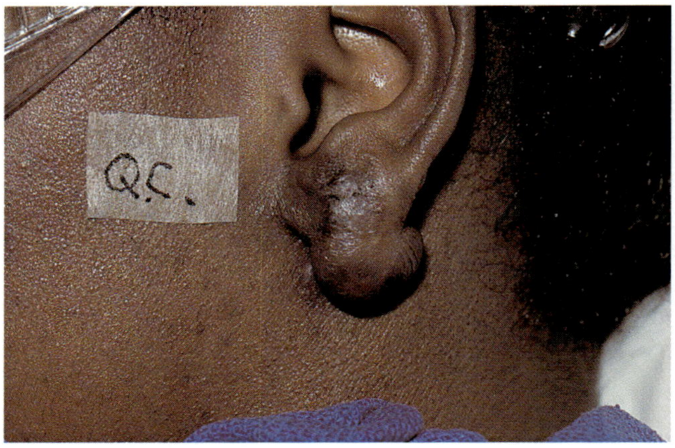

Figure 18–53. A characteristic location for a keloid lesion, which is caused by abnormal matrix deposition, is the site of earlobe piercing.

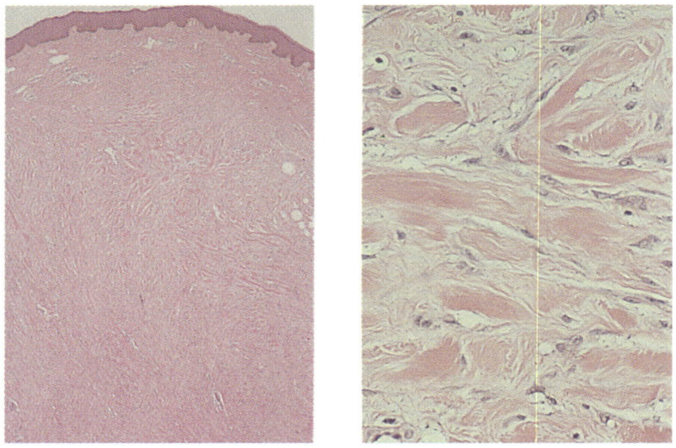

Figure 18–54. *Left,* The dermis is replaced by abnormal bundles of collagen, which consist of *(right)* thick, hyalinized bands intermingled with loose foci of fibroblastic proliferation.

Chondrodermatitis Nodularis Helicis

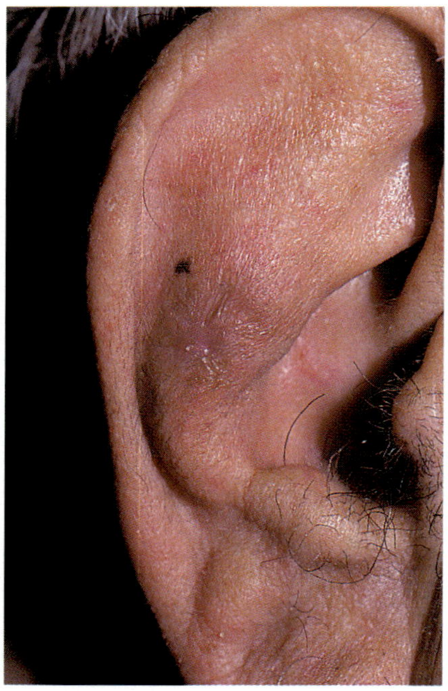

Figure 18–55. Chondrodermatitis. A hyperkeratotic nodule with central ulceration on the ear clinically mimics squamous cell carcinoma.

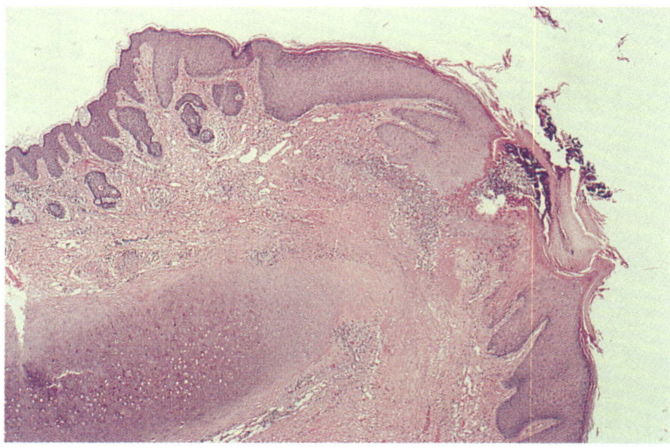

Figure 18–56. At scanning magnification, cartilage *(bottom left)* gradually merges with the fibrotic and inflamed dermis, which is surmounted by hyperplastic, focally ulcerated epidermis.

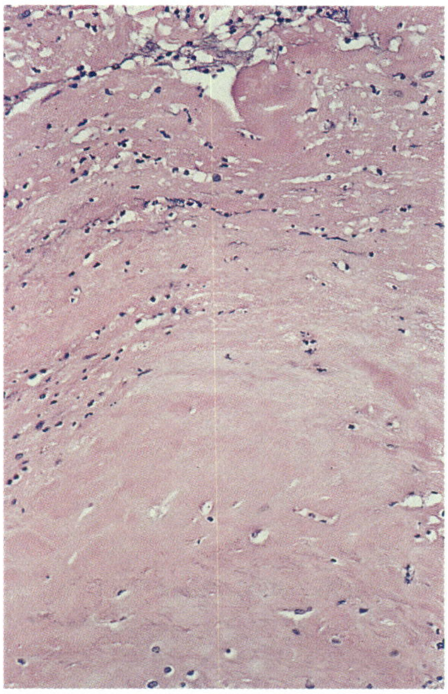

Figure 18–57. A zone of characteristic hyalinization and chondroid change persists within perichondral connective tissue *(top)*.

Stasis Dermatitis

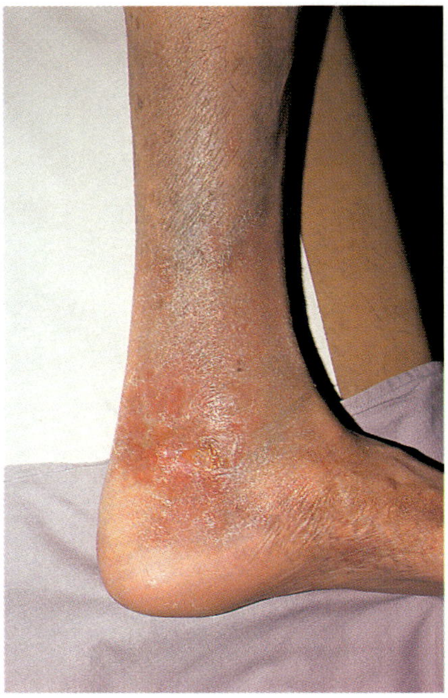

Figure 18–58. Stasis. Brawny, indurated edema of the ankle is present in a patient with chronic venous insufficiency.

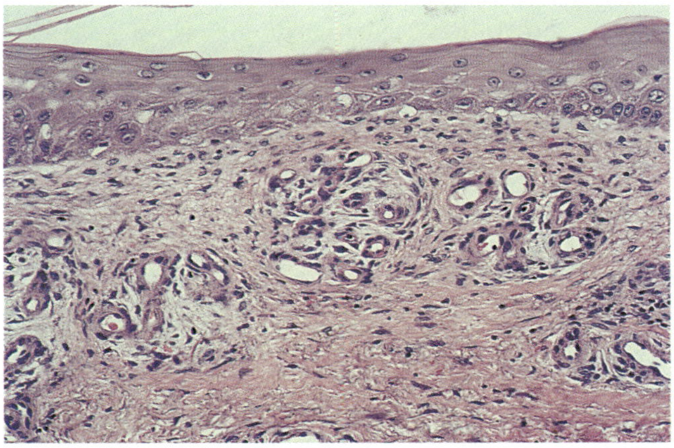

Figure 18–59. Histologically, there is abnormal deposition of collagen and almost tumoral proliferation of small vessels within the superficial dermis.

19

Dermatopathology of Systemic Disease

This section illustrates the more common cutaneous disorders that relate to the coexistence of systemic disease, thus permitting the skin biopsy to potentially reveal life-threatening yet covert metabolic, endocrine, or neoplastic disorders. The dermatopathology of systemic disease could easily be the sole subject of an atlas monograph, and therefore discussion is restricted to conditions that are occasionally seen in routine practice or fall within the limits of routine differential diagnostic considerations. Some manifestations of systemic disease already have been portrayed in chapters that emphasize their primary histologic patterns (*e.g.,* lupus erythematosus [Chapter 6]).

The staining characteristics of systemic disease involving the skin are exceedingly important for formulation of the most accurate diagnosis. Consider, for example, common descriptions of many of the disorders illustrated in this chapter: homogenized, pale, eosinophilic collagen bundles of scleroderma; deep-purple vascular encrustation in hypercalcemia; and diffuse blue-gray dermal pallor of mucinosis in thyrotoxicosis. As in the preceding chapters, attention to tinctorial properties, as well as architecture and cytology, is crucial to accurate distinction of conditions that may be histologically similar but biologically very different.

Scleroderma

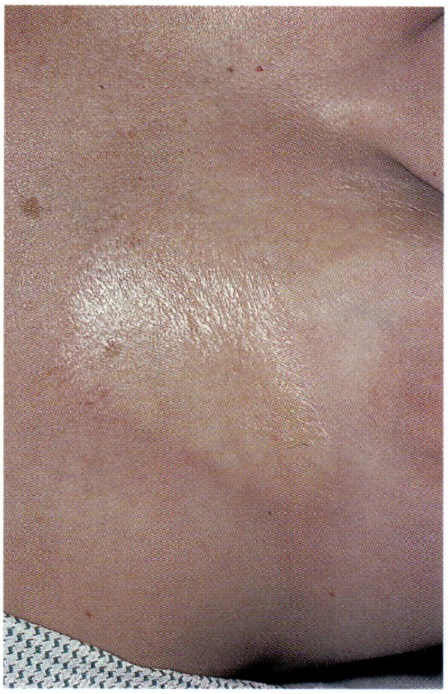

Figure 19–1. Scleroderma. An indurated plaque is anchored to the underlying fascia and covered by a glistening, atrophic epidermal layer. There is a violaceous hue at the perimeter of the lesion, where it has been expanding centrifugally.

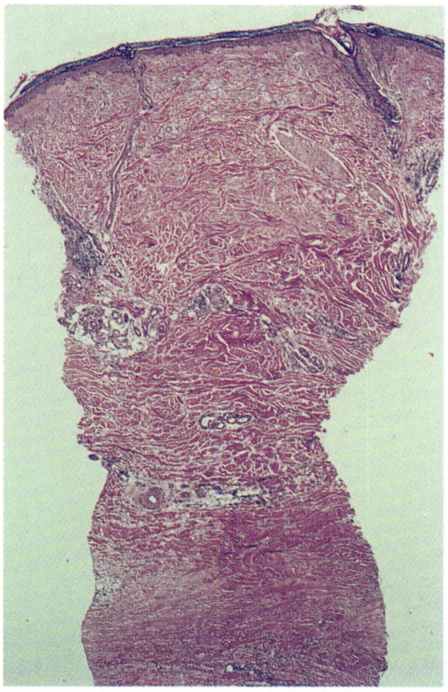

Figure 19–2. At scanning magnification, the biopsy specimen shows a markedly thickened dermis. Eccrine coils are atrophic and appear to be entrapped within the thickened deep dermal collagen bundles.

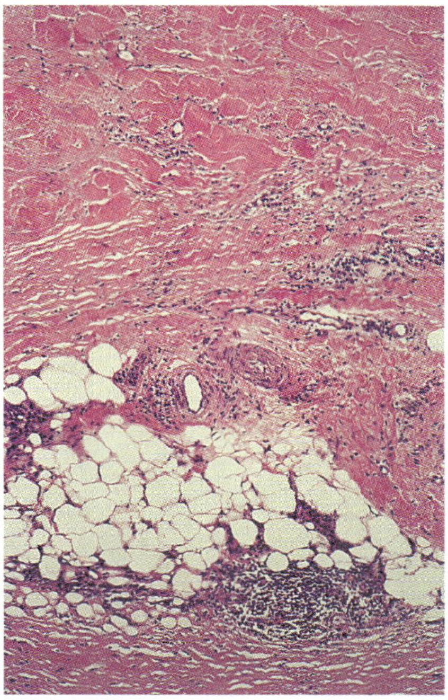

Figure 19–3. Higher magnification reveals sclerotic, thickened, hyalinized collagen bundles infiltrating and replacing subcutaneous adipose tissue. Angiocentric cuffs of lymphocytes and plasma cells are focally observed at the base of the panel.

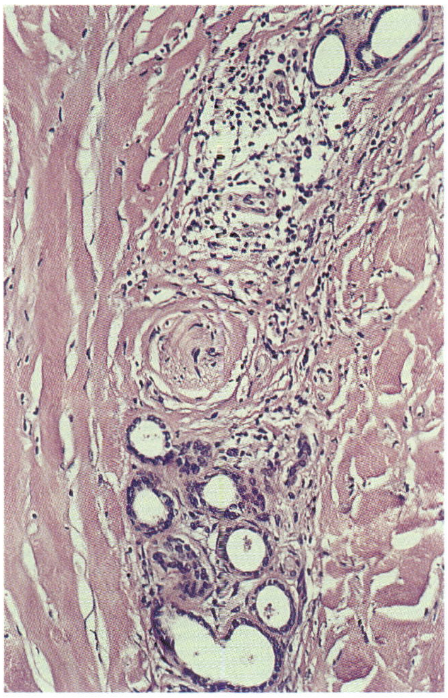

Figure 19–4. Entrapped eccrine coils and a dermal nerve twig. Note the pale, thickened collagen bundles.

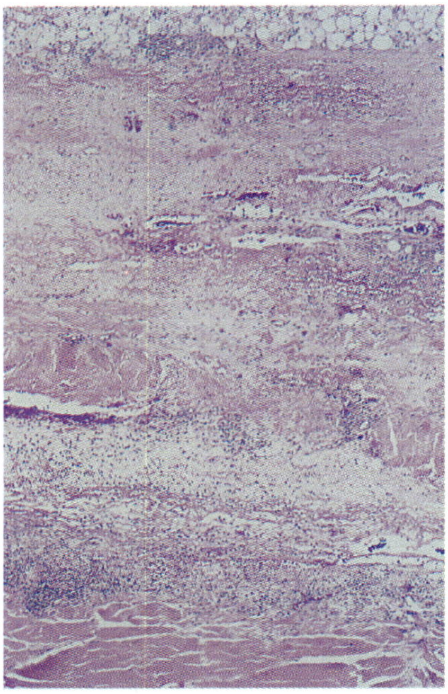

Figure 19–5. Eosinophilic fasciitis, a deep variant of scleroderma. Remnants of deep dermis and subcutis *(top center)* are bound to underlying fascia *(bottom)* by layers of focally edematous and inflamed fibrous tissue.

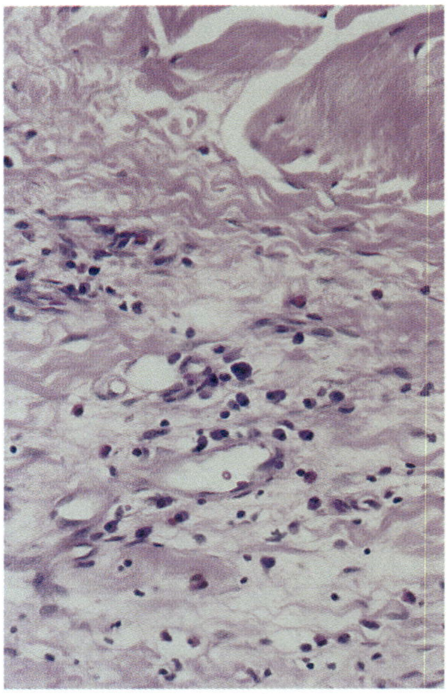

Figure 19–6. Thickened collagen bundles, similar to those seen in scleroderma, and perivascular and interstitial lymphocytic infiltrates with associated eosinophils are observed at higher magnification.

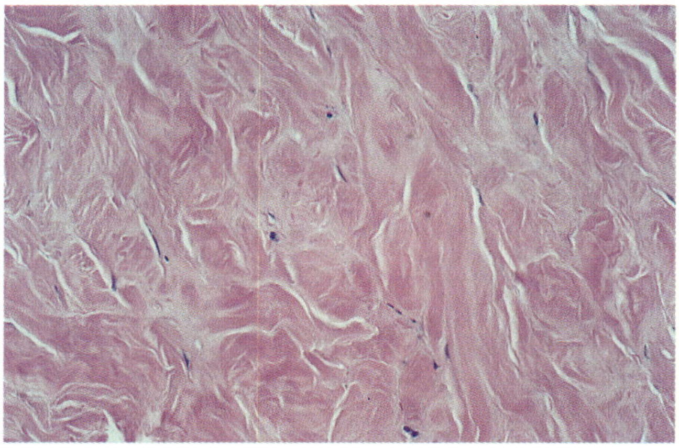

Figure 19–7. Although the dermal collagen bundles are thickened in scleroderma and scleredema (see Fig. 19–8), the spaces between bundles are reduced in scleroderma, whereas these spaces are widened by mucopolysaccharide deposits in scleredema (see Fig. 19–8).

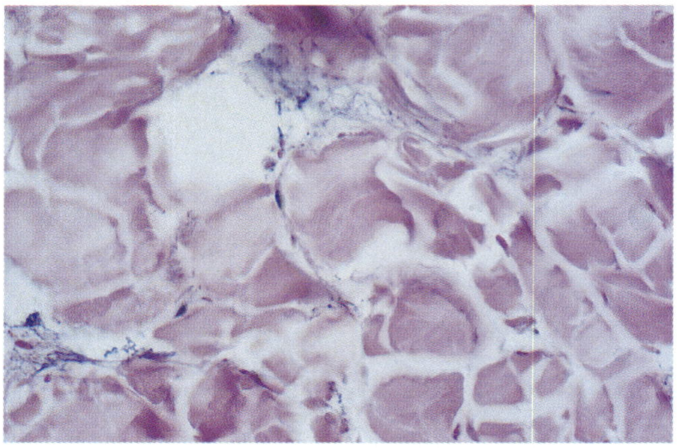

Figure 19–8. Scleredema. Compare with scleroderma in Figure 19–7.

Lymphocytic "Vasculitis" Associated with Collagen Vascular Diseases

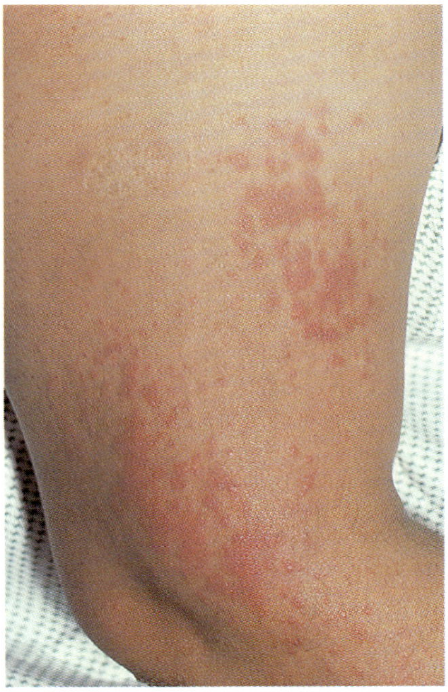

Figure 19–9. Deep lymphocytic venulitis: Rheumatoid arthritis. This patchy, maculopapular, deeply erythematous eruption in a patient with rheumatoid vasculitis revealed only deep perivenular cuffs of lymphocytes and plasma cells with mild endothelial degeneration in the biopsy specimen.

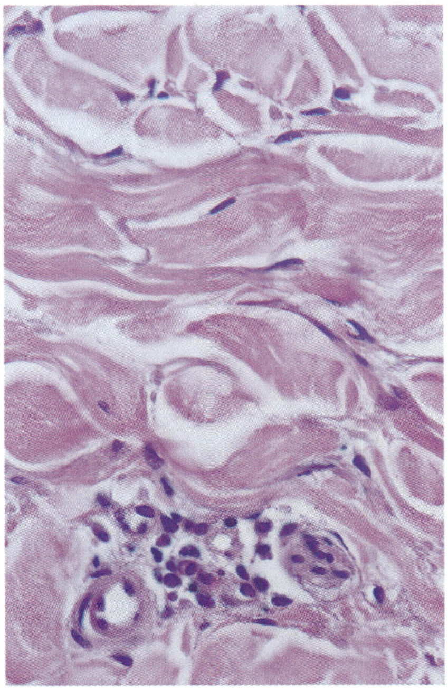

Figure 19–10. Although not entirely specific, deep angiocentric lymphoplasmacytic infiltrates may correlate with the presence of active collagen vascular disease.

Diabetes Mellitus

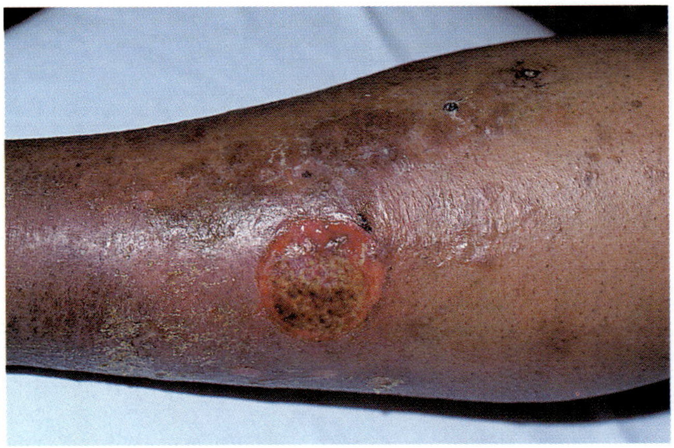

Figure 19–11. Bullous eruption of diabetes. Clinical examination discloses multiple bullae and shallow ulcers.

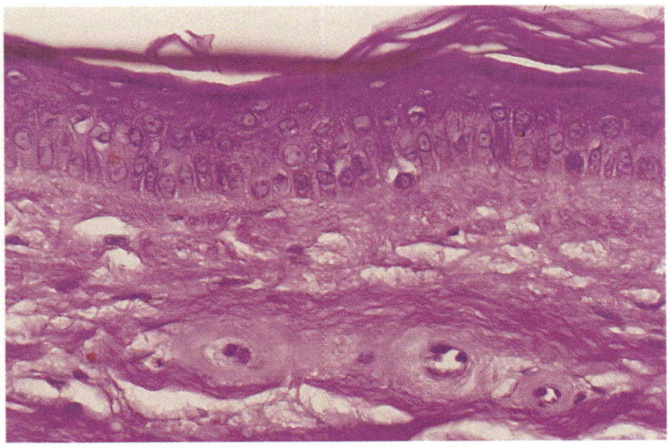

Figure 19–12. A biopsy specimen from perilesional skin where the epidermis is intact revea s striking basement membrane thickening about superficial dermal vessels. The blisters were relatively noninflammatory and subepidermal in location.

Pretibial Myxedema

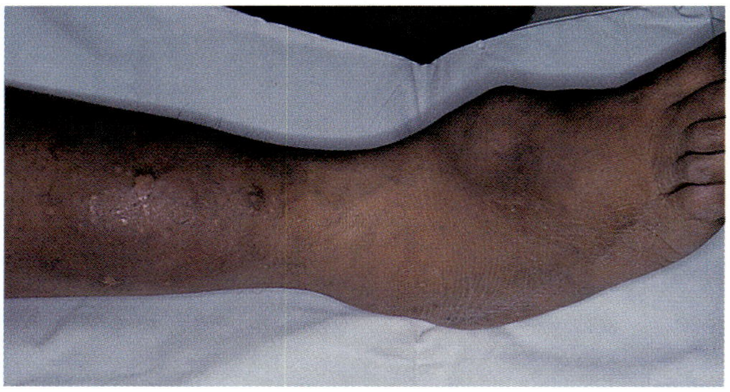

Figure 19–13. Pretibial myxedema: Thyrotoxicosis. Nodular, yellow, waxy plaques with follicular prominence are present on the anterior tibial skin of this patient who has severe hyperthyroidism.

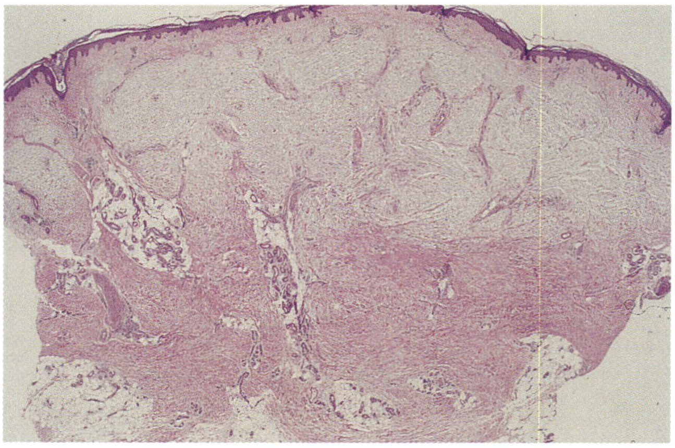

Figure 19–14. At scanning magnification, there is striking dermal thickening due to mucin deposition, which extends into the mid-dermis to deep dermis.

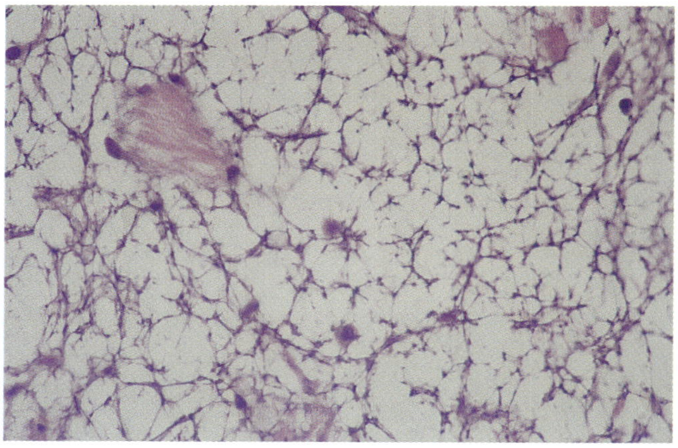

Figure 19–15. At high magnification, the mucin widely separates adjacent collagen bundles and appears as fine, blue-gray strands.

Lichen Myxedematosus

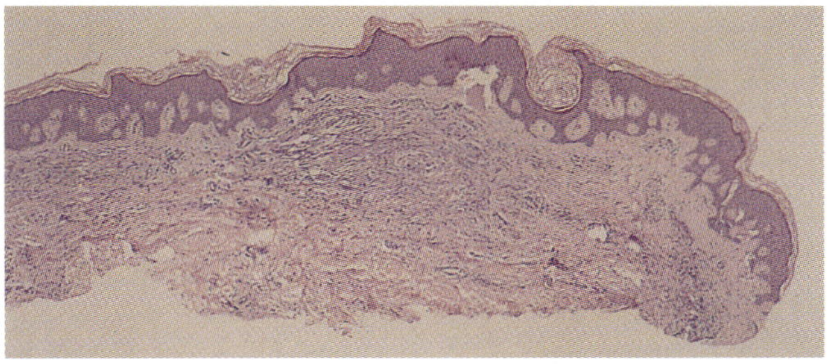

Figure 19–16. Lichen myxedematosus. Associated with paraproteinemia, this disorder has large quantities of pale blue-gray mucin in the upper dermis to mid-dermis.

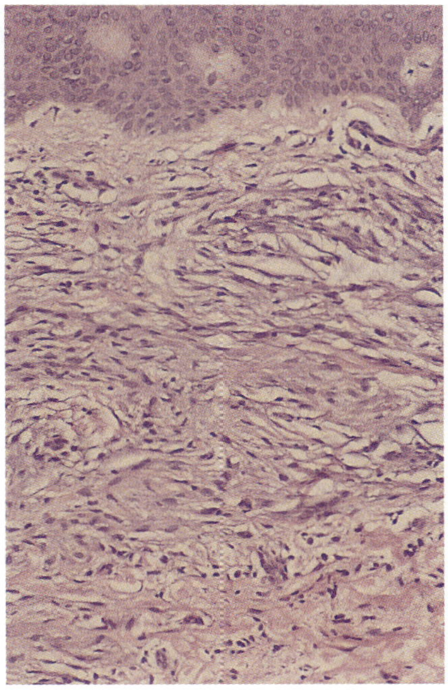

Figure 19–17. However, unlike pretibial myxedema, there is prominent associated proliferation of fibroblasts within the mucinous deposits in lichen myxedematosus.

Effects of Excessive Glucocorticoids

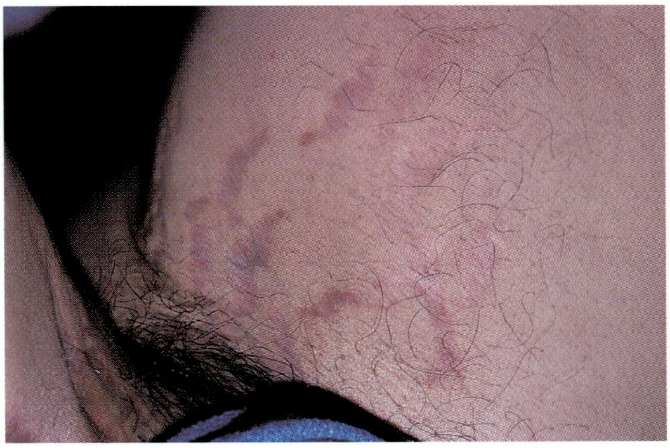

Figure 19–18. Gross pathologic manifestations of glucocorticoid overproduction. Striae distentia consist of erythematous, slightly depressed streaks, which show altered collagen bundles in biopsy specimens.

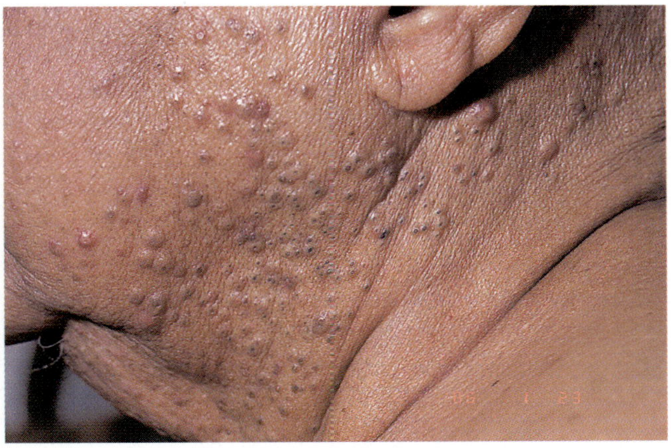

Figure 19–19. Steroid acne. Note that all lesions are synchronized with regard to evolutionary stage. Both steroid acne and striae distensae are generally diagnosed based on clinical appearance alone.

Porphyria Cutanea Tarda

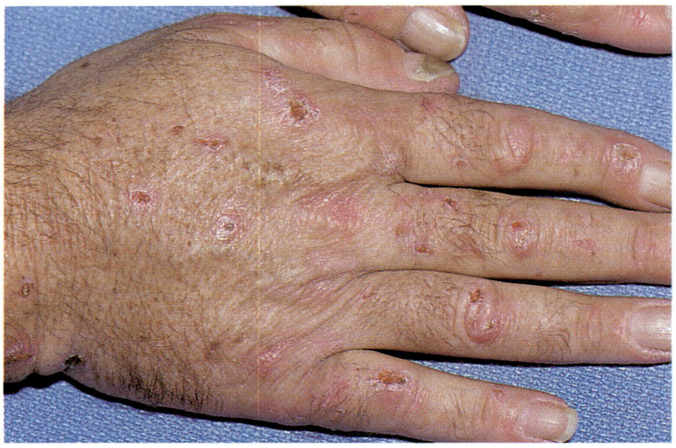

Figure 19–20. Porphyria cutanea tarda. Small blisters and shallow erosions occurred after sun exposure.

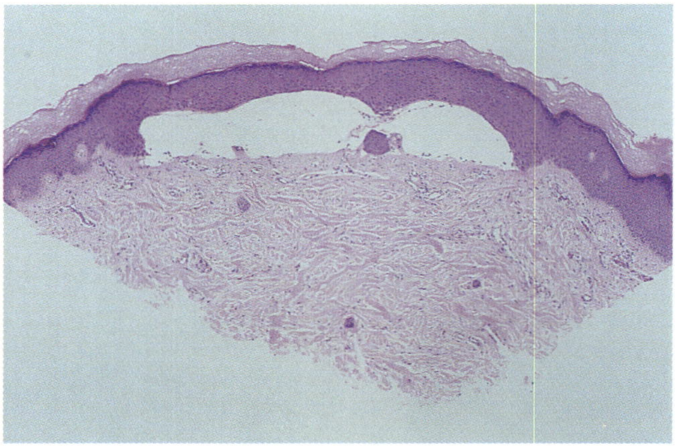

Figure 19–21. Scanning magnification reveals a noninflammatory subepidermal blister.

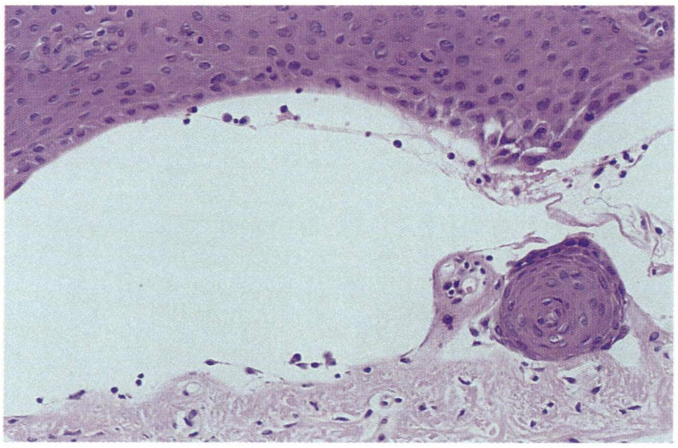

Figure 19–22. The blister base includes a rigid papilla containing vessels with thickened walls. The walls are composed of glassy pink material that stains for albumin and immunoglobulin by direct immunofluorescence (see Chap. 2).

Storage Disease

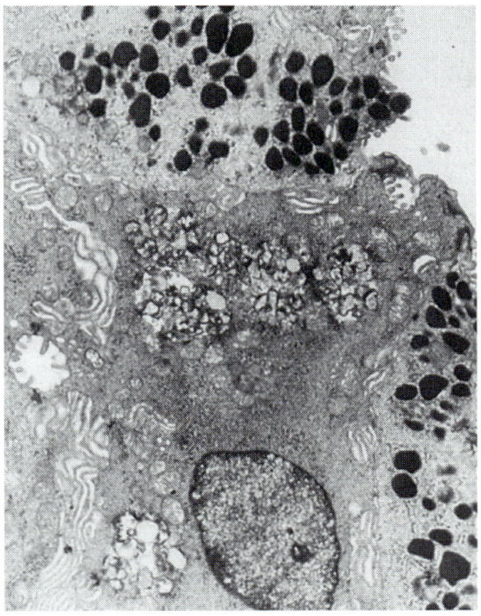

Figure 19–23. Storage disease: Lipofuscinosis. Electron micrograph of the secretory portion of a dermal sweat gland shows collections of variably electron-lucent cytosomes near the apical portion of a luminal cell.

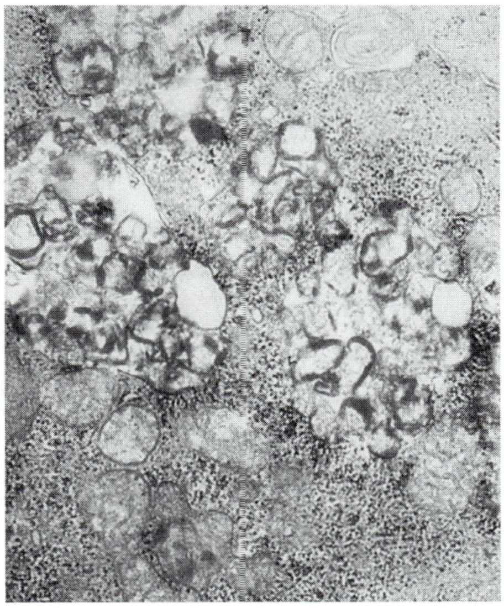

Figure 19–24. At higher magnification (×20,000), these inclusions have fingerprint profiles compatible with lipofuscinosis. Although skin biopsies occasionally may be useful for ultrastructural detection of abnormal deposits in various metabolic storage disorders, the routine histology is seldom abnormal or informative.

Acanthosis Nigricans

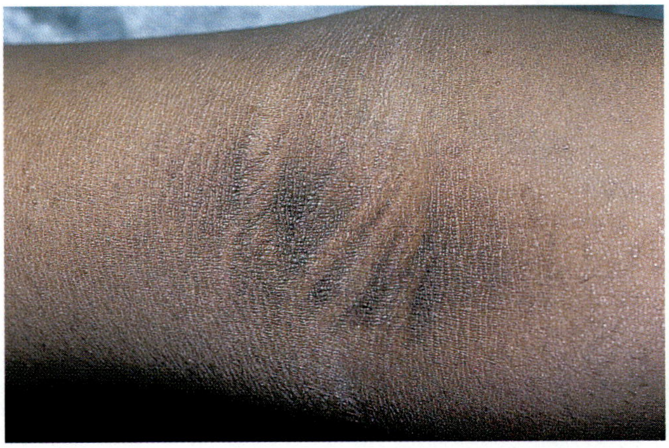

Figure 19–25. Early acanthosis nigricans. A potential harbinger of internal malignancy or endocrine (*e.g.*, pituitary) dysfunction, this disorder manifests as slightly verrucous hyperpigmented plaques, often involving flexural and intertriginous skin.

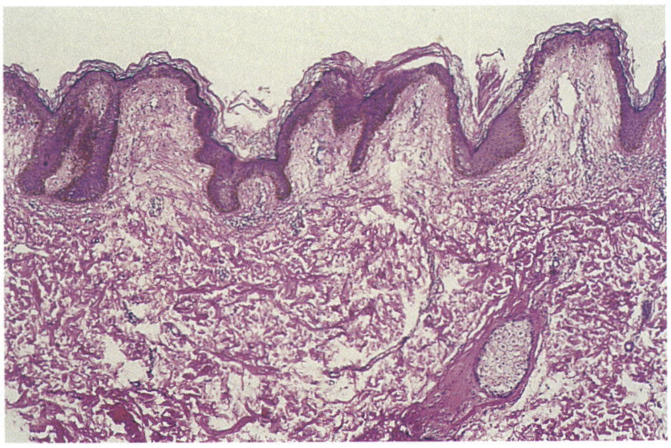

Figure 19–26. Histologically, there is papillomatous epidermal and superficial dermal hyperplasia.

Advanced Atherosclerosus

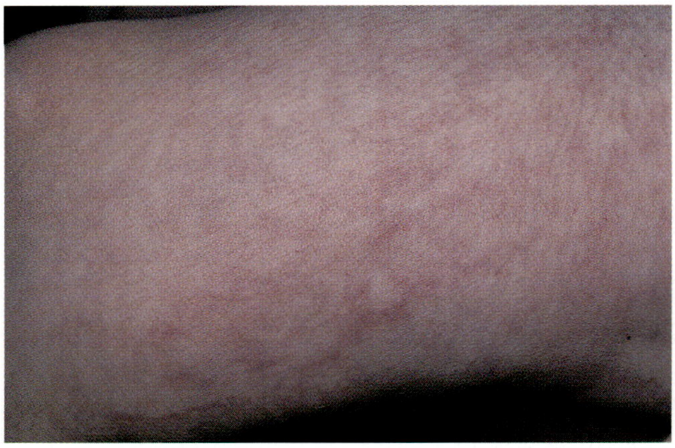

Figure 19–27. Systemic vascular disease: Livedo reticularis. Net-like, mottled erythema of the lower extremity is typical of the clinical appearance of livedo reticularis.

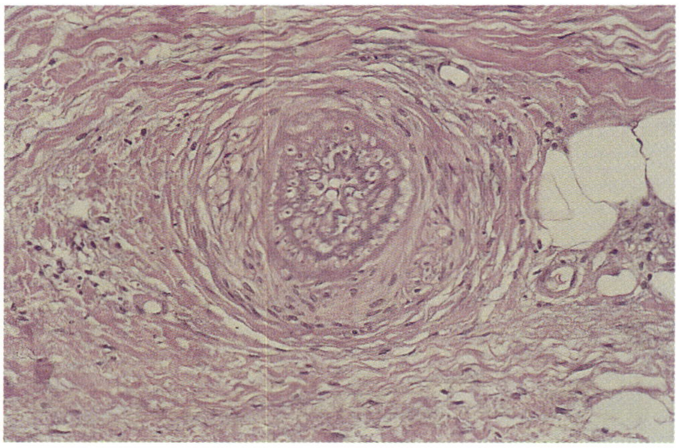

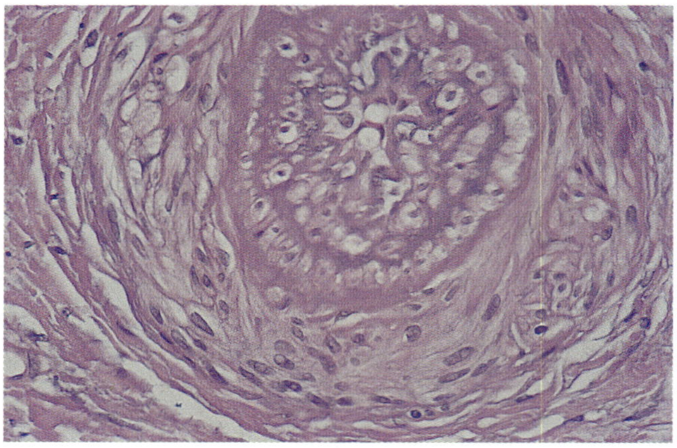

Figures 19–28 and 19–29. In this case, obliterative intimal hyperplasia of medium-sized vessels was responsible. In other patients, thromboembolic disease may result in a similar pattern, particularly in the case of atheromatous emboli to the lower extremities.

Hyperuricemia

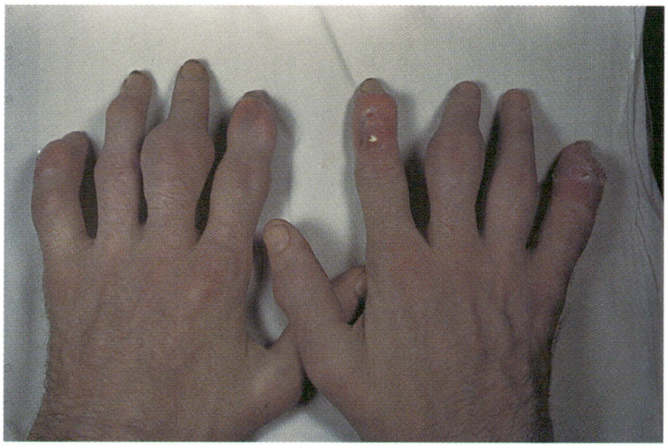

Figure 19–30. Hyperuricemia with tophi. The proximal and distal interphalangeal joints are deformed by urate deposits (*i.e.,* tophi).

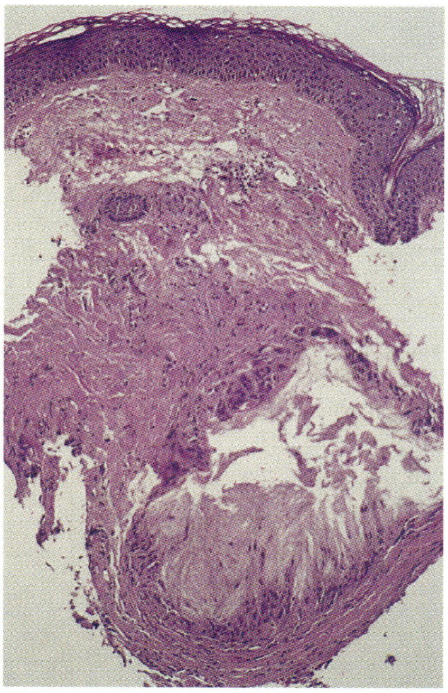

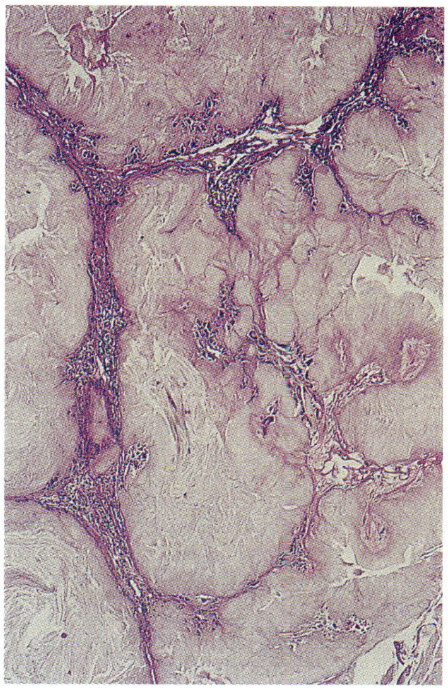

Figures 19–31 and 19–32. In alcohol-fixed material, urate deposits are seen as aggregates of thin, needle-shaped crystals surrounded by a foreign body giant cell response and fibrosis within the deep dermis. In Figure 19–32, the crystals are relatively clear and separated by trabeculae containing inflammatory cells.

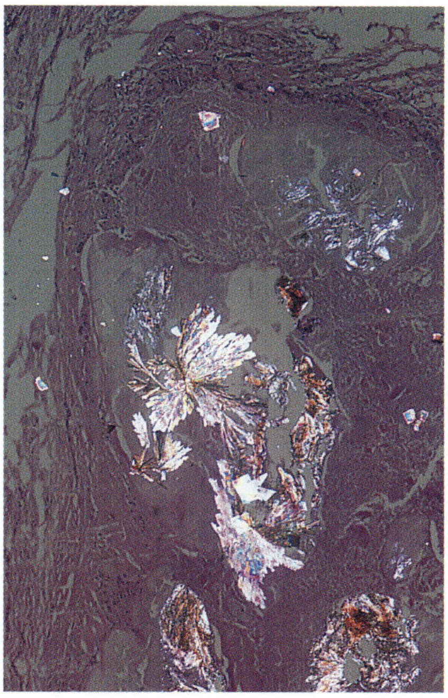

Figure 19–33. Examination by polarization microscopy reveals characteristic birefringence in these otherwise nondescript regions.

Hypercalcemia

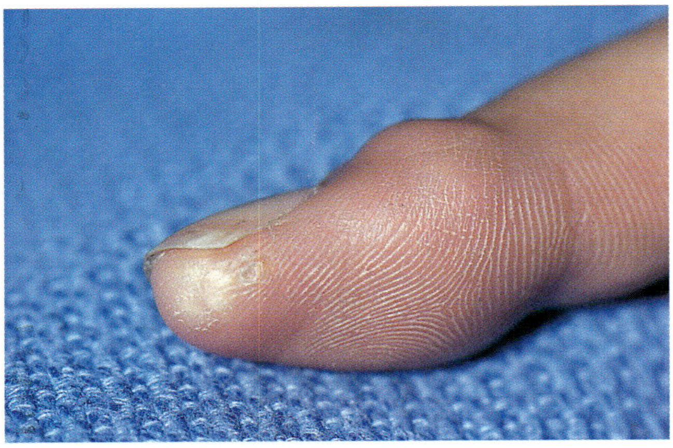

Figure 19–34. Dystrophic and metastatic calcification. Firm, calcified dermal and subcutaneous nodules in a patient with scleroderma. This phenomenon is likely to result from dystrophic calcification of abnormal matrix elements.

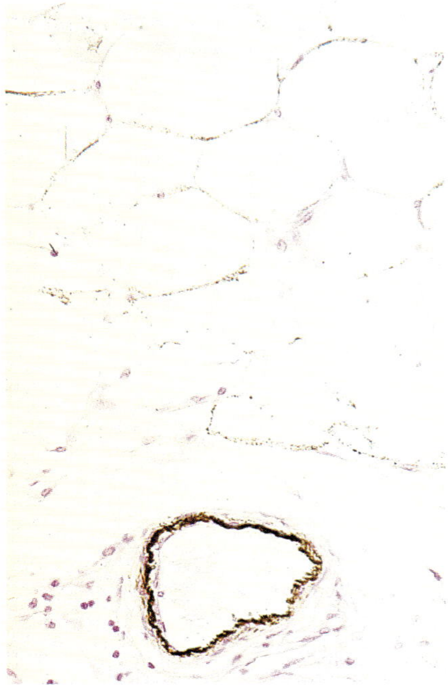

Figure 19–35. Metastatic calcification of normal vessel walls in a patient with hypercalcemia due to hyperparathyroidism. The majority of involved vessels are in the subcutaneous fat, and von Kossa stain for calcium confirms the nature of the deposit *(bottom).*

Amyloidosis

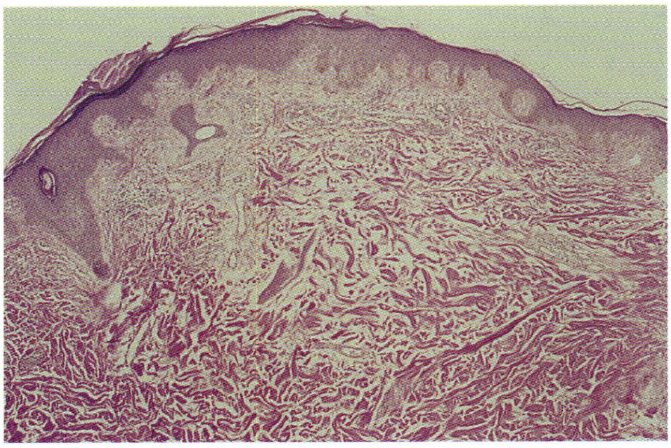

Figure 19–36. Systemic amyloidosis. At scanning magnification, the epidermis is slightly hyperplastic, but definite pathology is difficult to detect.

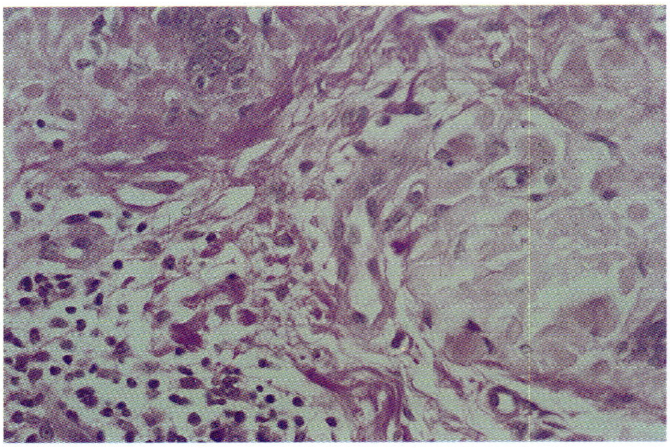

Figure 19–37. Careful scrutiny at higher magnification reveals pale-pink aggregates of amyloid about superficial and deep dermal vessels and around adnexae *(top left and right).* Amyloid restricted to dermal papillae, as is the case in lichenoid amyloidosis, is not detected.

Hyperlipidemia

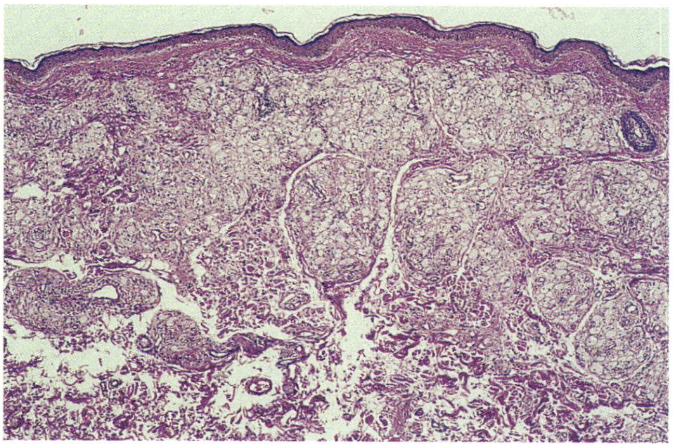

Figure 19–38. Xanthelasma. There are nodular aggregates of foam cells in the superficial dermis and mid-dermis.

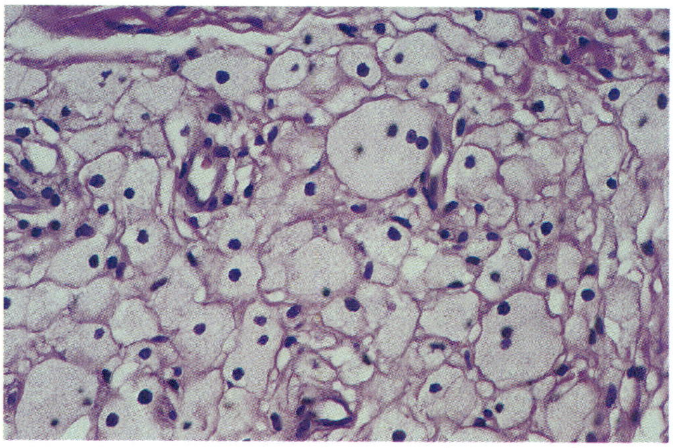

Figure 19–39. The cells have small, centrally located nuclei and abundant cytoplasm filled with small lipid vacuoles.

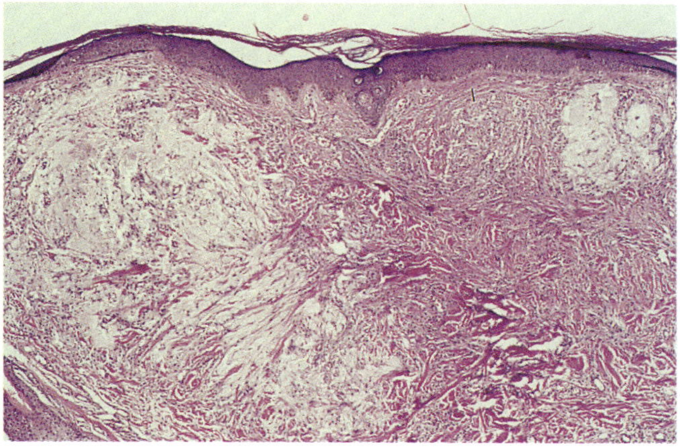

Figure 19–40. Tuberous xanthoma. This relatively late lesion shows poorly aggregated clusters of lipidized histiocytes admixed with fibroblasts.

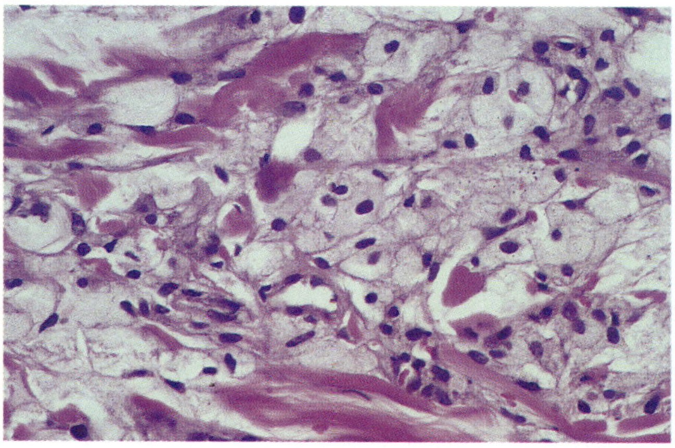

Figure 19–41. At higher magnification, the characteristic cytoplasmic vacuoles are apparent.

V

Regional Dermatopathology

20

Dermatopathology of Hair

Hair is the end-product of an actively growing and cycling population of terminally differentiated cutaneous structures. Although the structure of hair is known, its exact function in humans is uncertain. It may provide protection from the environment, enhance tactile senses, and contribute to thermoregulation. For the most part, however, it appears to have cosmetic value as an adornment, as demonstrated by the extensive demand for products that stimulate hair growth and procedures that minimize the appearance of hair loss.

The structure of hair is generally the same throughout the body: its major components are an outer root sheath, inner root sheath, hair shaft, and follicular bulb. The outer root sheath is a modified extension of the epidermis that descends from the skin surface to the most deeply placed portion of the hair follicle, the bulb. The bulb is composed of the follicular papilla, specialized condensation of connective tissue and vasculature, and follicular matrix keratinocytes. The follicular matrix contains germinative cells that produce an inner root sheath and a hair shaft that is centrally placed within the follicular canal. The outer root sheath forms an envelope that surrounds the inner root sheath and the hair shaft. The entire follicular unit, in turn, is surrounded by a delicate mantle of fibrous tissue that holds an elaborate network of arterioles, venules, cutaneous nerves, and resident perivascular mast cells, monocytes, and T lymphocytes. The adventitial sheath is most easily seen in sections as a delicate band of fibrovascular tissue surrounding an anagen hair or a collapsed tract trailing behind a telogen hair. Once a hair begins the anagen phase of its growth cycle, it descends in this tract into subcutaneous adipose tissue, where it normally resides for several years. The integrity of this support network is crucial to normal functioning of the follicular unit. Interruption, inflammation, or entrapment of hair in thickened collagen will likely compromise normal cycling and hair growth.

Although the structure of hair is similar throughout the body, its caliber and density vary from one anatomic site to the next. For example, the scalp and body of the neonate are covered by small-caliber miniature follicles with little or no pigment—vellus hairs. These hairs are eventually replaced by larger caliber hairs that are well endowed with pigment—terminal hairs. In adults, vellus hairs can still be found in limited areas, such as the forehead, the ears, and in women, the face. Knowledge of the normal distribution of hair throughout the body can provide clues to diagnosis. For example, finding a large number of vellus hairs in a scalp biopsy of a male patient would suggest a diagnosis of male pattern, or androgenic, alopecia.

Normal Anatomy

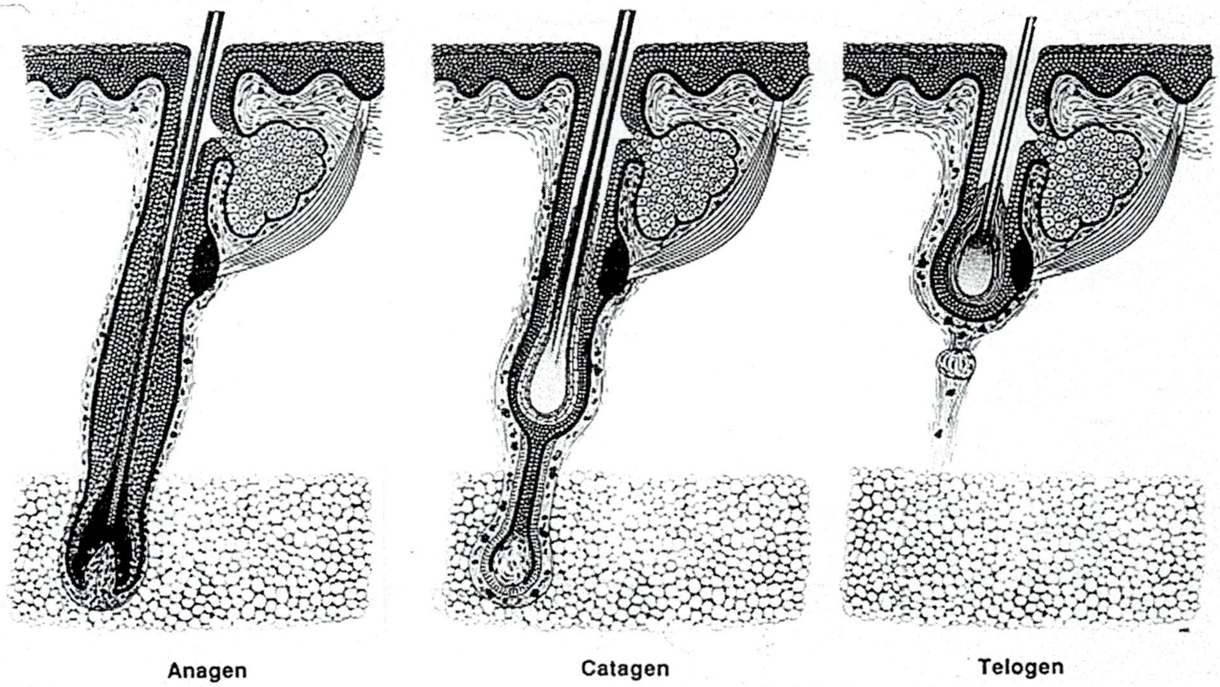

Figure 20–1. Schematic representation of the major components of a hair and of the hair cycle (*i.e.*, anagen, catagen, and telogen growth phases).

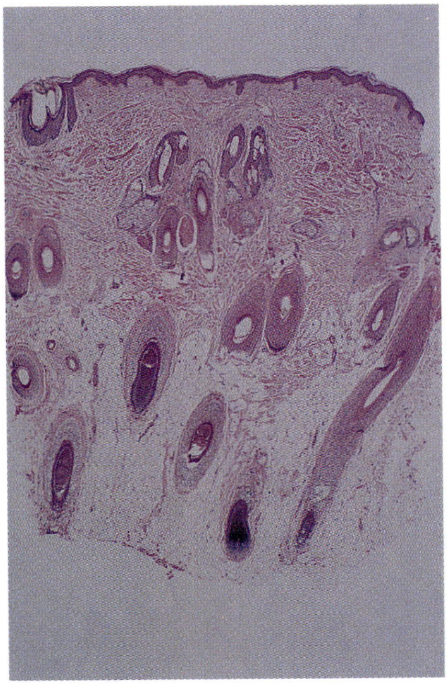

Figure 20–2. Normal hair density on the scalp.

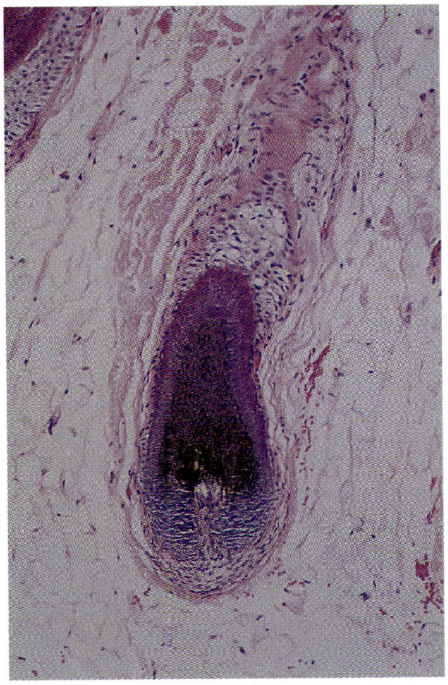

Figure 20–3. Anagen hair. The papilla is embedded deep in the subcutaneous adipose tissue of scalp skin.

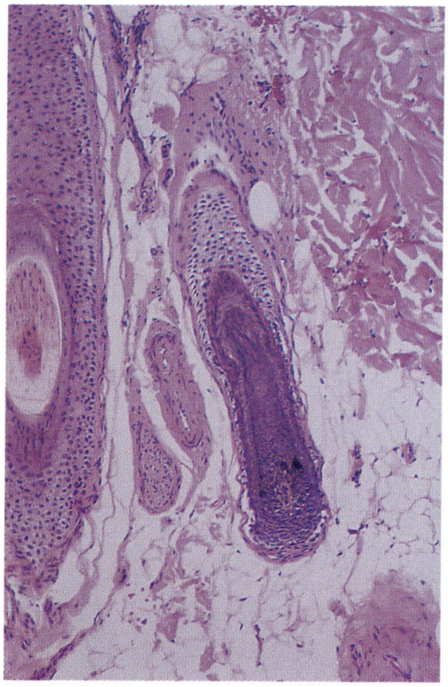

Figure 20–4. Hair in transition to catagen growth phase. The hair papilla ascends to the dermal-subcutaneous junction.

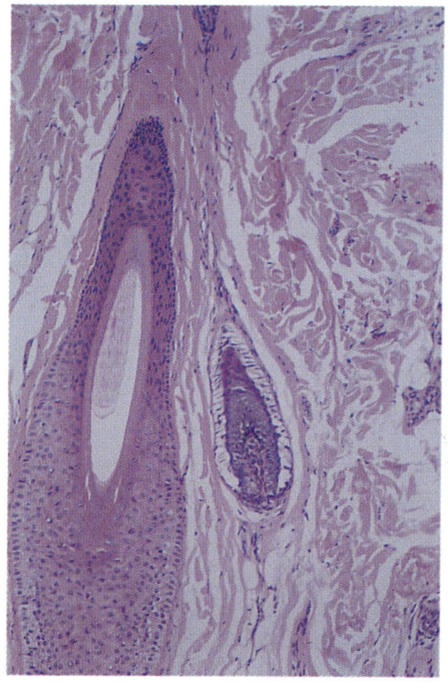

Figure 20–5. Telogen hairs in sections have their papillae entirely within dermal stroma.

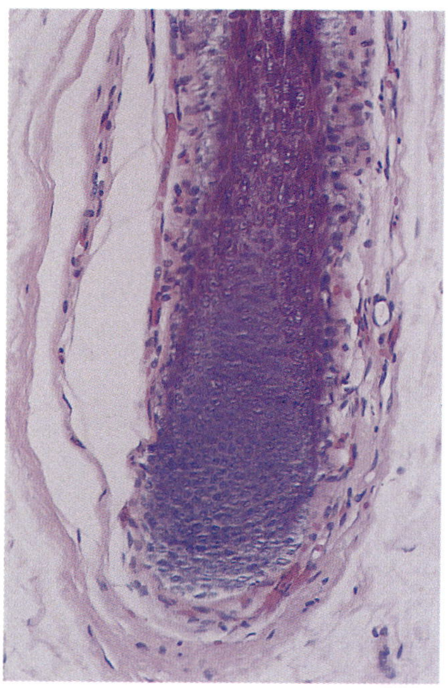

Figure 20–6. Perifollicular adventitial sheath. This delicate fibrovascular envelope surrounding the hair follicle carries a complex vascular network and resident mononuclear cells and mast cells.

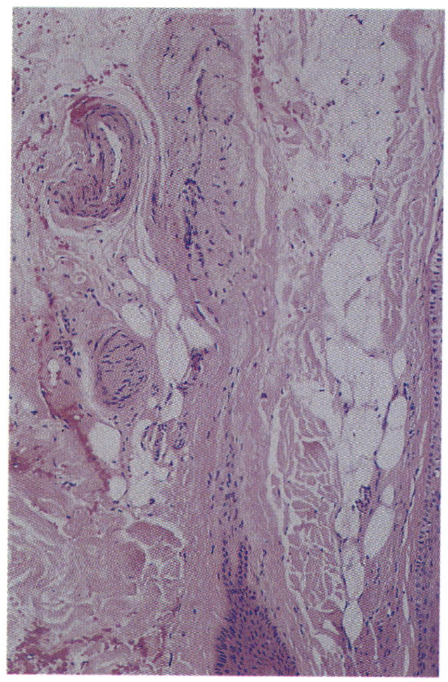

Figure 20–7. Collapsed adventitial sheath appears as a fibrous streamer left behind in the path of a hair in telogen growth phase.

Abnormalities of Hair Shaft

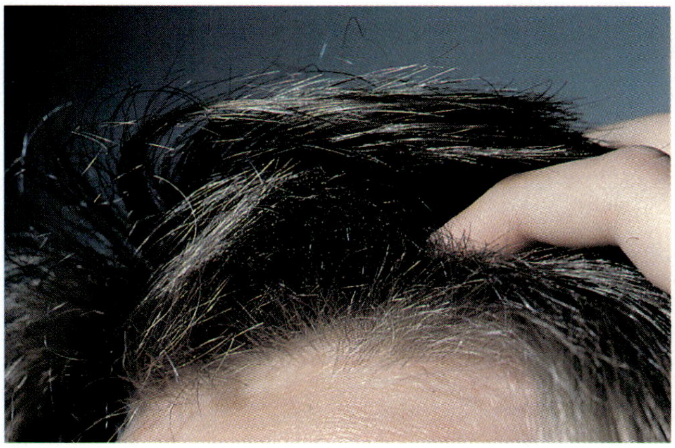

Figure 20–8. Clinical appearance of scalp hair in a patient with trichorrhexis nodosa. Note the beaded appearance of the hair shafts *(center)*.

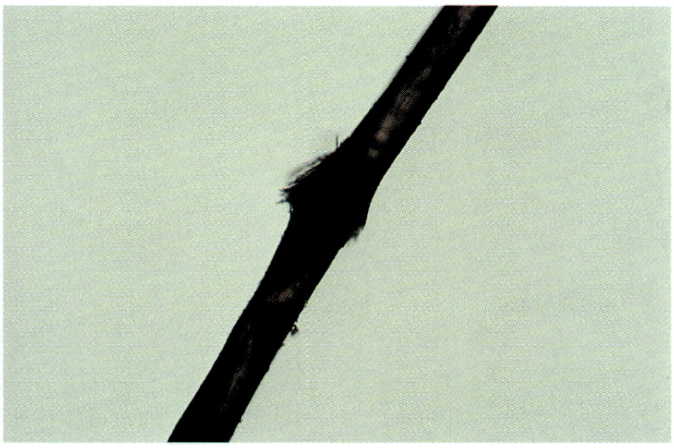

Figure 20–9. Hair mount of trichorrhexis nodosa. Along the hair shaft, there are zones of splaying of the hair cortex, similar to two paintbrushes being pushed together at their bristle ends.

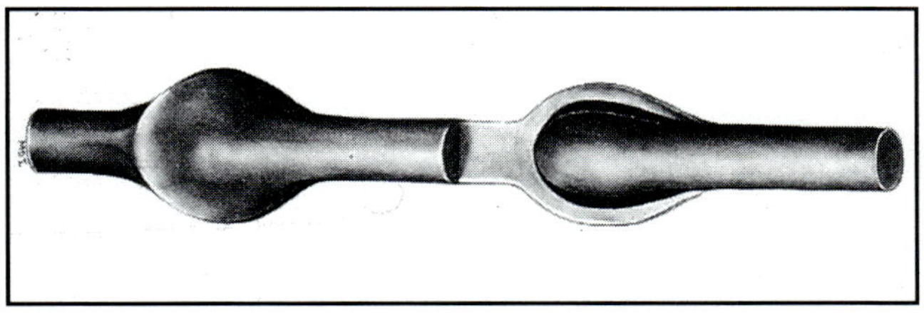

Figure 20–10. Trichorrhexis invaginata: Hairs have invaginations along their shafts, which have the appearance of a ball-and-socket. (Courtesy of Michael Ioffreda, MD.)

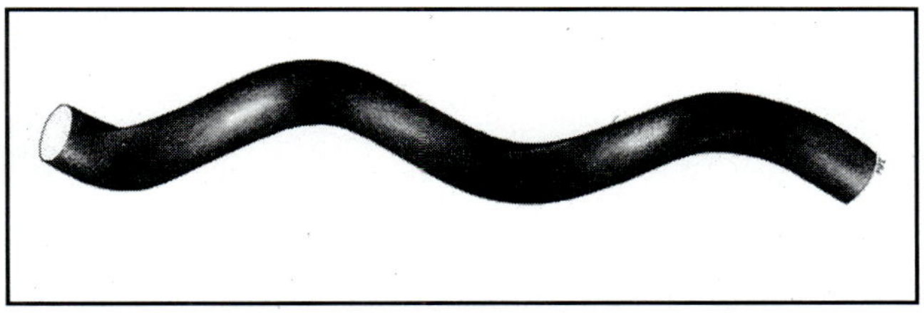

Figure 20–11. Pili torti: Multiple twists at irregular intervals occur along the hair shaft. (Courtesy of Michael Ioffreda, MD.)

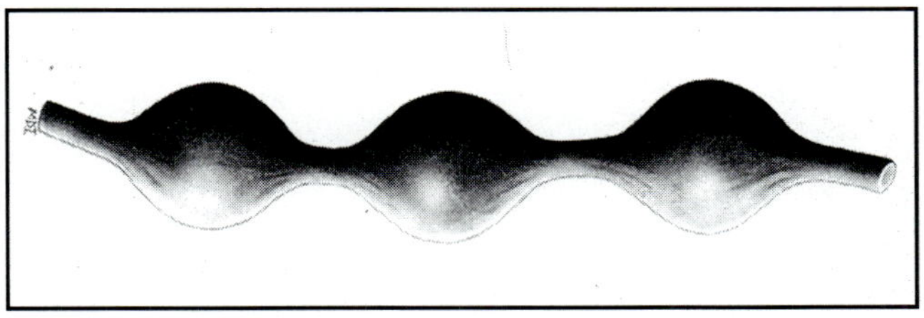

Figure 20–12. Monilethrix: Hair shafts have a beaded appearance. (Courtesy of Michael Ioffreda, MD.)

Traumatic Alopecia

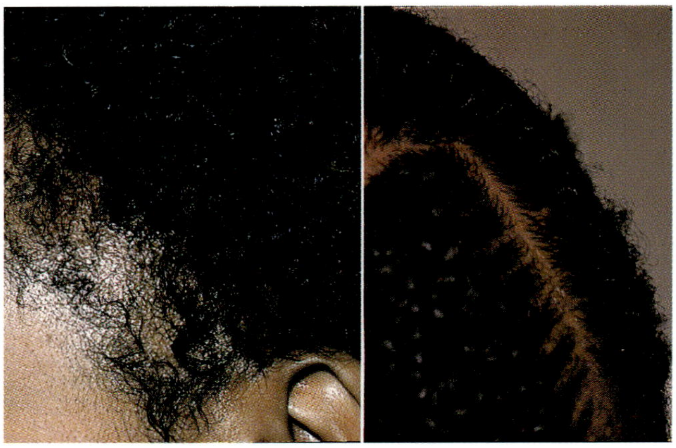

Figure 20–13. Traumatic alopecia. Widening of parts occurs as a result of chronic tension *(right)*. The marginal hairline recedes *(left)*. Greatest shortening of hair shafts occurs at the point of maximal tension.

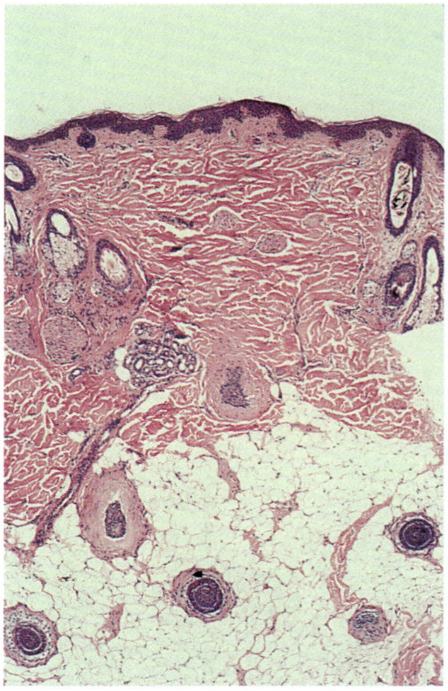

Figure 20–14. There is prominent thickening of perifollicular adventitial sheaths and an isolated hair cast in a follicular infundibulum.

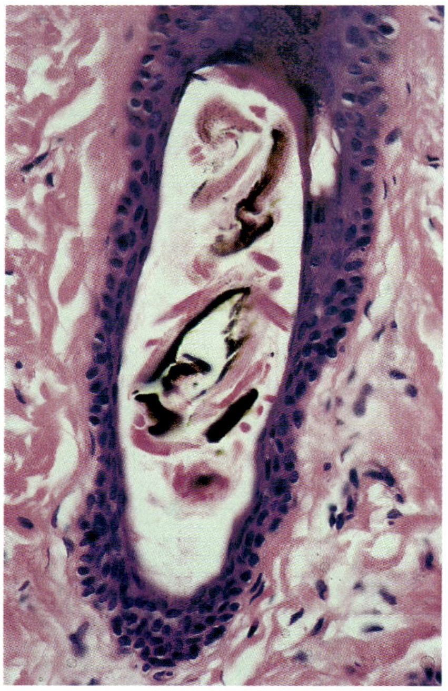

Figure 20–15. Corkscrew hair and hair cast are located in the follicular infundibulum.

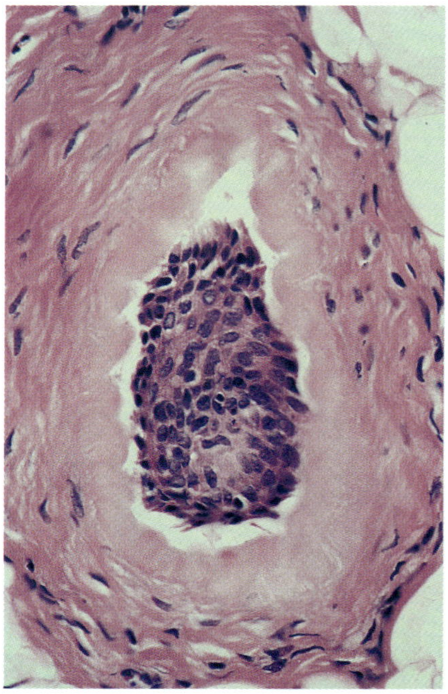

Figure 20–16. Fibrosis of the perifollicular sheath.

Folliculitis

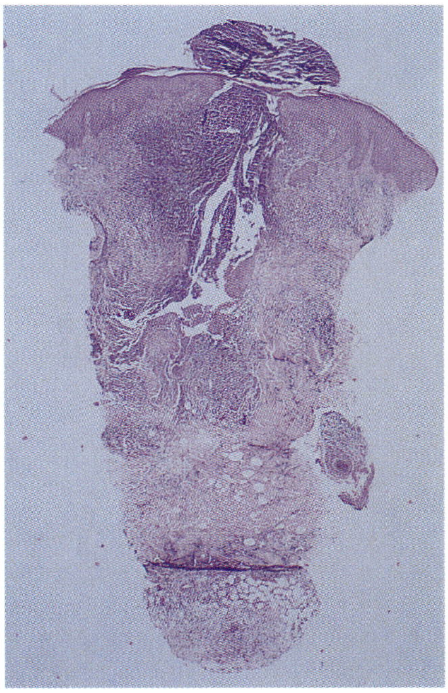

Figure 20–17. Furuncle. A dermal abscess surrounds a disrupted hair follicle along its length.

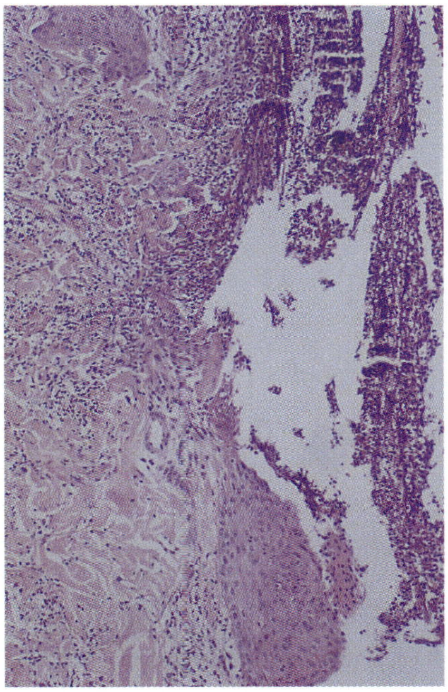

Figure 20–18. An intense, reutrophilic, inflammatory infiltrate completely disrupts portions of the follicular epithelium in this furuncle.

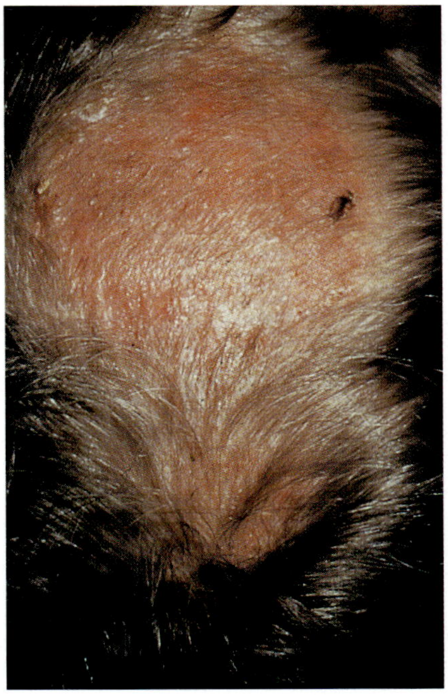

Figure 20–19. Tinea capitis. Pronounced breakage and hair loss have resulted from fungal infection. The erythema and scaling seen here may be absent in some cases.

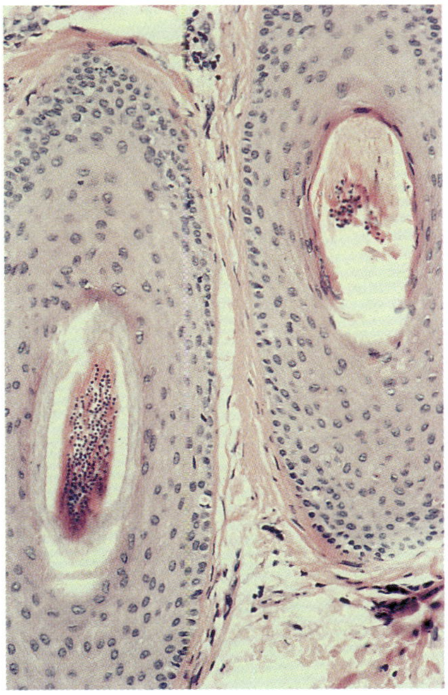

Figure 20–20. In tinea capitis, there are large numbers of basophilic spores in hair shafts, with only sparse dermal inflammatory infiltrates.

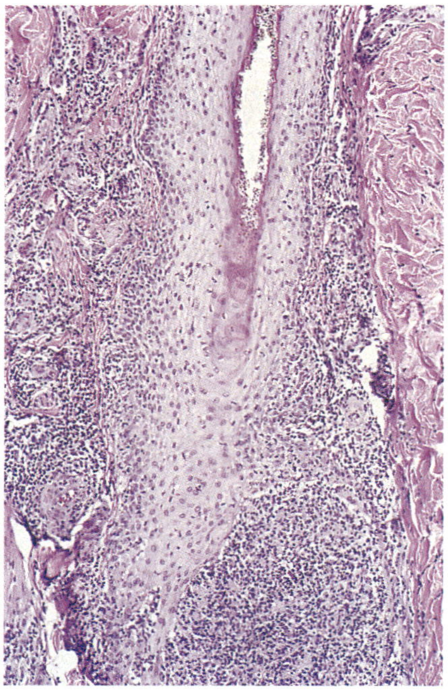

Figure 20–21. Inflammatory tinea capitis. The perifollicular abscess is composed of large numbers of neutrophils.

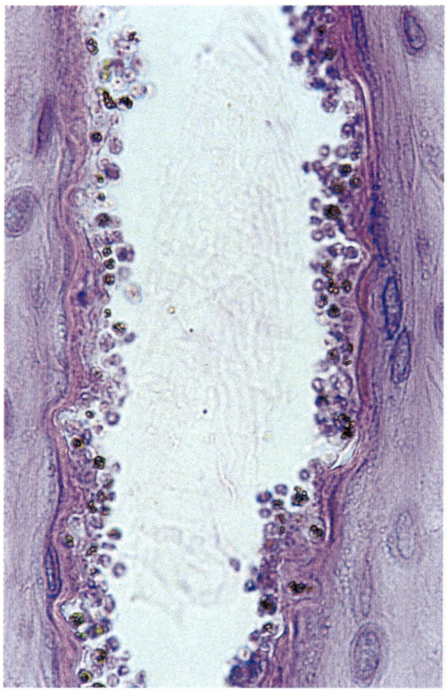

Figure 20–22. Higher magnification of Figure 20–21 shows large numbers of spores in the follicular canal.

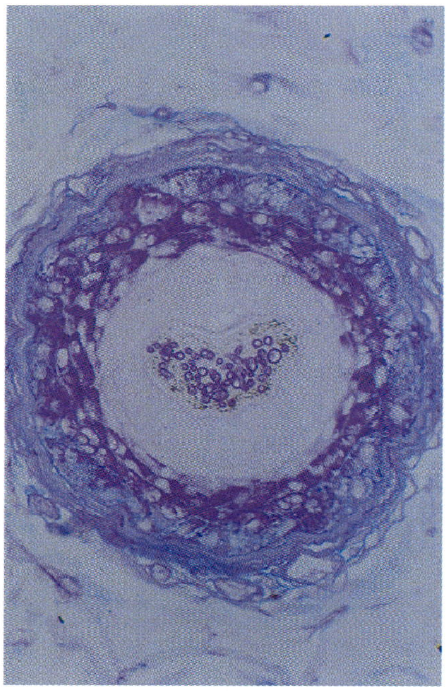

Figure 20–23. In endothrix infection, spores are found in the center of the hair shaft (periodic acid–Schiff stain).

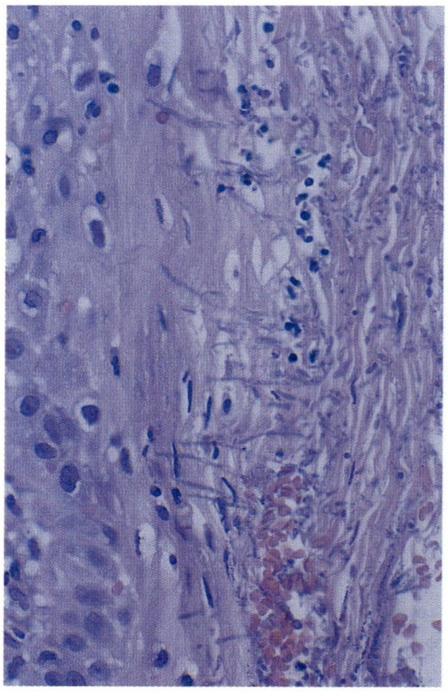

Figure 20–24. In ectothrix infection, large numbers of branching hyphae can be seen traversing the follicular epithelium and entering adjacent dermal stroma (hematoxyin and eosin stain).

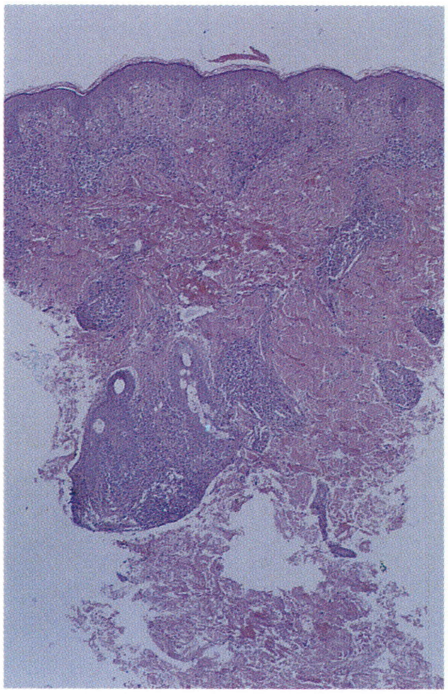

Figure 20–25. Secondary syphilis. Low magnification shows a perivascular, perifollicular, lichenoid inflammatory infiltrate.

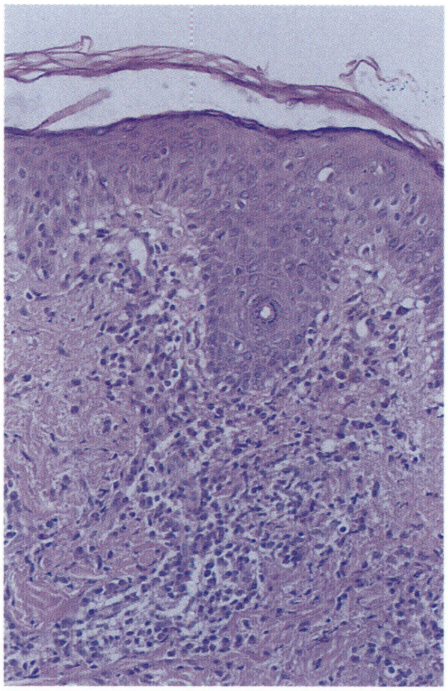

Figure 20–26. High magnification of secondary syphilis discloses a lymphoplasmacytic infiltrate with occasional histiocytes that infiltrates epithelium. Special stains revealed the presence of spirochetes.

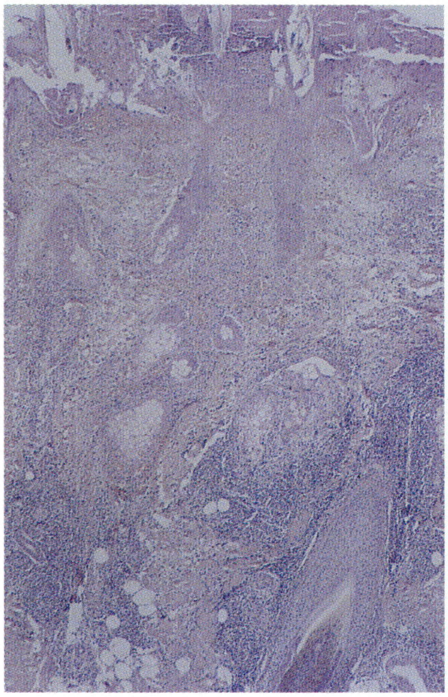

Figure 20–27. Herpes zoster of the scalp. There are broad zones of epidermal and superficial follicular necrosis. Note the depth of the inflammatory infiltrate.

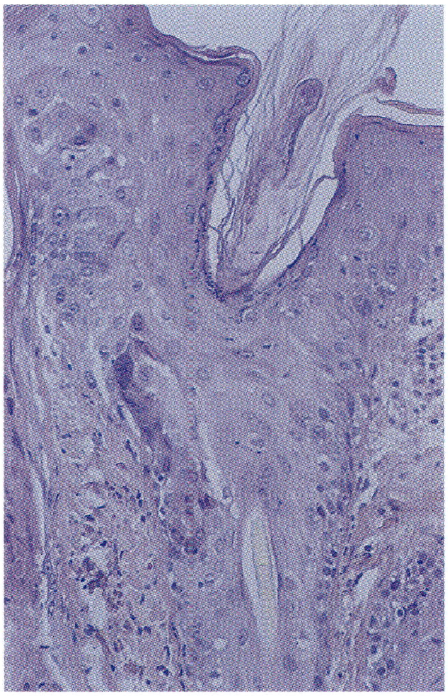

Figure 20–28. Follicular keratinocytes in herpes zoster acquire a wind-blown, disarrayed appearance. Note the early formation of multinucleated keratinocytes with nuclear molding *(center right)*. These changes are characteristic of the herpesvirus cytopathic effect.

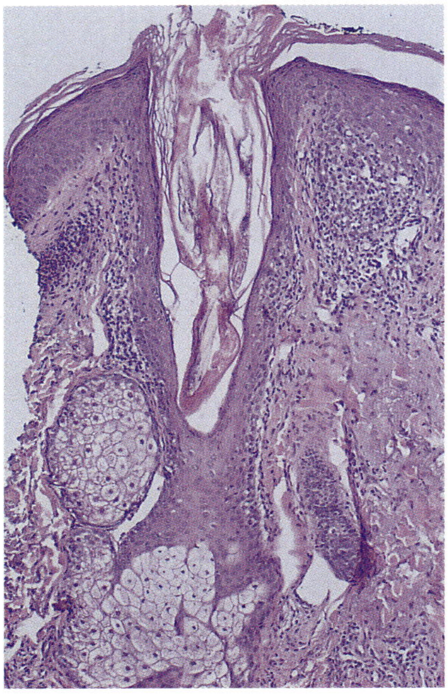

Figure 20–29. *Demodex folliculorum.* The mite is embedded head-first into an ectatic follicular orifice.

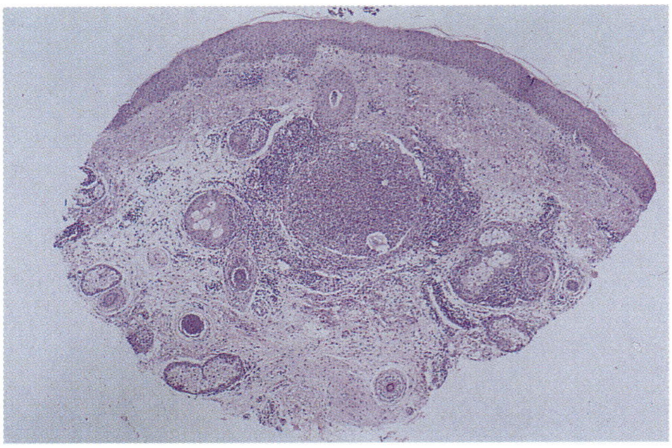

Figure 20–30. A dermal abscess is produced at the level of a follicular infundibulum infected with *Demodex.*

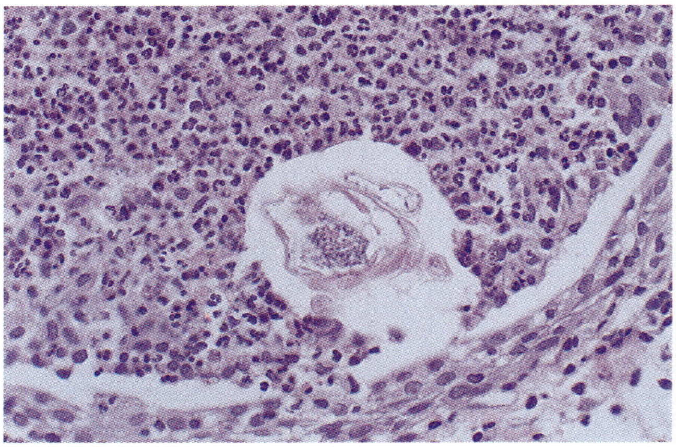

Figure 20–31. High magnification of Figure 20–30 shows the abscess abutting remnant follicular epithelium and surrounding a *Demodex* organism.

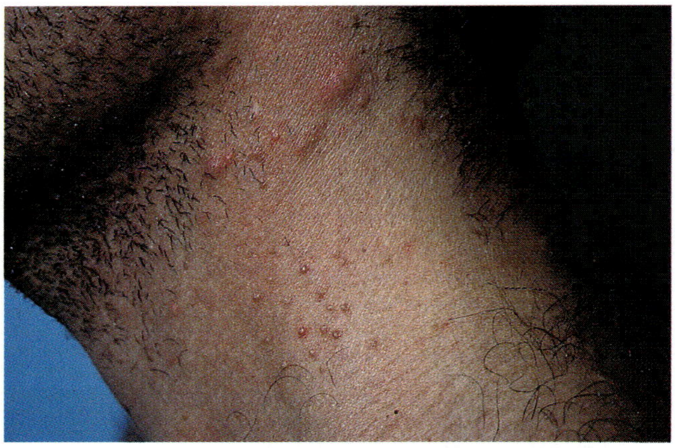

Figure 20–32. Eosinophilic pustular folliculitis. Erythematous perifollicular papules are seen on the neck and beard area of an HIV-infected patient.

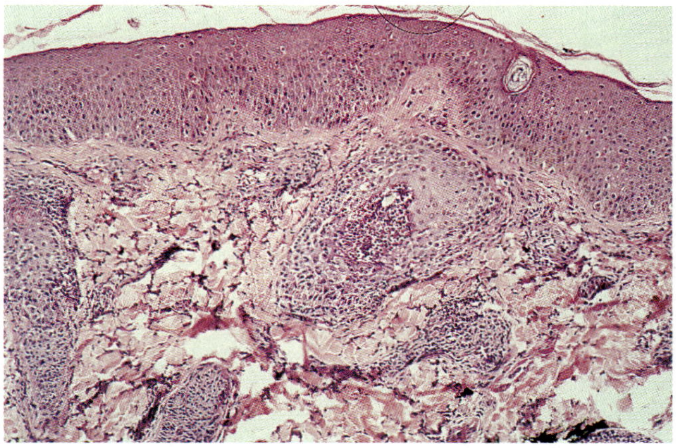

Figure 20–33. Eosinophilic pustular folliculitis. Discrete zones of inflammation are concentrated around hair follicles.

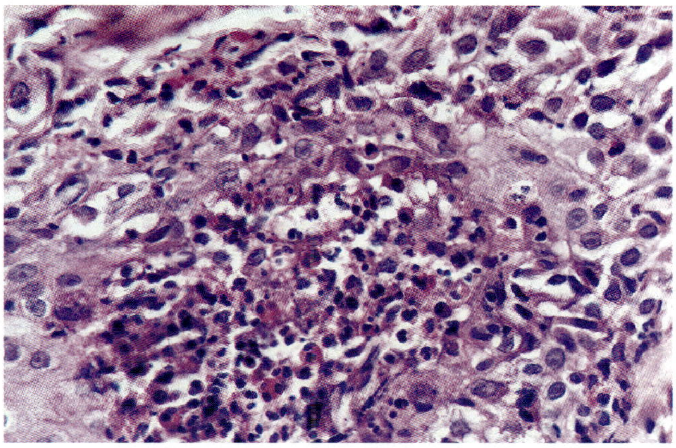

Figure 20–34. Higher magnification of Figure 20–33 discloses that follicular epithelium is disrupted by collections of eosinophils admixed with rare lymphocytes. Special stains are negative for fungal elements.

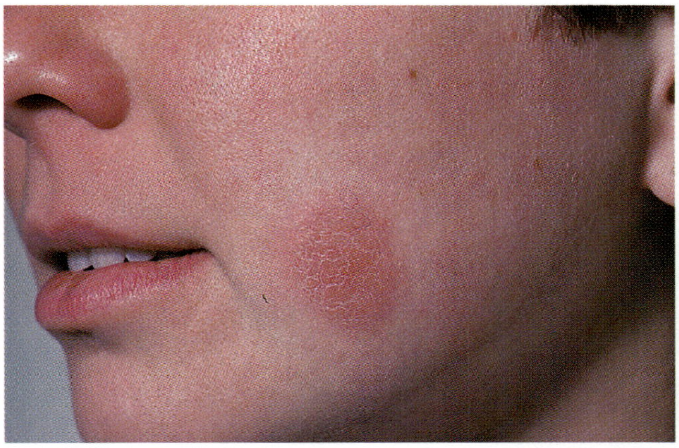

Figure 20–35. Follicular mucinosis. A discrete plaque of erythema and crusting is present on the cheek of a young woman.

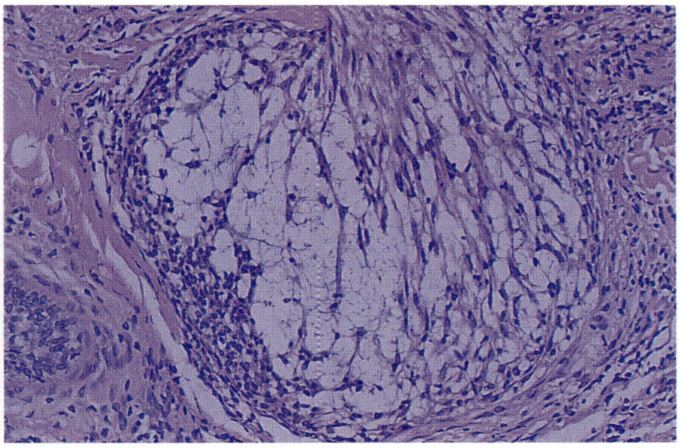

Figure 20–36. The reticulated pattern of follicular and sebaceous epithelium in follicular mucinosis is caused by deposition of mucopolysaccharides (*i.e.*, mucin) between epithelial cells. Mucin forms cyst-like cavities in these areas. There is a perifollicular and intrafollicular lymphocytic infiltrate with occasional eosinophils.

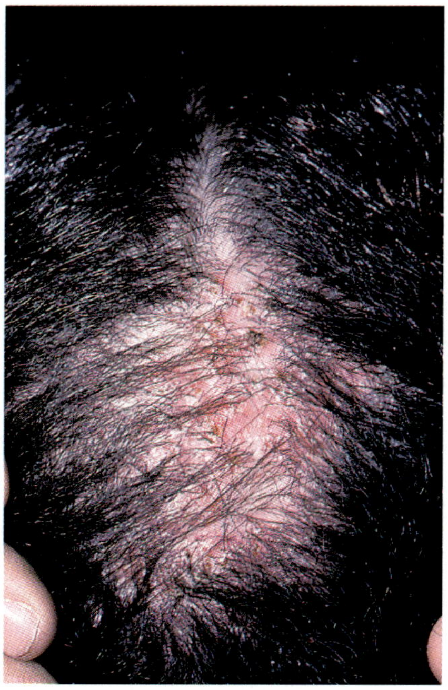

Figure 20–37. Follicular decalvans. Perifollicular pustules and crusting surround intact hair follicles. There is a background of erythema and a localized decrease in hair density.

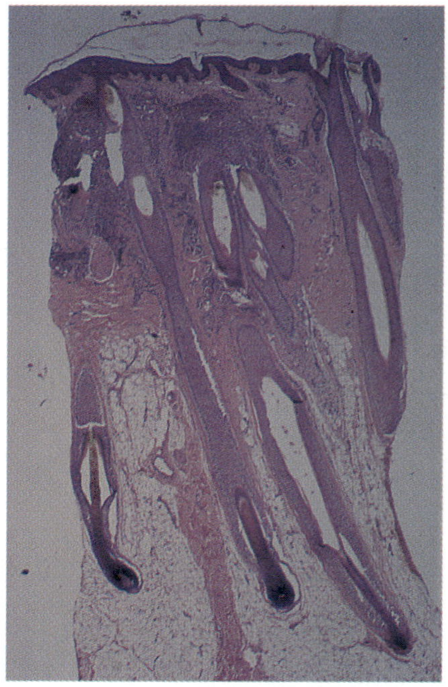

Figure 20–38. Dense inflammation is present about the superficial portions of hair follicles in folliculitis decalvans.

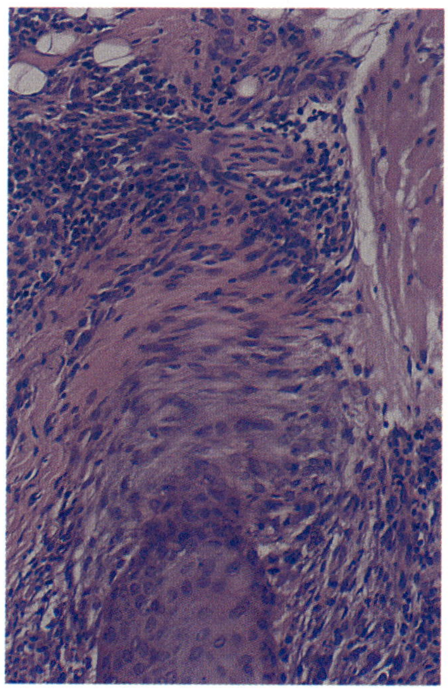

Figure 20–39. Advanced lesions of folliculitis decalvans show perifollicular fibrosis and lymphoplasmacytic infiltrates enmeshed in scar.

Reversible Alopecia: Alopecia Areata

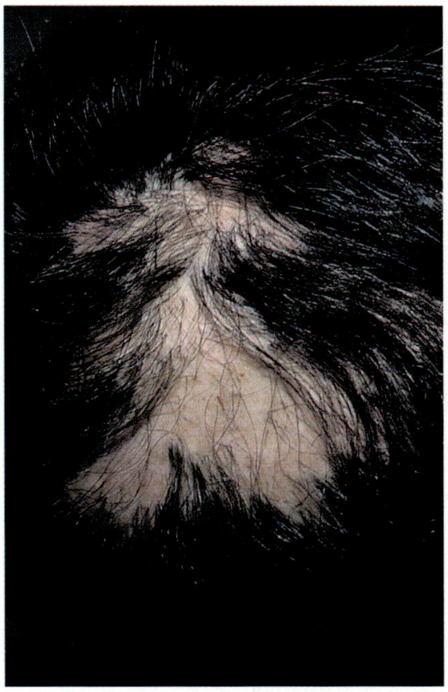

Figure 20–40. Alopecia areata. Areas of hair loss, within which are hair shafts with tapered ends known as "exclamation-point hairs."

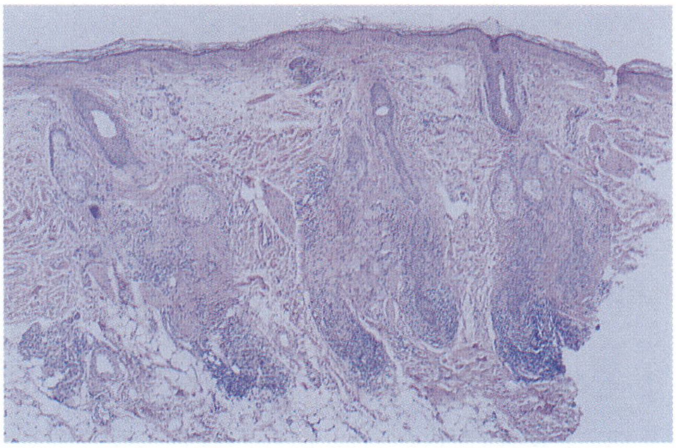

Figure 20–41. Alopecia areata. Intense inflammatory infiltrates are seen around multiple follicular papillae.

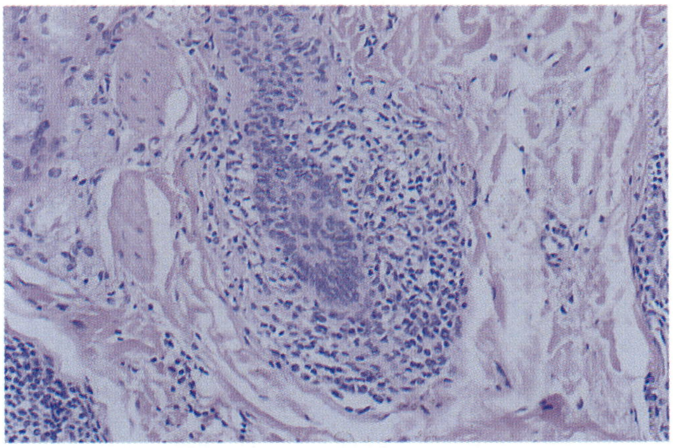

Figure 20–42. The intense lymphocytic infiltrate of alopecia areata surrounds a hair papilla, mimicking a swarm of bees.

Irreversible Alopecia

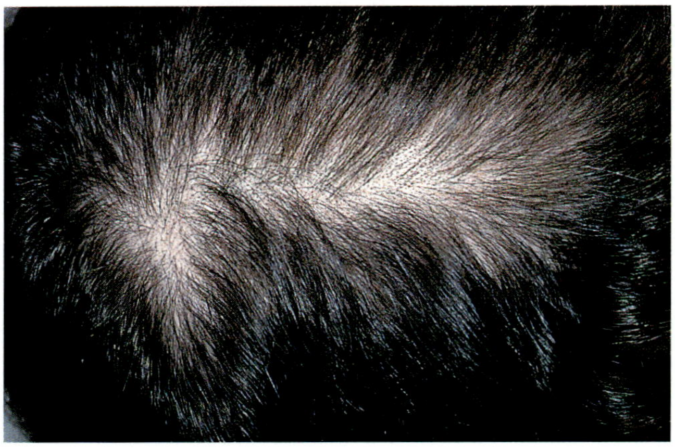

Figure 20–43. Androgenic alopecia. Thinning of the crown has occurred in an adult woman.

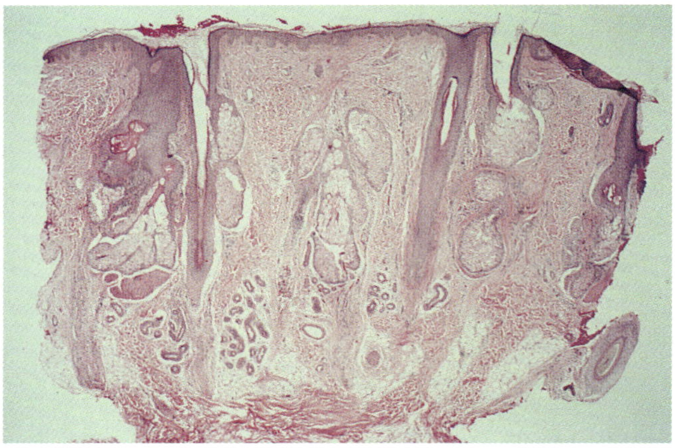

Figure 20–44. Two terminal anagen hair follicles are present in this biopsy of androgenic alopecia. Centrally, there are mature sebaceous glands around a miniaturized hair follicle.

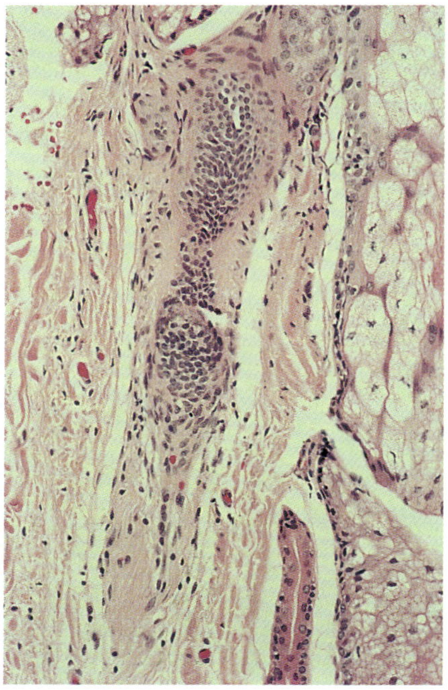

Figure 20–45. In androgenic alopecia, there is marked diminution of the caliber of a telogen hair follicle and thickening of the perifollicular sheath.

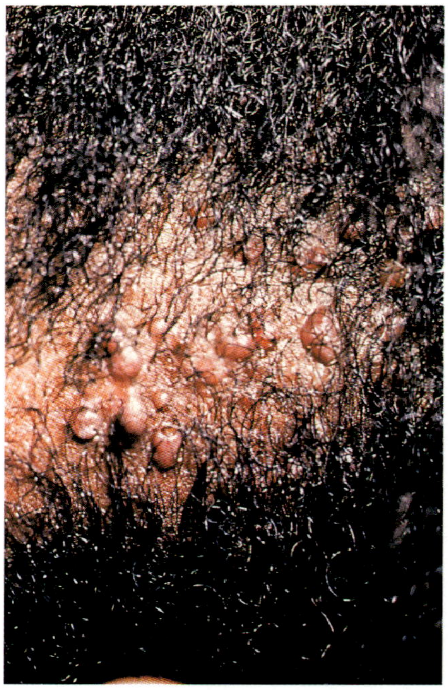

Figure 20–46. Acne keloidalis: Firm, flesh-colored, perifollicular papules stud the nape of the neck.

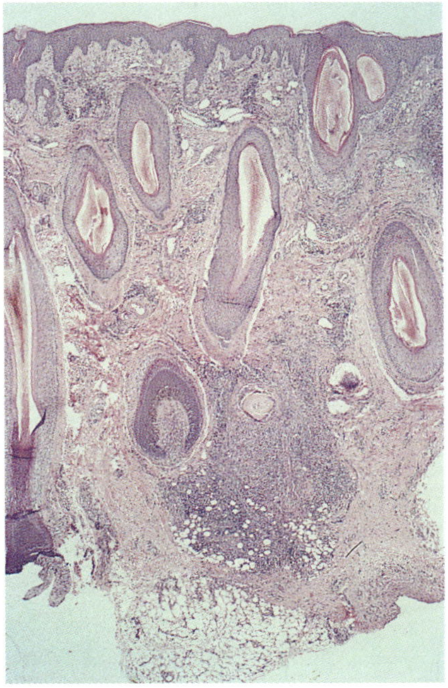

Figure 20–47. Pseudofolliculitis barbae: Biopsy specimen from the beard area shows a focus of intense inflammation in the deep dermis.

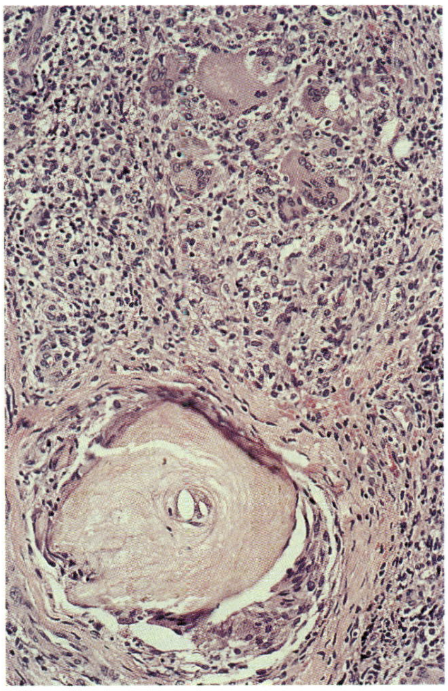

Figure 20–48. Higher magnification of Figure 20–47 shows a granulomatous infiltrate surrounding a hair shaft with an attached remnant of follicular epithelium.

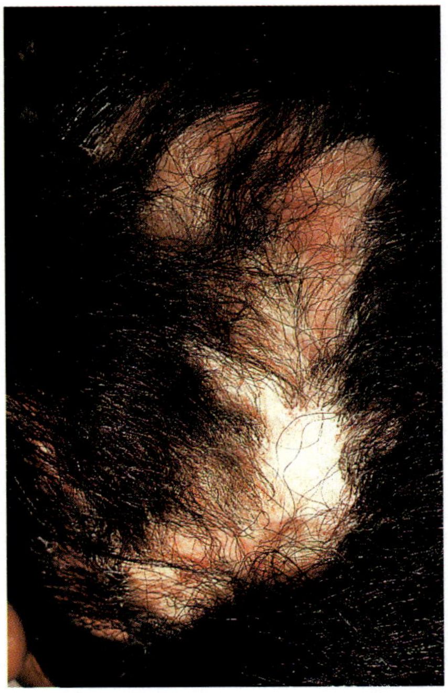

Figure 20–49. Lupus erythematosus alopecia. Multiple patches of hair loss are present in the scalp. Many show prominent erythema; centrally, the white areas correlate with zones of scarring.

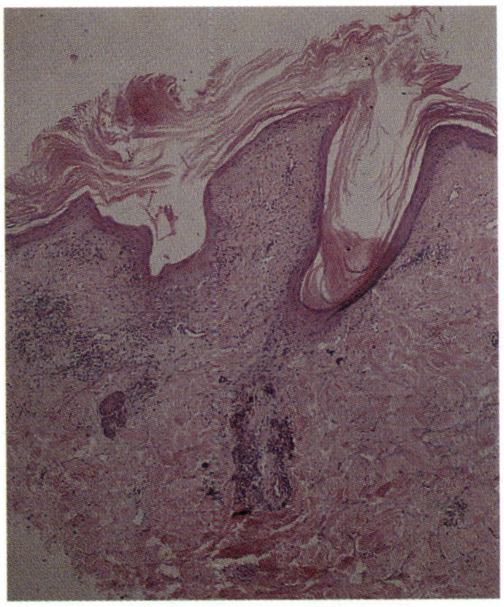

Figure 20–50. In lupus erythematosus alopecia, there is prominent follicular ectasia and plugging. The undulating rete ridge pattern of the epidermis is lost, and hyperkeratosis is present.

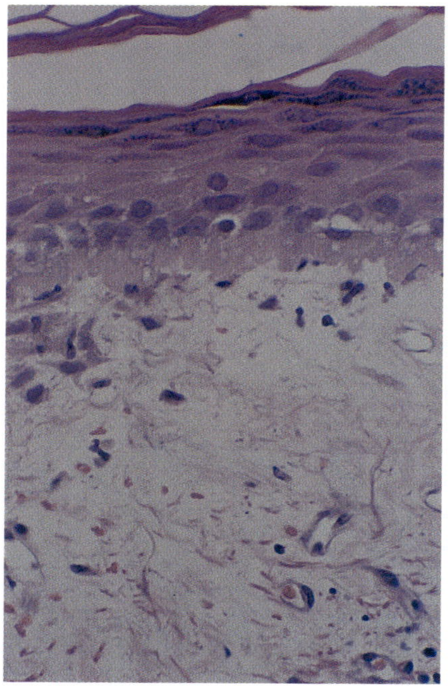

Figure 20–51. There is prominent thickening and tortuosity of the basement membrane in lupus erythematosus alopecia. The dermis contains abundant mucin.

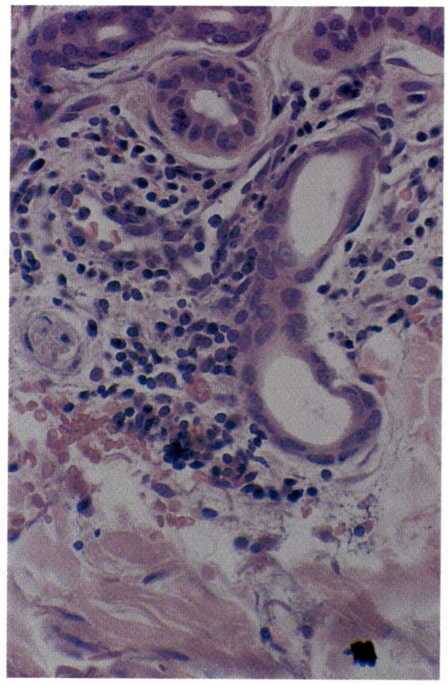

Figure 20–52. A lymphoplasmacytic inflammatory infiltrate commonly surrounds eccrine glands in the deep dermal stroma, an important clue to the diagnosis of lupus erythematosus alopecia.

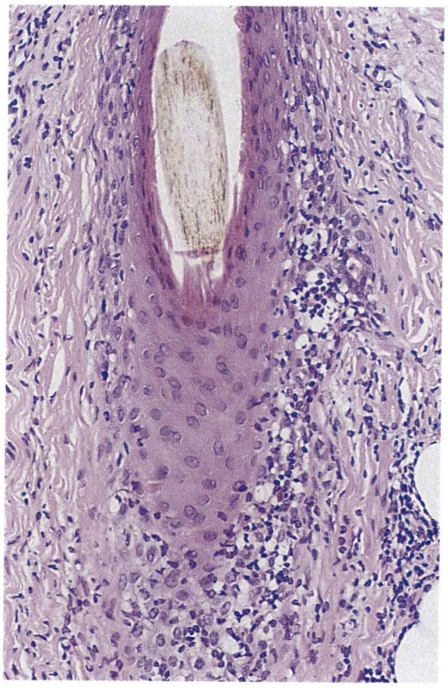

Figure 20–53. Lichen planopilaris. A band-like infiltrate surrounds the upper half of a hair follicle and extends along adjacent interfollicular epithelium.

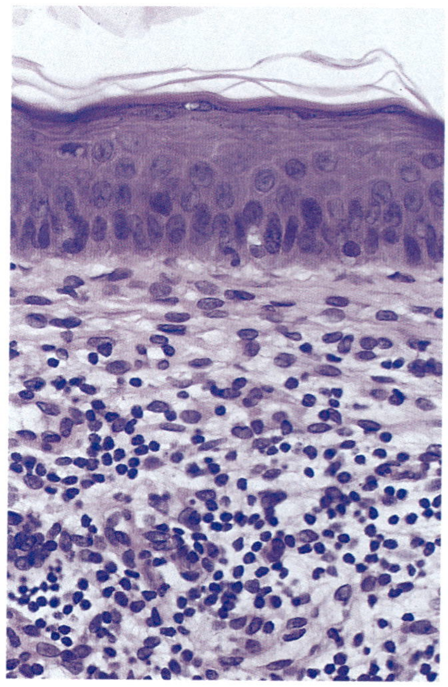

Figure 20–54. Interfollicular epithelium in lichen planopilaris shows loss of the rete ridge pattern but no thickening of the basement membrane as in lupus erythematosus alopecia.

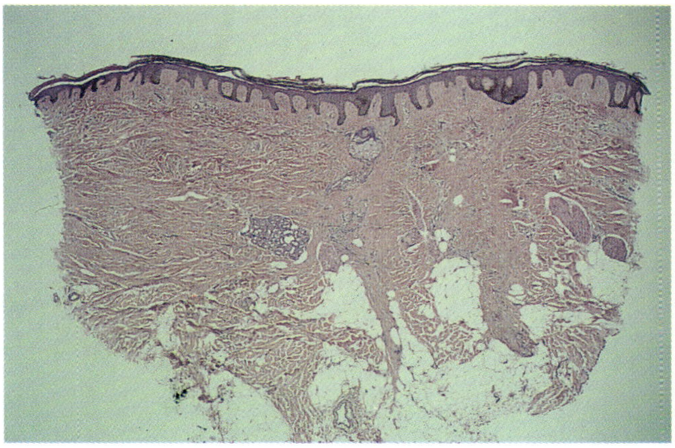

Figure 20–55. Pseudopelade. Complete loss of hair follicles has occurred. Only follicular tracts remain as indicators of previously cycling hairs at this site.

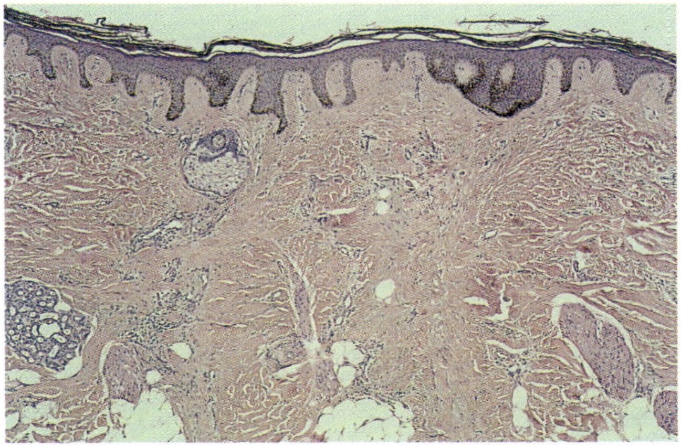

Figure 20–56. Rare appendages (*i.e.,* a sebaceous gland and pilar muscle) surround fibrotic tracts in pseudopelade. Note the absence of inflammation.

21

Dermatopathology of Nails

Nails are similar to hair in that they are terminally differentiated cutaneous structures composed in part of keratin. Nails are usually found on the dorsal surface of each digit and have, at least in part, a protective function for the specialized tactile units of fingers and toes. They may also enhance tactile sensitivity and the ability to perform precise mechanical functions. Unlike hair, however, the growth of nails has not been categorized into different phases of a growth cycle.

The most apparent portion of the nail, the nail plate, is synthesized by the nail matrix, much like the hair shaft is synthesized by the hair matrix. The nail matrix is located beneath the proximal nail fold, or cuticle. It is composed of germinative cells and variable numbers of melanocytes. The germinative cells divide and differentiate into cells that keratinize to form the nail plate, and the melanocytes contribute melanin granules to keratinocytes.

As it grows, the nail plate moves along the surface of the subjacent nail bed. The nail bed has a longitudinally grooved configuration that supports a rich supply of blood vessels and nerves. The elongated appearance of splinter hemorrhages correlates with the orientation of blood vessels within these longitudinal grooves. Dermal blood flow is carefully regulated by arteriovenous anastomoses known as glomus bodies. Glomus bodies function as thermoregulators as well as pressure regulators that maintain arterial blood pressure in the digits.

Changes in the nails and surrounding soft tissues may be clues to cutaneous or systemic diseases. Examples of the latter include ragged-appearing nail folds with tortuous capillary loops in systemic lupus erythematosus and dermatomyositis. Firm brown-yellow papules and nodules near the proximal nail fold and dorsal aspect of the distal interphalangeal joint suggest the possibility of multicentric reticulohistiocytosis. Half-and-half nails (the distal half of the plate is red to brown and the proximal half is white) are seen with renal failure. Many hereditary diseases have associated nail changes, including psoriasis, alopecia areata, and lichen planus. Usually, changes characteristic of these disorders are present concurrently elsewhere on the integument, so with these disorders, nail biopsies are performed infrequently.

In general, nail biopsies are performed much less often than biopsies elsewhere on the skin. Nail biopsy or surgery requires technical expertise, because in many instances it requires removal of the nail plate and care in manipulation of the nail matrix. If the nail matrix is unaltered by the procedure, the nail plate will slowly regenerate over the course of several months. If it is injured, permanent nail deformity will result. For these reasons, nail surgery is not undertaken for trivial reasons.

Normal Anatomy

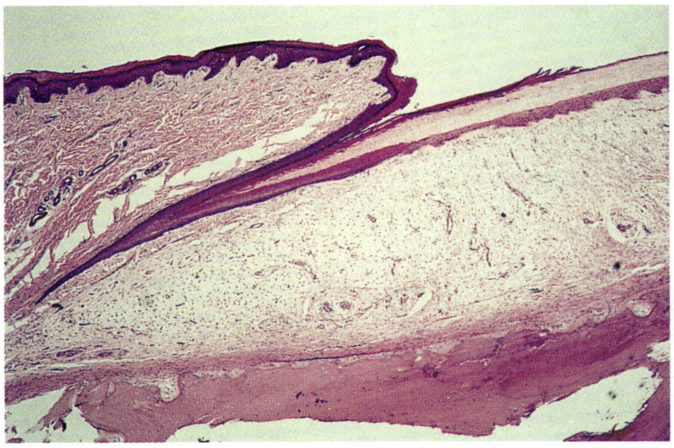

Figure 21–1. Panoramic view of a normal nail. The nail plate exits from beneath the proximal nail fold. Beneath the nail plate is the nail matrix proximally *(left)* and nail bed distally *(right)*. Bone is present at the deep portion of the specimen *(bottom)*.

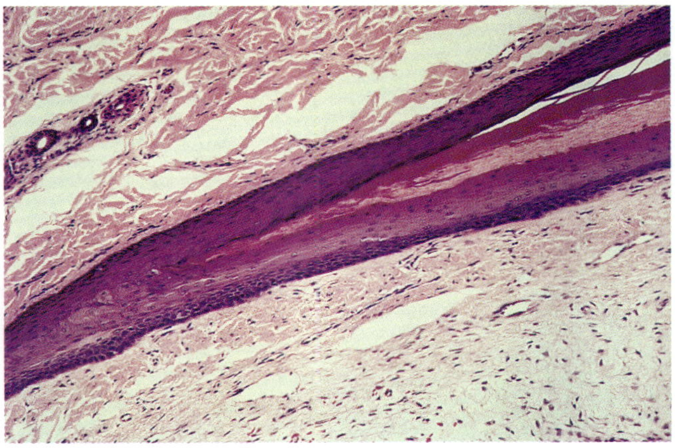

Figure 21–2. Synthesis of the nail plate occurs in the area of the proximal nail fold and nail matrix.

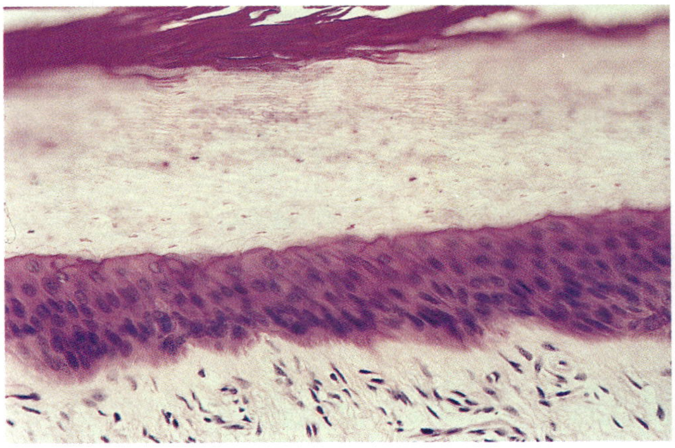

Figure 21–3. The nail bed is seen with its undulating dermal-epithelial junction *(bottom)* and overlying nail plate *(upper half)*.

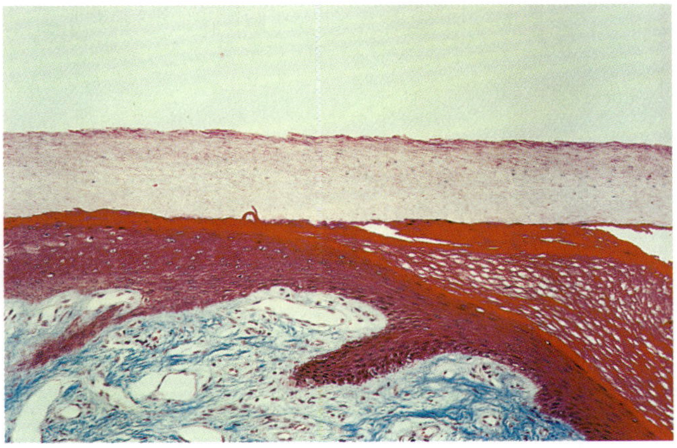

Figure 21–4. The hyponychium is the place where the nail plate meets the stratum corneum at the distal end of the nail *(central horizontal plane)*. Subungual keratotic debris collects in the hyponychium in pathologic states *(trichrome stain)*.

Mechanical Injury

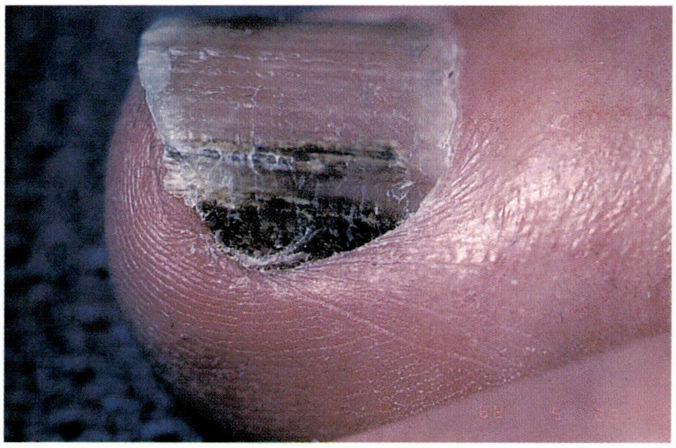

Figure 21–5. Subungual hemorrhage: A pigmented band on the lateral edge of the great toe nail.

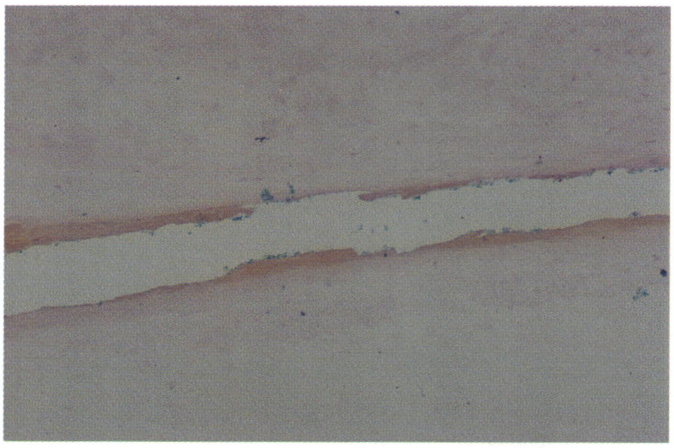

Figure 21–6. The removed nail plate seen in Figure 21–5 shows a split in the plate, which contains erythrocytes. Prussian blue stain confirms the presence of iron (hemosiderin) in the nail plate from prior hemorrhage.

Infection

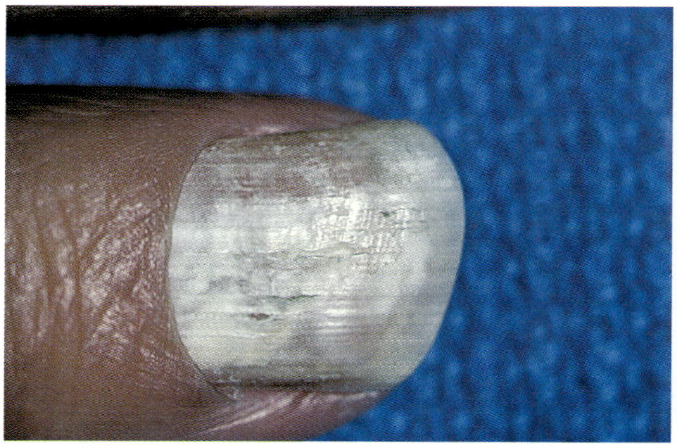

Figure 21–7. Onychomycosis. An opaque nail plate has ridging on the surface and yellow discoloration laterally. Periodic acid–Schiff stain reveals septate branching hyphae in the nail plate.

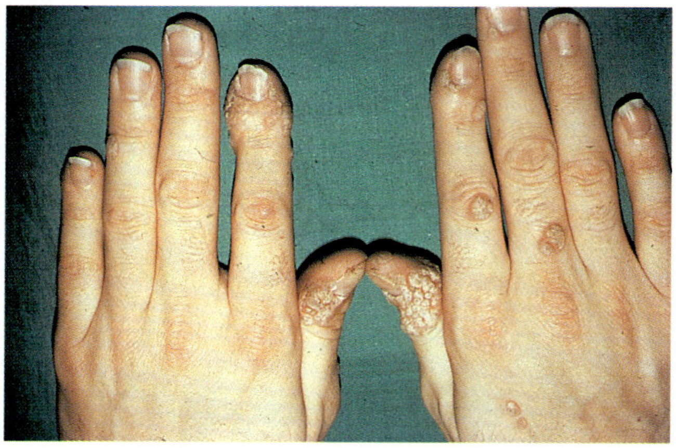

Figure 21–8. Verruca vulgaris of the fingers and nails. Multiple verrucous scaly nodules on slightly erythematous bases are present around the nails and on the knuckles.

Lichen Planus

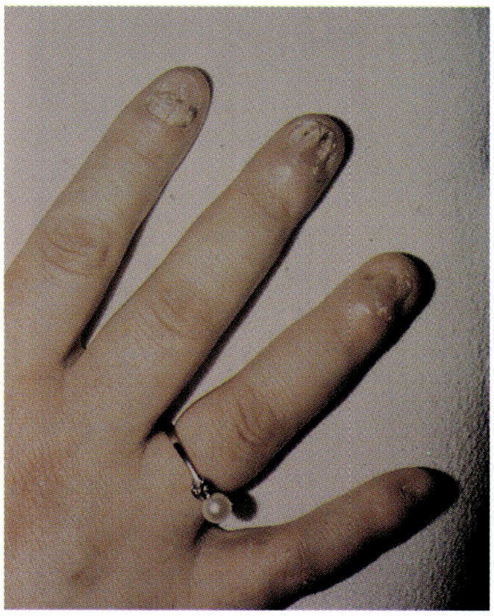

Figure 21–9. Lichen planus of the nails. Marked dystrophy of the nail plate and pterygium formation are present.

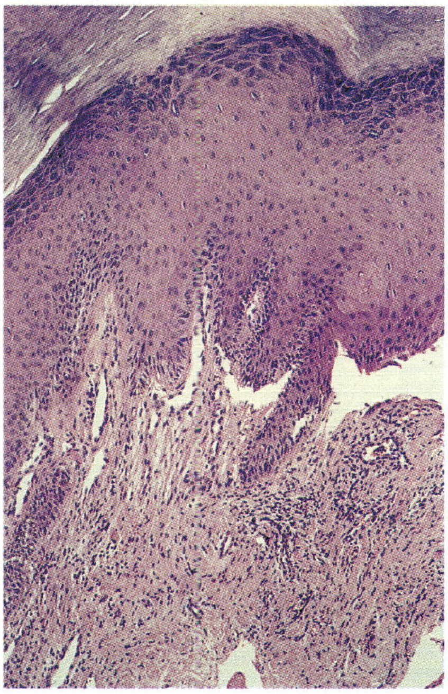

Figure 21–10. There is focal separation of the nail bed epithelium from the dermis and an inflammatory infiltrate in the dermal stroma.

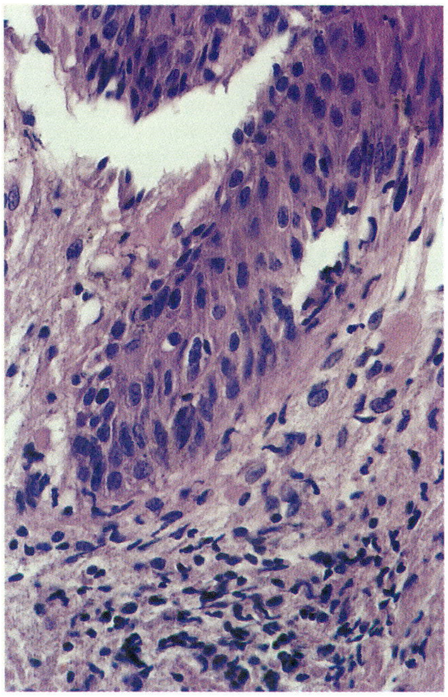

Figure 21–11. Lymphocytes tag the basilar layer of the nail bed. Focal basilar keratinocyte necrosis can be seen. These changes are similar to those of lichen planus located elsewhere on the skin.

Psoriasis

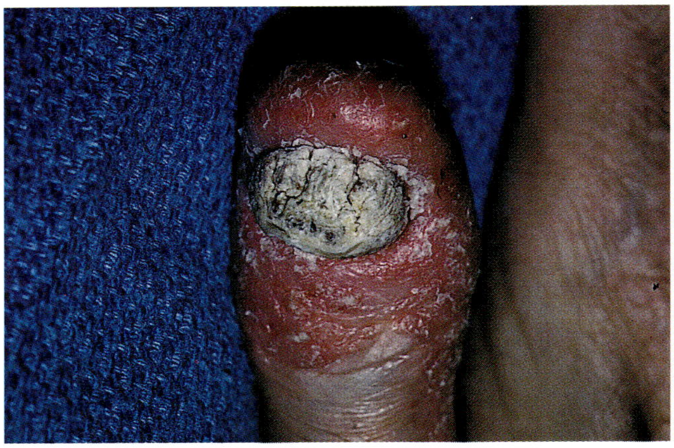

Figure 21–12. Psoriasis of the nail. The nail plate is yellow, friable, and raised by subungual debris. The surrounding skin is scaly and erythematous.

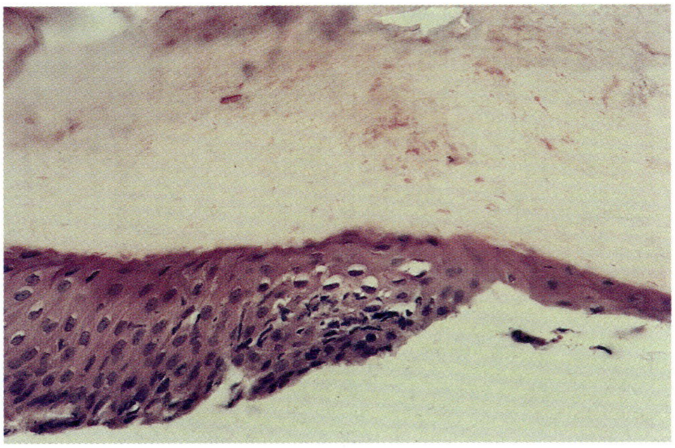

Figure 21–13. The nail bed is focally infiltrated by inflammatory cells.

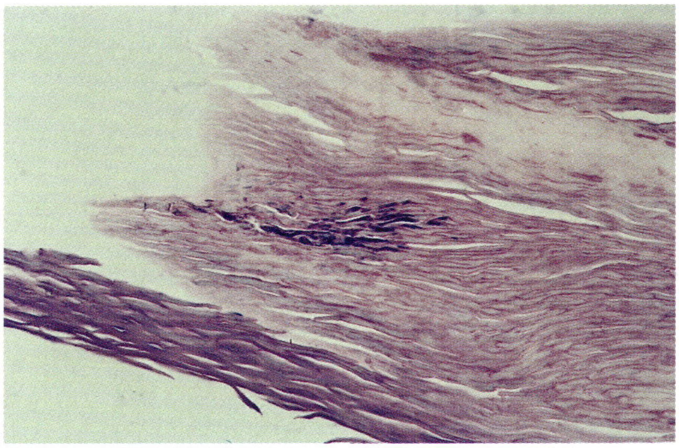

Figure 21–14. A collection of neutrophils is present in a parakeratotic focus of the nail plate. Periodic acid–Schiff stain was negative.

Neoplasms Affecting the Nail Bed, Matrix, or Plate

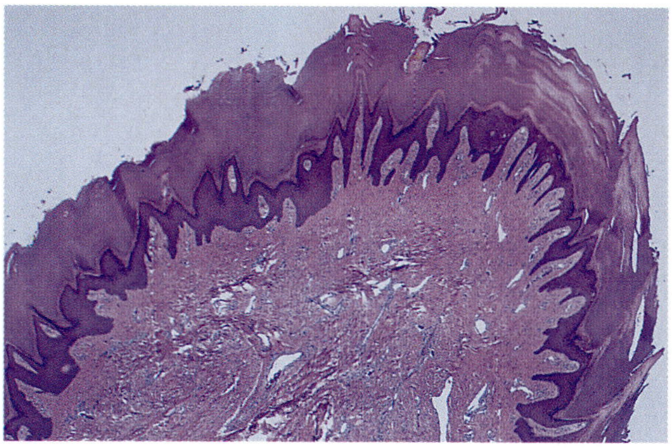

Figure 21–15. Acquired fibrokeratoma. An exophytic nodule is surrounded by hyperplastic epithelium and hyperorthokeratotic scale. The stroma contains collagen bundles and ectatic blood vessels.

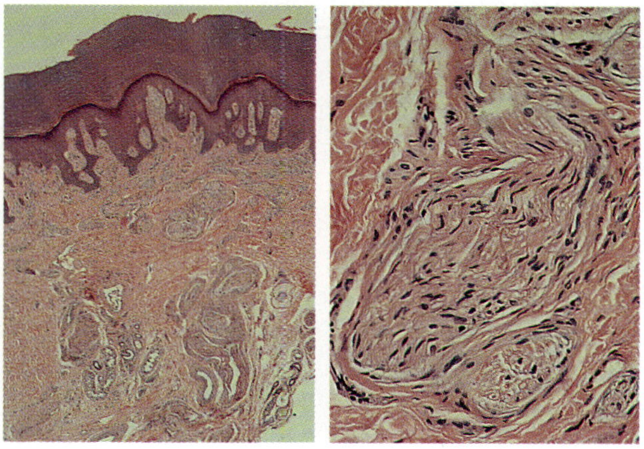

Figure 21–16. Accessory digit. Hyperplastic epithelium and hyperorthokeratotic scale surmount a dermis that contains collections of tortuous nerves *(left)*. Close-up of nerves in different planes of cross section *(right)*.

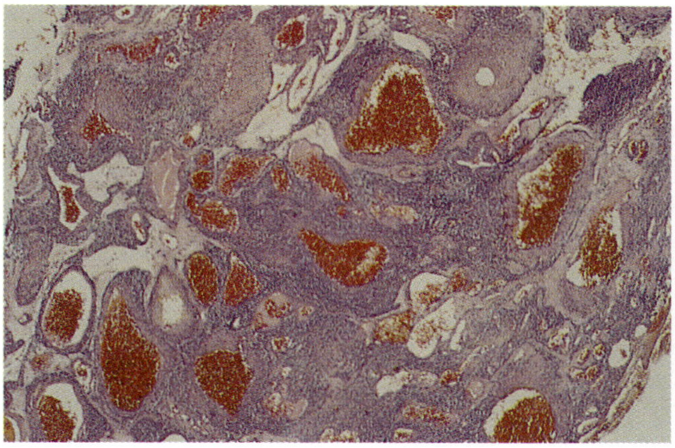

Figure 21–17. Glomus tumor. A collection of vascular spaces is surrounded by large numbers of basophilic cells.

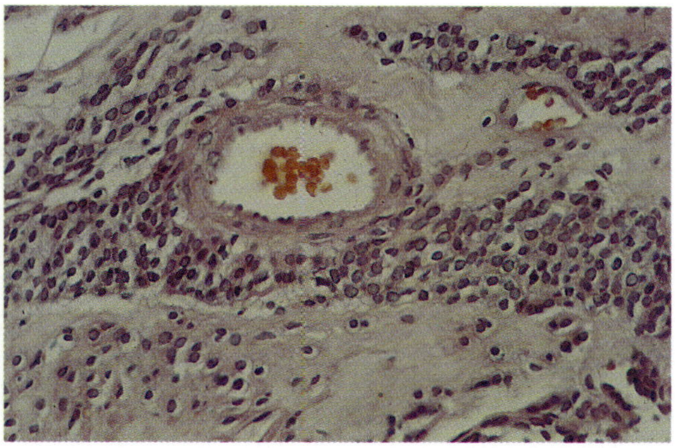

Figure 21–18. The blood vessels of glomus tumors are lined by endothelial cells and surrounded by a monotonous population of cells with round, basophilic nuclei.

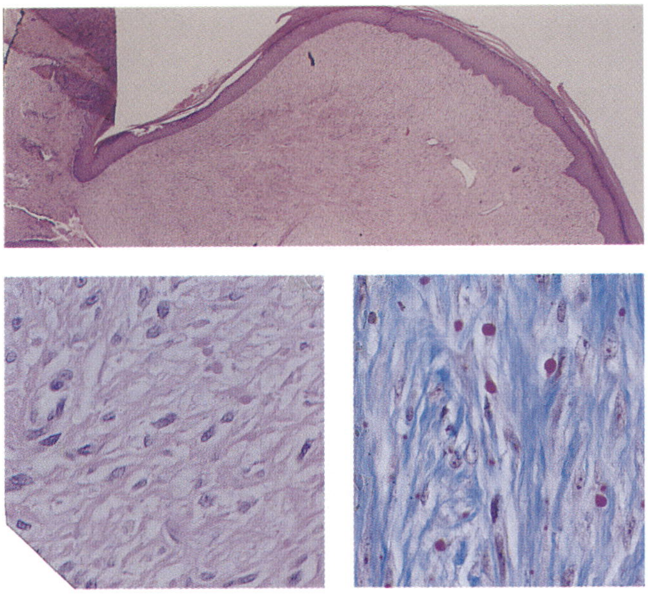

Figure 21–19. Infantile digital fibromatosis. A large exophytic nodule is surrounded by an epithelial collarette *(top of lesion to the right)*. In the stroma, there is a proliferation of fibroblast-like cells with intracytoplasmic, eosinophilic inclusion bodies *(bottom left)*. These inclusion bodies are easily discerned with Masson trichrome stain *(bottom right)*.

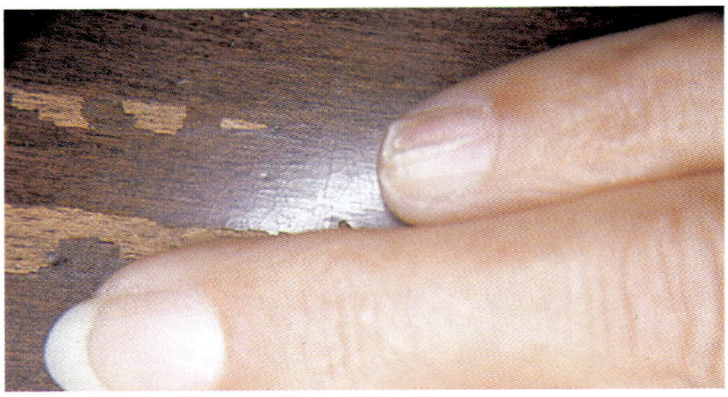

Figure 21–20. Digital myxoid cyst. An erythematous, dome-shaped nodule is present at the base of the nail on the fifth digit. The longitudinal groove in the nail plate occurred because the cyst impinges on the nail matrix.

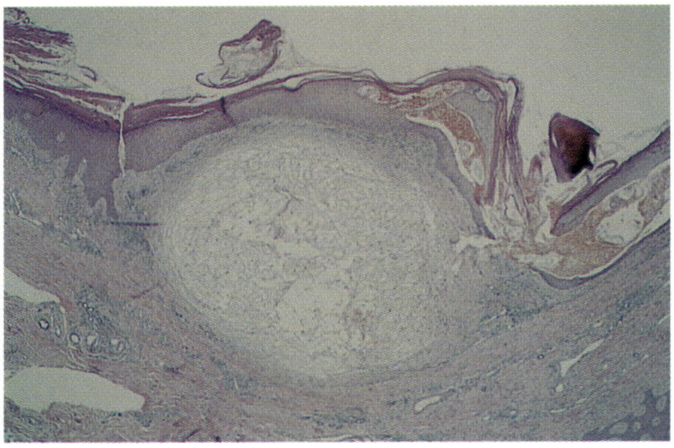

Figure 21–21. Digital myxoid cyst. A large, nodular collection of basophilic material expands the dermal stroma. Mucin is eliminated through the epidermis and into the stratum corneum.

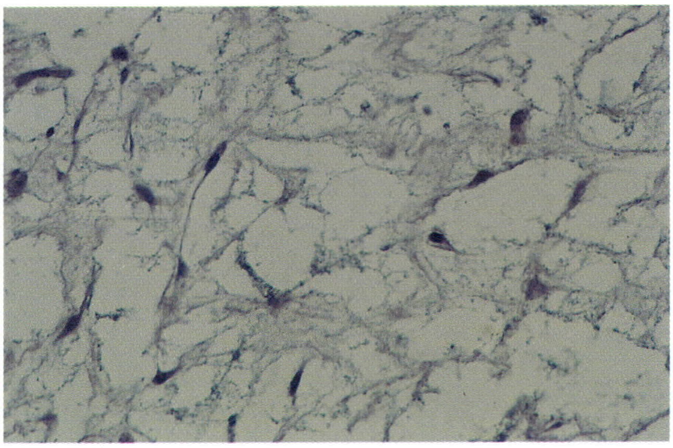

Figure 21–22. Dermal deposits of stringy, granular basophilic material characteristic of mucin are separated by stellate fibroblasts in a digital myxoid cyst.

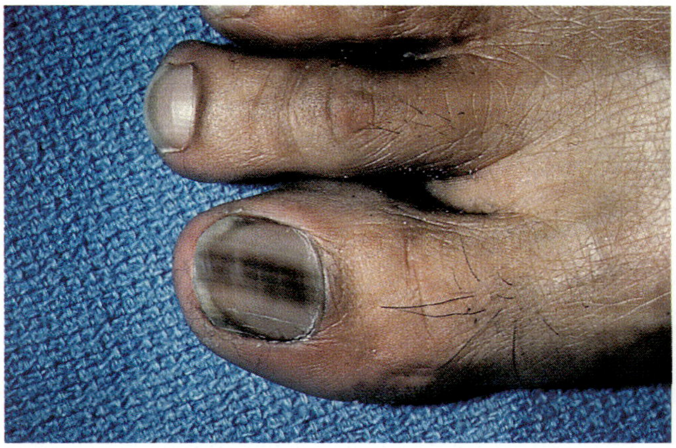

Figure 21–23. Lentigo of nail bed. A pigmented band in the nail of the great toe represents a lentigo of the nail bed.

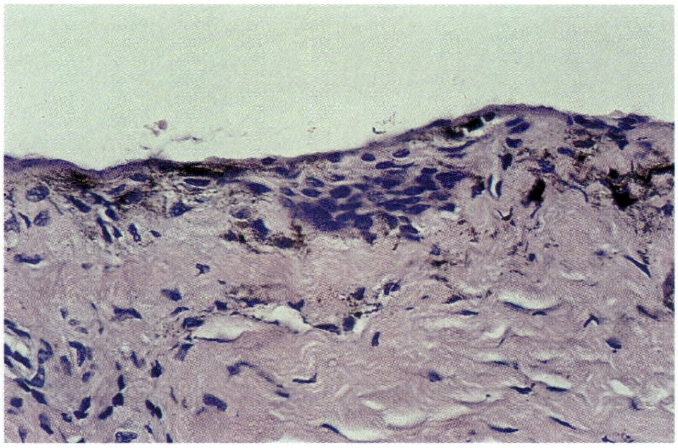

Figure 21–24. The basilar layer of nail bed epithelium in a lentigo shows increased numbers of melanocytes. There are melanophages in the superficial dermal stroma.

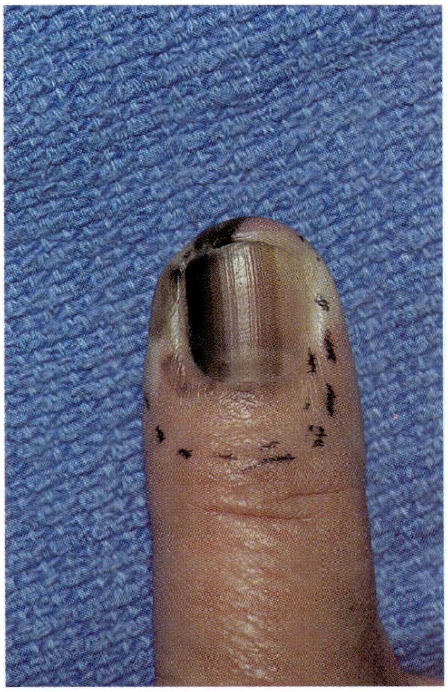

Figure 21–25. Acral lentiginous melanoma. A variegate band of brown-black pigment runs the length of the nail plate. Note the spillage of pigment onto the proximal and lateral nail folds.

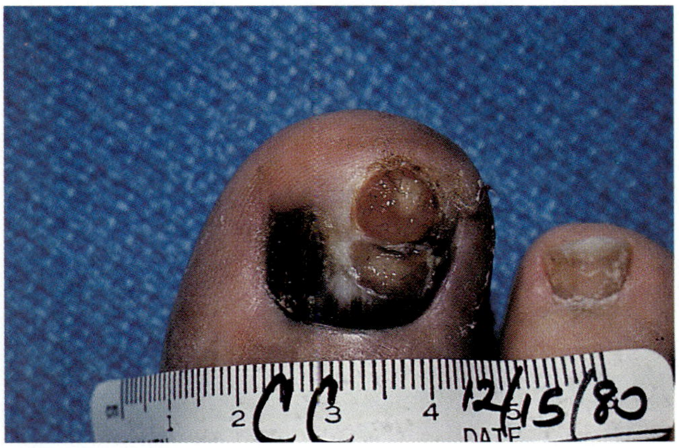

Figure 21–26. Complete loss of the nail plate in acral lentiginous melanoma. The nail bed is black. Centrally, there are two exophytic nodules representing the vertical growth phase. (Courtesy of the Pigmented Lesion Group at the University of Pennsylvania.)

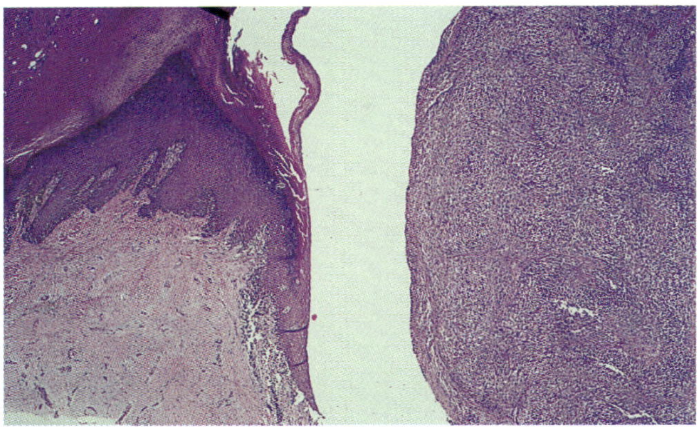

Figure 21–27. Scanning magnification of acral lentiginous melanoma shows a continuous proliferation of melanocytes along the basilar layer of the nail bed (*left:* radial growth phase) and a large exophytic nodule (*right:* vertical growth phase).

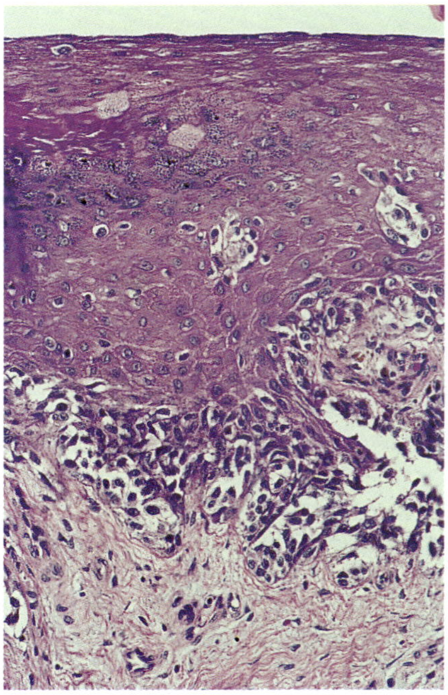

Figure 21–28. Pleomorphic melanocytes in the radial growth phase of acral lentiginous maligna melanoma grow in a continuous fashion along the basilar layer of epithelium with little tendency for upward growth of individual cells.

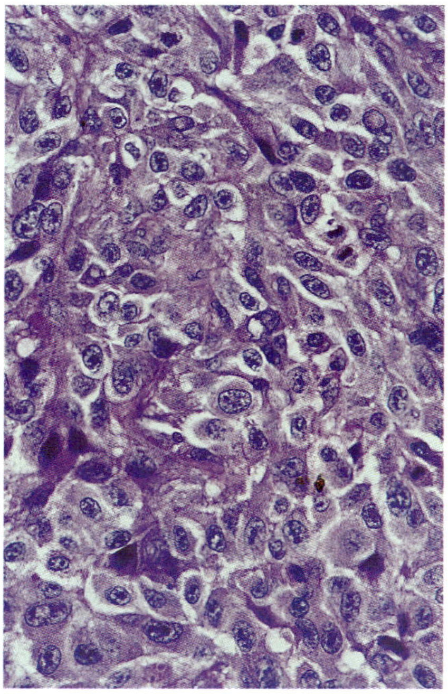

Figure 21–29. Cells of the vertical growth phase in acral lentiginous melanoma display a high degree of cytologic pleomorphism, abundant mitotic activity, and minimal pigment in their cytoplasms.

22

Dermatopathology of Anogenital Skin

Anogenital skin, especially the vulva, is prone to affliction by a variety of lesions that rarely affect other skin areas, probably because of local environmental factors. Clothing contributes to the unusual environment of anogenital skin by trapping heat and restricting air circulation; this creates a very moist environment with an increased hydrophilic state of the stratum corneum. Because the absorptive power of the skin is dependent on its state of hydration, the wet anogenital area is far more absorptive of extrinsic, and often irritating, substances than is extragenital skin. The apposition of anogenital skin folds, particular in obese persons, leads to skin friction and consequent chronic irritation in a mucosa that is inherently easily irritated. All of these factors lead to an environment conducive to the growth of bacteria and fungi. Because many sexually transmitted organisms also affect the anogenital skin, diagnostic confusion concerning otherwise characteristic histopathologic entities may result from both a gross and microscopic perspective because of the superimposed changes of sexually transmitted diseases and local environmental factors.

The skin of the labia majora is identical to extragenital skin. Hair follicles are present on the lateral aspects of the labia majora but are absent on the medial aspects. Because squamous vulvar intraepithelial neoplasia (VIN), Paget cells, and melanoma cells may extend into the hair sheaths and its associated pilosebaceous unit, these structures must be encompassed in any treatment modality for VIN; consequently, the excision or ablation must be of sufficient depth (at least 3 to 4 mm) to ensure their destruction. Hart line marks the demarcation between the skin and mucous membrane of the vulva. This line extends in a curvilinear fashion, starting anteriorly from the medial aspect of the labia majora, extending to the most inferoposterior aspect of the labia minora, and ending posteriorly at the vaginal fourchette. Sebaceous glands are present medial and posterior to the labia minora at the junction with Hart line, and these open directly onto the epithelial surface, resulting in small, pale-yellow elevations known as Fordyce spots. The vulvar epithelium contains melanocytes, and increased pigmentation may result from hormonal influences. Langerhans cells and Merkel cells are present in the vulva, as in other skin sites.

The vulvar vestibule is that portion of the vulva demarcated by the clitoris anteriorly, fourchette posteriorly, labia minora anterolaterally, and Hart line posterolaterally. The skin in this area is of endodermal origin; the remainder is of ectodermal origin. The squamous epithelium of the vestibule is predominantly nonkeratinized, whereas that of the labia minora, fourchette, and prepuce is thinly keratinized. In women of reproductive age, the squamous epithelium is well glycogenated. The high moisture content of this area may affect the appearance of dermatoses; in particular, scaling may be much less obvious.

The mucous membrane of the glans penis is composed of nonglycogenated stratified squamous epithelium that is keratinized in the circumcised male and nonkeratinized in the uncircumcised male. A lamina propria and the corpus spongiosum lie beneath the epidermis; normal skin adnexal structures are not present in the glands. The outer surface of the foreskin has a dermis containing a few sebaceous and sweat glands. The inner surface of the foreskin is lined by a mucosa identical to that of the glands. The epidermis of the penile shaft is thin and minimally keratinized. Few sebaceous and sweat glands are present, and hair follicles are present in the proximal portion. As in the vulva, the skin is relatively hyperpigmented.

Perianal skin is keratinized and contains sweat glands as well as apocrine glands, sebaceous glands, and hair follicles.

Most dermatologic conditions affecting extragenital skin can also affect anogenital skin. Herpes virus infection and specific dermatoses such as psoriasis and lichen planus are illustrated elsewhere in this atlas and are repeated in this section. Benign melanocytic lesions such as freckles and nevi, as well as adnexal tumors, occurring on anogenital skin are identical grossly and microscopically to those elsewhere; of the adnexal tumors, the most common is the papillary hidradenoma, a benign eccrine tumor seen more frequently in the vulva. Consequently, the lesions covered in this section are restricted to those characteristically found in anogenital skin or those that have a prognosis or presentation that is altered by this location. In addition, because the preponderance of non-neoplastic, infectious, and intraepithelial and invasive carcinomas that afflict the anogenital skin affect women, the illustrations emphasize those that involve the female genital tract.

Lichen Sclerosus

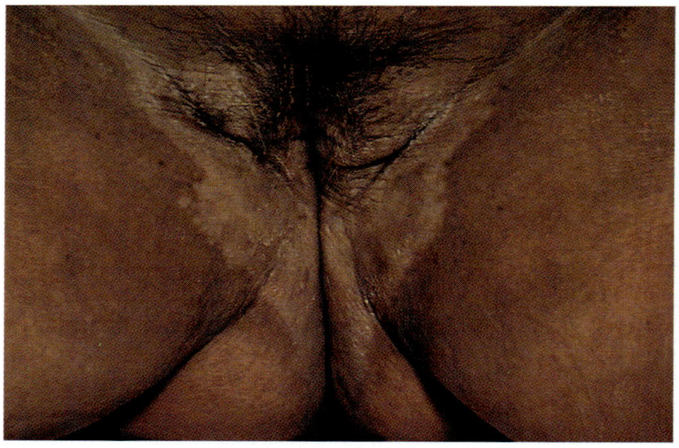

Figure 22–1. Lichen sclerosus. This whitish plaque has a characteristic bilaterally symmetric pattern (*i.e.,* butterfly pattern).

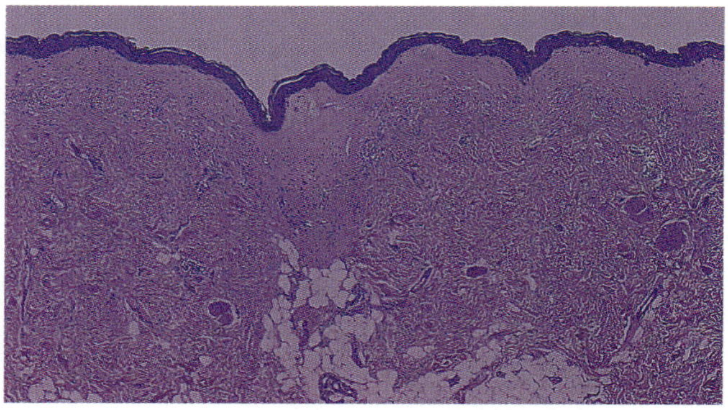

Figure 22–2. At scanning magnification, there is epidermal atrophy with loss of rete ridges and a pale band of hyalinized collagen within the superficial dermis.

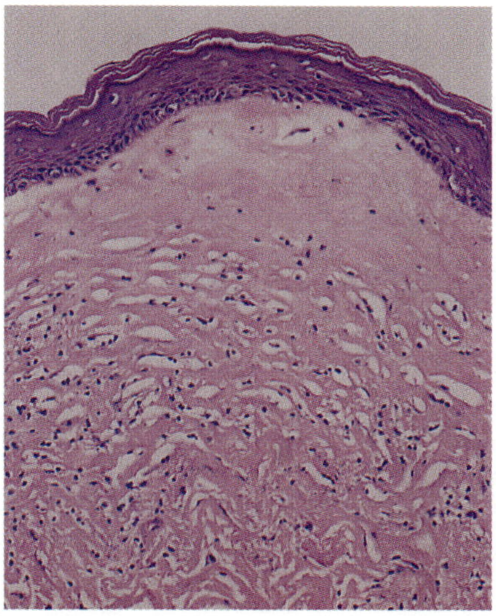

Figure 22–3. The hypocellular zone of hyalinization is better appreciated at higher magnification; note the absence of cellular atypia in the overlying epidermis.

Squamous Cell Hyperplasia

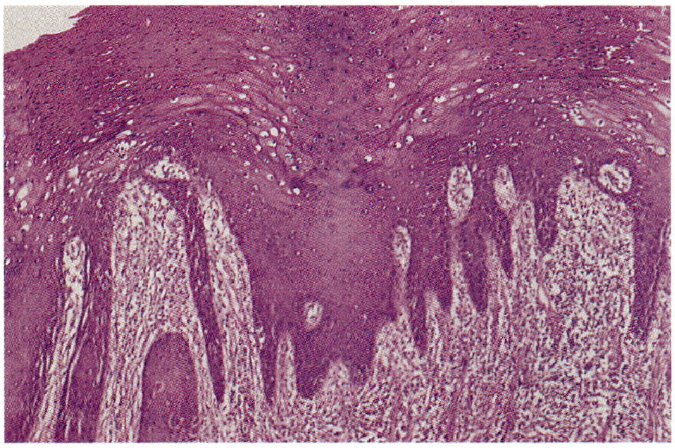

Figure 22–4. Squamous cell hyperplasia. There is marked irregular elongation of rete ridges in association with hyperkeratosis and parakeratosis.

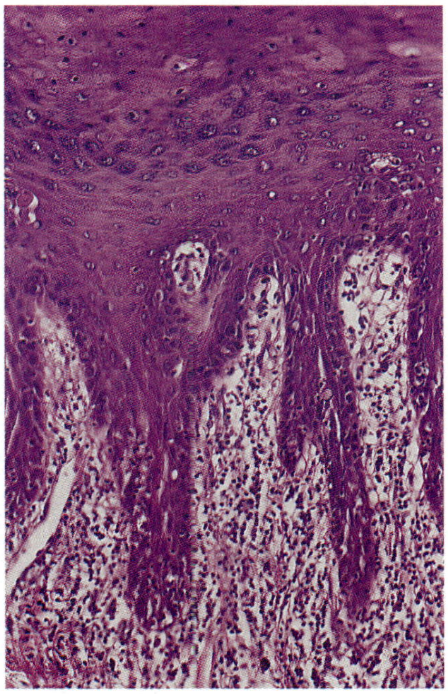

Figure 22–5. The dermis contains a nonspecific inflammatory infiltrate composed of lymphocytes and plasma cells; dysplasia is not present within the hyperplastic epidermal layer.

Condyloma Acuminatum

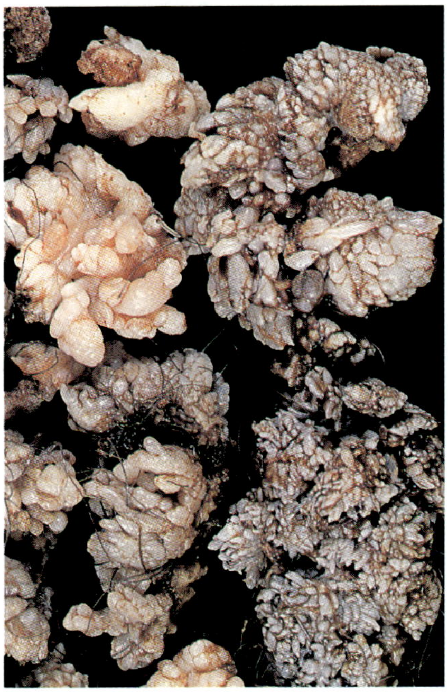

Figure 22–6. Condyloma acuminatum. These multiple cauliflower-like, endophytic lesions were surgically removed from the vulva.

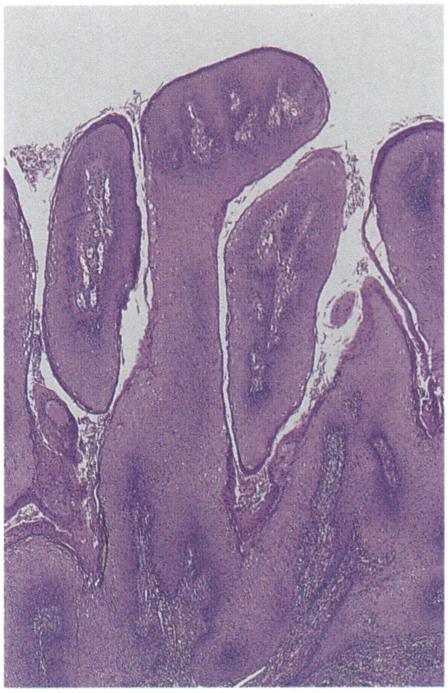

Figure 22–7. At scanning magnification, papillary fronds formed by delicate fibrovascular cores covered by acanthotic epithelium are seen.

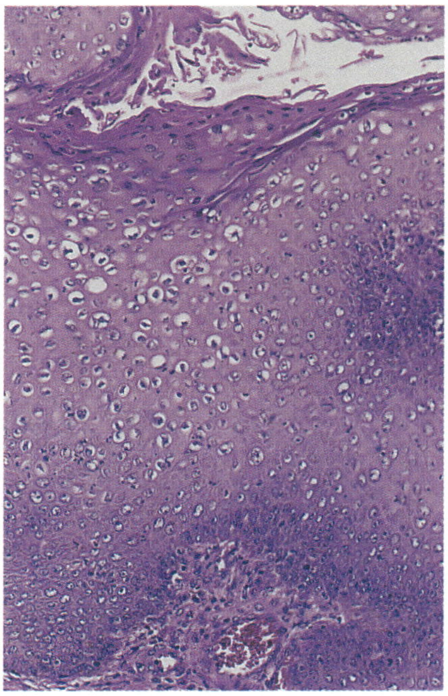

Figure 22–8. Higher magnification demonstrates superficial koilocytes with irregular nuclear contours and characteristic perinuclear clear spaces.

Vulvar Intraepithelial Neoplasia

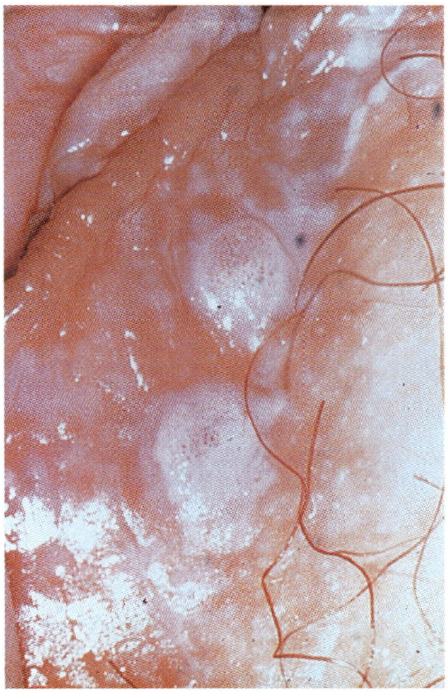

Figure 22–9. Vulvar intraepithelial neoplasia (VIN). Roughened, red-to-white lesions are present on the vulva and the vaginal introitus. Central white areas with punctate surface characteristics have been accentuated by the use of topical acetic acid.

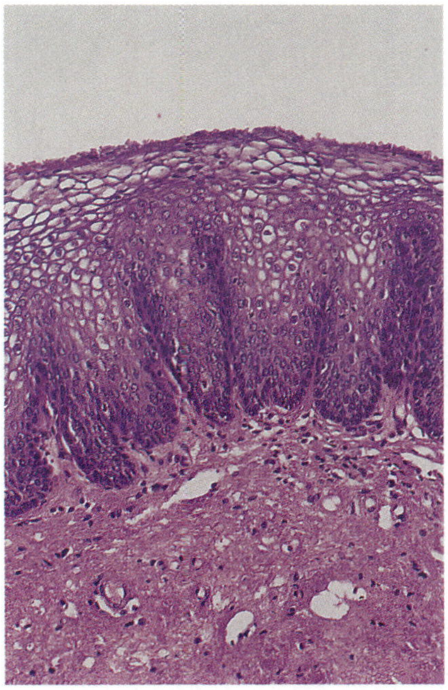

Figure 22–10. VIN I (*i.e.,* mild dysplasia) consists of dysplasia affecting cells confined to the lowermost third of the epithelial layer.

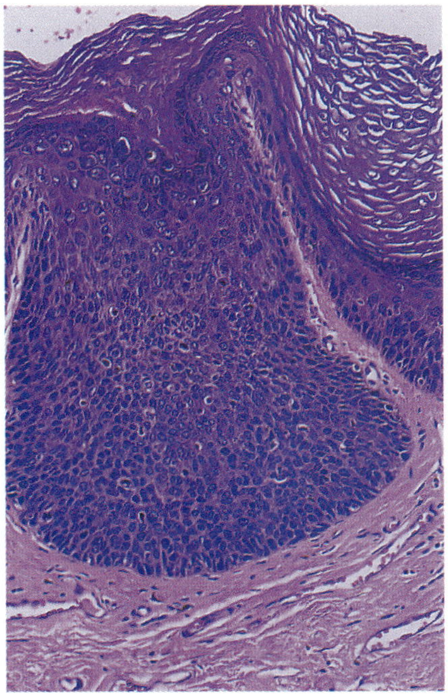

Figure 22–11. VIN III (*i.e.,* severe dysplasia). Small uniform cells with a high nuclear-to-cytoplasmic ratio and coarsely clumped chromatin.

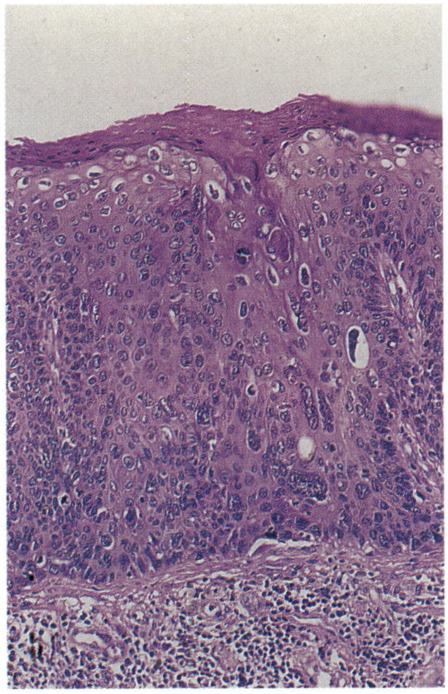

Figure 22–12. VIN III (*i.e.,* severe dysplasia). Multiple large multinucleated cells.

Squamous Cell Carcinoma

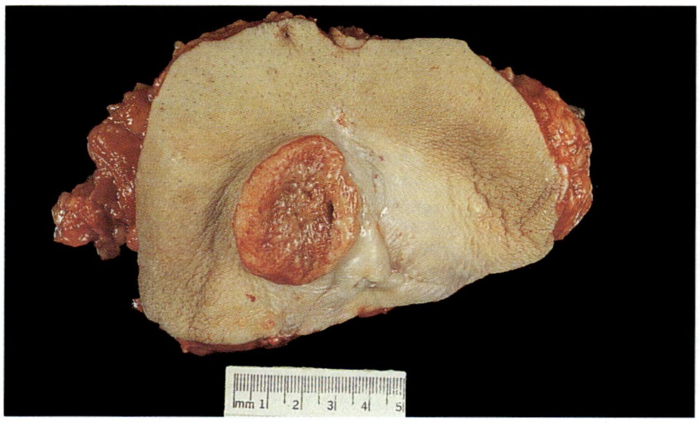

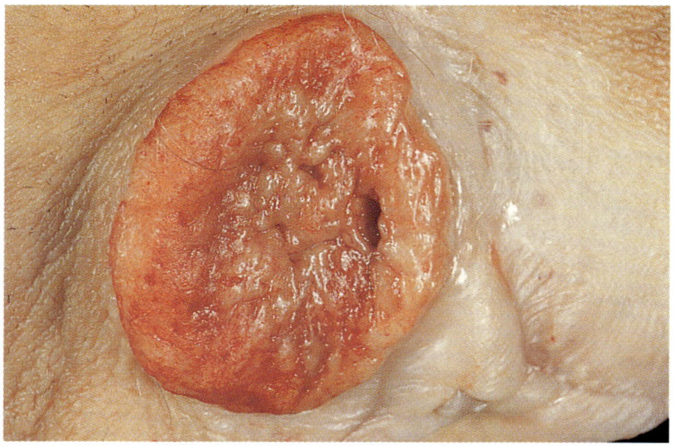

Figures 22–13 and 22–14. Vulvar squamous cell carcinoma. A large, ulcerated lesion is present in a vulvectomy specimen.

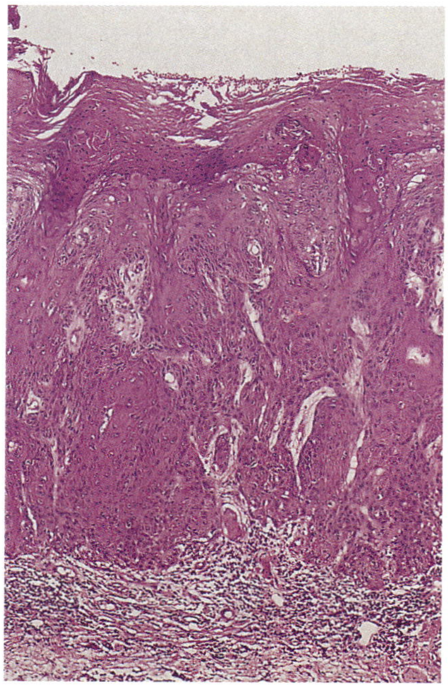

Figure 22–15. Moderately well-differentiated invasive carcinoma with anastomosing, finger-like extensions into underlying inflamed connective tissue is seen.

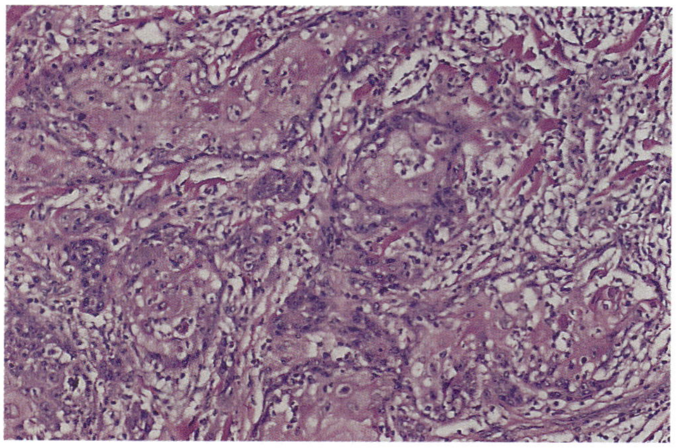

Figure 22–16. Nonkeratinizing, invasive nests of vulvar carcinoma are seen at higher magnification.

Verrucous Carcinoma

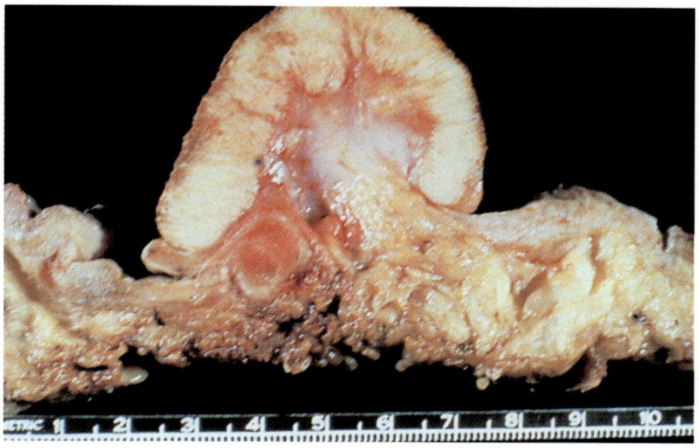

Figure 22–17. Verrucous carcinoma. On cross section, this bulky, exophytic tumor has a well-defined inferior border, which appears to compress the underlying stroma rather than invade it.

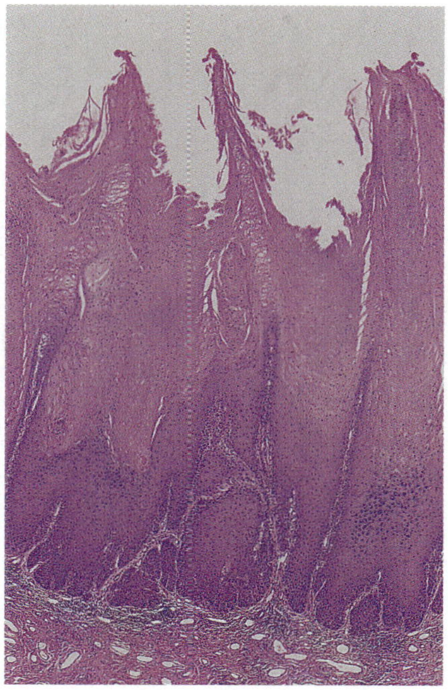

Figure 22–18. Histologically, the lower border is composed of rounded, bulky, club-like rete pegs that extend into the underlying stroma.

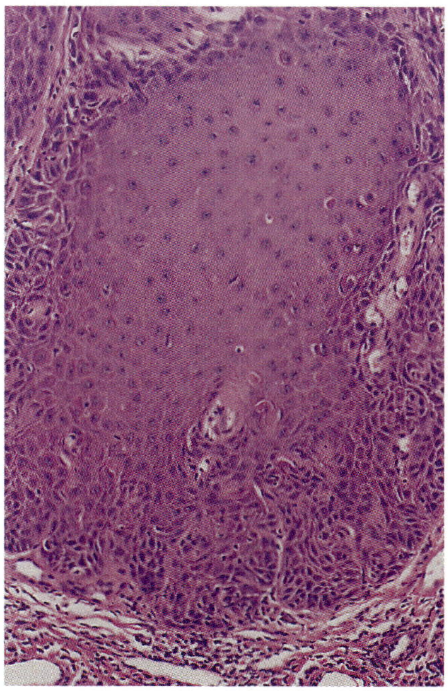

Figure 22–19. The cells of the verrucous carcinoma are well differentiated with uniform nuclei, a low nuclear-to-cytoplasmic ratio, and rare mitoses.

Paget Disease

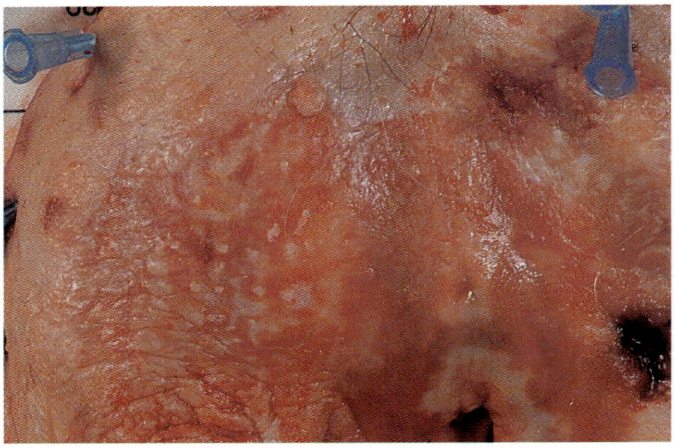

Figure 22–20. Paget disease is a nonsquamous type of VIN. A moist, map-like region on the labia is composed of erythema with interposed islands of tan-white hyperkeratosis.

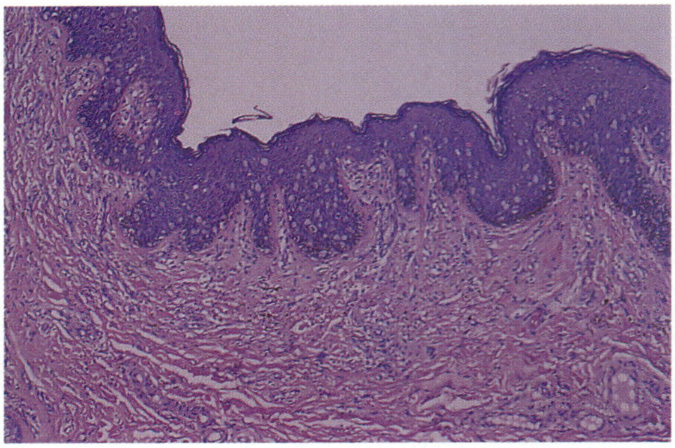

Figure 22–21. Pale staining Paget cells are present as single cells and as small clusters within the epidermal layer.

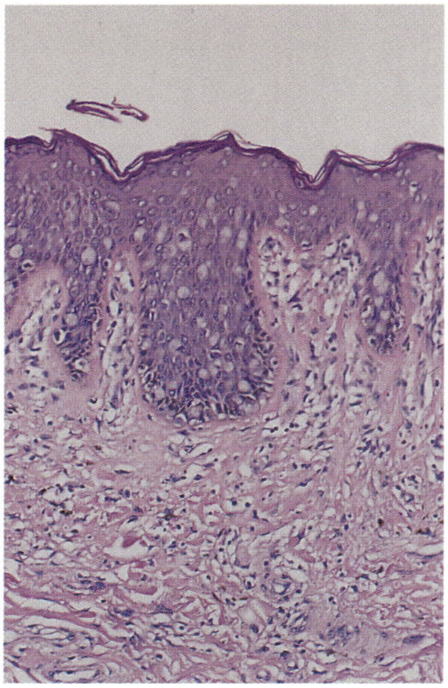

Figure 22–22. Some of the Paget cells have a signet-ring quality to their cytoplasm, with nuclei compressed at the cell periphery.

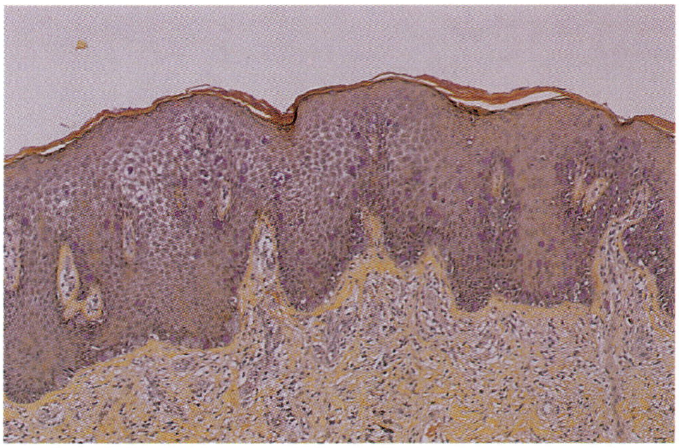

Figure 22–23. Mucicarmine staining reveals that many of the Paget cells contain intracytoplasmic mucin (orange-red cells scattered throughout the epithelium).

Vulvar Melanoma

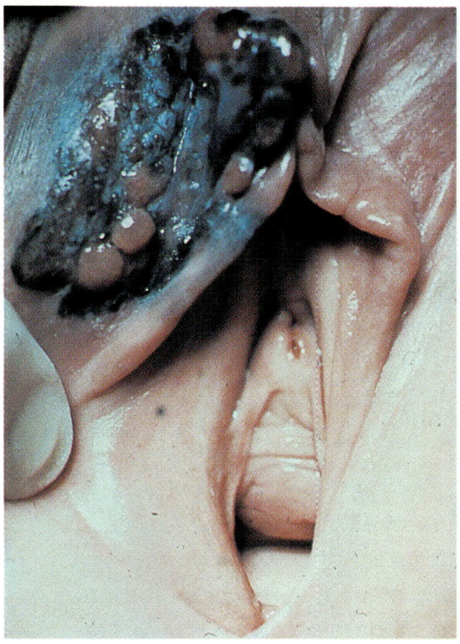

Figure 22–24. This deeply pigmented vulvar tumor shows both macular areas of brown-black discoloration corresponding to the radial growth phase and nodular regions of vertical growth phase.

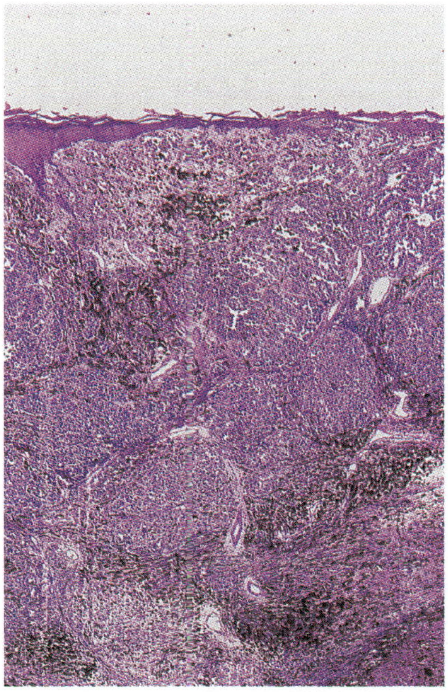

Figure 22–25. The vertical growth phase is characterized by expansile, nodular growth of cells, ranging from relatively nonpigmented cells to zones of heavily pigmented cells and melanophages.

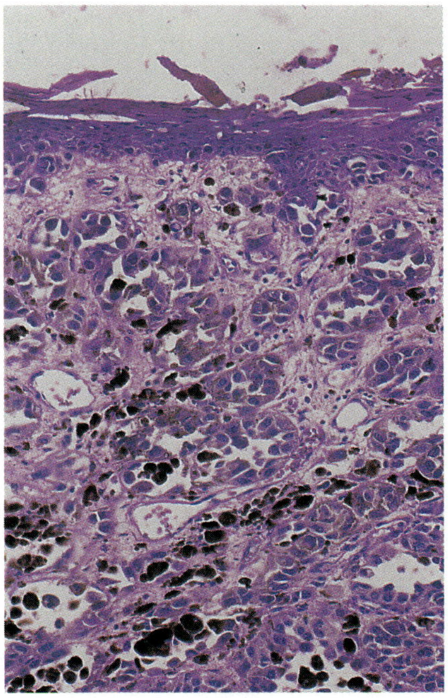

Figure 22–26. On higher magnification, the tumor cells in this field are predominantly epithelioid and contain obvious cytoplasmic melanin. The overlying epithelium retains lentiginous growth of malignant cells, residua of the radial growth phase that gave rise to this potentially metastasizing subepithelial component.

23

Dermatopathology of Oral Mucosa

Dermatopathologists are frequently confronted with oral mucosal biopsies. This is in part the result of the occasional occurrence of oral manifestations in certain dermatoses (*e.g.,* lichen planus, pemphigus). Moreover, the development of a white region on the oral mucosa *(leukoplakia)* generally raises the possibility of squamous cell carcinoma, a condition that has a similar histologic appearance, whether it occurs on the skin or mucosa. On the other hand, many conditions are unique to the oral cavity, such as forms of gingivitis, periodontitis, disorders of salivary glands, and specific forms of glossitis. In these situations, conventional dermatopathology often fails to consider the salient differential diagnostic points that permit accurate diagnostic evaluation. Accordingly, the specific disorders illustrated are those most frequently encountered in oral biopsies by the dermatopathologist and oral pathologist.

As in keratinizing epithelium, perception of colors and staining nuances is also of critical importance in evaluating the oral mucosal biopsy. Detection of organisms and viral cytopathic changes, dysplasia and anaplasia within nuclei, deposits, trauma, and patterns of inflammatory cell infiltration all depend on the ability to discriminate shades of color at both scanning and higher magnifications. Clinical detection of pathology in the oral epithelium also relies heavily on alterations in hue, since palpation often is not as accessible as on the cutaneous surface. Accordingly, both clinical and histologic manifestations of common disorders of the oral cavity are emphasized.

Traumatic Ulceration

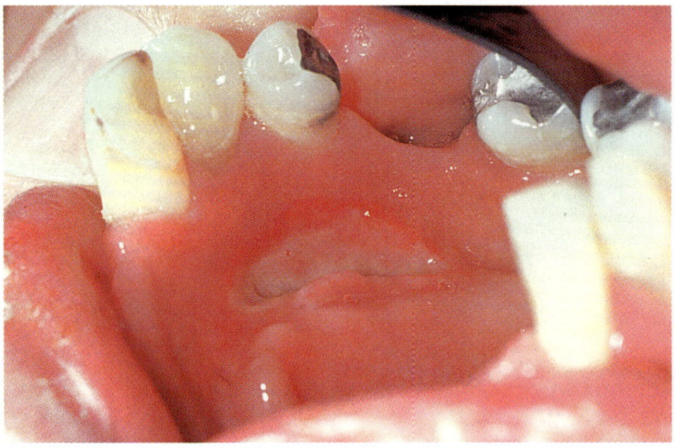

Figure 23–1. A traumatic ulcer on the lingual aspect of the mandible *(center)* was caused by a denture flange.

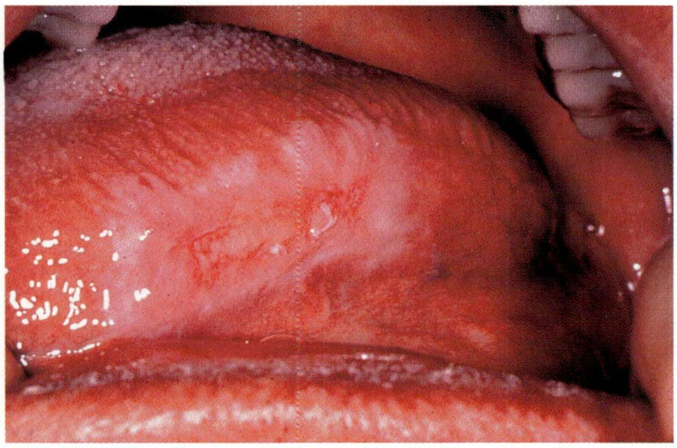

Figure 23–2. A chronically traumatized zone on the lateral lingual margin shows central linear ulceration and surrounding hyperkeratosis.

Aphthous Stomatitis

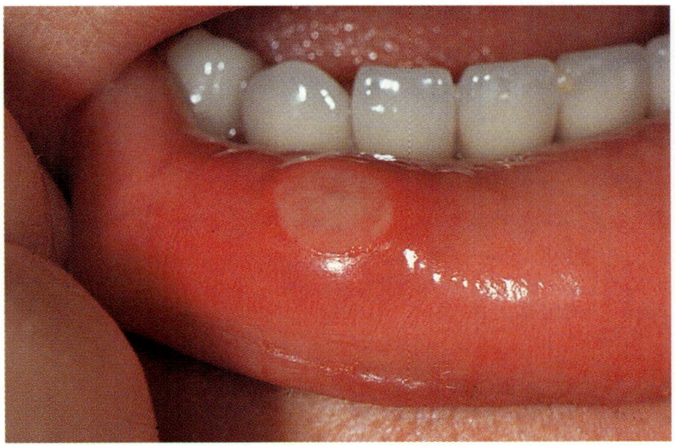

Figure 23–3. A minor aphthous ulcer is present on the lower lip. The lesion is less than 1 cm in diameter and typically circular.

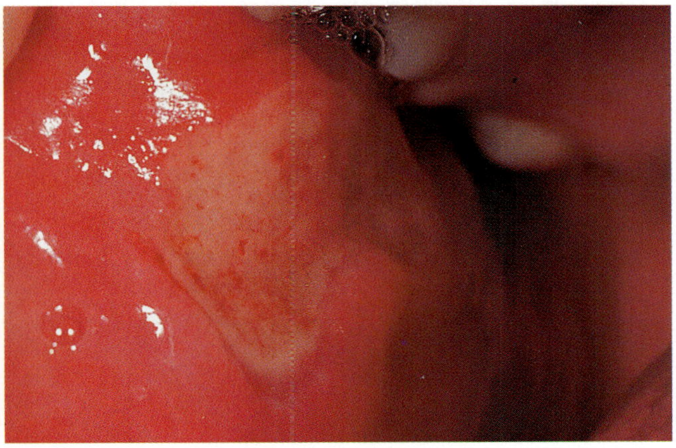

Figure 23–4. A major aphthous ulcer of the buccal mucosa, which was present for 4 months before treatment.

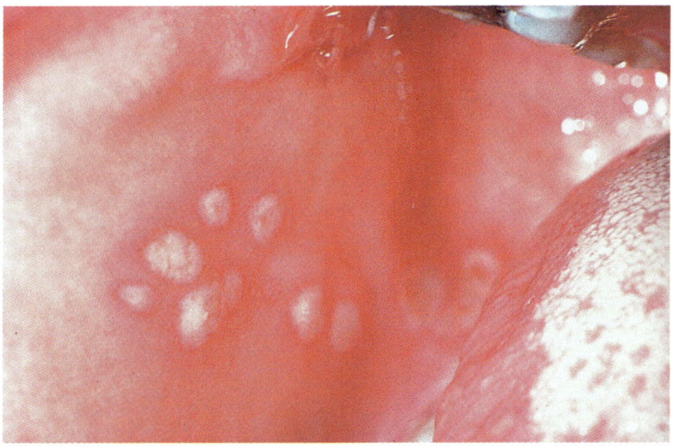

Figure 23–5. Nonvesicular, cluster-pattern, herpetiform, aphthous ulcerations.

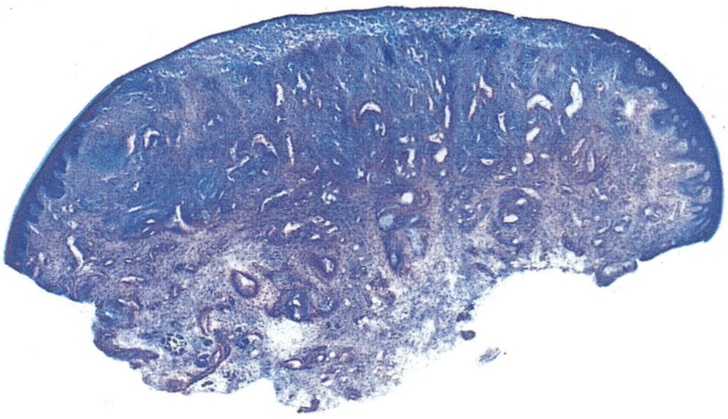

Figure 23–6. Histopathology of recurrent aphthous stomatitis. An excisional biopsy specimen of a minor aphthous lesion shows a central surface defect and intense cellularity with deeper, focal, perivascular cell aggregations (periodic acid–Schiff stain).

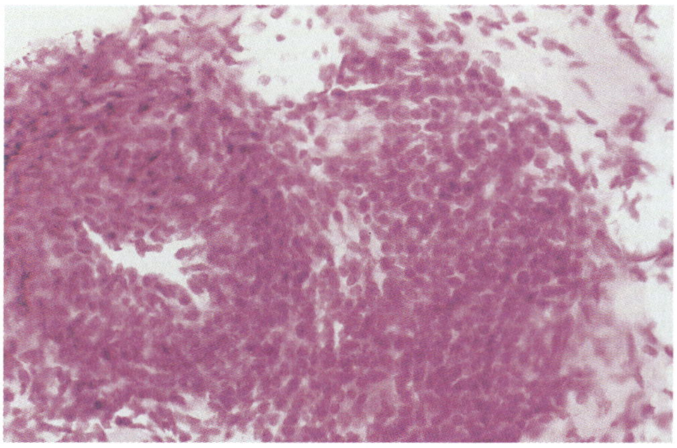

Figure 23–7. High-power magnification of the intense perivascular lymphocytic clusters in aphthous lesions.

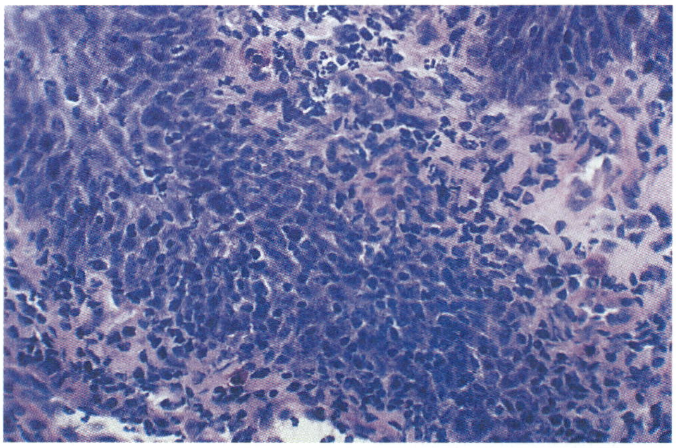

Figure 23–8. The epithelium in aphthous lesions is infiltrated with large numbers of lymphocytes that, in the ulcerative phase, are predominantly CD8-positive.

Oral Lichen Planus

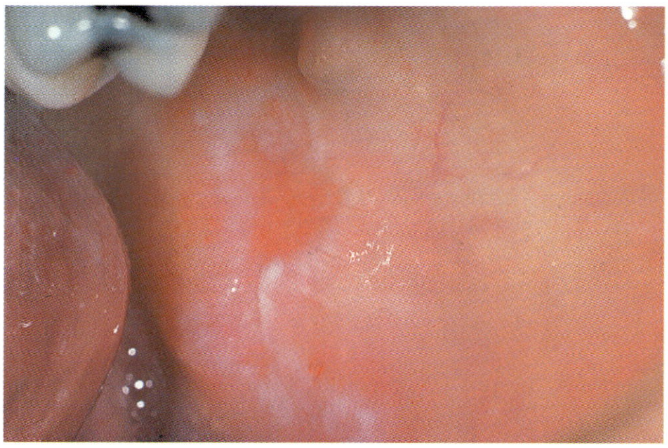

Figure 23–9. Clinical variants of oral lichen planus. A lesion of lichen planus is present on the buccal mucosa. The central atrophic zone is surrounded by radiating linear and reticular striae. The parotid papilla is at the upper pole of the lesion.

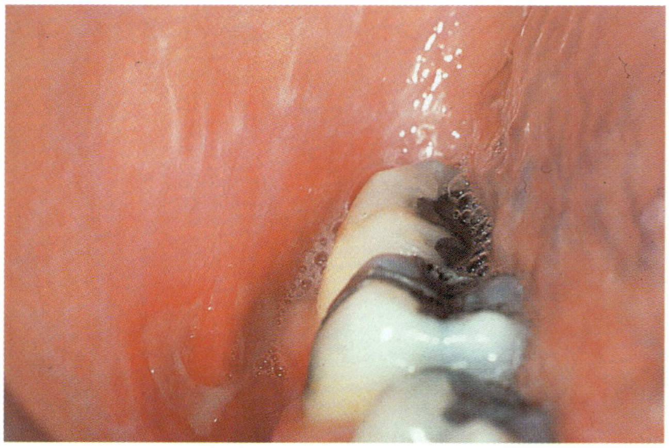

Figure 23–10. Reticular Wickham striae on the posterior buccal mucosa run through the reflection of the buccal sulcus and onto the gingiva. Erosive areas in this site are frequent and may be associated with adjacent amalgam restorations.

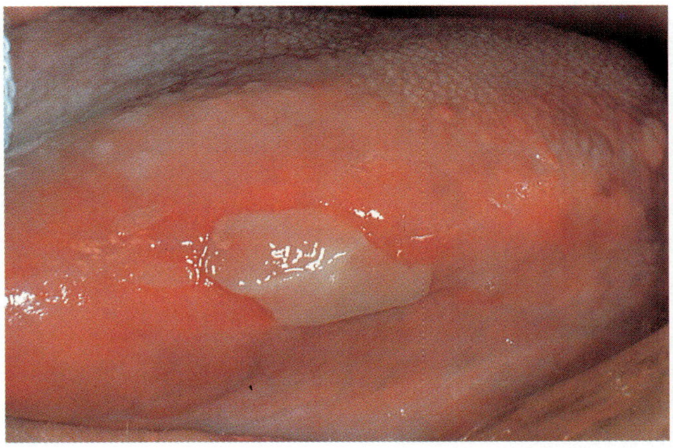

Figure 23–11. A bullous lesion on the lateral lingual margin is present in a patient with drug-related lichen planus. There is marked peripheral depapillation and small annular lesions on the dorsum.

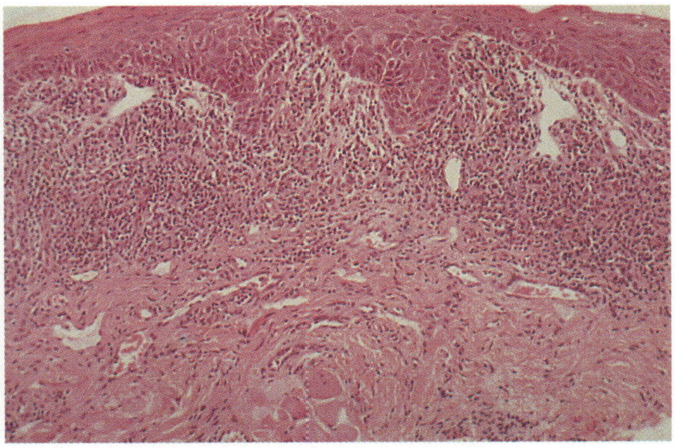

Figure 23–12. Histopathology of oral lichen planus. Lichen planus shows the characteristic juxtaepithelial, lymphohistiocytic infiltrate below an acanthotic, parakeratinized epithelium.

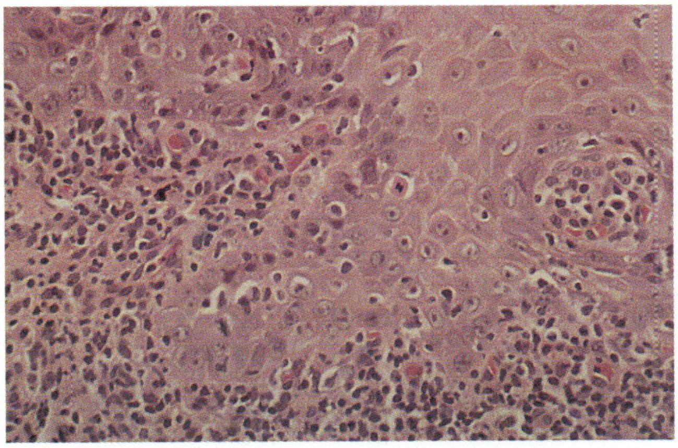

Figure 23–13. Higher magnification shows intraepithelial lymphocytes, disruption of the basal cells, and the presence of intraepithelial, eosinophilic, apoptotic bodies.

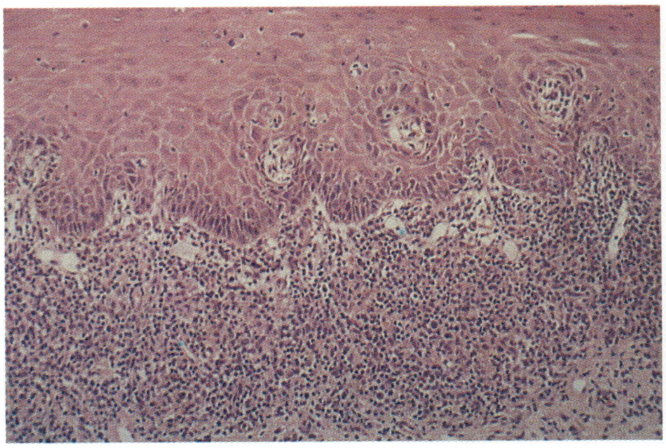

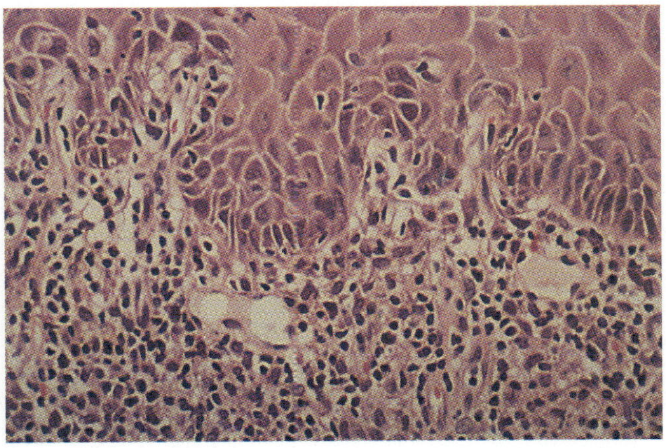

Figures 23–14 and 23–15. In lichenoid dysplasia, the typical histologic features of lichen planus are combined with epithelial dysplasia. Hyperchromaticity, irregularity in nuclear size and shape, and drop-shaped rete pegs are present.

Oral Lupus Erythematosus

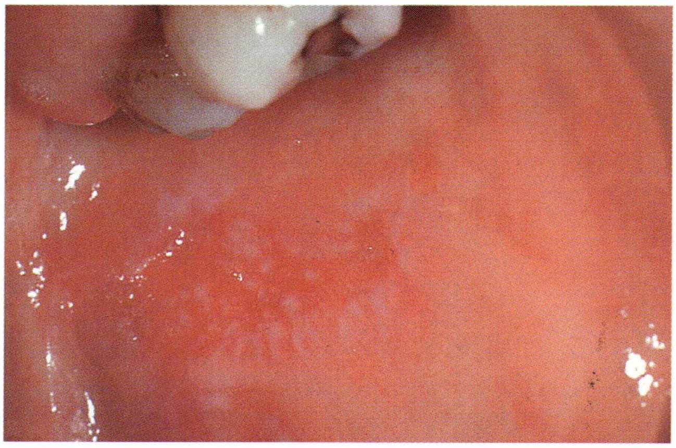

Figure 23–16. Clinical and histologic features of oral lesions of lupus erythematosus. A discoid lupus erythematosus lesion is present on the buccal mucosa. The central, depressed atrophic zone contains keratotic papules and telangiectases. The margin shows radiating striae.

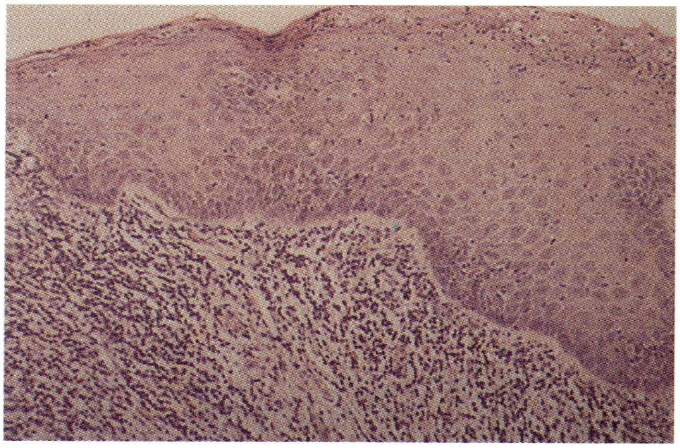

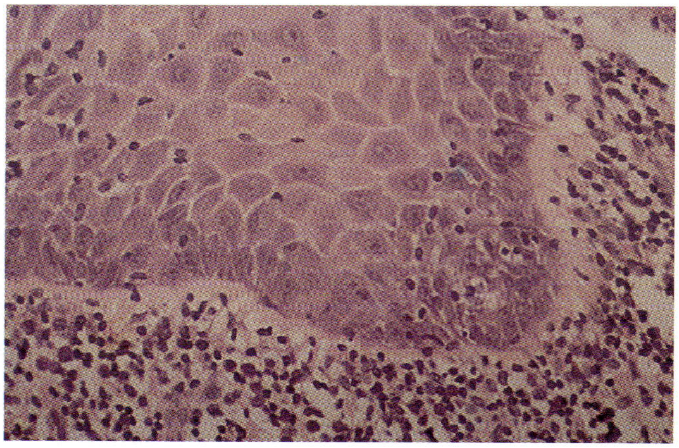

Figures 23–17 and 23–18. Discoid lupus erythematosus produces parakeratosis with plugging, a mixed inflammatory infiltrate, and thickening of the basement membrane zone.

Oral Mucosal Pemphigoid

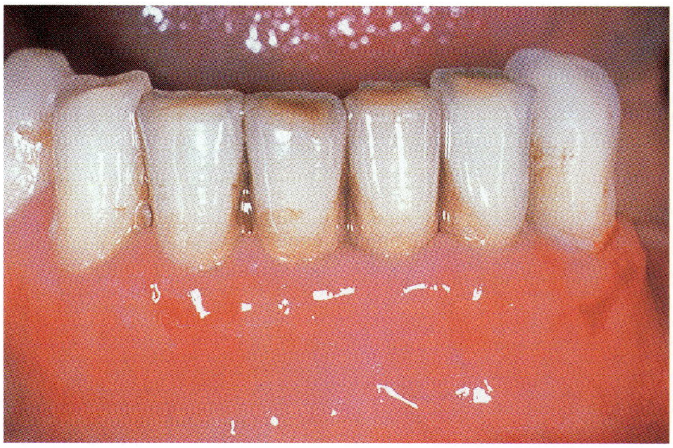

Figure 23–19. Oral mucosal pemphigoid. Typical gingival appearance in active cicatricial pemphigoid. There is superficial erosion of an intensely erythematous gingiva with moderate local pain.

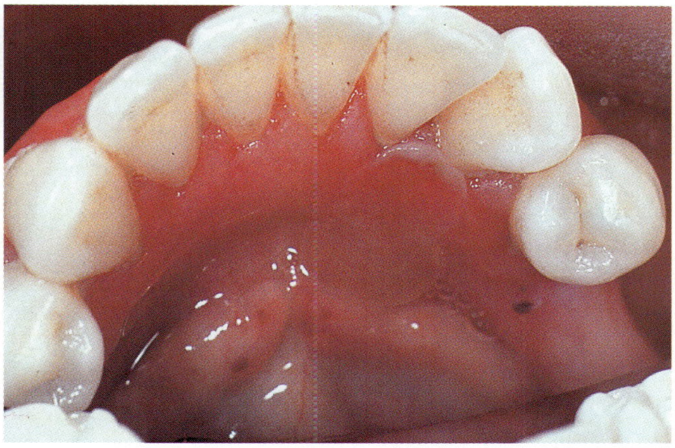

Figure 23–20. A collapsed bulla is present on the lingual aspect of the lower anterior teeth in a pemphigoid patient. The bulla was caused by local trauma during a dental prophylaxis procedure.

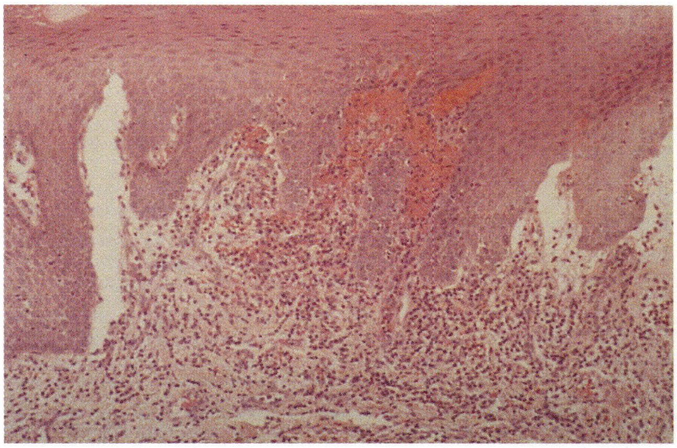

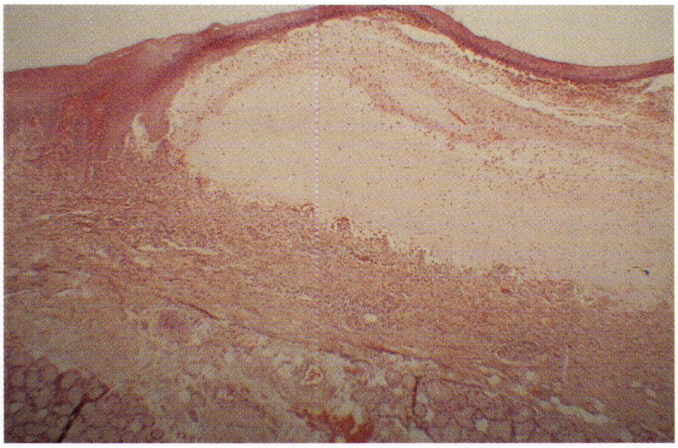

Figures 23–21 and 23–22. Cicatricial pemphigoid demonstrates the characteristic separation of the epithelium from the lamina propria at the basement membrane zone, forming a subepithelial bulla.

Plasma Cell Gingivitis

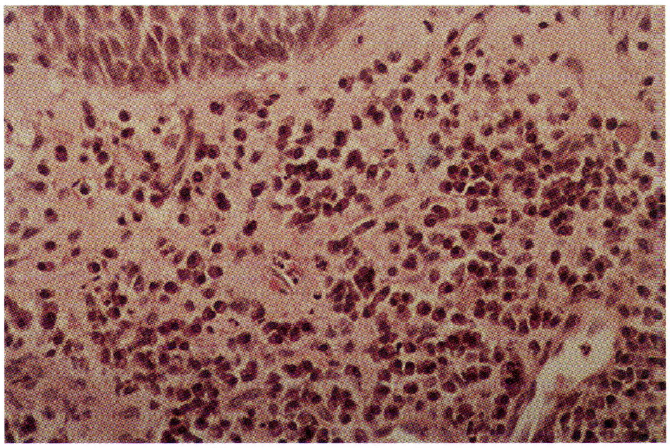

Figure 23–23. Plasma cell gingivitis. Large numbers of plasma cells are present in a vascular lamina propria.

Fibroepithelial Hyperplasia

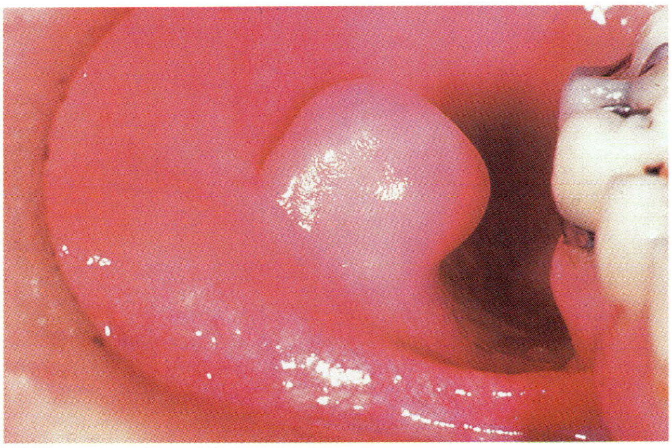

Figure 23–24. Fibroepithelial hyperplasia. A firm, smooth-surfaced uninflamed fibroepithelial polyp is located on the buccal mucosa. These lesions are usually caused by local dental trauma.

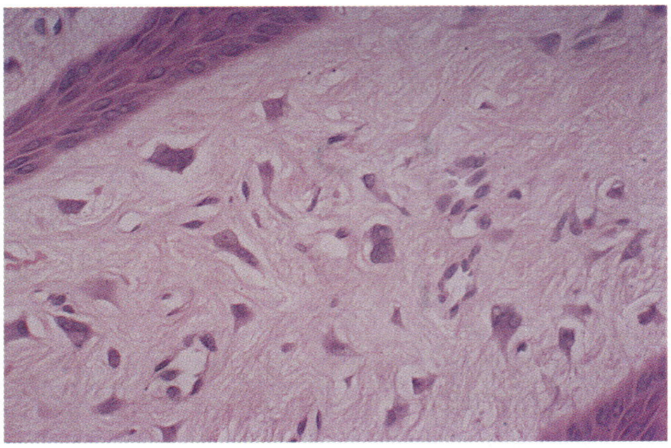

Figure 23–25. Some reactive hyperplastic polyps have large stellate and multinucleated cells in a loosely textured fibrous tissue band immediately subjacent to the epithelium. These polyps have been termed giant cell fibromas.

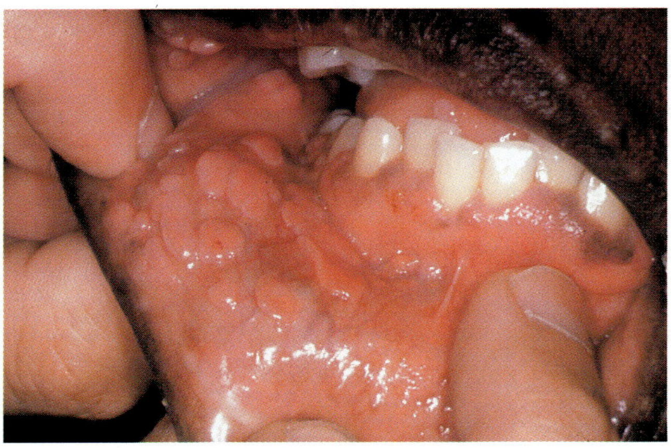

Figure 23–26. Fibroepithelial hyperplasia. Numerous flattened papules are present on the inner aspect of the lower lip in an aboriginal patient with Heck disease.

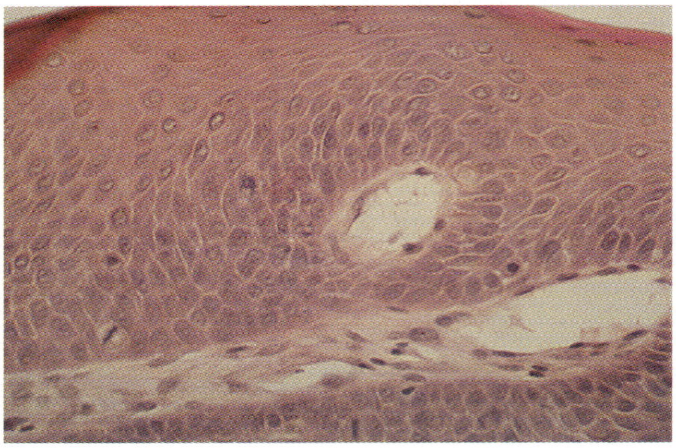

Figure 23–27. Mitosoid bodies (large, clear cells containing mitosis-like nuclear formations) in an acanthotic epithelium are typical of Heck disease.

Papillary and Verrucous Lesions

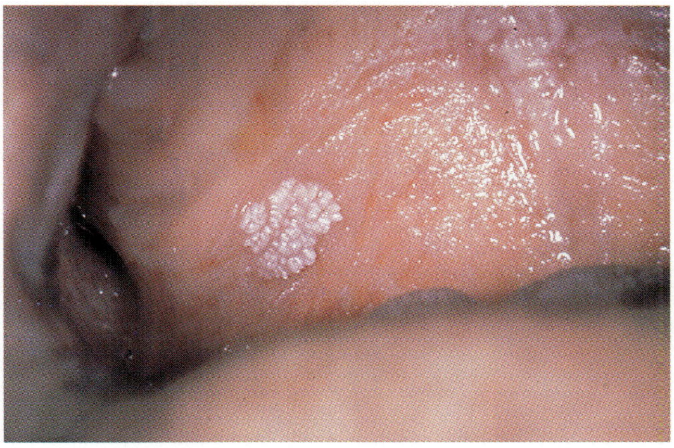

Figure 23–28. Papillary lesions. A flattened sessile papilloma with heavy hyperkeratosis of the surface projections is present on the lateral aspect of the posterior hard palate.

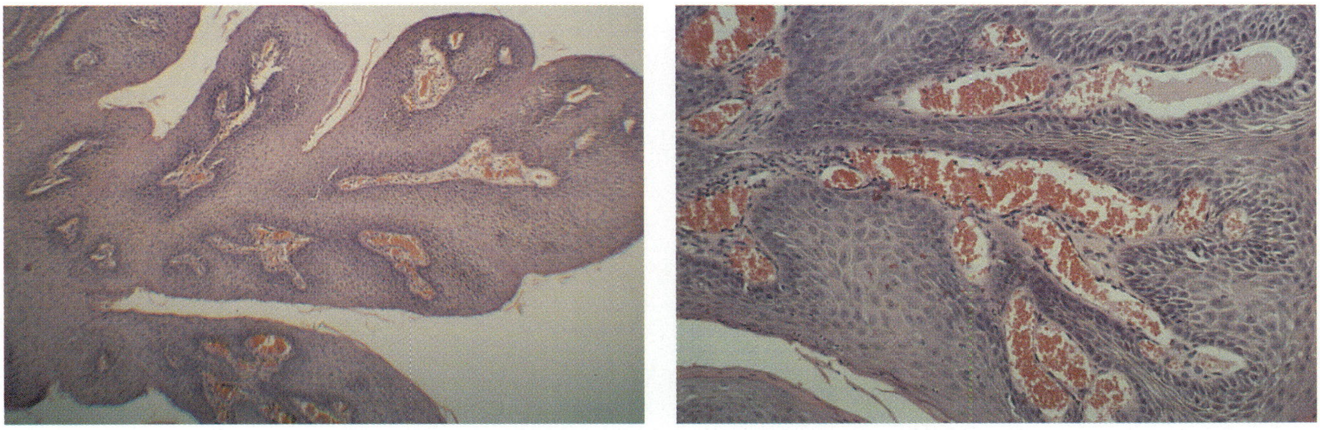

Figures 23–29 and 23–30. This squamous papilloma consists of finger-like projections of acanthotic epithelium supported by thin, highly vascular connective tissue cores.

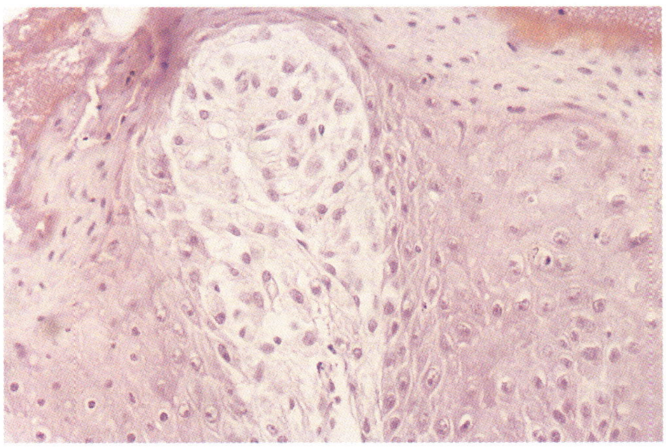

Figure 23–31. In verruciform xanthoma, typical large, clear xanthoma cells fill the clefts between epithelial rete pegs.

Glossitis

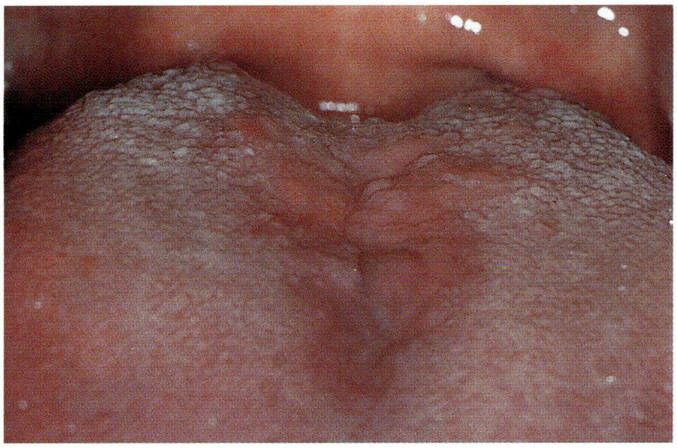

Figure 23–32. Lesions of the tongue. Median rhomboid glossitis shows a central depapillated zone with some surface irregularity immediately anterior to the foramen caecum on the dorsum of the tongue.

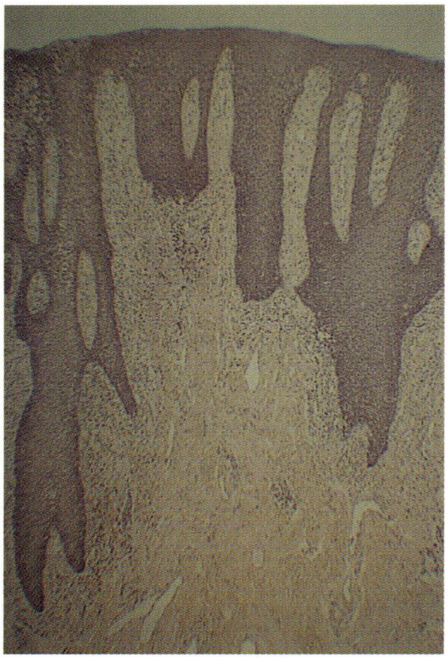

Figure 23–33. Median rhomboid glossitis is histologically unremarkable but often shows pseudoepitheliomatous hyperplasia with hyalinization in the subjacent tissues.

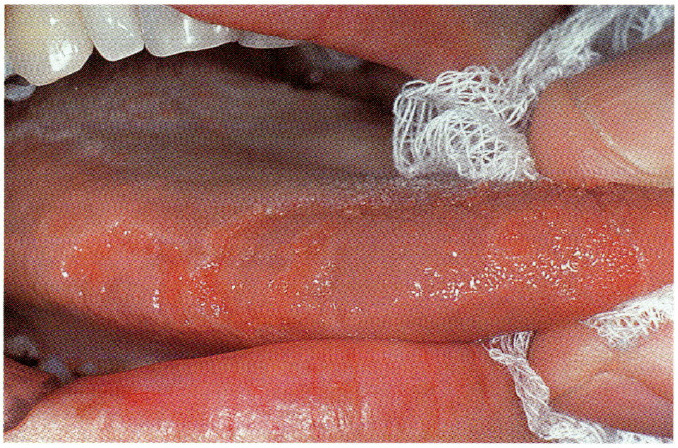

Figure 23–34. Typical circinate lesions of benign migratory glossitis. A depressed area shows papillary atrophy and is surrounded by a raised white border.

Crohn Disease

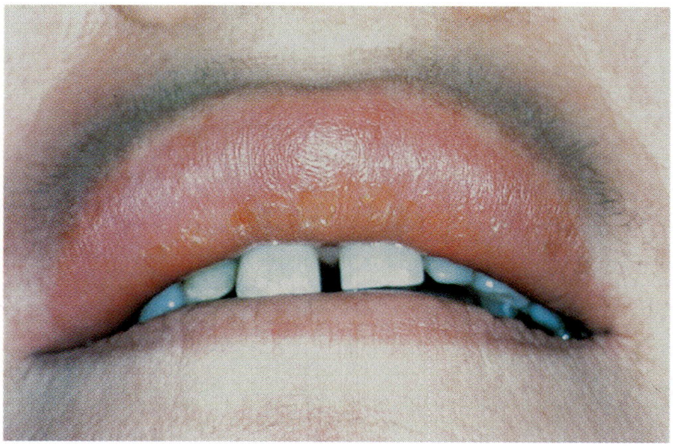

Figure 23–35. Crohn disease and orofacial granulomatosis. Enlargement of the upper lip occurred in a patient with Crohn disease.

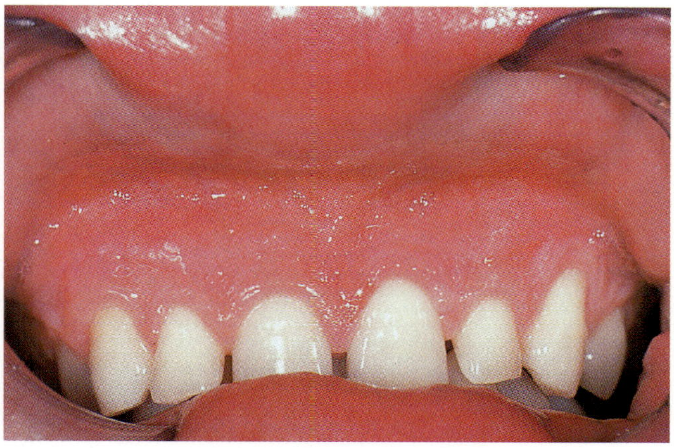

Figure 23–36. Hyperplastic gingival lesions are present in a patient with oral Crohn disease. This patient also had cobblestoning of the buccal mucosa and recurrent ulcerations.

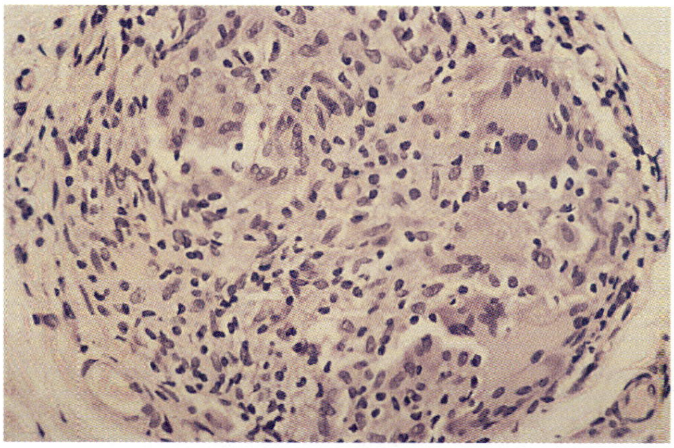

Figure 23–37. The discrete, noncaseating granuloma of orofacial granulomatosis contains small numbers of epithelioid cells and multinucleated giant cells.

Fordyce Granules

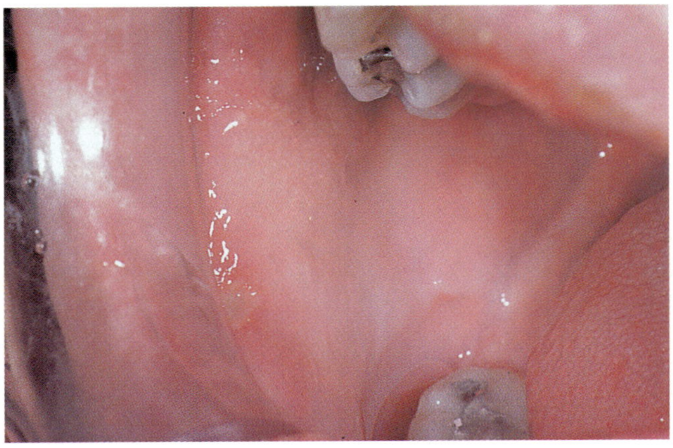

Figure 23–38. Fordyce granules. Numerous small, whitish-yellow, subepithelial sebaceous glands comprise Fordyce granules.

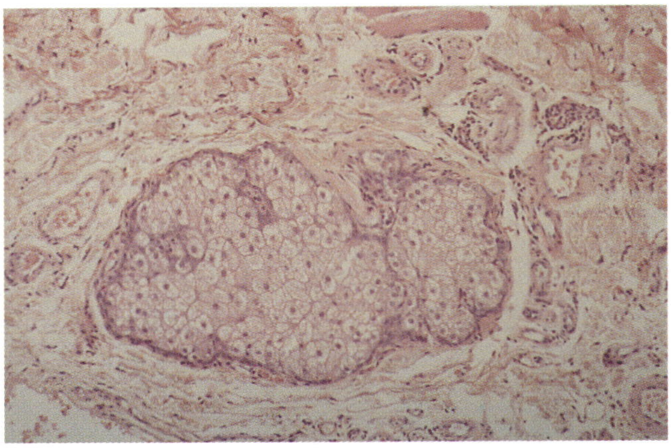

Figure 23–39. Histologically, Fordyce granules show a normal sebaceous gland structure without other associated skin adnexae.

White Sponge Nevus

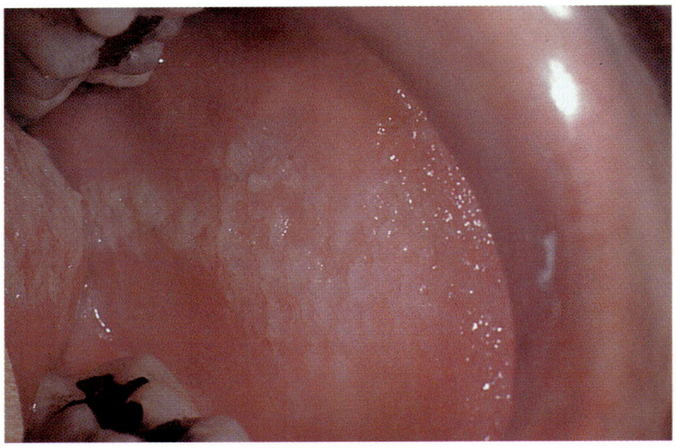

Figure 23–40. This white sponge nevus involves the buccal mucosa and lateral lingual margins and has a thickened, irregular, white, folded surface.

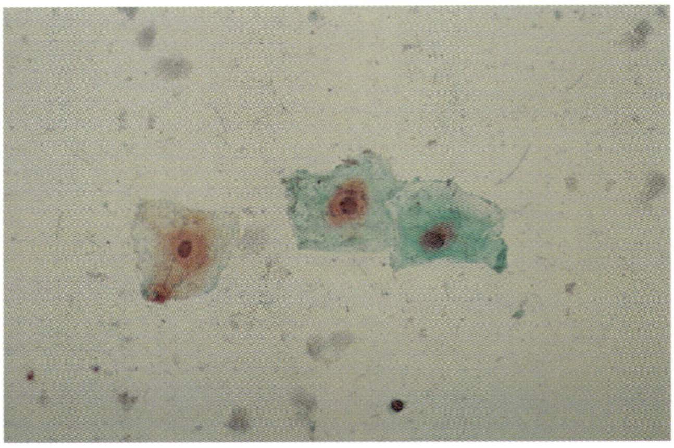

Figure 23–41. A Papanicolaou-stained smear from a white sponge nevus shows the characteristic red-pink perinuclear halo.

Mucocele

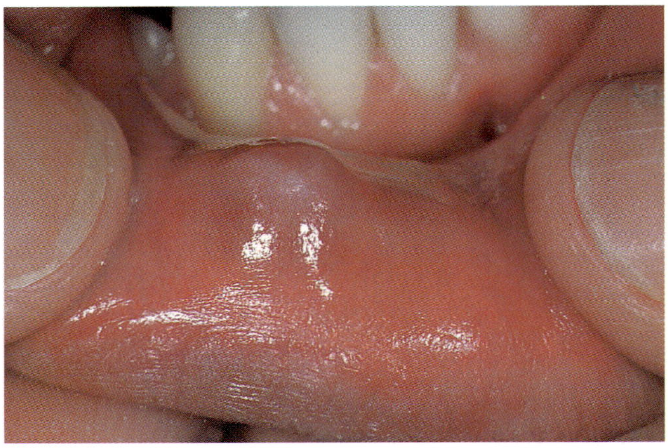

Figure 23–42. Mucocele of the lower lip. The bluish lesions are freely movable and nonindurated.

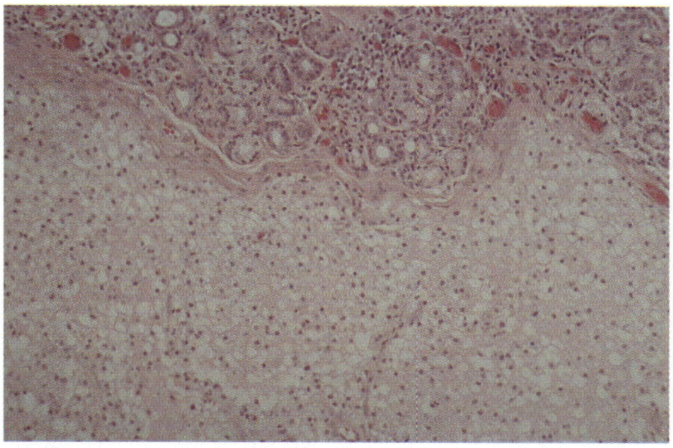

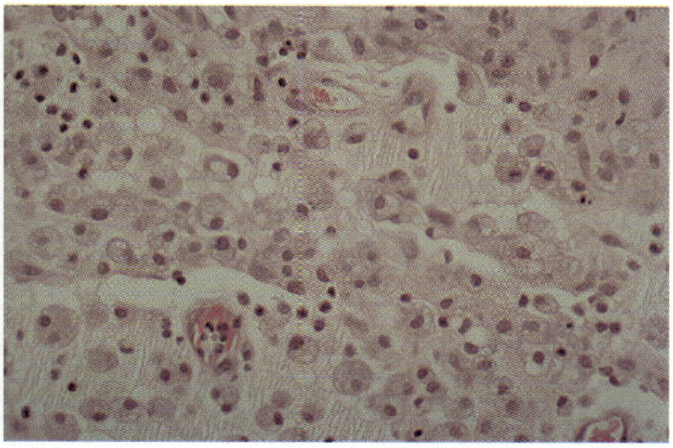

Figures 23–43 and 23–44. A mucous extravasation cyst shows the distinct walling-off of the mucous pool and the presence of large numbers of macrophages and foam histiocytes.

Necrotizing Sialometaplasia

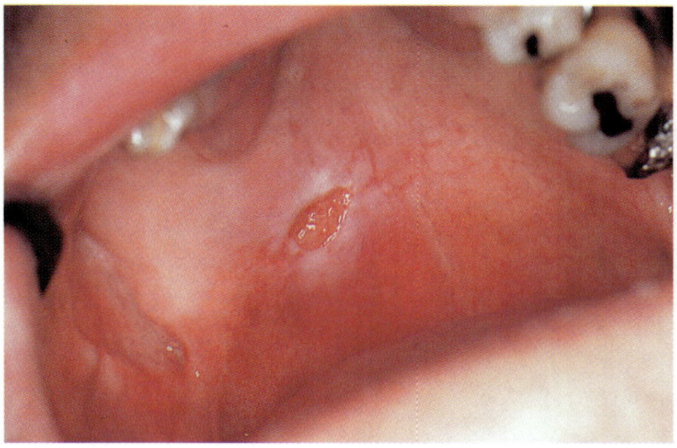

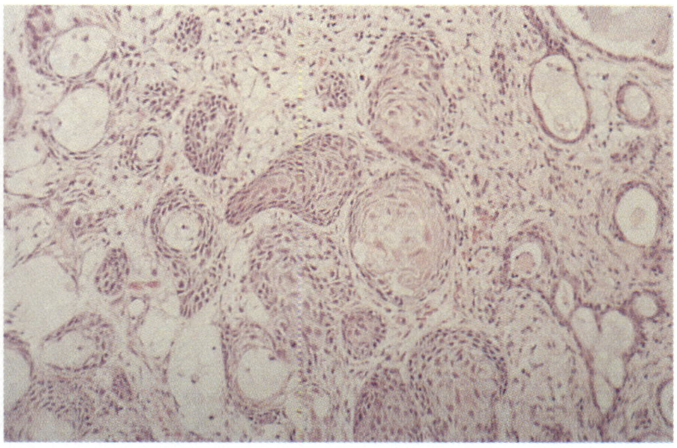

Figures 23–45 and 23–46. A lesion of necrotizing sialometaplasia shows marked squamous metaplasia of the acinar and ductal elements and pseudoepitheliomatous hyperplasia.

Sjögren Syndrome

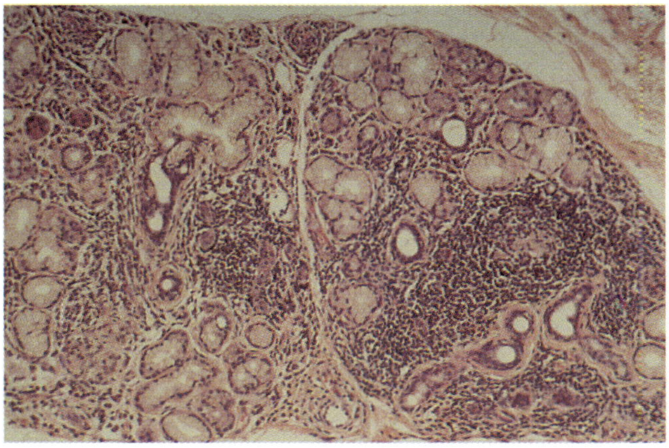

Figure 23–47. Minor mucous salivary gland from a patient with Sjögren syndrome shows extensive (grade 4) infiltration by lymphocytes and loss of acini.

Gingival Hyperplasia

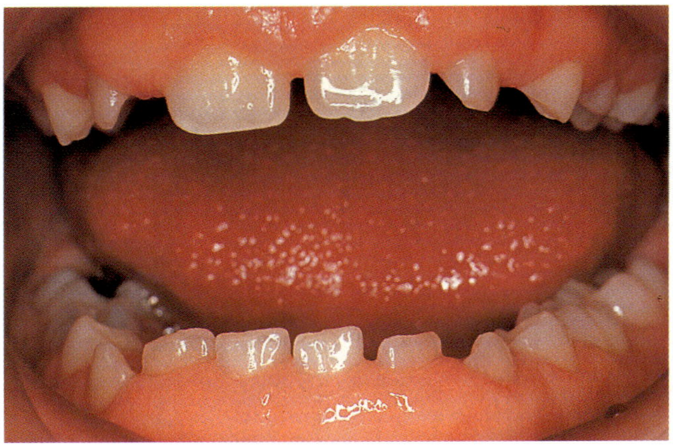

Figure 23–48. Bulky, dense, fibrous overgrowth of the gingivae occurs in fibromatosis gingivae, particularly around the lower anterior teeth.

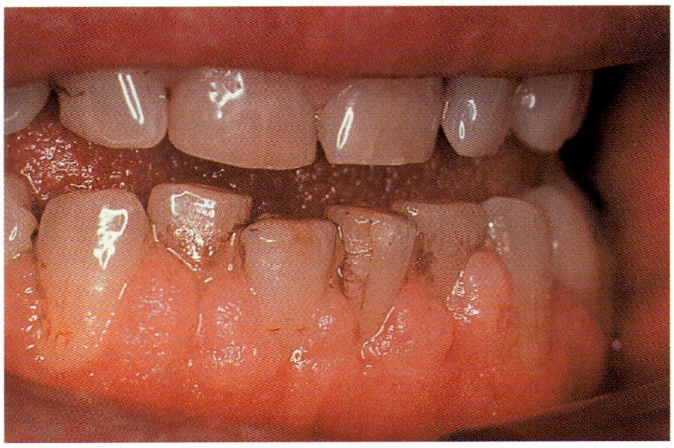

Figure 23–49. Cyclosporin-induced gingival overgrowth occurred in a cardiac allograft recipient. The drug-related gingival overgrowth tends to involve the interdental papillae, in contrast to fibromatosis gingivae.

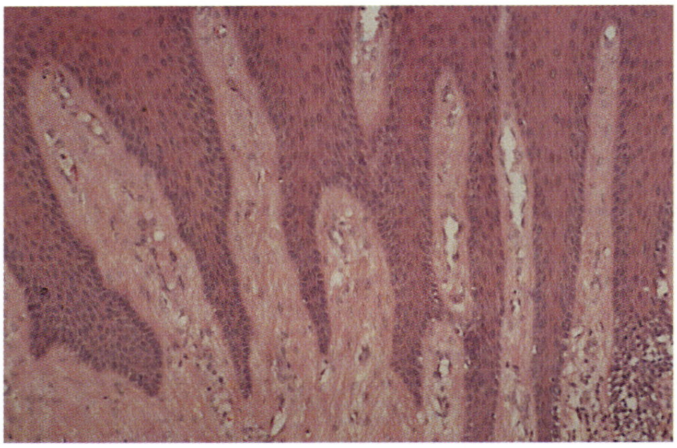

Figure 23–50. Phenytoin-induced gingival overgrowth shows a dense, fibrous tissue mass with elongation of rete pegs often in a test-tube pattern.

Gingival Fibroma

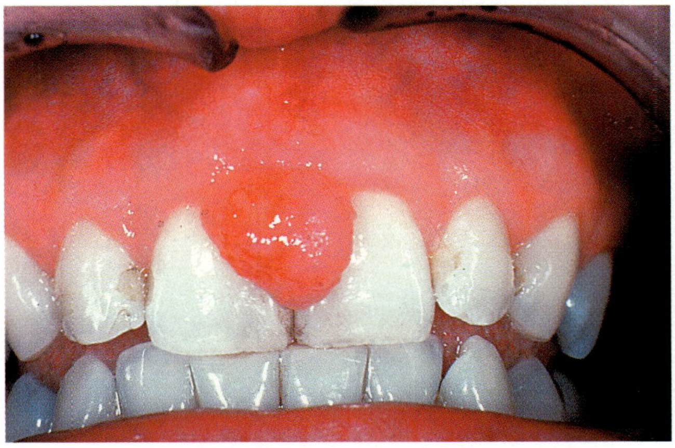

Figure 23–51. Localized gingival enlargement. A peripheral fibroma extends from the gingival margin. The surface has been traumatized secondarily.

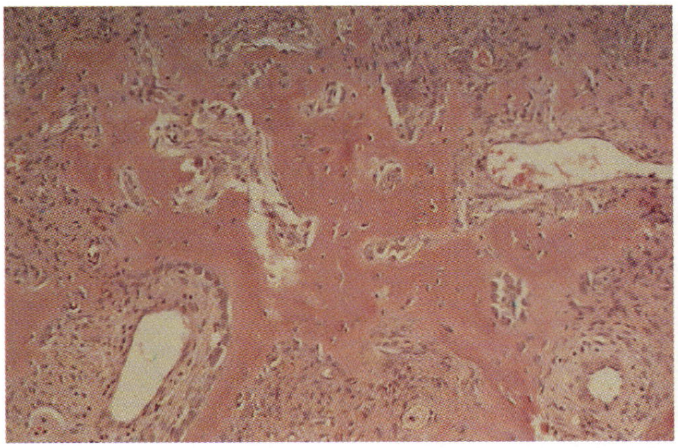

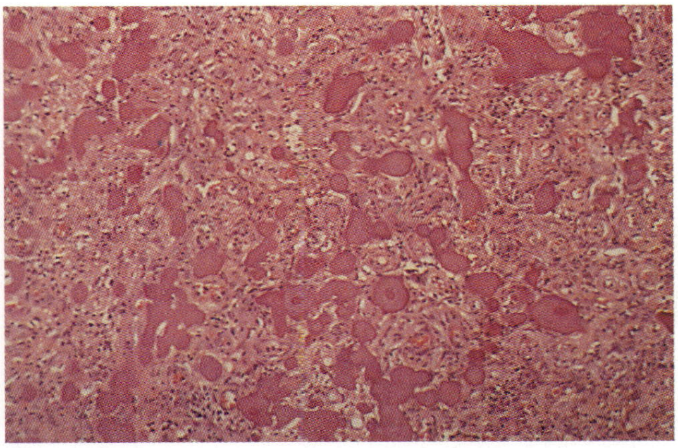

Figures 23–52 and 23–53. A peripheral fibroma shows the typical fibroplastic tissue response with the deposition of bone, calcific structures, and cementum spheres, some of which show concentric Liesegang rings.

Gingival Pyogenic Granuloma

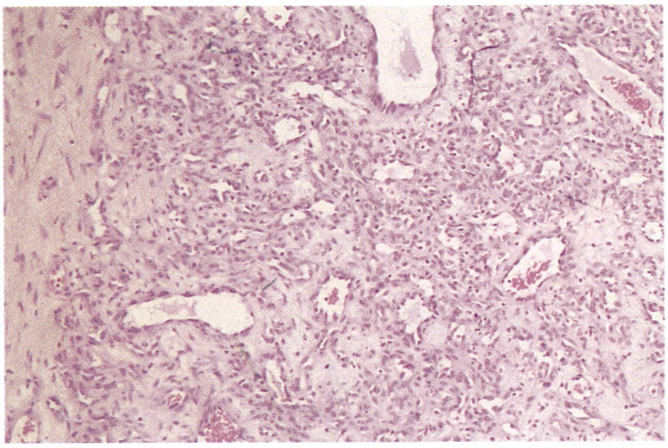

Figure 23–54. This "angiogranuloma" consists of numerous small vascular channels and noncanalized endothelial cell clusters in variably inflamed connective tissue.

Peripheral Giant Cell Lesion

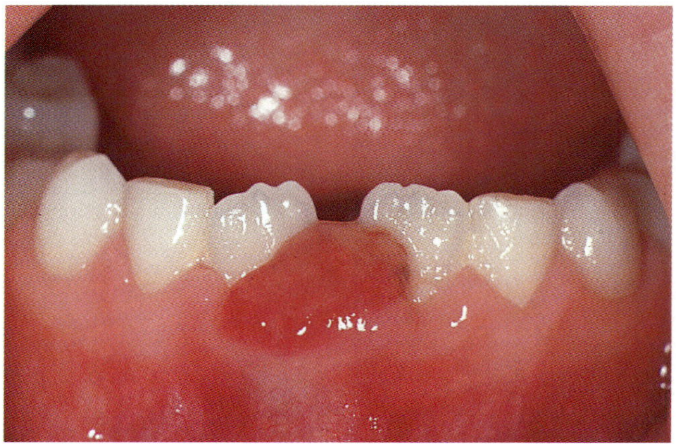

Figure 23–55. Typical cyanotic appearance of a peripheral giant cell lesion. This lesion has eroded the underlying alveolar bone and is causing displacement of the lower central incisor teeth.

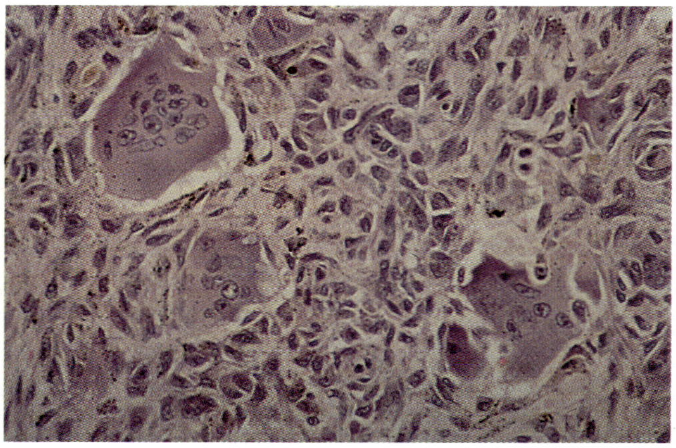

Figure 23–56. A giant cell lesion contains a variable mononuclear cell component. Multinuclear giant cells are frequently seen in association with blood vessels.

Gingivitis and Periodontal Disease

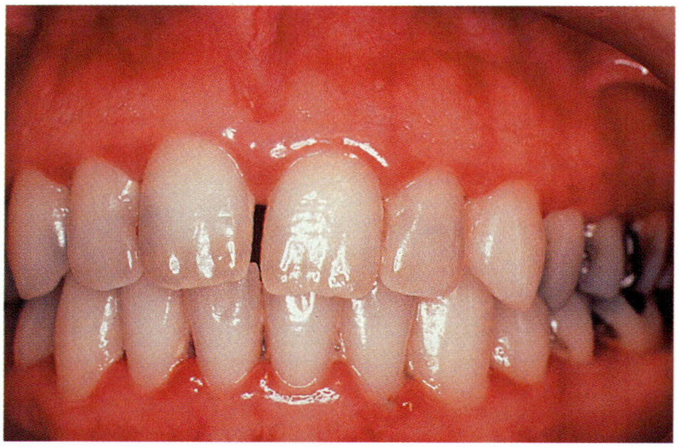

Figure 23–57. Marginal gingivitis is characterized by erythema, edema, loss of stippling, and bleeding in response to probing.

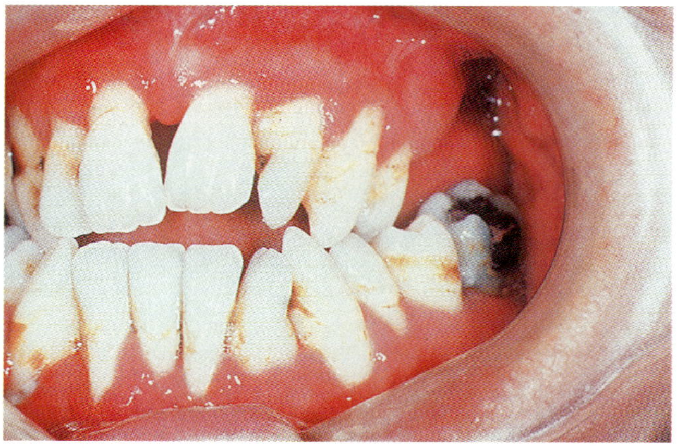

Figure 23–58. Progressive adult periodontitis shows extensive inflammation of the periodontal tissues and loss of tooth support.

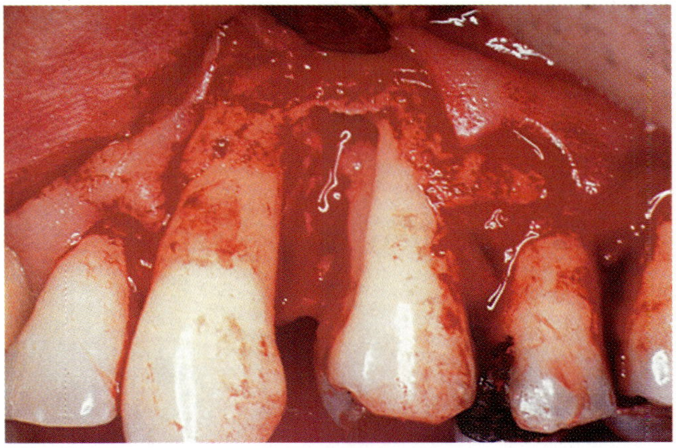

Figure 23–59. Direct visualization of the supporting alveolar bone by raising a mucoperiosteal flap shows the extent of alveolar bone loss in a patient with adult periodontitis.

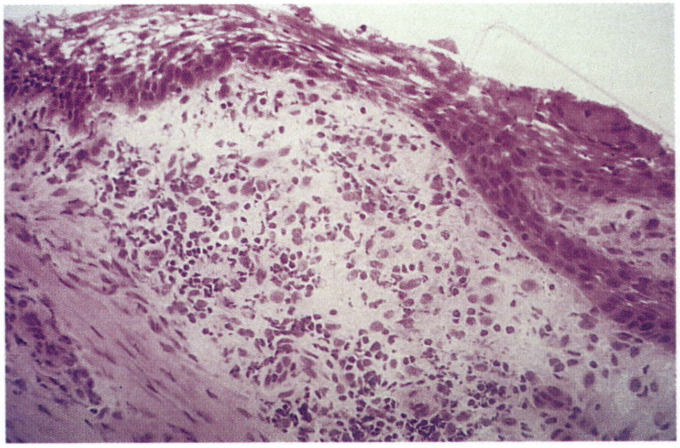

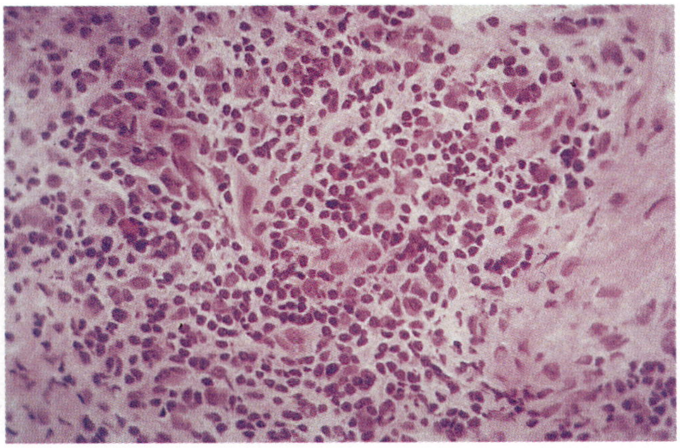

Figures 23–60 and 23–61. A histologic specimen from a patient with adult periodontitis shows extensive infiltration of the gingival connective tissues by mononuclear cells, particularly lymphocytes.

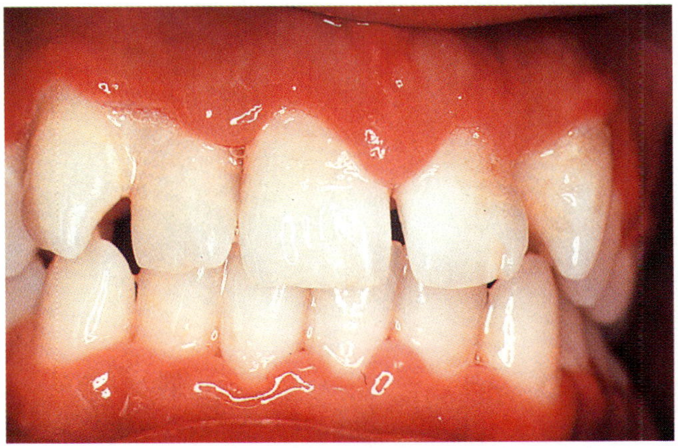

Figure 23–62. Acute necrotizing ulcerative gingivitis shows cratering of the gingival soft tissues.

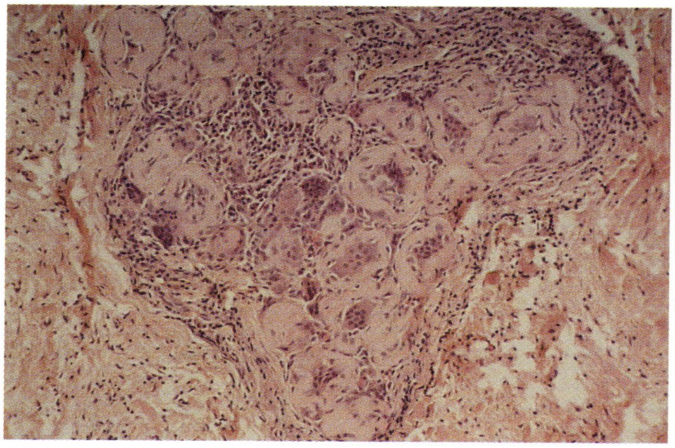

Figure 23–63. Pulse granuloma due to retained food particles. The pulse granuloma contains discrete, foreign body giant cells within gingival connective tissue and associated rings of hyalinized material.

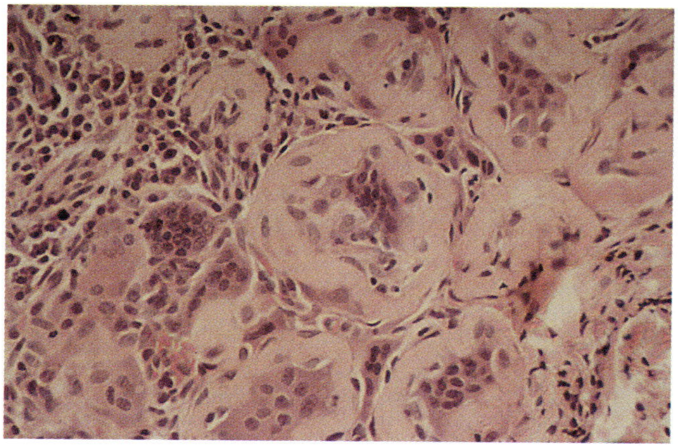

Figure 23–64. Higher magnification shows the pale hyalin rings, some of which are incomplete and contain cellular connective tissue coils.

24

Dermatopathology of Ocular Adnexae

The ocular adnexal region is anatomically complex because skin, muscle, fat, connective tissue, and glandular tissues coexist. Nearly any type of tumor may develop in this area. In the orbital region, it is important to emphasize that the primary purpose of the eyelids is to provide protection for the eye. Thus, the eyelids have both a dynamic and a functional role. In the treatment of lesions in this area, any alteration of the anatomic structure must not disturb the functional and protective role of the eyelids, or significant ocular complications may occur. The anatomies of the eyelids and lacrimal system are reviewed and serve as a base for appreciating the origins of the diverse array of pathologic lesions that arise there. Although many of the lesions described are similar dermatopathologically to lesions elsewhere in the body, they are discussed because their appearance in the eyelids occasionally differs. The rare lesions unique to the eyelids are also described, but these are not seen as often in practice.

This section focuses on the dermatopathology of lesions of the external eyelid and adnexae. The diseases that arise from the conjunctiva (mucous membrane), lacrimal system, orbit, and ocular surface disorders are beyond the scope of this chapter.

Normal Anatomy

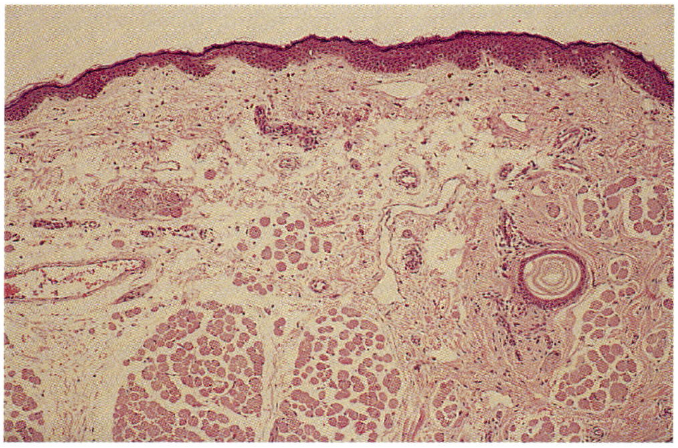

Figure 24–1. Normal adult eyelid skin. The epidermis is thin, and the dermis contains blood vessels, lymphatics, and nerves. Glandular structures are present in the subcutaneous layer.

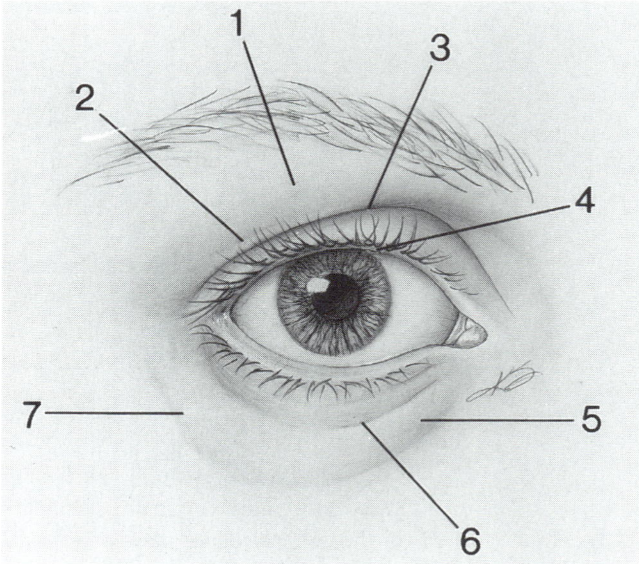

Figure 24–2. External eyelid anatomy. *1,* Superior orbital sulcus; *2,* upper lid fold; *3,* upper lid crease; *4,* highest point of lid curve; *5,* nasojugal fold; *6,* lower lid crease; *7,* malar fold.

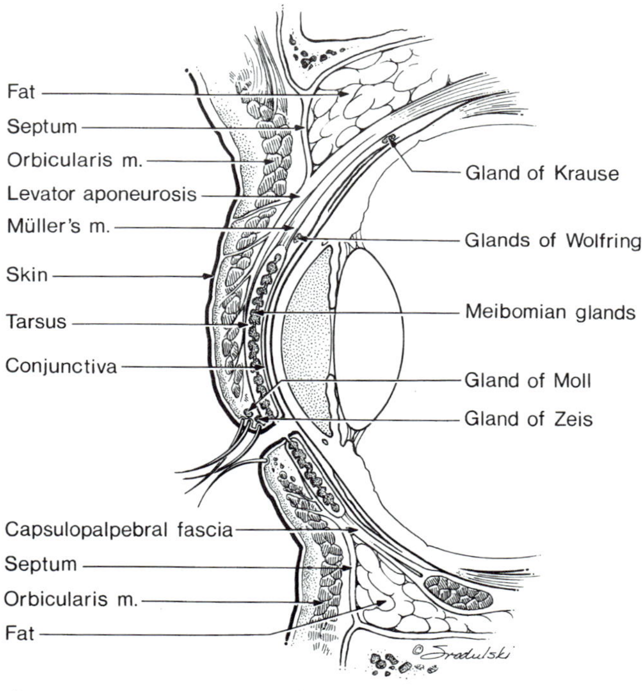

Figure 24–3. Cross-sectional anatomy of the normal eyelid.

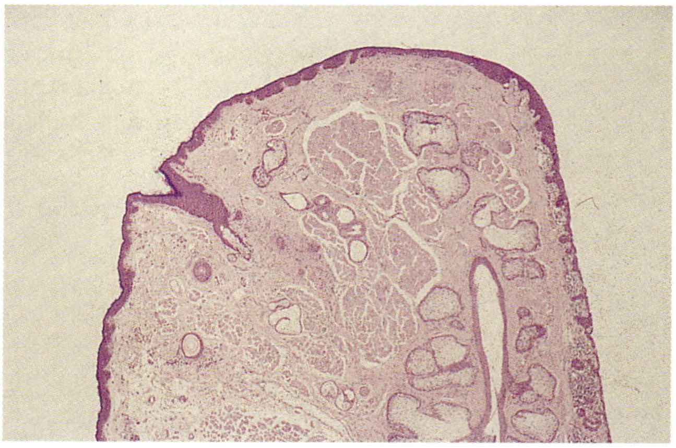

Figure 24–4. Cross section of the normal eyelid.

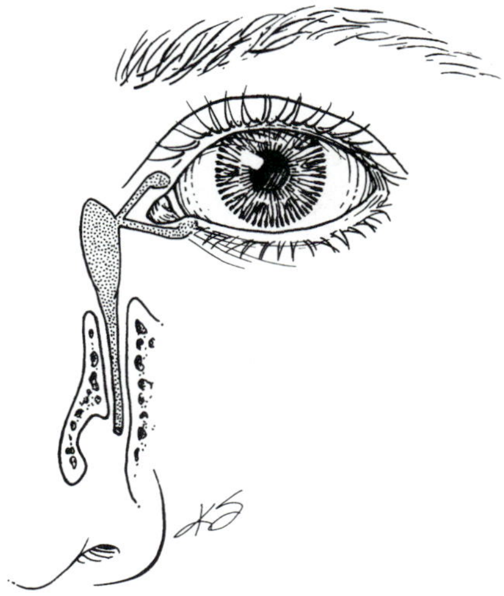

Figure 24–5. Location and anatomy of the nasolacrimal drainage system.

Squamous Papilloma

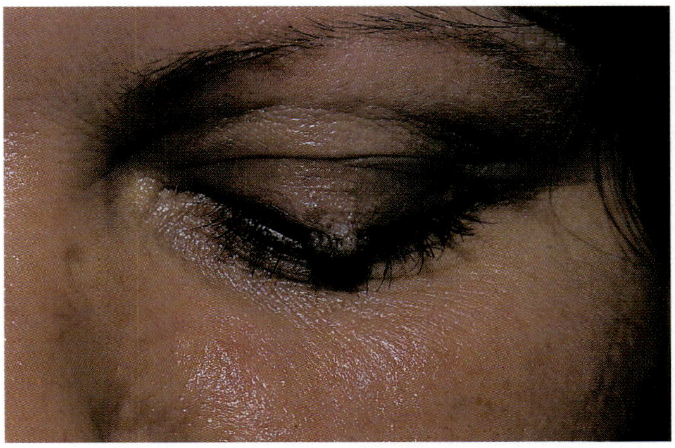

Figure 24–6. Squamous papilloma of left upper eyelid.

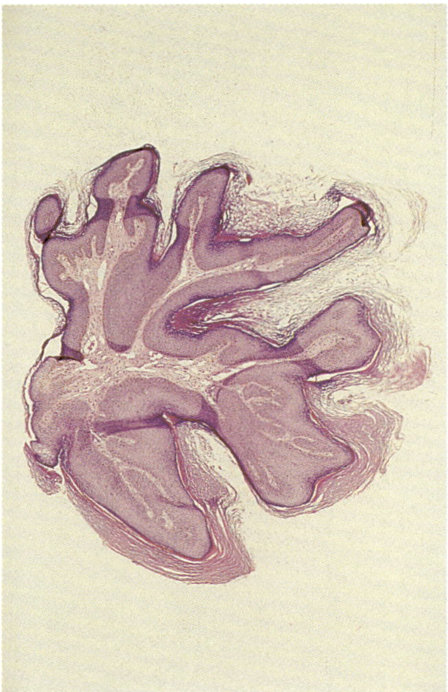

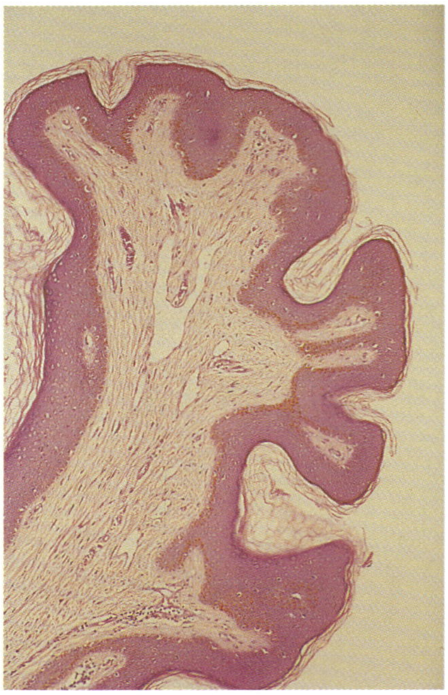

Figures 24–7 and 24–8. A pedunculated skin growth exhibits hyperkeratotic and acanthotic epithelium, which surrounds a fibrovascular core.

Inverted Follicular Keratosis

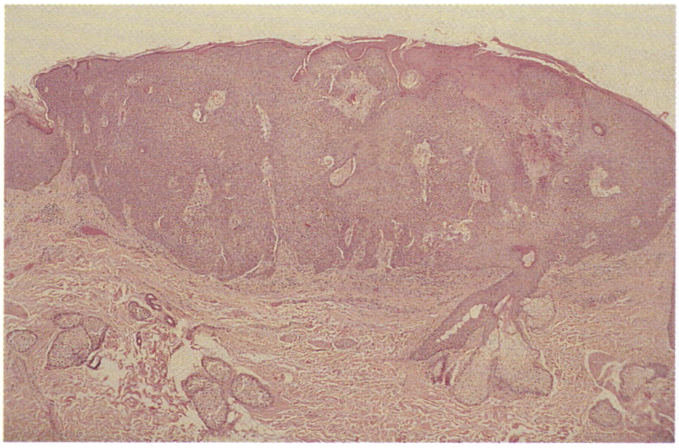

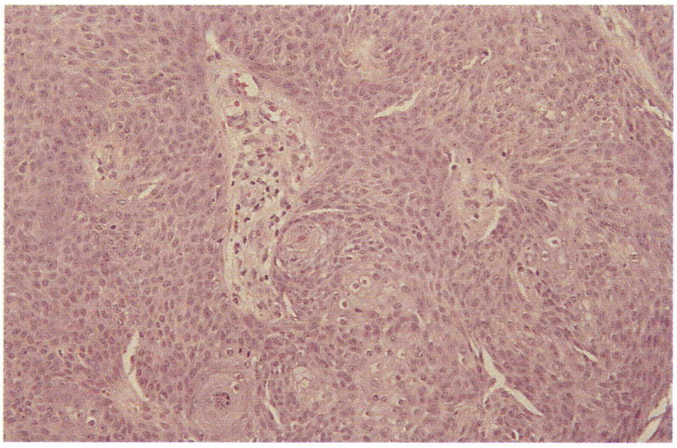

Figures 24–9 and 24–10. Inverted follicular keratosis. Marked hyperkeratosis, parakeratosis, and basilar acanthosis are present. Note the flattened base of the lesion, which resembles a seborrheic keratosis. These lesions are sometimes referred to as irritated seborrheic keratosis, although generally the latter are less endophytic.

Keratoacanthoma

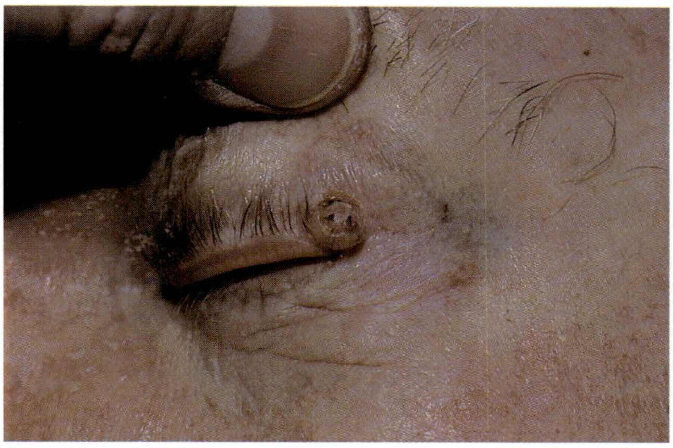

Figure 24–11. Keratoacanthoma. Dome-shaped lesion of the left upper lid with a keratin-filled central crater.

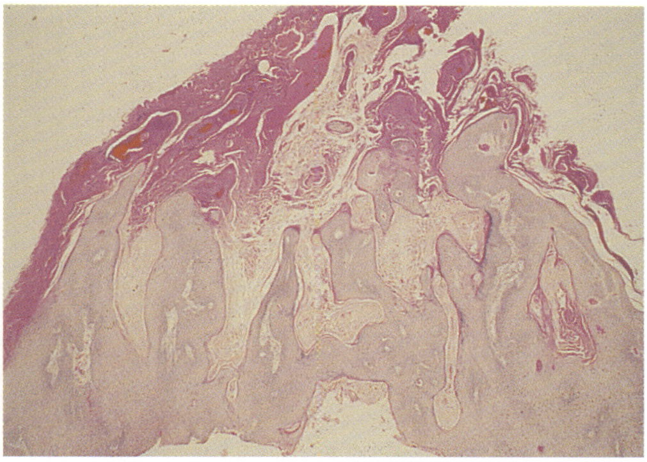

Figure 24–12. The cup-shaped mass is filled with keratin and lined by a hyperplastic proliferation of squamous epithelium.

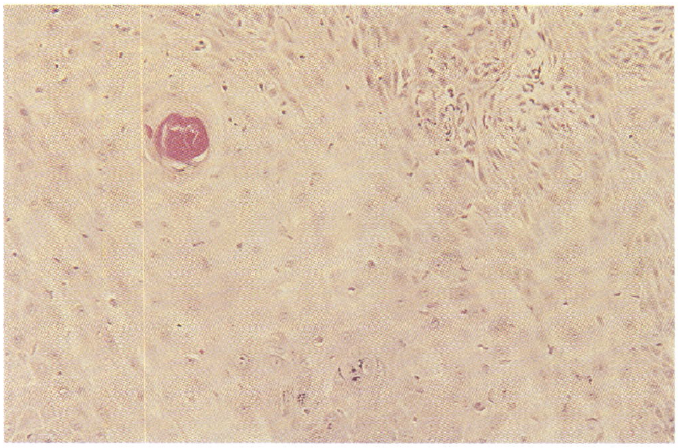

Figure 24–13. Higher magnification shows many atypical dyskeratotic cells.

Seborrheic Keratosis

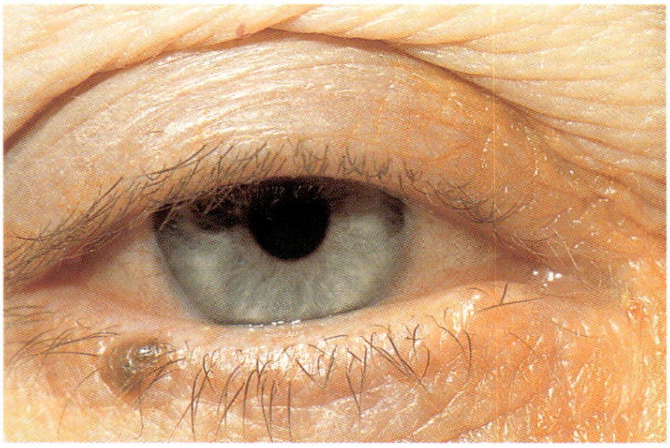

Figure 24–14. Seborrheic keratosis.

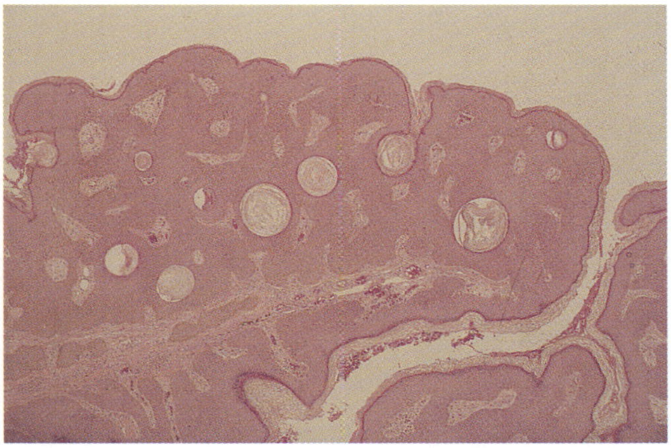

Figure 24–15. This lesion may also occur as a variant of squamous papilloma that exhibits an additional finding—intraepithelial horn cysts. These lesions show varying degrees of pigmentation.

Actinic Keratosis

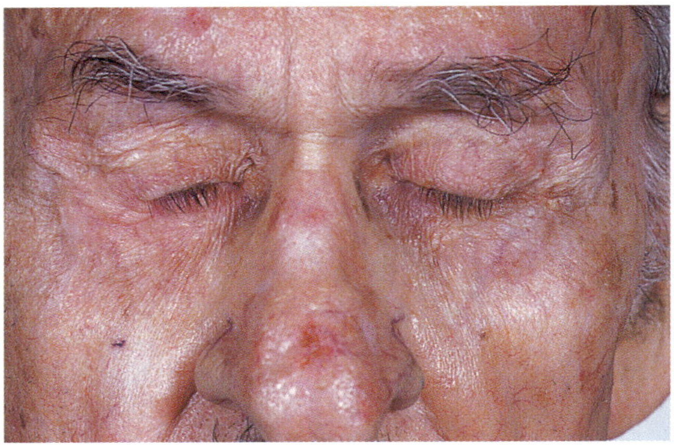

Figure 24–16. Actinic keratosis. Multiple erythematous, flat, scaly lesions cover the entire midface region.

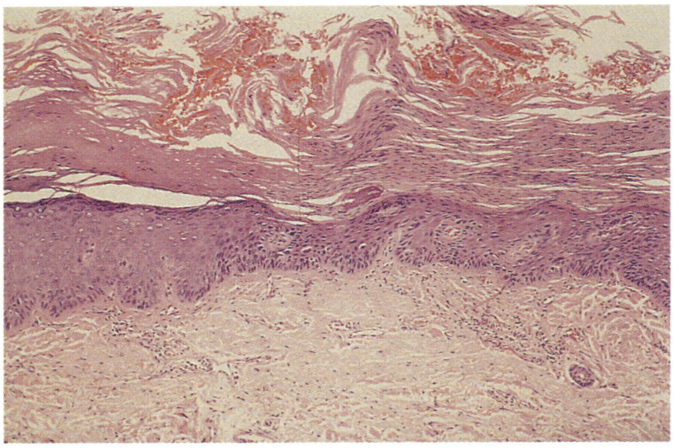

Figure 24–17. This potentially precancerous skin lesion is characterized by hyperkeratosis, parakeratosis, dyskeratosis, and focally intense inflammation at the base of the lesion. The epithelial basement membrane is intact.

Squamous Cell Carcinoma

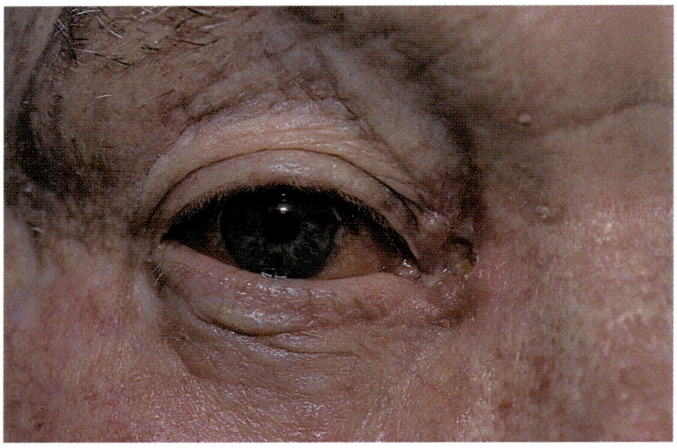

Figure 24–18. This squamous cell carcinoma lesion of the right medial canthal area exhibits raised, erythematous, irregular borders with a central area of ulceration. Surface crusting is apparent over the inferior half of the lesion.

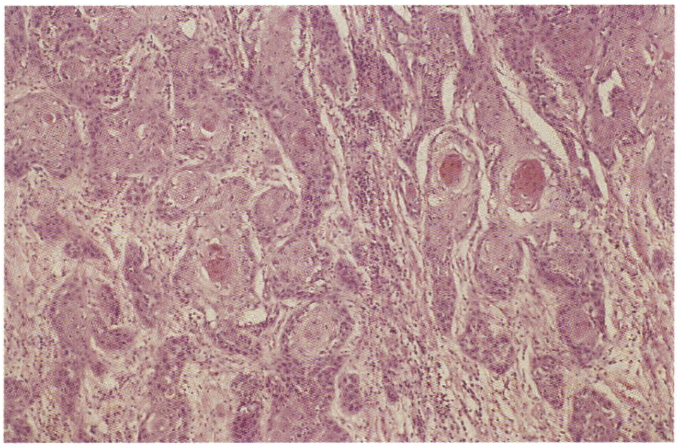

Figure 24–19. The lesion is a centrally ulcerated mass with anaplastic squamous cells with abundant eosinophilic (*i.e.*, keratin-filled) cytoplasm, dyskeratotic pearls, and circular aggregates of tumor cells.

Basal Cell Carcinoma

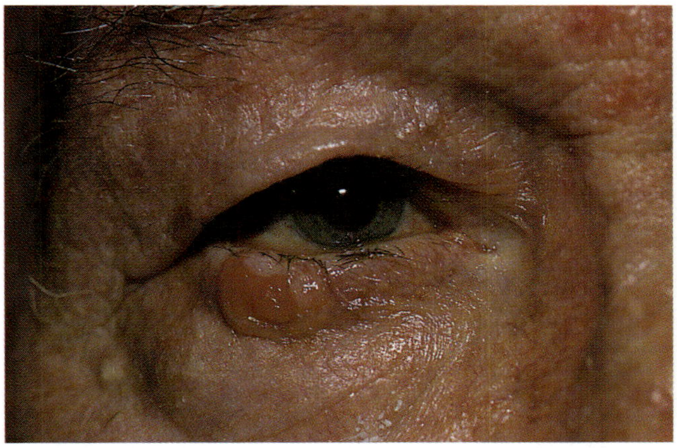

Figure 24–20. Basal cell carcinoma. A large, elevated nodule with a central area of ulceration is present on the right lower eyelid.

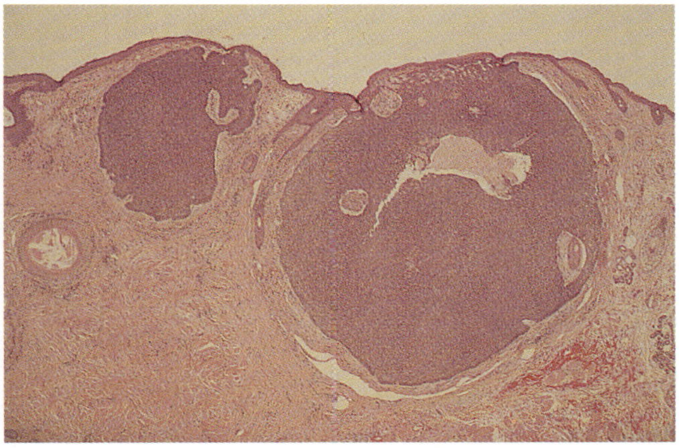

Figure 24–21. Nodular basal cell carcinoma.

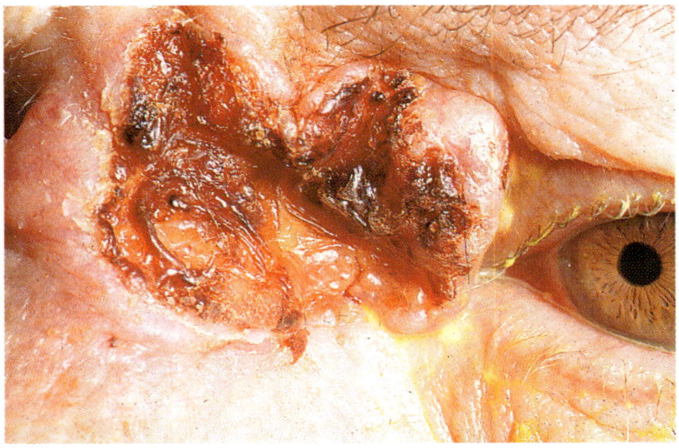

Figure 24–22. Morpheaform basal cell carcinoma.

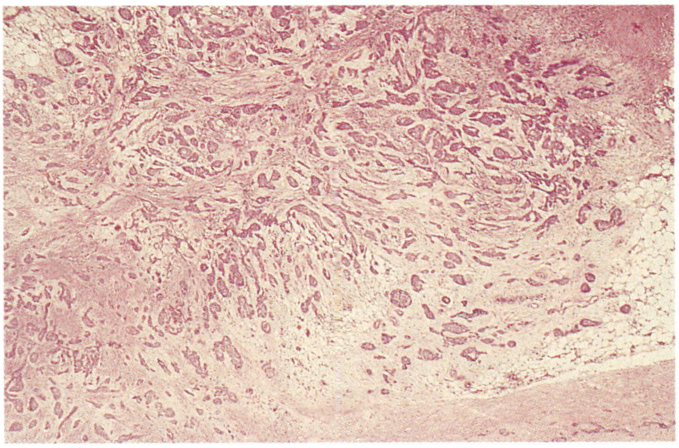

Figure 24–23. Strands and tendrils of tumor cells infiltrate the surrounding tissue in morpheaform or sclerosing basal cell carcinoma. A discrete mass is not present.

Melanocytic Nevi

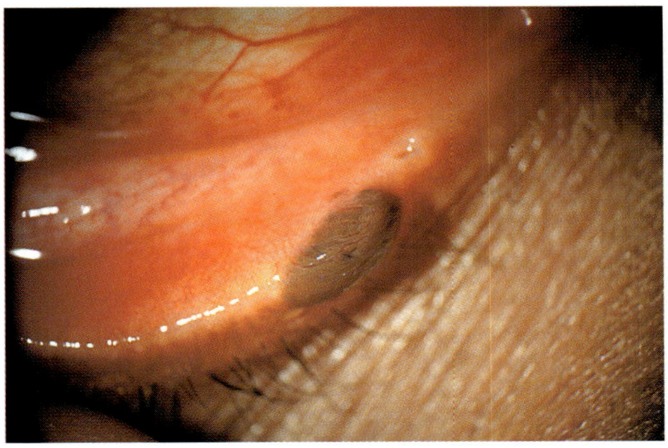

Figure 24–24. A nevus of right lower lid margin is present.

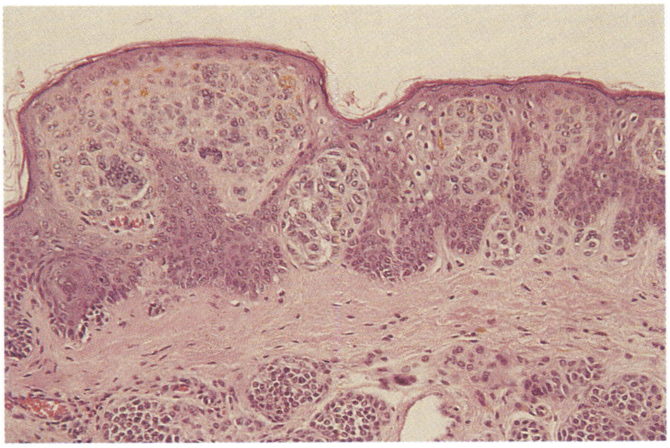

Figure 24–25. Compound nevus. Nevus cells are present both within and beneath the epithelium. More mature nevus cells deep in the dermis lose cytoplasm, pigment, and nesting pattern and resemble aggregated lymphocytes *(bottom)*.

Melanoma

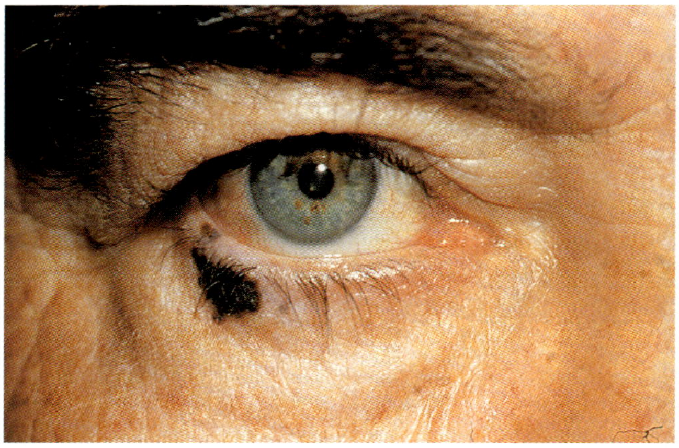

Figure 24–26. Malignant melanoma. A deeply pigmented lesion of the right lateral lower lid is present. Note the additional pigmented area on the lid margin. (Courtesy of Charles R. Leone, MD.)

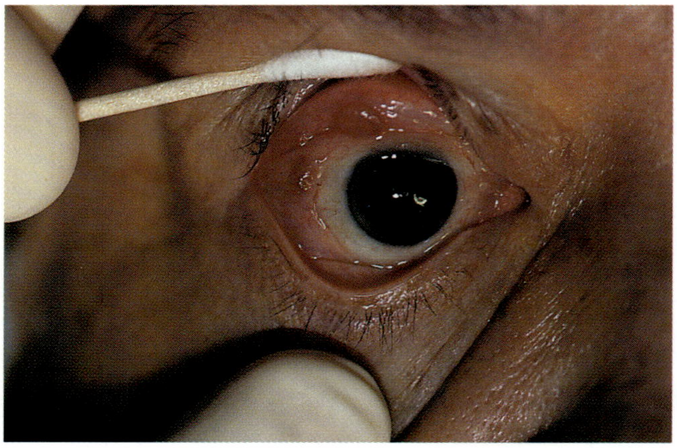

Figure 24–27. This tumor invades the right upper lid margin and conjunctival surface.

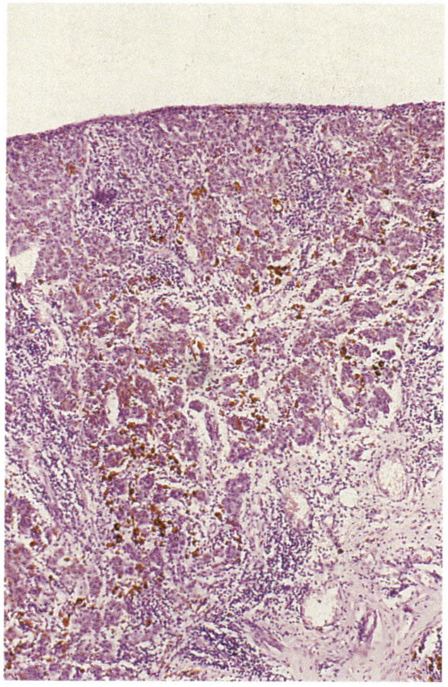

Figure 24–28. Microscopic examination reveals a richly pigmented tumor composed of invasive, atypical melanocytes that arose from a pre-existing junctional nevus that had been followed for many years.

Hordeolum and Chalazion

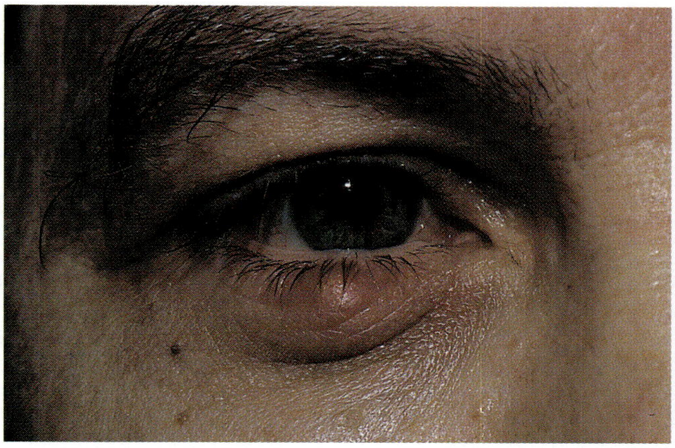

Figure 24–29. External hordeolum. Note the erythema surrounding the lesion. It has already begun to localize and is beginning to point toward the skin surface.

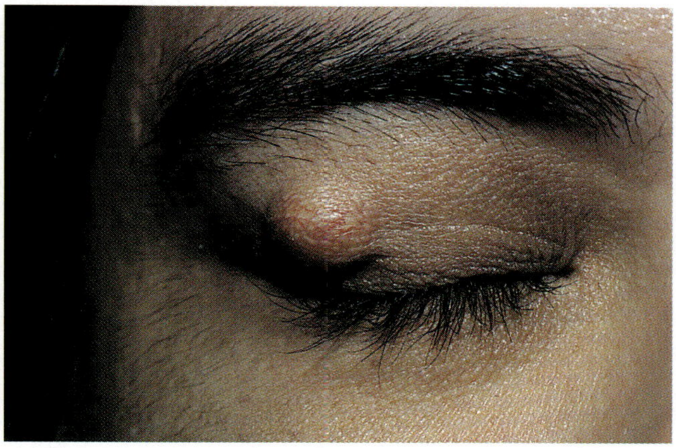

Figure 24–30. In this chronic chalazion, no inflammation of the skin is present.

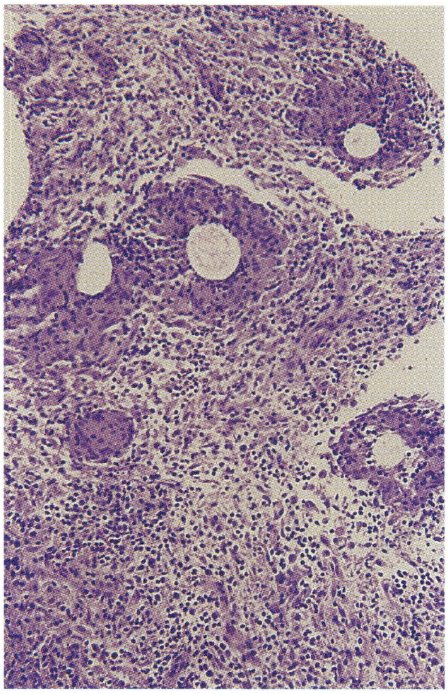

Figure 24–31. A chronic, noncaseating, granulomatous, inflammatory infiltrate surrounds lipid vacuoles in this chalazion.

Sebaceous Carcinoma

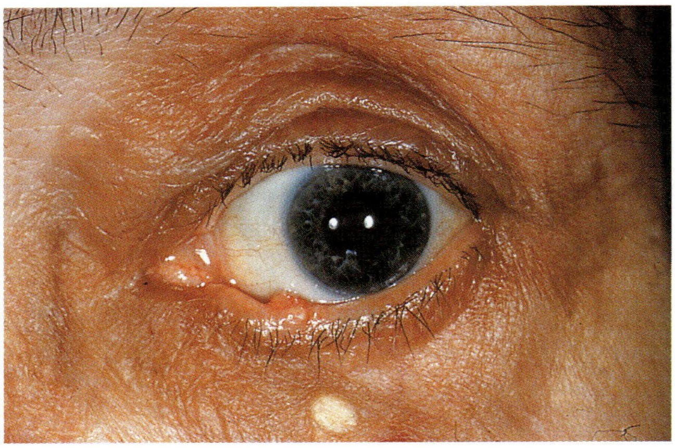

Figure 24–32. Sebaceous cell carcinoma of the left lower eyelid, located at the medial third of the lid margin, has a very nonspecific appearance. (Courtesy of Charles R. Leone, MD.)

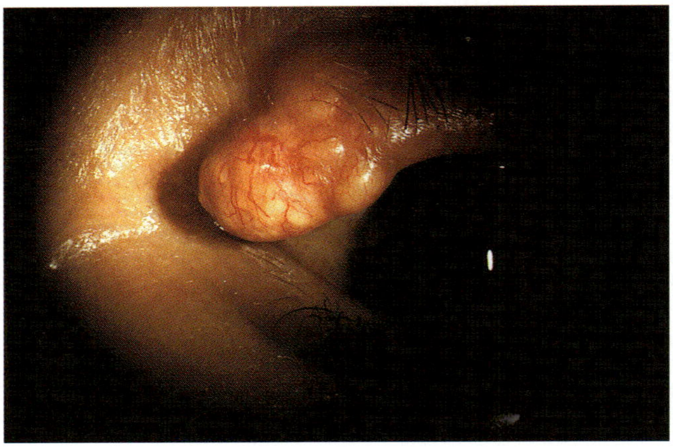

Figure 24–33. Sebaceous cell carcinoma of the left lower lid in the lateral canthal area is a large, yellowish lesion with a papillomatous-like growth pattern. Telangiectatic vessels are present on the surface, and there is a loss of eyelashes in the area of the tumor.

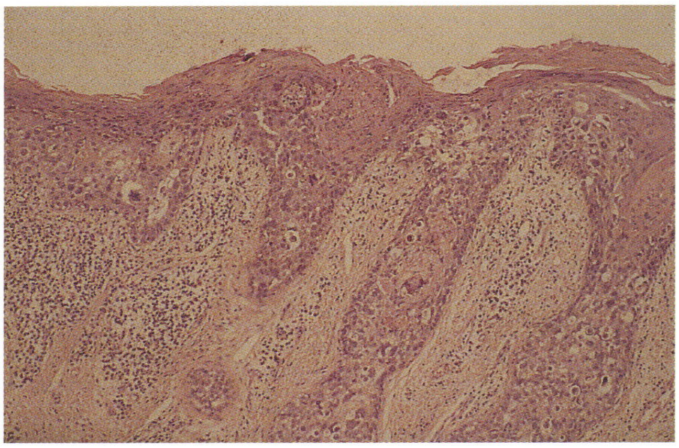

Figure 24–34. Sebaceous carcinoma exhibiting primarily intraepithelial growth by malignant lipidized cells.

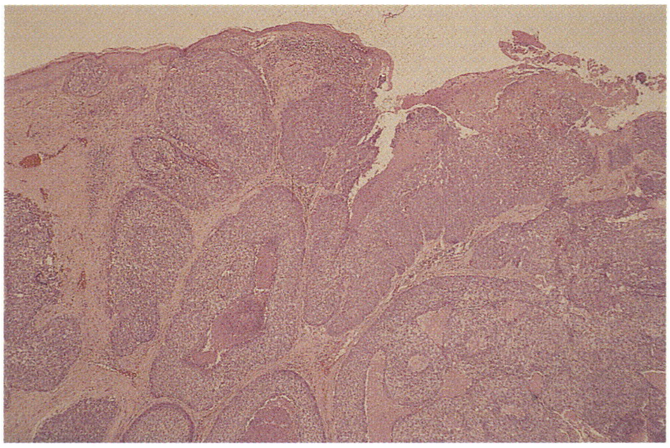

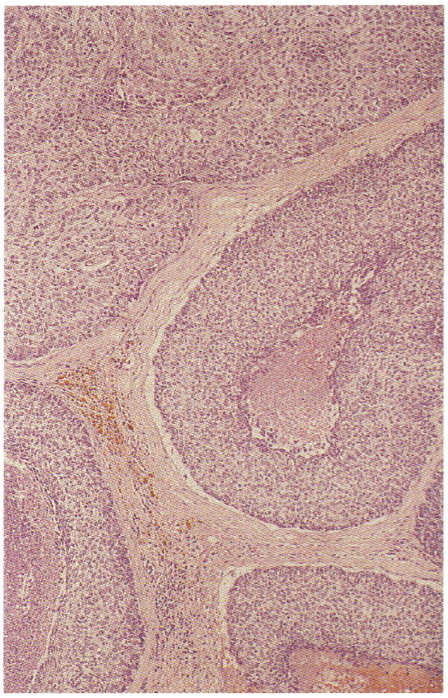

Figures 24–35 and 24–36. Sebaceous cell carcinoma. Normal sebaceous elements are replaced by malignant epithelial cells. At first glance, the tumor lobules appear to have peripheral palisading. This appearance may falsely masquerade as a basal cell carcinoma.

Syringoma

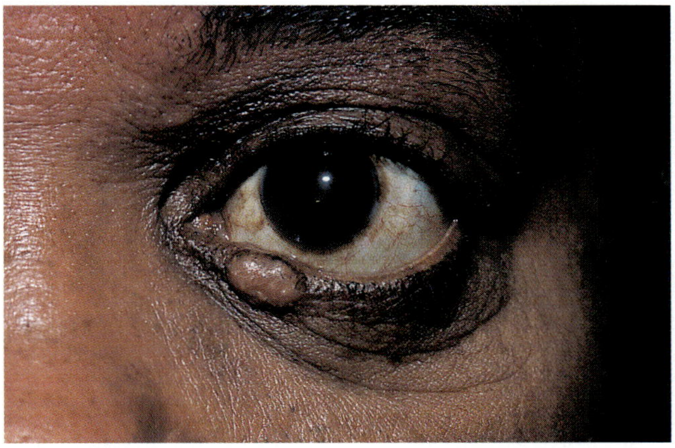

Figure 24–37. Syringoma. A waxy, yellowish lesion is present on the lower lid of a middle-aged woman.

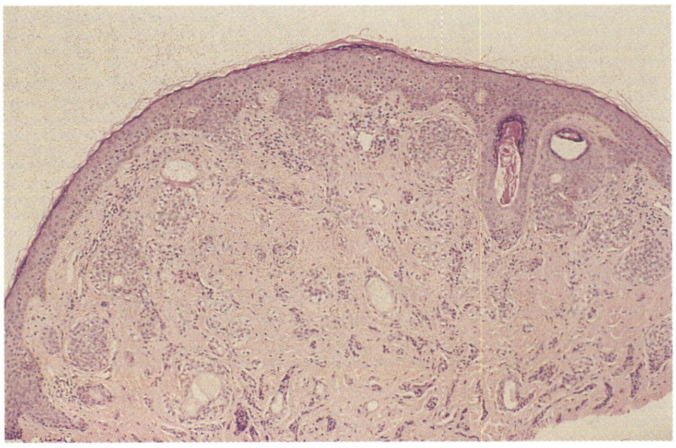

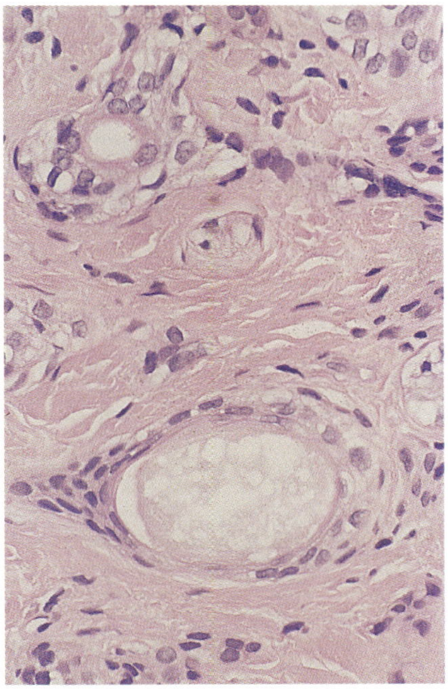

Figures 24–38 and 24–39. In this benign tumor of eccrine differentiation, there is a proliferation of cystic ductules and epithelial strands set within a fibrous stroma, showing a typical tadpole-like configuration.

Neurofibroma and Neurilemmoma

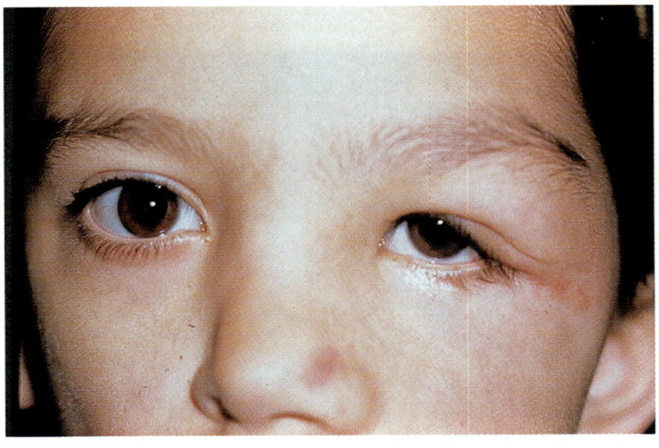

Figure 24–40. Neurofibroma. Typical S-shaped configuration of the upper eyelid is characteristic of neurofibroma.

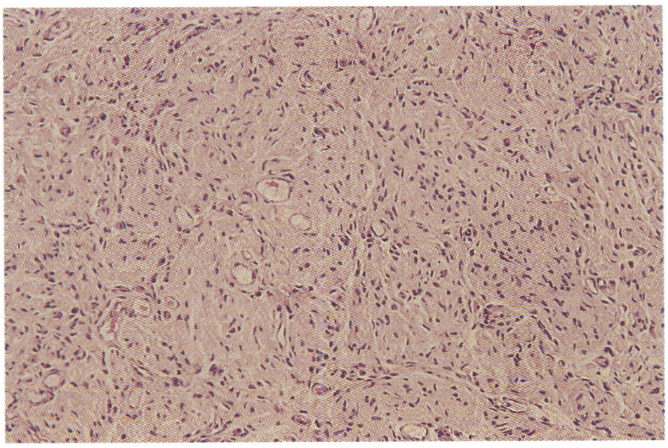

Figure 24–41. The tumor mass is composed of bland, spindle-shaped cells arranged about nerve bundles incorporating endoneurium and Schwann cells.

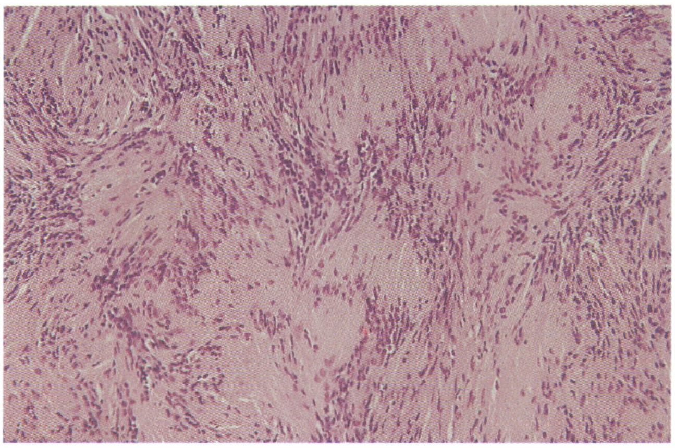

Figure 24–42. Two different morphologic patterns of neurilemmoma are found. Antoni A pattern exhibits a fascicular arrangement surrounded by collagenous sheath. The Antoni B pattern (not shown) consists of a loose network of more poorly organized cells.

Pyogenic Granuloma

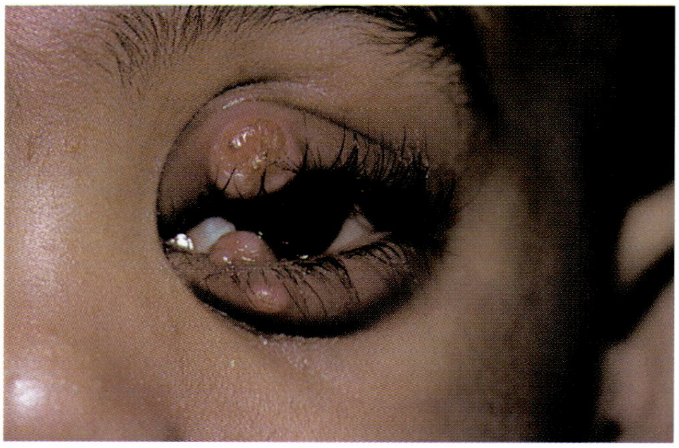

Figure 24–43. Pyogenic granuloma. Multiple pyogenic granulomas of all four eyelids occurred after multiple recurrent chalazion. On the right lid, all of the lesions are on the inner aspect (not shown). The left lid has lesions on both the external and internal surfaces.

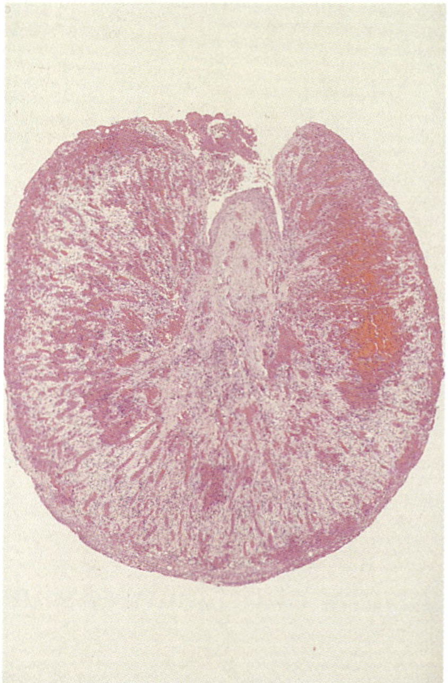

Figure 24–44. This benign, reactive mass is an exuberant proliferation of granulation tissue with a chronic inflammatory infiltrate. Capillaries, endothelium, fibroblasts, plasma cells, and lymphocytes are present.

Capillary Hemangioma

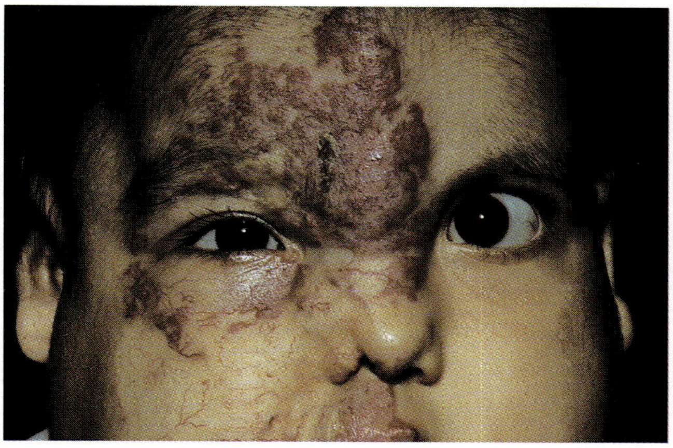

Figure 24–45. Capillary hemangioma. Extensive involvement of the facial area is seen on this patient.

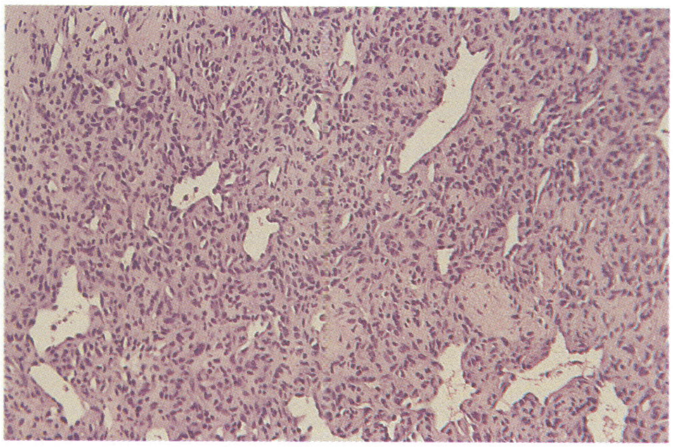

Figure 24–46. The lesion removed from the eyelid exhibits incomplete regression. The bulk of this tumor is a monotonous proliferation of capillaries, larger collecting vessels, and fibrosis.

Apocrine Hidrocystoma

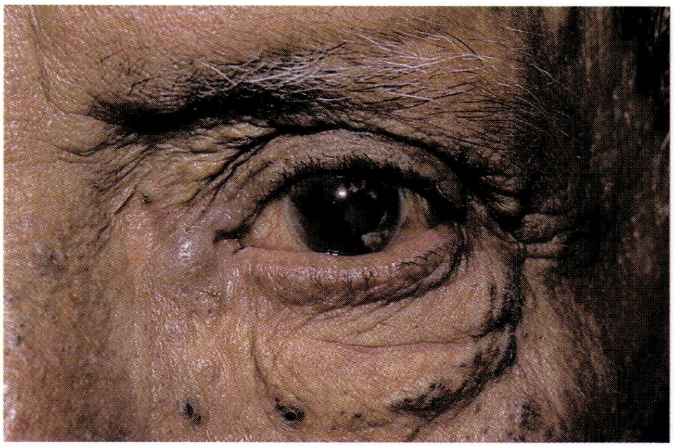

Figure 24–47. Apocrine hidrocystoma. There is a translucent, cystic nodule adjacent to the lid margin in the left medial canthal area.

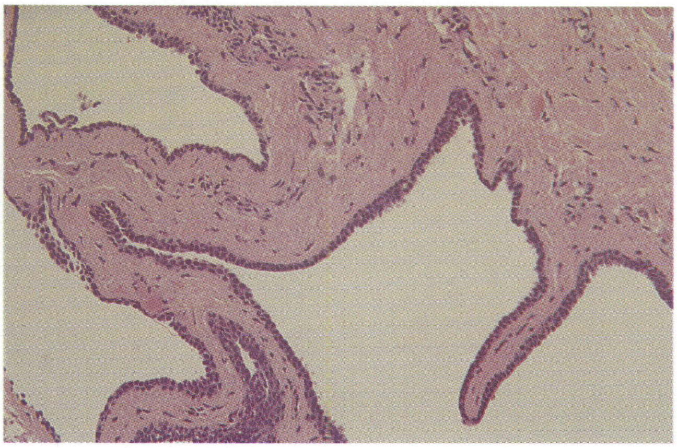

Figure 24–48. Apocrine hidrocystoma. A clear, arborizing cyst is lined by a bilayer of low cuboidal epithelium. The inner cell layer elaborates its products by apical decapitation secretion.

Dermoid Cyst

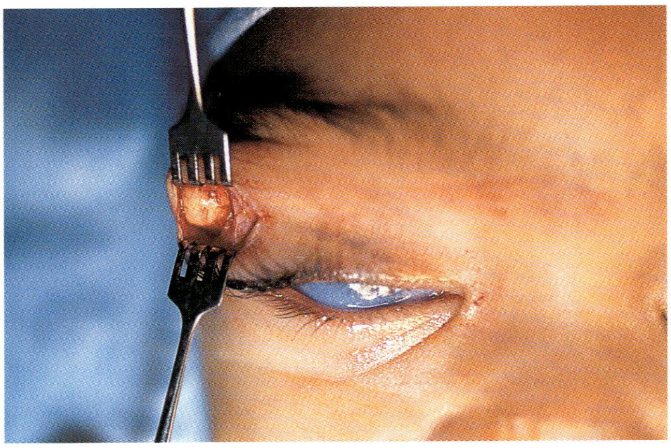

Figure 24–49. Dermoid cyst. Gross appearance of the lesion at the time of removal. Dermoid cysts are generally firm, encapsulated, ovoid, yellowish-white lesions.

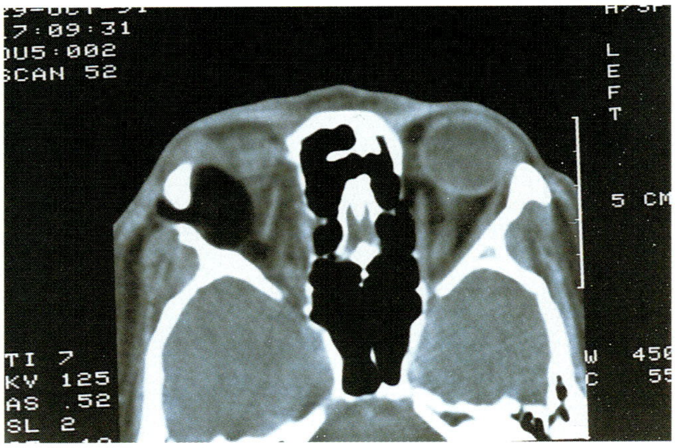

Figure 24–50. Computed tomography scan demonstrates a dermoid cyst of the right orbit extending through the frontozygomatic suture area and giving off an external component, which renders it dumbbell shaped. There is an air density mass in the temporal aspect of the right orbit.

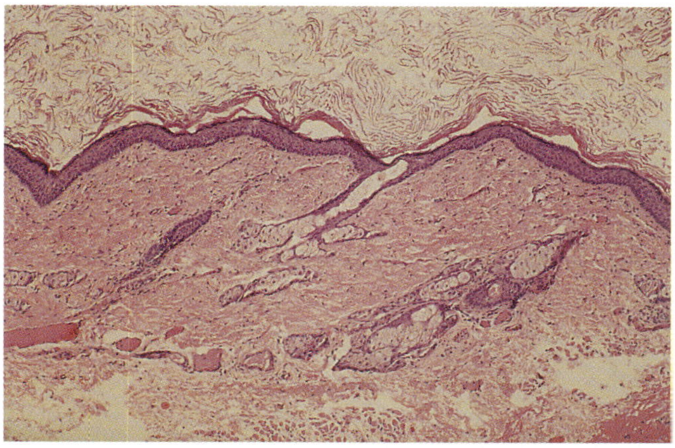

Figure 24–51. The cystic lesion is lined by cutaneous epithelium that rests on dermal tissue containing skin appendages such as hair follicles, sebaceous glands, and sweat glands. These structures communicate with the cyst lumen and fill it with debris.

Xanthelasma

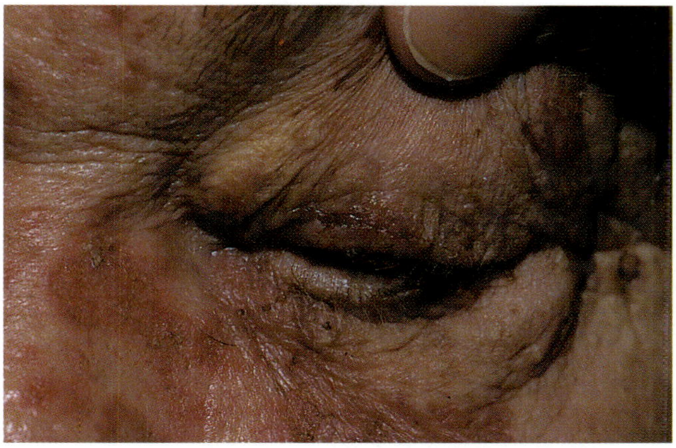

Figure 24–52. Xanthelasma. A yellowish, flat plaque is seen in the medial portion of the right upper eyelid. Lateral to the xanthelasma, near the lid margin, is an ulcerated basal cell carcinoma. In the surrounding tissue, there are multiple areas of erythematous, scaly, actinic keratotic lesions. The histology is identical to a xanthoma depicted in Chapter 19 of this atlas.

25

Comparative Dermatopathology

Veterinary dermatopathology is an evolving discipline that covers a wide range of species. Dermatopathology of animals is not a recognized subspecialty, as it is in humans, but remains part of the broader discipline of veterinary pathology. However, the field of veterinary dermatopathology has evolved as a specialty in recent years, and the number of individuals with expertise in this area continues to grow.

The range of diseases in veterinary dermatopathology is immense, as are the species in which these diseases occur. In experimental dermatopathology, the mouse and rat are the most commonly used species. However, our companion animals, the dog and the cat, display the greatest diversity of diseases, as well as afford the pathologist the largest number of specimens for histopathologic evaluation.

This chapter represents a very brief and general overview of the skin of the dog and cat and provides examples of the complicated responses of this skin to injury. Because practicing pathologists and dermatopathologists occasionally receive biopsies of animal skin for diagnostic evaluation, it is hoped that this section may be of practical significance. Humans and nonhuman vertebrates share a number of common or analogous mechanisms of inflammatory and neoplastic change affecting their integuments. Therefore, it also is hoped that this effort will stimulate thought concerning the comparative dermatopathology of humans and animals, and that from this new diagnostic and therapeutic approaches for both may evolve.

Non-neoplastic Disorders Affecting the Epidermis

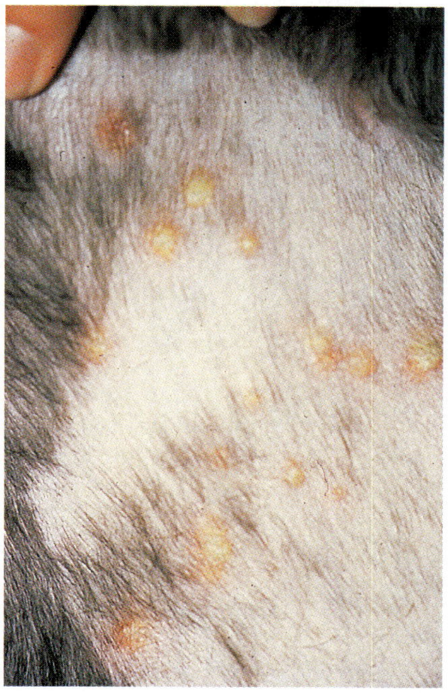

Figure 25–1. Pustular diseases: Canine pemphigus foliaceus. Clinically, there are multiple intraepidermal pustules that bridge several hair follicles.

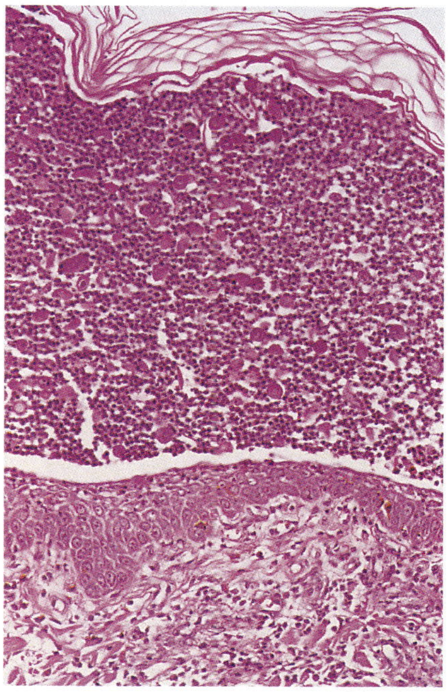

Figure 25–2. Subcorneal pustules contain numerous acantholytic cells, neutrophils, and eosinophils in pemphigus foliaceus.

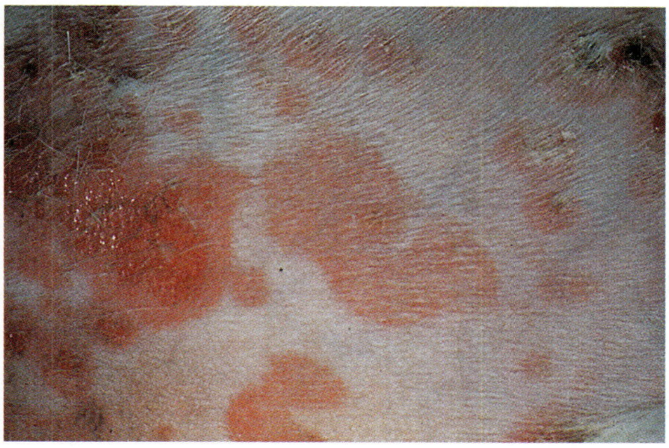

Figure 25–3. Necrotizing diseases of the epidermis. Erythema multiforme is present in a dog with severe erythema and occasional target-like lesions.

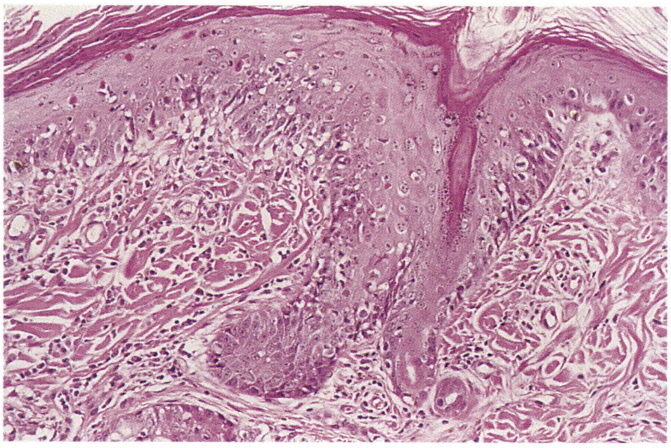

Figure 25–4. The epidermis in canine erythema multiforme is hyperplastic with parakeratosis, diffuse dyskeratosis, and spongiosis, and there is a mild lymphoid infiltrate of the epidermis and dermis. Early vacuolar changes are seen within the basal cell area.

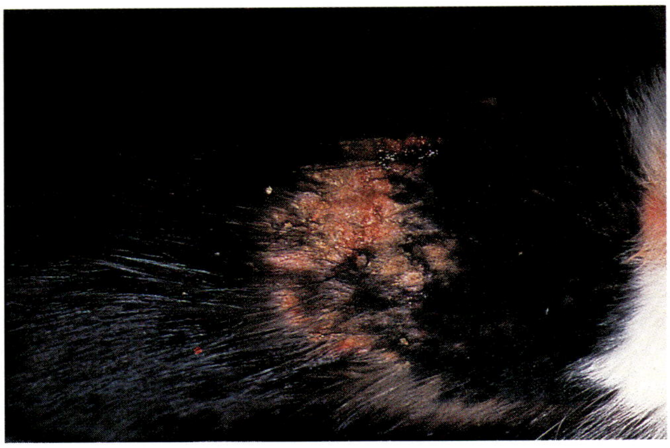

Figure 25–5. Exudative and ulcerative diseases of the epidermis. Multifocal papular, pustular, and crusting dermatitis characterize this allergic condition in a cat.

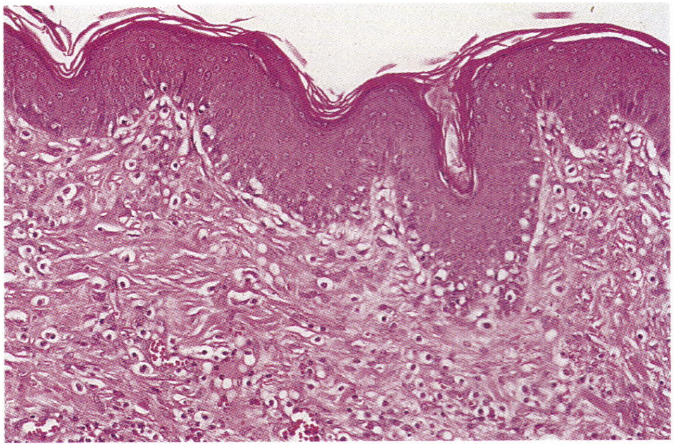

Figure 25–6. In a biopsy from the animal depicted in Figure 25–5, epidermal hyperplasia is seen with infiltration of the epidermis and dermis by mast cells and superficial dermal linear fibrosis.

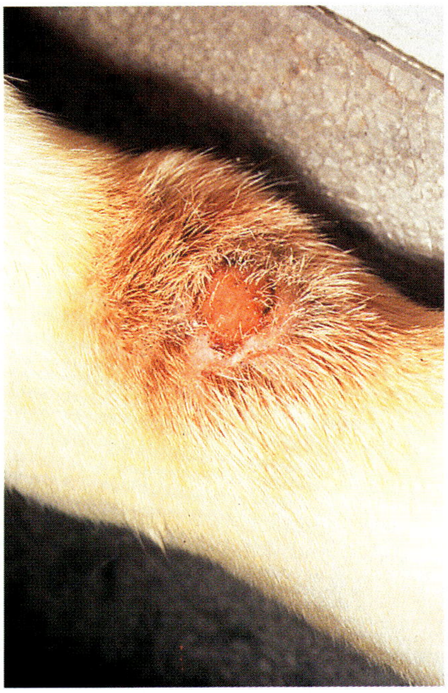

Figure 25–7. Hyperplastic diseases of the epidermis. Acral lick dermatitis is present with a central ulcer and marked peripheral skin thickening. (Courtesy of Kevin Shanley, DVM.)

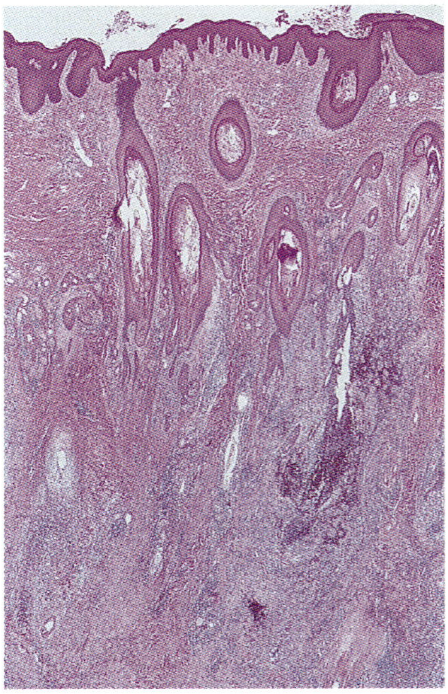

Figure 25–8. Epidermal hyperplasia, dermal fibrosis, periadnexal inflammation, and a perforating folliculitis are seen in acral lick dermatitis.

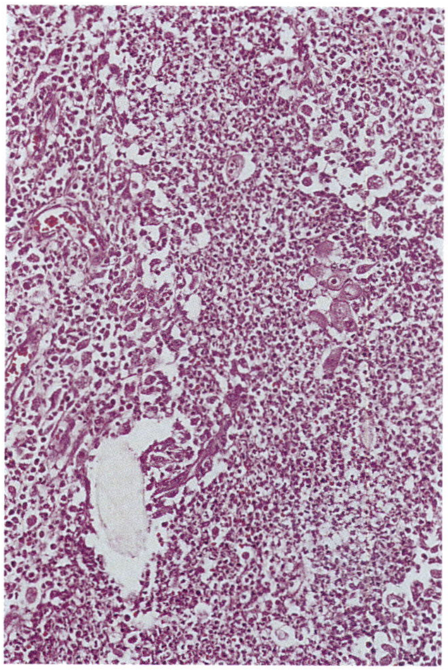

Figure 25–9. Higher magnification of the biopsy shown in Figure 25–8; naked pieces of hair have evoked an infiltrate of neutrophils and eosinophils.

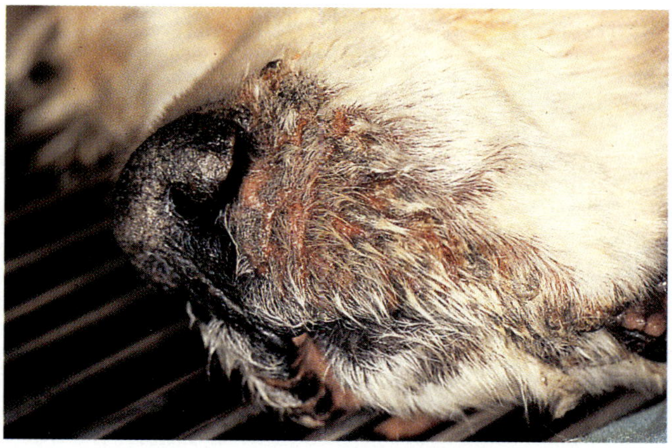

Figure 25–10. Hyperkeratotic diseases of the epidermis. Hepatocutaneous syndrome (*i.e.,* superficial necrolytic dermatitis) has produced an extensive, hyperplastic, crusting dermatitis involving the nasal skin. (Courtesy of Kevin Shanley, DVM.)

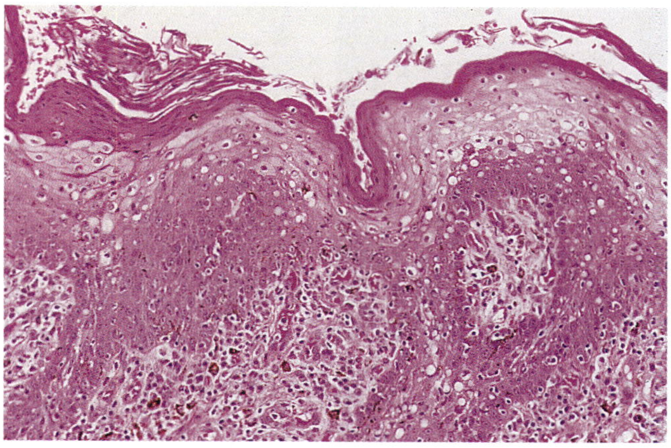

Figure 25–11. Parakeratosis, spongiosis and pallor of the upper portion of the epidermis, and epidermal hyperplasia with melanin drop-off and dermal inflammation are seen in the cross section of a biopsy from the lesion in Figure 25–10. This histology resembles toxic epidermal necrolysis in humans.

Non-neoplastic Disorders Affecting the Dermis

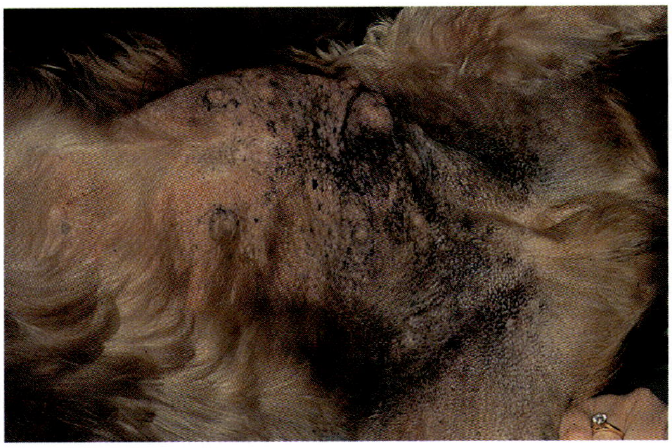

Figure 25–12. Perivascular diseases of the dermis. Atopic dermatitis is seen with hyperemia, hyperpigmentation, and thickening of the epidermis in the inguinal area of this dog.

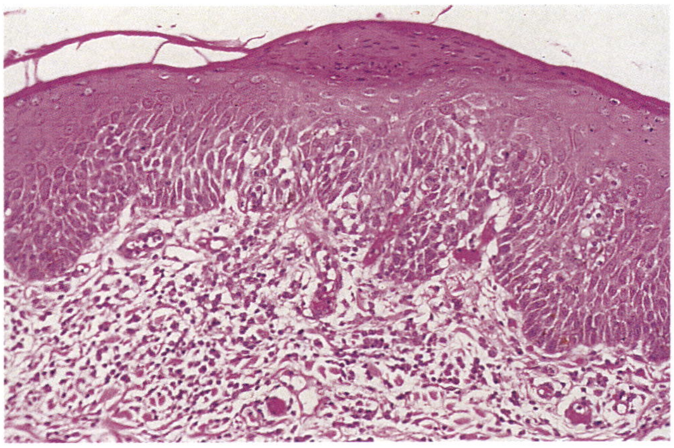

Figure 25–13. Superficial parakeratosis at the site of self-induced trauma, epidermal and dermal edema, vascular dilation with margination of granulocytes, and perivascular infiltration by lymphocytes, plasma cells, and mast cells are seen in atopic dermatitis.

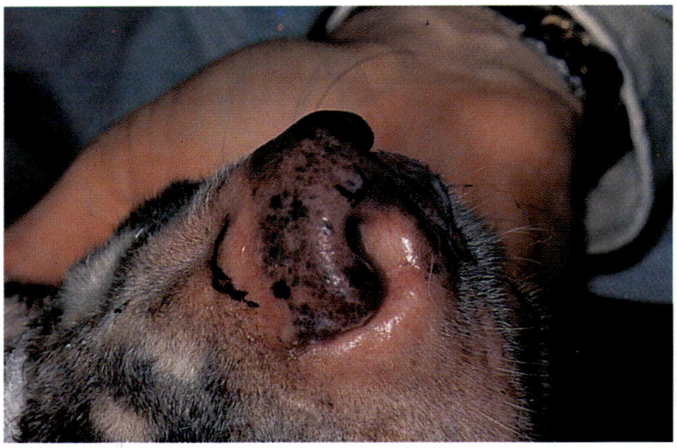

Figure 25–14. Lichenoid (*i.e.,* interface) diseases of the dermis. Nasal depigmentation is present in a case of Vogt-Koyanagi-Harada–like disease, a syndrome characterized by depigmenting dermatitis and uveitis. (Courtesy of James Jeffers, VMD.)

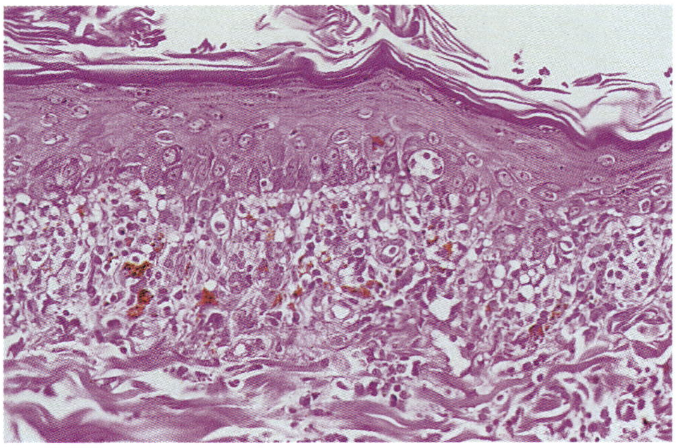

Figure 25–15. Interface lichenoid dermatitis with melanin drop-off is seen in a biopsy; the cellular infiltrate consists of histiocytes and melanophages, with a lesser number of lymphocytes and plasma cells.

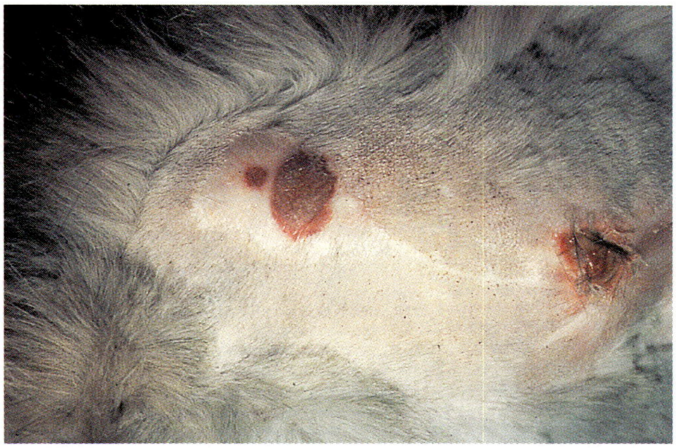

Figure 25–16. Infectious nodular granulomatous and pyogranulomatous disease of the dermis. The large, erythematous intradermal masses are the aggregates of *Microsporum canis* infection. (Courtesy of William Miller, VMD.)

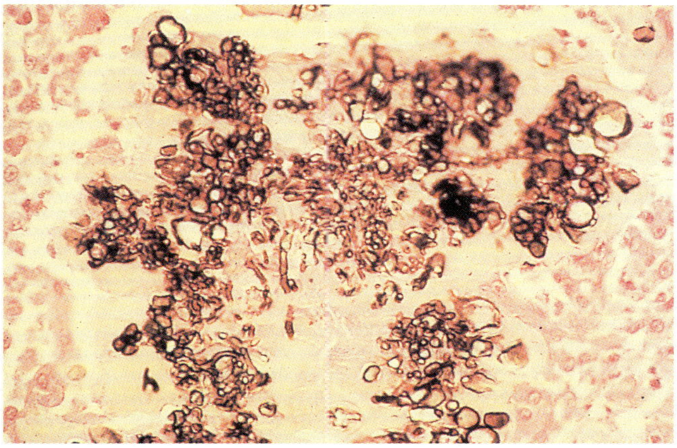

Figure 25–17. Fungal pseudomycetoma and the associated granulomatous inflammation are present in the dermis in infectious nodular granulomatous and pyogranulomatous disease.

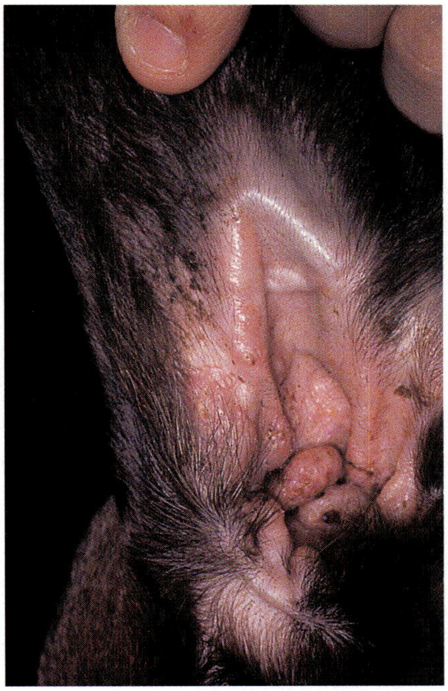

Figure 25–18. Noninfectious nodular and diffuse granulomatous and pyogranulomatous disease of the dermis. Swelling, hyperemia, vesicles, and pustules involve the outer ear of this young dog with juvenile cellulitis. (Courtesy of James Jeffers, VMD.)

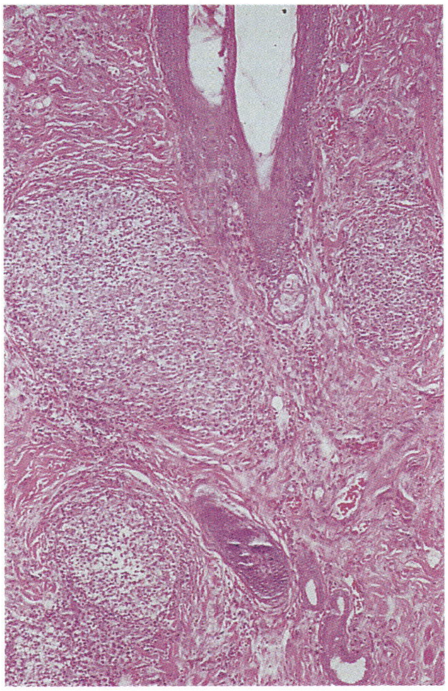

Figure 25–19. Numerous pyogranulomatous foci are seen within the dermis and are often associated with adnexa in this biopsy of the lesion depicted in Figure 25–18.

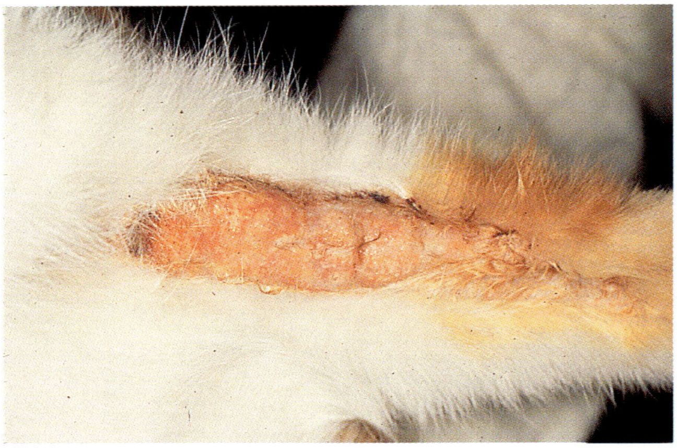

Figure 25–20. Nodular and diffuse diseases of the dermis with prominent eosinophils and plasma cells. Collagenolytic granulomas involve the rear leg of a cat. (Courtesy of James Jeffers, VMD.)

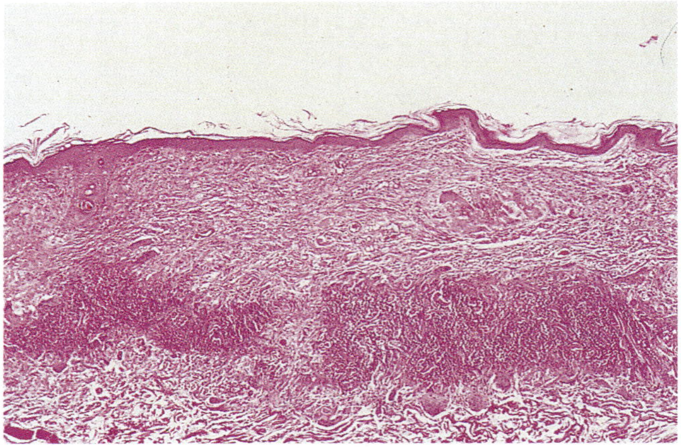

Figure 25–21. A large band of degenerate collagen is seen in the deep dermis in collagenolytic granuloma, and a small focus is present in the superficial dermis. A marked infiltrate by multinucleated giant cells surrounds these foci. The histology is reminiscent of palisaded granulomatous dermatitis in humans.

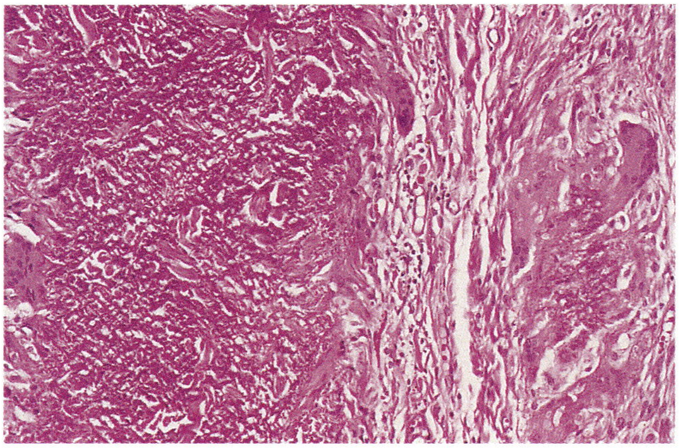

Figure 25–22. Higher magnification of the lesion depicted in Figure 25–21 shows degenerated collagen (*left*) surrounded by giant cells (*far right*).

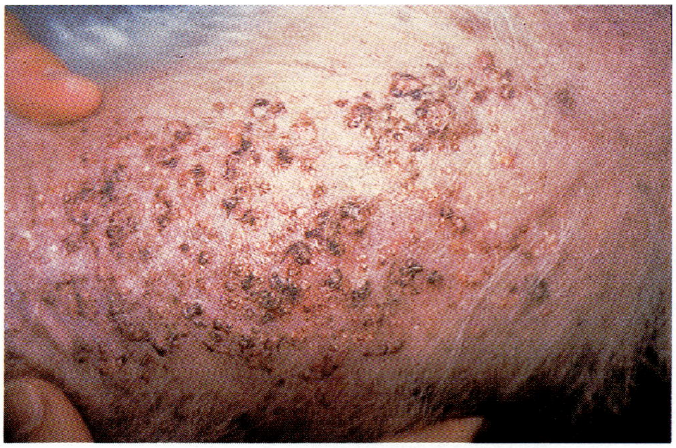

Figure 25–23. Dysplastic and depositional diseases of dermal connective tissue. Alopecia, multifocal epidermal hyperplasia, and numerous pustules characterize this case of calcinosis cutis due to hyperadrenocorticism. (Courtesy of Kevin Shanley, DVM.)

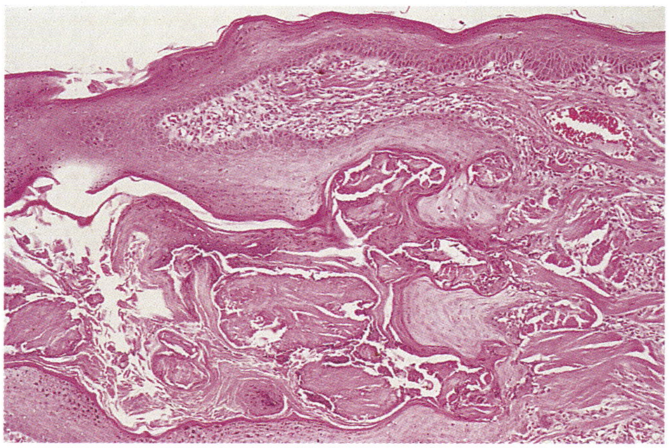

Figure 25–24. The mineralized foci in calcinosis cutis are being surrounded by the outer root sheath of the hair follicle, allowing the material to be removed from the dermis.

Non-neoplastic Disorders Affecting Adnexae

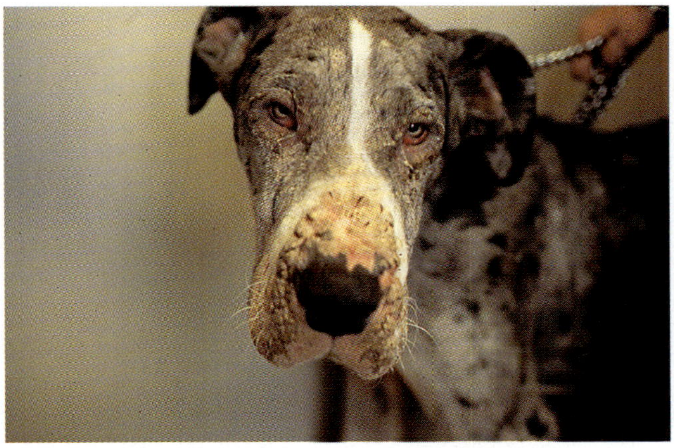

Figure 25–25. Pustular and nodular diseases, with and without follicular destruction. Canine demodicosis is localized to the head of this dog.

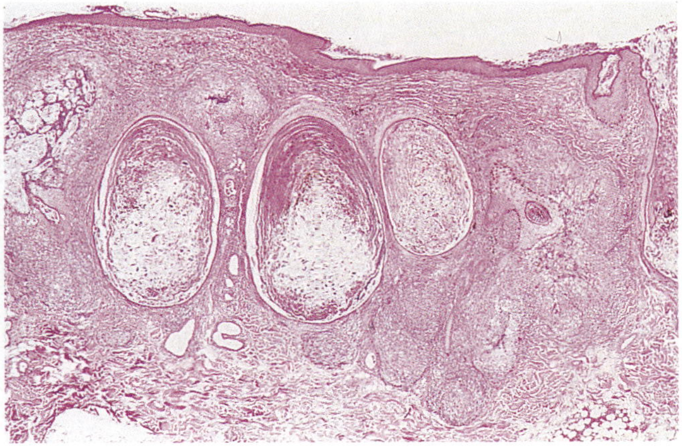

Figure 25–26. Canine demodicosis with severe follicular hyperkeratosis, numerous *Demodex* mites within the dilated infundibulum, and several perifollicular granulomas are seen.

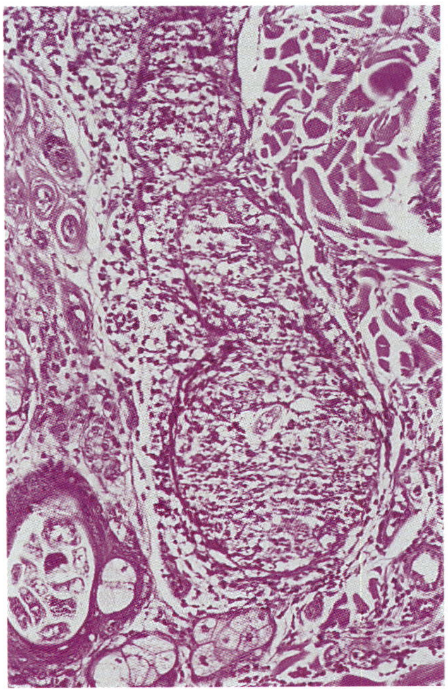

Figure 25–27. Higher magnification of Figure 25–26 demonstrates intrafollicular mites (*bottom left*) and perifollicular granuloma with a central mite.

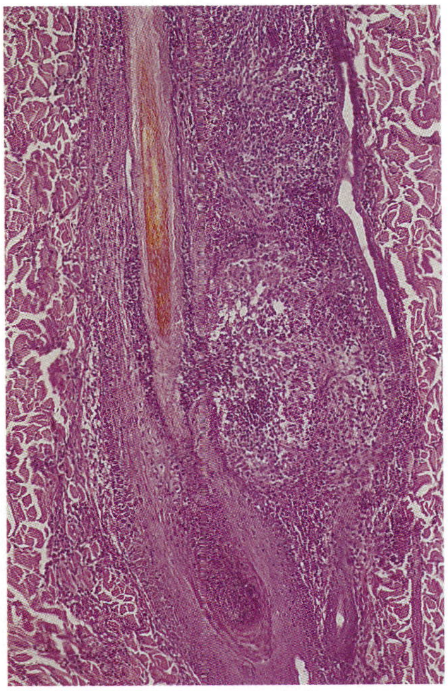

Figure 25–28. Dermatophytosis is present in a dog with a perforating folliculitis and numerous arthroconidia around the hair shaft.

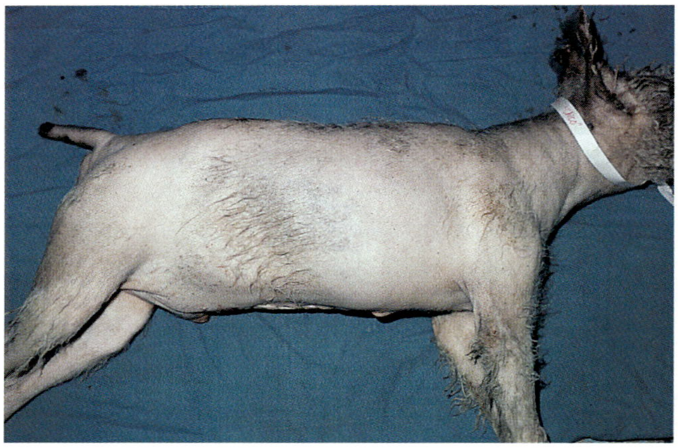

Figure 25–29. Atrophic diseases of the hair follicle. Canine hyperadrenocorticism. This dog shows extensive alopecia and a pendulous abdomen.

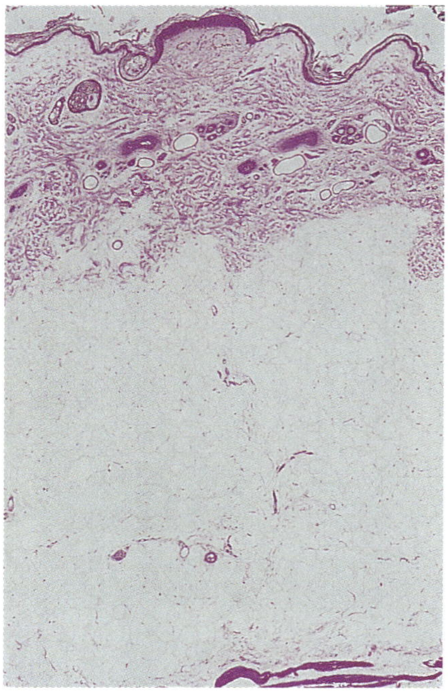

Figure 25–30. Histologic specimen of hyperadrenocorticism includes epidermal thinning, hyperkeratosis and infundibular hyperkeratosis, decreased dermal collagen, and a lack of any inflammatory cells. Note the difference in histologic appearance from Figures 25–23 and 25–24, which also are caused by hyperadrenocorticism.

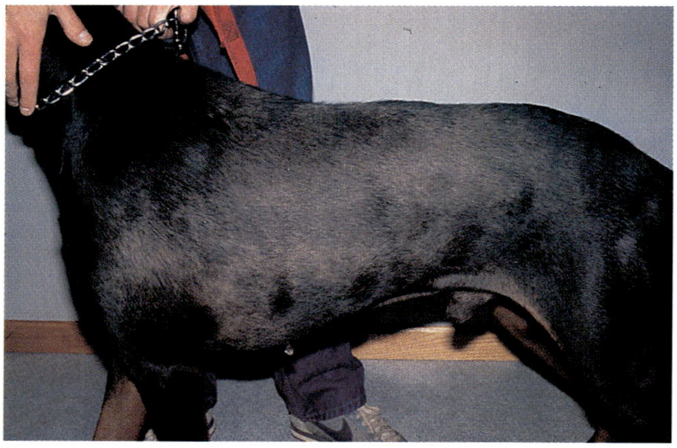

Figure 25–31. Dysplastic diseases of the hair follicle. Color dilution alopecia involves the thoracic and abdominal area. (Courtesy of Richard Long, DVM.)

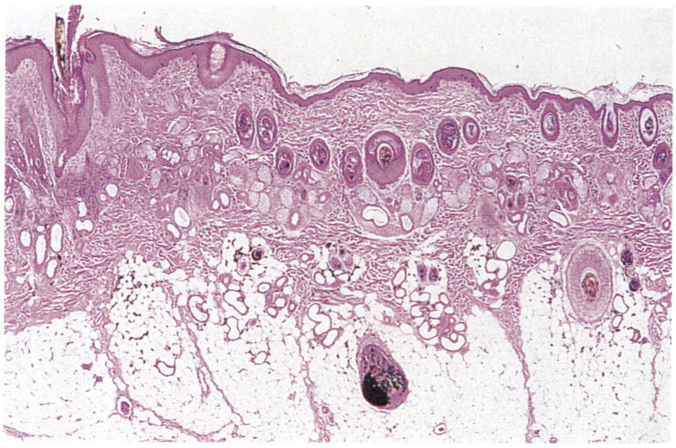

Figure 25–32. A biopsy of color dilution alopecia reveals hair loss and aggregation of melanin within the bulbar region, shaft of the hair, and within melanophages around hair follicles.

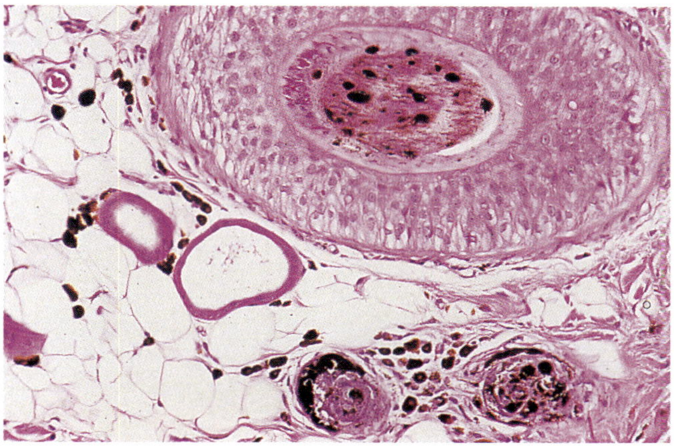

Figure 25–33. Higher magnification of Figure 25–32.

Disorders of the Panniculus

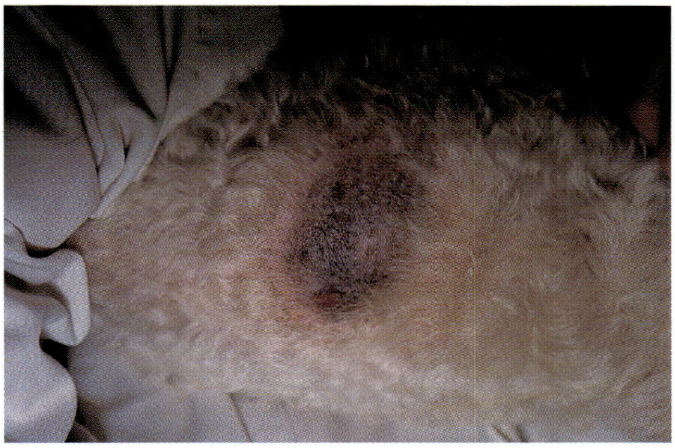

Figure 25–34. Diseases of the panniculus. Alopecia and hyperpigmentation occurred at the site of a rabies vaccination.

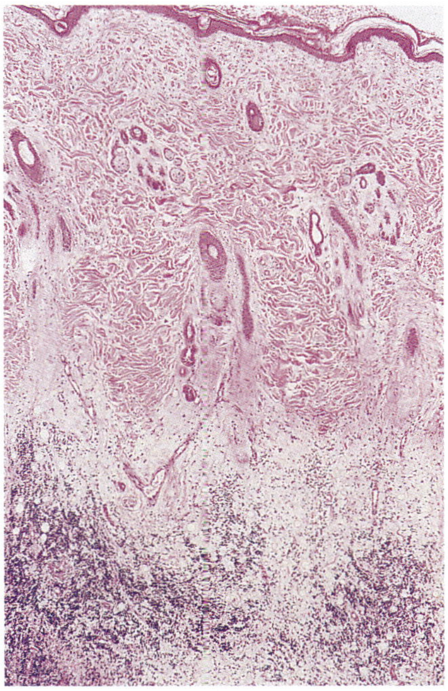

Figure 25–35. Alopecia and dermal fibrosis are seen in a biopsy of the lesion depicted in Figure 25–34, particularly around the remnants of hair follicles. A marked lymphoid infiltrate obliterates the panniculus adiposus.

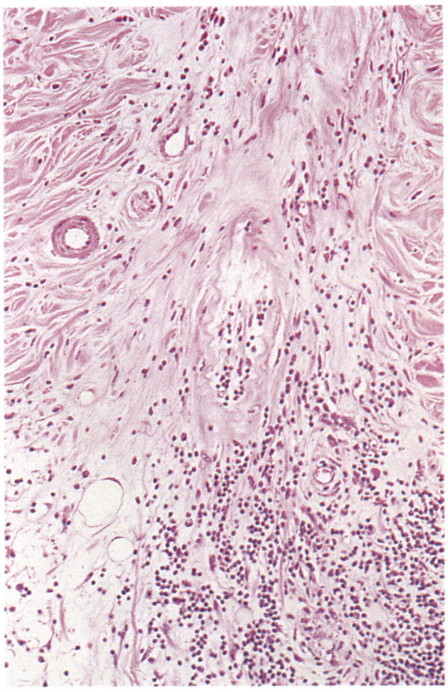

Figure 25–36. The inflammatory infiltrate of lymphocytes and plasma cells surrounds the remnants of the hair follicle.

Basal Cell Tumor

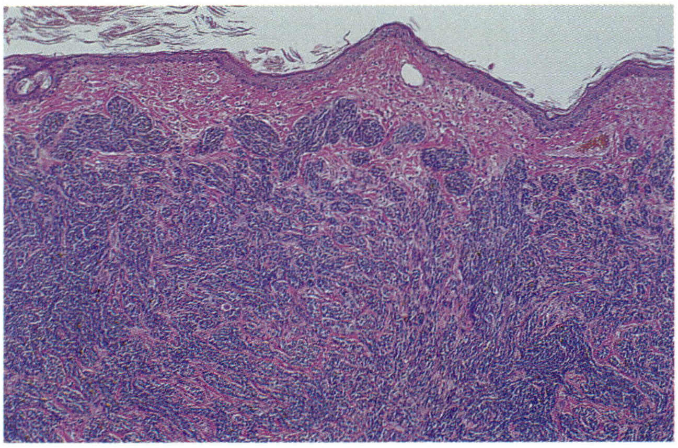

Figure 25–37. Basal cell tumor. Feline basal cell carcinoma extends from the superficial to the deep dermis.

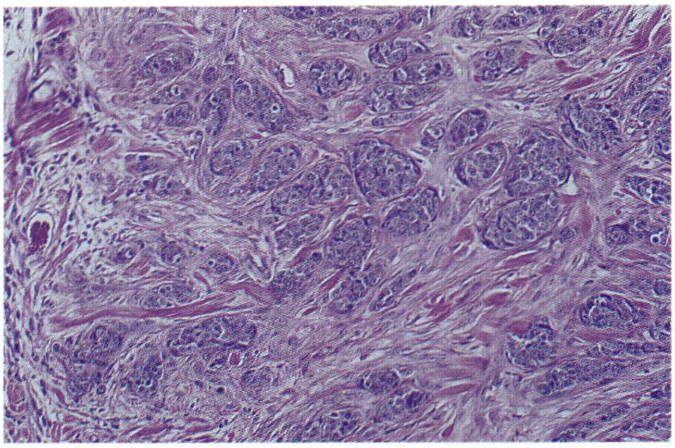

Figure 25–38. Deep edge of Figure 25–37 shows infiltrating carcinoma cells and a modest desmoplastic host response.

Squamous Cell Carcinoma

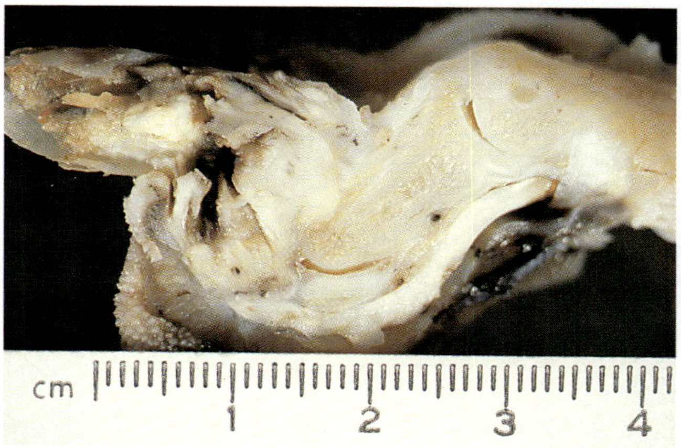

Figure 25–39. Squamous cell carcinoma. Subungual squamous cell carcinoma with destruction of the third phalanx in a dog.

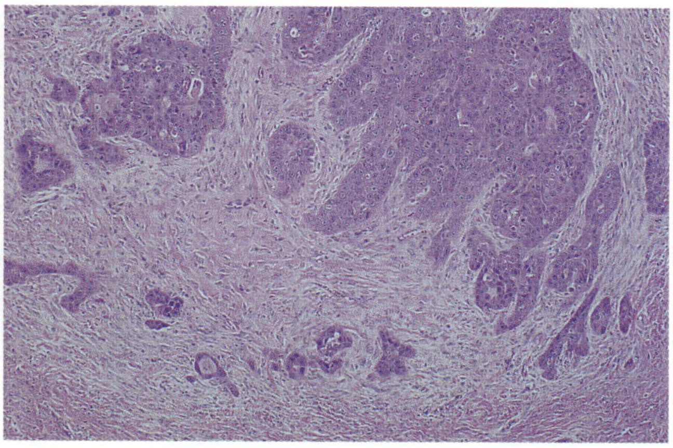

Figure 25–40. Infiltrative squamous cell carcinoma with desmoplasia.

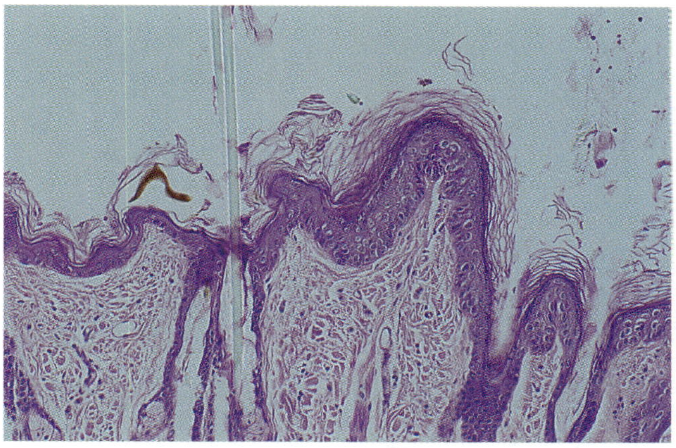

Figure 25–41. Bowen disease in a cat.

Sebaceous Tumors

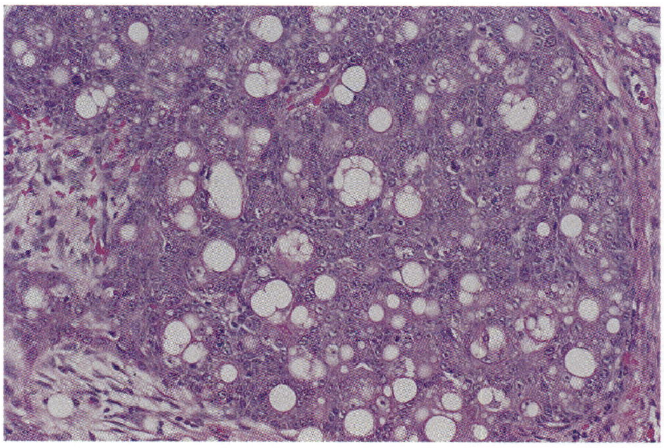

Figure 25–42. Sebaceous adenoma. There is marked mitotic activity but little nuclear pleomorphism associated with the reserve cells.

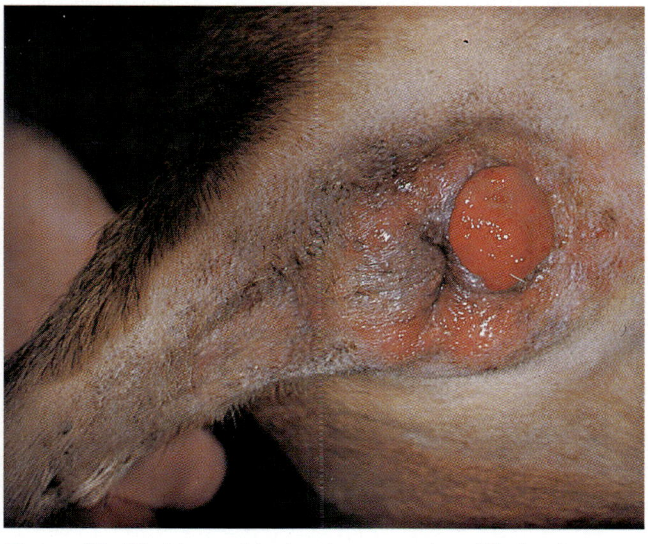

Figure 25–43. Hepatoid gland tumors (modified sebaceous glands of the dog). Hepatoid gland tumor with extensive ulceration arose in the perianal area of a dog.

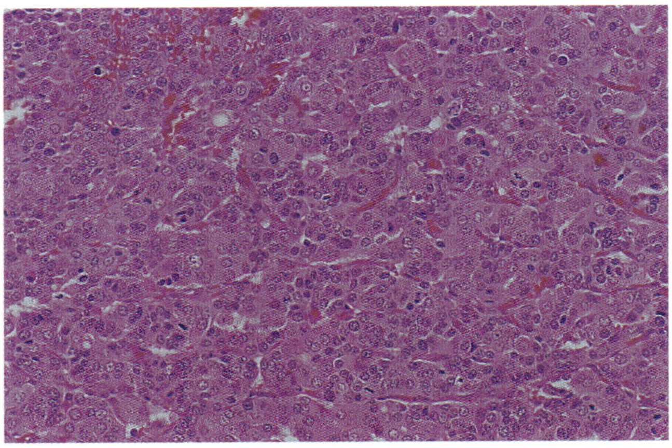

Figure 25–44. Hepatoid gland adenoma with multiple small lobules, small peripheral reserve cells, and large cells with an abundant eosinophilic cytoplasm (*i.e.,* hepatoid cells).

Apocrine Adenoma and Carcinoma

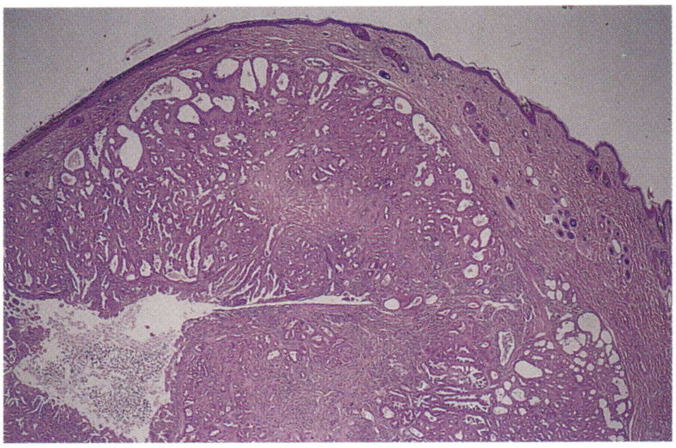

Figure 25–45. Apocrine gland tumors. Apocrine cystadenoma occurred in a dog.

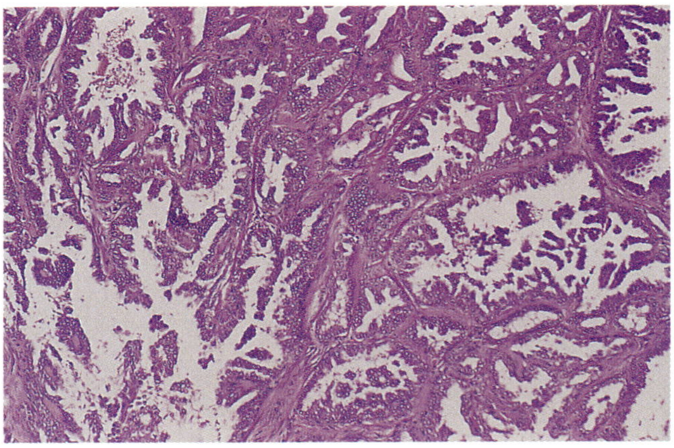

Figure 25–46. Apocrine carcinoma with papillary architecture arose in the inguinal area of a dog.

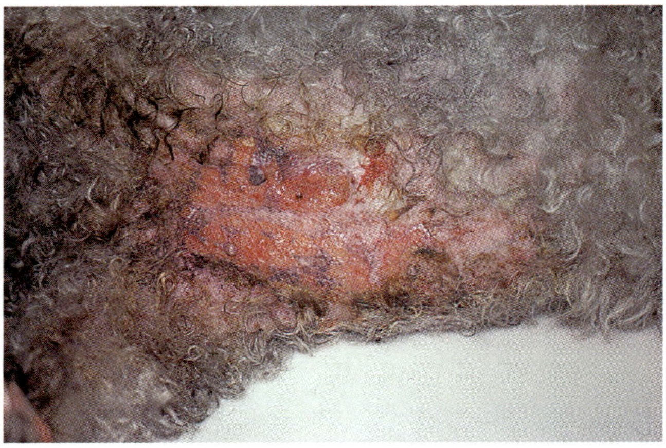

Figure 25–47. Ulceration of the skin overlies an apocrine carcinoma.

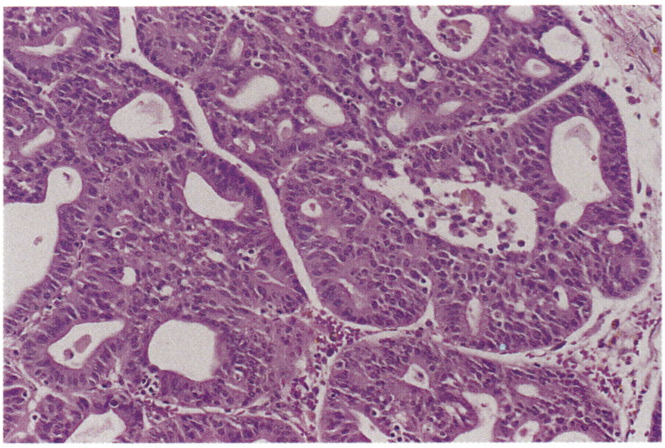

Figure 25–48. Anal sac gland adenocarcinoma occurring in a tubular pattern.

Keratoacanthoma

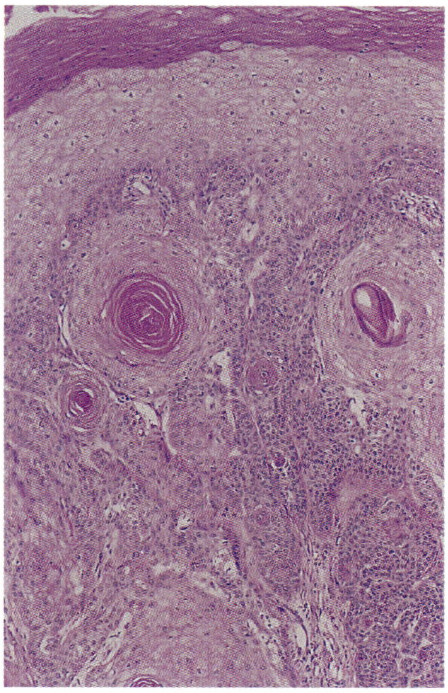

Figure 25–49. Intracutaneous cornifying epithelioma (keratoacanthoma) is represented by a lining of large cells with an extensive eosinophilic cytoplasm and anastomosing cords of epithelial cells at the periphery of the tumor.

Trichoepithelioma

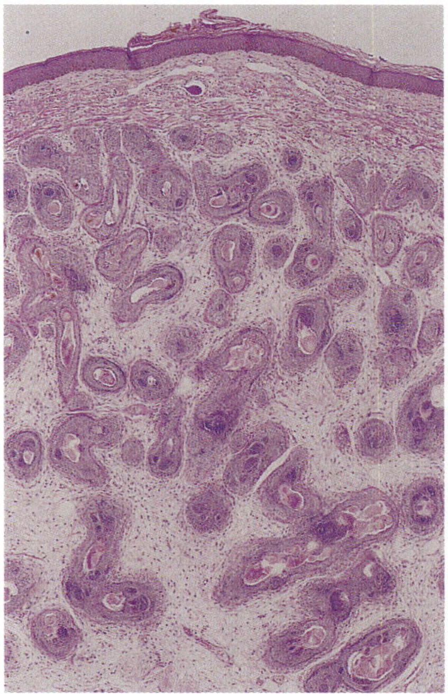

Figure 25–50. Trichoepithelioma. The multiple islands of neoplastic cells show differentiation to the external root sheath and a central aggregation of shadow cells.

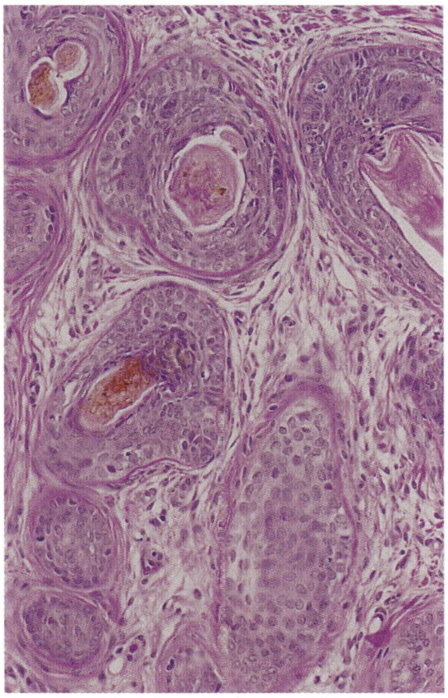

Figure 25–51. Trichoepithelioma. Higher magnification of Figure 25–50.

Pilomatrixoma

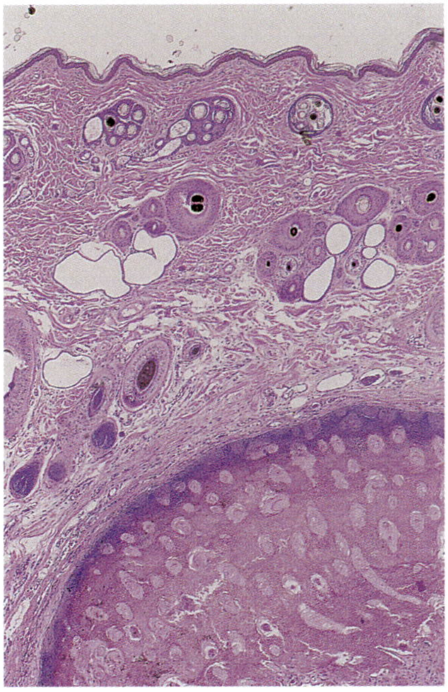

Figure 25–52. Pilomatrixoma. Pilomatrixoma in the deep dermis has a peripheral rim of basophilic cells and large central aggregates of shadow cells.

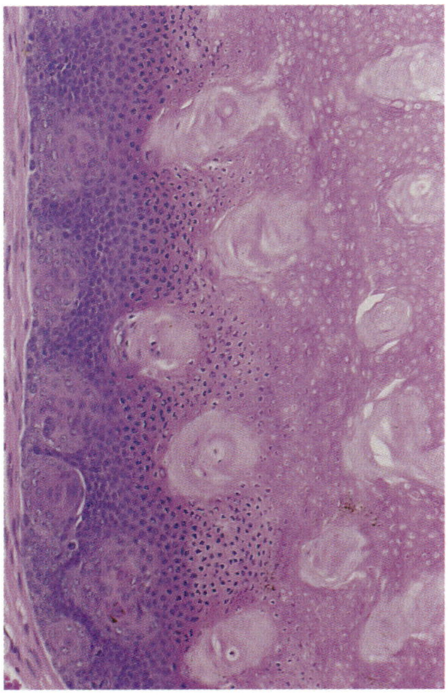

Figure 25–53. Pilomatrixoma. Higher magnification of Figure 25–52.

Melanoma

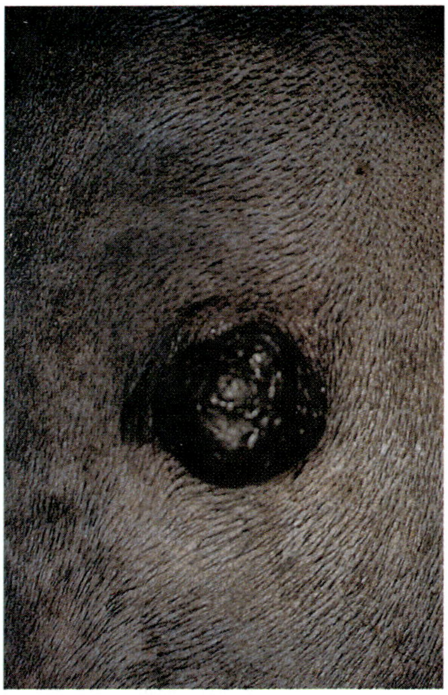

Figure 25–54. Melanoma. Dermal melanoma arising on the haired skin of a dog.

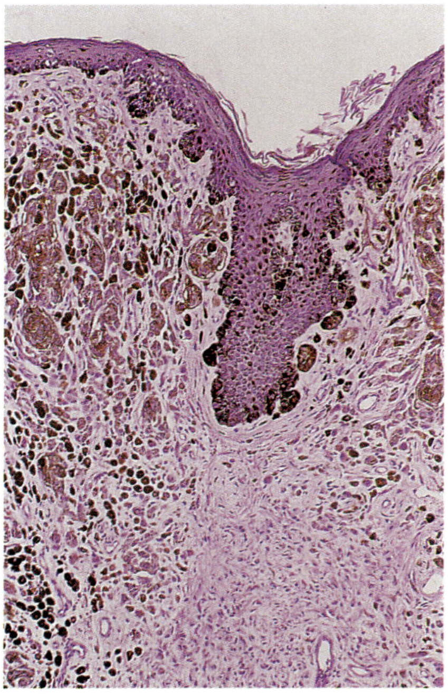

Figure 25–55. Dermal melanoma with minimal junctional activity, a population of highly pigmented round cells in the upper dermis, and sheets of poorly pigmented tumor cells in the deeper zones in a dog.

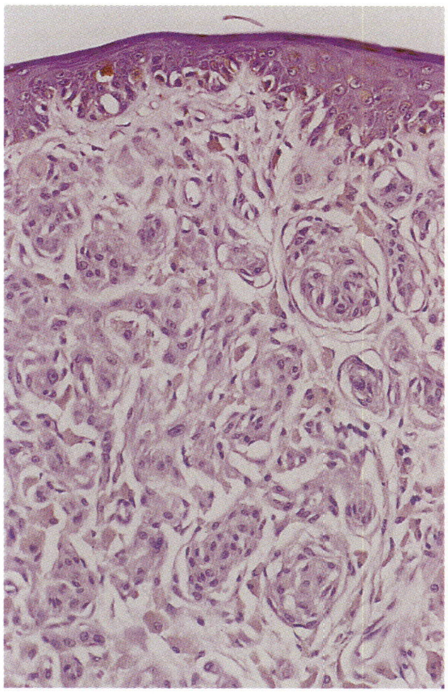

Figure 25–56. Melanoma. Higher magnification of the upper portion of Figure 25–55.

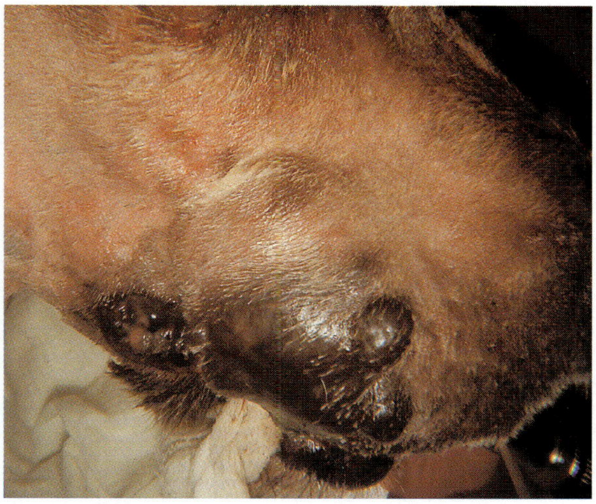

Figure 25–57. Malignant melanoma arising at the mucocutaneous junction of the lip.

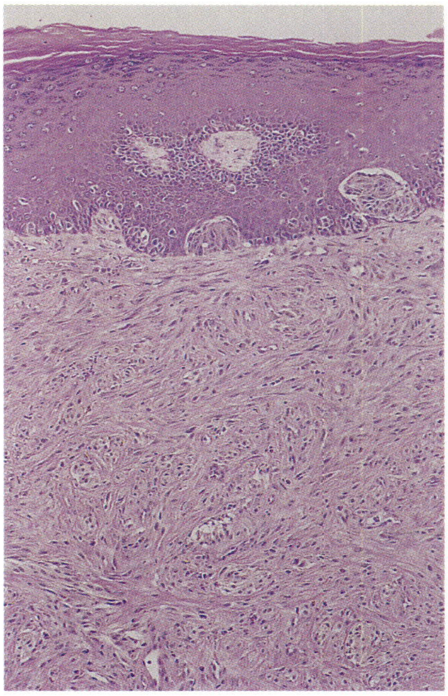

Figure 25–58. Malignant melanoma of the lip with a nest of neoplastic cells in the epithelium and extensive invasion of the subepithelial tissue.

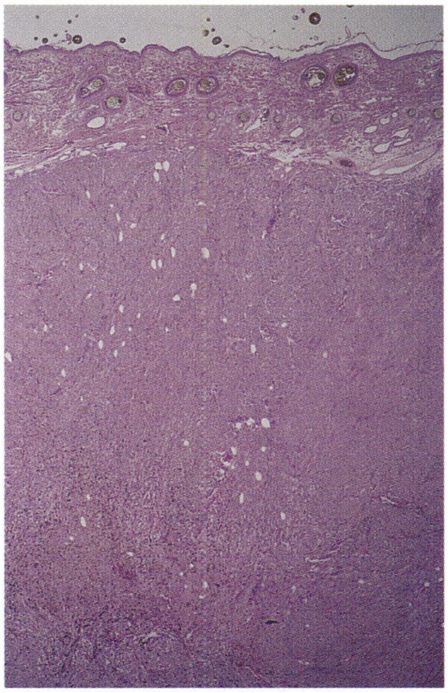

Figure 25–59. Malignant melanoma arising as a nodular mass in the skin.

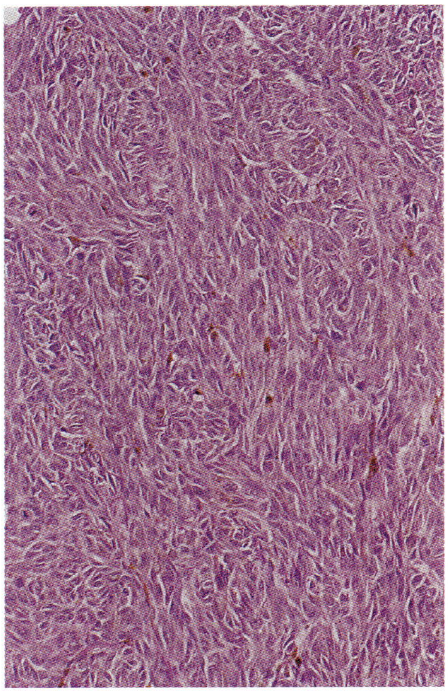

Figure 25–60. Higher magnification of Figure 25–59 reveals proliferation of spindle-type melanoma cells.

Hemangiopericytoma

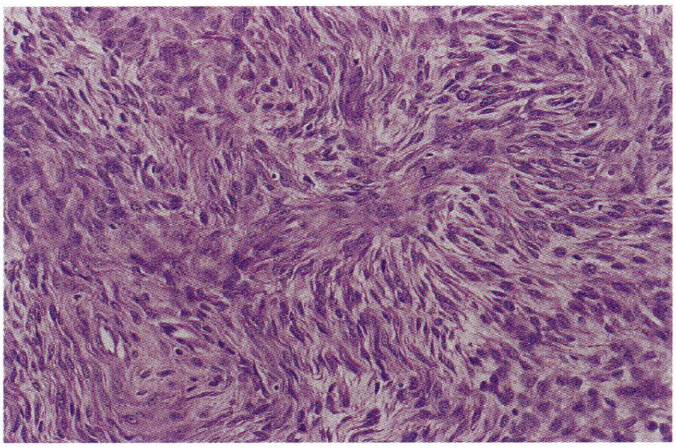

Figure 25–61. Canine hemangiopericytoma, storiform pattern.

Histiocytoma

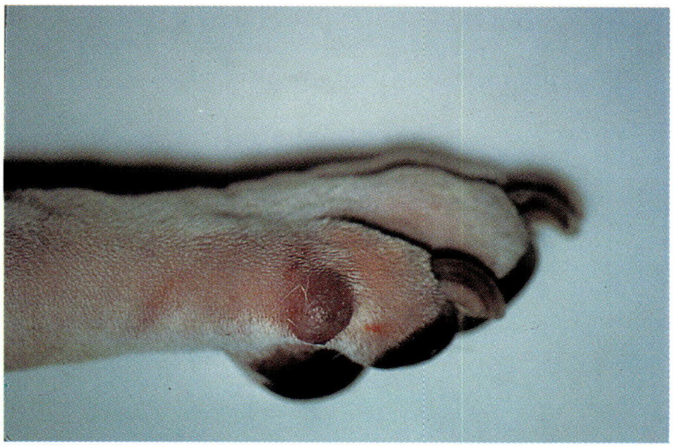

Figure 25–62. Canine cutaneous histiocytoma. The lesion appears as an elevated, erythematous mass on the digit of a dog. (Courtesy of Barbara Kummel, DVM.)

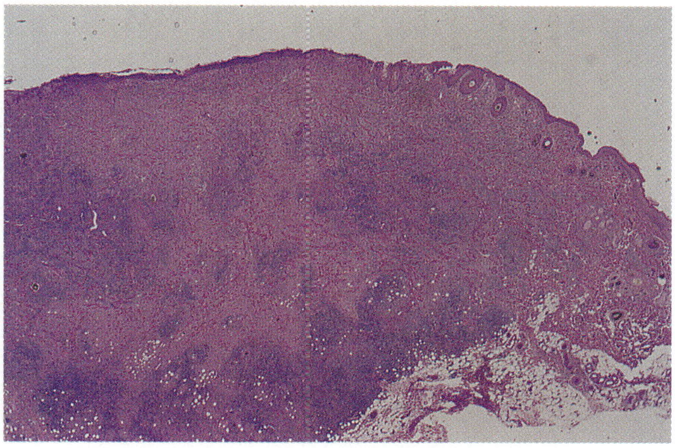

Figure 25–63. Tumor cells infiltrate the dermis and panniculus adiposus, with extensive lymphoid infiltration into the tumor.

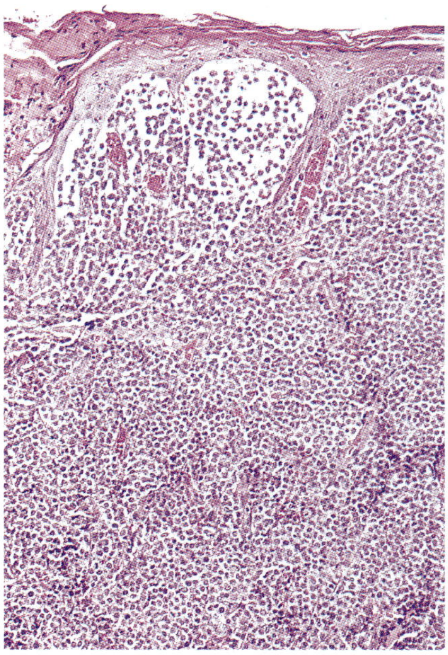

Figure 25–64. Sheets and cords of neoplastic cells are present in the dermis.

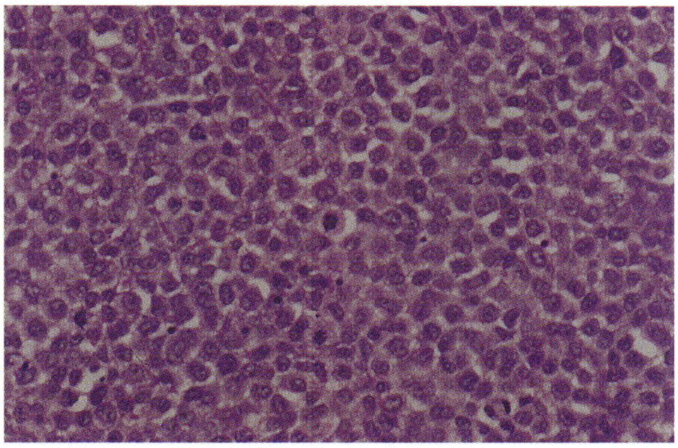

Figure 25–65. Neoplastic cells have ovoid nuclei, some of which have nuclear clefts. Mitoses are numerous.

Mast Cell Tumor

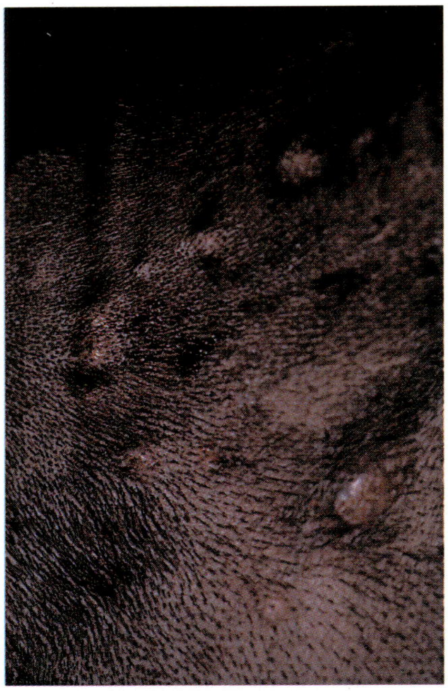

Figure 25–66. Mast cell tumor. Multiple nodular intradermal masses are present in a dog. (Courtesy of Barbara Kummel, DVM.)

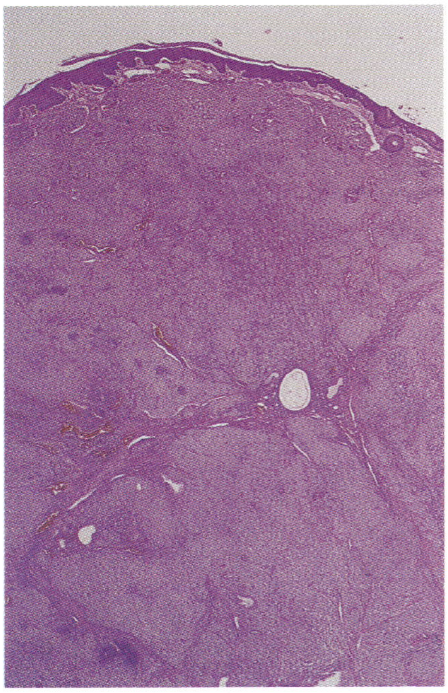

Figure 25–67. Dermal collagen has been obliterated by sheets of tumor cells.

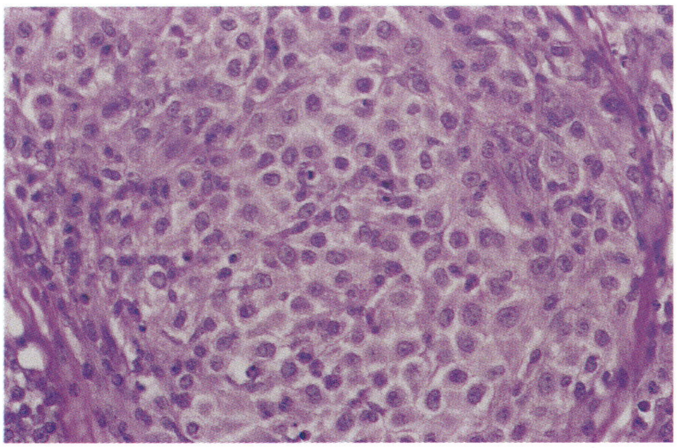

Figure 25–68. High magnification reveals tumor cells and eosinophils.

Lymphoma

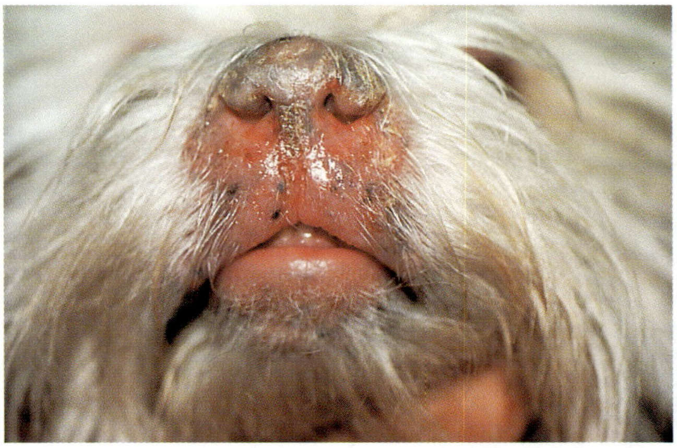

Figure 25–69. Cutaneous lymphosarcoma, erythematous type, involves skin and mucous membranes in a dog. (Courtesy of Barbara Kummel, DVM.)

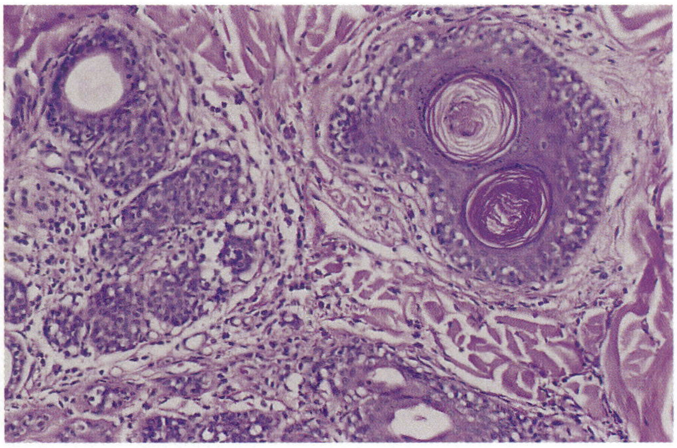

Figure 25–70. Cutaneous lymphosarcoma, epidermotropic type, with extensive involvement of the follicular epithelium.

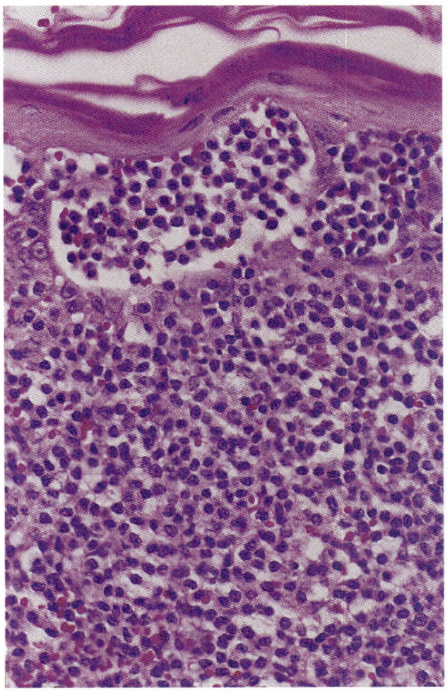

Figure 25–71. Cutaneous lymphosarcoma, with Pautrier microabscesses. The tumor cells appear plasmacytoid.

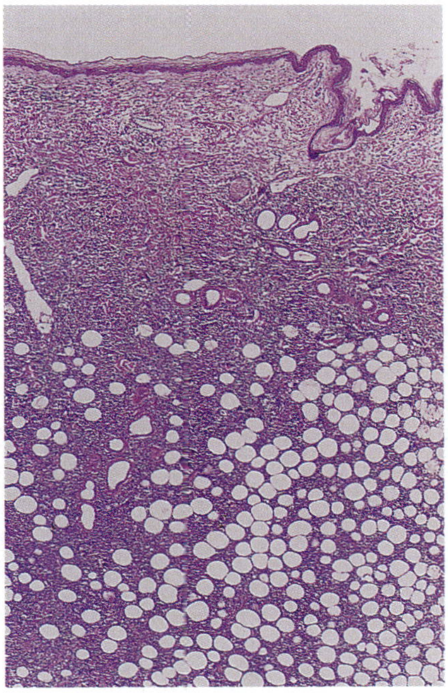

Figure 25–72. Cutaneous lymphosarcoma, nonepidermotropic type.

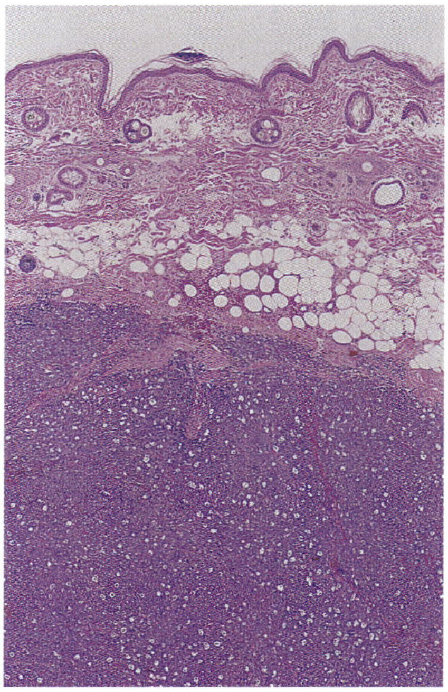

Figure 25–73. Cutaneous lymphosarcoma, subcutaneous nodule, Burkitt type, with numerous tingible-body macrophages in the tumor.

Plasmacytoma

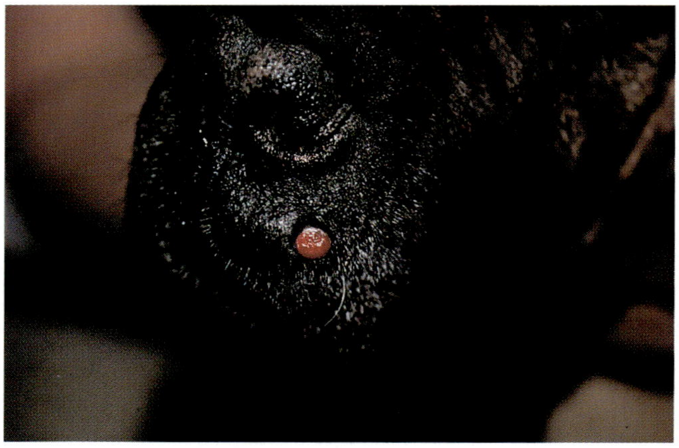

Figure 25–74. Cutaneous plasmacytoma on the lip. (Courtesy of Barbara Kummel, DVM.)

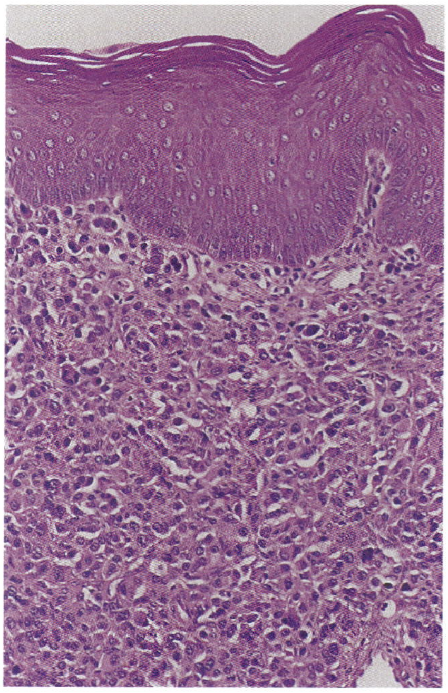

Figure 25–75. There is extensive infiltration of dermal tissue by plasmacytoid tumor cells.

Index

Page numbers in *italics* refer to illustrations; numbers followed by t indicate tables.